Textbook of Nasal Tip Rhinoplasty

Natarajan Balaji

Textbook of Nasal Tip Rhinoplasty

Open Surgical Techniques

Springer

Natarajan Balaji
NHS Lanarkshire
University Hospital of Monklands
Airdrie, Lanarkshire, UK

ISBN 978-3-030-48156-8 ISBN 978-3-030-48157-5 (eBook)
https://doi.org/10.1007/978-3-030-48157-5

This Springer imprint is published by the registered company Springer Nature Switzerland AG
The registered company address is: Gewerbestrasse 11, 6330 Cham, Switzerland

Foreword

It is a pleasure and honour to introduce this textbook on nasal tip rhinoplasty. Surgeons practicing rhinoplasty are acutely aware that whilst it may seem simple to many, they are far from straightforward. It is difficult to achieve consistently good results, with both minimal need for revision and pleasing long-term outcomes which are aesthetically balanced, and blend well with other facial features. The nasal tip is a particularly volatile area, and absolute mastery is a goal we must always strive for but may never achieve. However, by understanding the assessment of the tip, surgical principles, application of the correct techniques and resultant outcomes, surgeons may gain near mastery of this coveted field.

Any surgeon who intends to become accomplished in rhinoplasty will experience a significant learning curve, particularly with regards to the nasal tip. Improved outcomes in nasal tip surgery may be achieved by harbouring in-depth knowledge. Successful senior surgeons, in my opinion, have the absolute obligation to impart their knowledge for the younger generation. This is what exactly Mr. Balaji has done in this publication.

The book illustrates clear learning objectives, details on aetiology, pathology and pathogenesis of tip deformities and lays the foundation for the assessment of the tip during consultation in the clinic. This is followed by discussion on surgical principles, detailed exploration of suture techniques, grafting techniques and then non-suture and non-grafting tip techniques. The nasal septum is discussed in depth, leading into the control of the dorsum and management of the alar base. Particular attention is drawn to cleft rhinoplasty, closure of skin flap as well as management of the nasal valves. I urge the readers to read thoroughly the discussion on the algorithm for nasal tip management. Case studies and ethical considerations, which often get less attention, are also well addressed.

This is a masterpiece, in which a single surgeon has delivered his knowledge, skill and love for nasal tip surgery with unparalleled insight. It outlines his thinking and lifetime of surgical experience. I congratulate Mr. Balaji for all his work and recommend this book to all surgeons interested in rhinoplasty surgery, regardless of experience, as it is a valuable reference guide, full of practical pointers for developing and improving rhinoplasty, particularly nasal tip surgery.

Mr. Alwyn R. D'Souza
FRCS(ORL-HNS), FRCS Eng.
Past President: British Society of Facial Plastic Surgery.
President Elect: European academy of facial plastic surgery.
Consultant ENT/Facial Plastic Surgeon,
University Hospital Lewisham, London, UK

Preface

To start with, I am happy to be born in a country where the earliest nasal reconstructive techniques were performed by the ancient Hindu sage Sushruta in 800 BC, never forgetting the ancient Egyptian texts dating back to the Old Kingdom (3000 BC). Equally, I am more than happy to be living in my adopted Scottish land, which taught me the art of rhinoplasty. Nasal tip surgery involves lot of "thinking" and "reasoning" and "problem-solving" skills. I find no two operations the same, requiring different skill sets with different expected outcomes, which make this operation so special. My book is intended to cover the nuances of open approach nasal tip rhinoplasty. Although there are various approaches to the nasal tip, "open" or "external" approach gives excellent access. The debate of "closed" versus "open" goes on, but as long as the outcome is good, the approach does not matter.

In attempting to write on nasal tip rhinoplasty, it is impossible to cover this complex topic in a comprehensive way and I am in no way able to cover the entire length and breadth of the topic, but at least able to cover the nuances of nasal tip surgery based on my personal journey and experience. To my knowledge there is no textbook available dedicated only to nasal tip surgery in the current literature and I have set out to fill this void. The techniques mentioned in this book are accepted techniques in the mainstream literature described by various experts in the field. Throughout the book, I have mentioned and referenced various experts in the field, who have described these techniques as much as I have. However, this list is not exhaustive and I may have inadvertently missed some and can only apologise for the oversight. This book represents my way of approaching the topic, how to arrive at a surgical algorithm in nasal tip deformities and how to execute various techniques in a "sequence" to achieve meaningful results, based on my personal experience with over 1700 patients over the years. The majority of the book (around 80%) involves actual description of each surgical technique stepwise -of "how I do it" with as many illustrations as possible. The art of nasal tip surgery is to identify the "Key" factor that will make the patient happy and be "conservative" in executing the "minimum" necessary intervention to achieve the "maximum" outcome as quickly and effectively as possible with "minimal" tissue trauma.

I am grateful to Prof. Tardy who allowed me to visit him in Chicago during the early 1990s, which triggered my interest in rhinoplasty. My book on tip work will not be complete without mentioning the names of a few doyens in the field who have pushed boundaries in rhinoplasty and from whom I have acquired knowledge, in both North America and Europe, notably Prof. Tardy, Dr. Tebbetts, Dr. Daniel, Dr. Adamson, Prof. G. J.Nolst Trenité and Dr. Fazil Apayddin. My list is not an exhaustive one, but again apologies if I have left some key figures. Also, over the years, I have learnt a lot through lectures, meetings and informal discussions from my colleagues in the UK, notably Mr. White, Mr. Sheikh, Mr. Calder, Mr. A.D'Souza and Prof. Woolford. I am extremely thankful for that knowledge. I would like to thank Mr. Simon

Ravichandran for his constructive comments on the hierarchy of chapters. I feel nasal tip surgery is about "thought process", and surgical skills are only secondary factors in achieving a good outcome. Discussions with teachers, colleagues and even trainees contribute to this "thought" process.

Finally, most of the financial proceeds and royalties from the sale of this book will be donated to the Scottish Otolaryngological Society for the advancement of teaching and training in facial plastic surgery for overseas fellows in Scotland.

Natarajan Balaji
Airdrie, Lanarkshire, UK

Acknowledgement

The first person I would like to thank is my wife Meena who has been a constant source of support and encouragement over the last 10 years. Without her words of motivation, I doubt this project would have been possible. I am extremely grateful to my two daughters Anita and Priya, both in the medical field, who have kept me focussed. Also to my late parents and uncle for their tireless efforts in supporting my endeavour to become a doctor.

I am extremely thankful to all my patients in both the NHS Lanarkshire and private sector for allowing me to use their clinical photographs for publication. I would like to thank Dr. Jane Burns, the Medical Director, and Dr. Rory Mackenzie, Chief of Medical Services at the University Hospital of Monklands, NHS Lanarkshire, for their kind permission in allowing me to use the clinical photographs of NHS Lanarkshire patients. I would like to thank Eric, John and Christine from the Medical Illustrations Department at the University Hospital of Monklands, Scotland, for their excellent help and support in taking high quality pictures. Some of the photographs have already been published by me over the years in various journals and have been reproduced in this book with the kind permission of the editors of the respective journals, and I offer my sincere gratitude to them. The articles have been referenced accordingly to the best of my knowledge.

I would like to thank Mr. Nicholas Calder, my colleague who has done a thorough review of the manuscript. I am indebted to the editorial and production staff, particularly Ms. Smitha Diveshan and Ms. Daniela Heller, at Springer for their professionalism and commitment towards this publication. Finally, I dedicate this work to my teachers, notably Mr. A. Baxter, Mr. B. W. Irvine, Mr. B. O. Reilly and Mr. A. Johnston, for being who I am today.

Contents

Introduction to Nasal Tip Rhinoplasty

Contents

N. Balaji, *Textbook of Nasal Tip Rhinoplasty*, https://doi.org/10.1007/978-3-030-48157-5_1

Learning Objectives

- To learn when, what and how to reconstruct nasal tip deformities.
- To learn how to assess the deformity, identify the pathology and relate that to the anatomical structures.
- To learn how to arrive at a surgical algorithm to correct various tip deformities.
- To learn how to execute the various techniques and in a "sequence".

1.1 Introduction

Nasal tip rhinoplasty is one of the most demanding and complex surgical procedures within the gamut of rhinoplasty surgery. The surgical skills needed are similar to that of a sculptor, and only the surgeon can envisage the final results before it is complete. This type of surgery also needs lot of thinking, reasoning and manual dexterity executing the procedure with minimal soft tissue trauma to achieve the maximum outcome. The major issue with this type of surgery is the lack of any radiological investigating tools to assess the shape, size and integrity of the tip cartilages, particularly after nasal trauma or previous surgery. Imagine doing a laparotomy without knowing what the diagnosis is! This operation demands not only creating ideal structural changes in the cartilaginous skeleton of the nasal tip, but also the overlying soft tissue envelope should re-drape on the cartilaginous skeleton for the aesthetic outcome to be externally visible to the patient and the family, something similar to a mannequin in a shop window. Most rhinoplasty surgeons will agree that despite the skills of the surgeon, the results can be unpredictable. This is due to various patient- and surgeon-related factors. While the patient-related factors would continue to present a certain degree of variability in the outcomes, the surgeon-related factors can be formalised and standardised to a significant extent with adequate knowledge and training. The aim of this book is to address this issue partially by providing knowledge in the pathogenesis and the surgical techniques available at present to address various nasal tip issues. There is no substitute for practical surgical experience and interaction with different patients in helping to understand the various principles of nasal tip reconstruction. When "not" to operate or whom "not" to operate is equally or more important than when and whom to operate. There is no yardstick to decide these factors. But over the years the surgeon will gradually acquire this knowledge subconsciously. The surgeon should also learn to listen to inner thoughts rather than relying on the assessment of a psychologist. The book is predominantly on Caucasian rhinoplasty, as around 85% of the author's patients are Caucasians. The rest of the patients are from the northern Indian subcontinent and Pakistan, which is somewhat similar to Caucasian pathology with larger noses requiring reduction.

The book is divided into various chapters starting from surgical anatomy, aetiology and pathogenesis of various tip deformities, be it acquired by trauma or congenital. This is followed by assessment of deformities, patient selection and how to arrive at an algorithm for correcting various tip deformities, followed by detailed step-by-step discussion of the practical aspects of various tip plasty procedures concentrating on "how" to execute the various procedures stepwise with colour illustrations. About 80% of the contents of the book deals with the practical aspects of executing the various surgical techniques in nasal tip plasty. In this book, the actual surgical techniques have been grouped into three major chapters, namely "suture techniques", "grafting techniques" and "non-suture and non-grafting" techniques. Generally these techniques done either in isolation or in combination would alter the definition, rotation and projection of the nose. Generally the rationale is to consider the non-aggressive approaches using mainly sutures in primary rhinoplasty and to use grafting techniques in secondary procedures, although in practice we tend to use both in various combinations. Roughly 90% of the Caucasian noses would require standard techniques of bulk reduction of the lateral crus and the use of sutures to achieve favourable results. Hence the word "sequence" is the key. When considering more than one surgical procedure in a patient, it is important not only in arriving at what procedures to do, but also in "what sequence" to do as well. The major sequence in tip surgery would be to start the work on the caudal septum first, then move to medial crus, then move to intermediate crus and then the dome and then finally to lateral crus. Also an important factor apart from sequence is relative "speed" by avoiding repetition and also avoiding too many techniques in the same patient. *The "mantra" for this surgery is to identify the "key" factor which will make the patient happy and be "conservative" in executing the "minimum" necessary techniques to achieve "maximum" outcome as quickly and effectively with minimal tissue trauma.* Doing all the available techniques in the same patient has become a new fad in "live surgery" meetings across the world these days, giving false impression to the trainees that they have to be aggressive and complex.

Doing a rhinoplasty is like sculpting; the final outcome is not definite and is envisaged by the surgeon after thorough examination and repeated consultations with the patient. A word of caution is using modern computer graphics software in projecting the expected outcomes. This can be counter-productive to the surgeon in increasing the patient's expectations rather than decreasing the expectations. Instead, it is preferable to show them pre- and post-op photographs of consented patients, so that they can envisage the outcomes and help in developing confidence in the surgeon. The final outcome of the surgery depends on the perception of beauty by the surgeon. "A thing of beauty is a joy for ever" says the opening line of a famous poem by the nineteenth century English poet Keats. But there is no perfect definition of beauty. Another famous quote being "beauty is in the eye of the beholder" and to a greater extent this is true. It has been found that beauty is related to symmetry and proportions. Many leading figures of the past, including Da Vinci, Pythagoras and Mozart, believed in symmetry and harmony in nature. It does seem to occur in nature a ***"golden ratio"*** which is pleasing to the eye and hence of relevance in aesthetic surgery [1]. This ratio seems to be around 1:1.618, first described by the Greeks. This ratio is also called "Phi" ration named after the Greek sculptor Phidias. This ratio is seen in various biological systems like plants and humans. For example, in an aesthetically beautiful face, the width of the nose to the width of the mouth is roughly around this ratio. In Leonardo da Vinci's Vitruvian Man (or "Man in a Circle"), the distance from the bottom of the foot to the navel is 1.618 times the distance from the navel to the top of the head, and the distance from the navel to the thyroid cartilage is 1.618 times the distance of the thyroid cartilage to the top of the head. So the "key" for achieving beauty would be to try and achieve symmetry.

This book is based on the personal experience of the author over 24 years in open septorhinoplasty and tip plasty (0ver 1700 patients) mostly in Caucasians (around 85%). The smaller percentage (around 15%) of the patients are Asian Indian and Pakistani origin, who are ethnically different, mostly requiring reduction rhinoplasty, associated with increased skin thickness, thinner cartilages, associated turbinate hypertrophies and increased thickness of mucosal flaps of the septum, all of which have an impact on the final outcome of the surgery. About 2% of the patients are of oriental origin, who have thinner skin requiring augmentation rhinoplasty with techniques requiring increasing tip projection and definition. There is no gross difference in males and females, although anecdotal evidence experience suggests that septal cartilage is thinner in younger males than females. Trauma is a major impact factor in the deformities and outcomes of rhinoplasty. Around 95% of the author's patients have post-traumatic noses and most of them (around 90%) had medial crural fractures with or without lateral crural scaring or weakness, altering the tip anatomy requiring nasal tip reconstruction.

Conclusion

Assessment of the nasal tip deformities, adequate examination, thorough repeated consultations and discussion with a "cool off" period of what is possible and what is not possible and staying with in the ethical realms are important keys to a successful rhinoplasty. As mentioned before, this book will concentrate only on open approach techniques and not discuss the pros and cons of various approaches. There are internal (closed) techniques the reader may be familiar with. This book does not claim that open approach is the best, as access is only the initial step and does not matter as long as the outcomes are good [2]. This book is based on the author's personal experience of over 1700 open rhinoplasty procedures over 24 years. There has been an honest endeavour to put the whole thought process of nasal tip reconstruction in a clear and concise form. The techniques described in this book are "the author's way" of doing things and pretty much all these techniques have been described by various rhinoplasty surgeons. The author has made an honest endeavour to acknowledge and reference the surgeons who initially described these techniques to the best of his knowledge.

References

1. Singh P, Vijayan R, Mosahebi A. The golden ratio and aesthetic surgery. Aesthet Surg J. 2019;39(1): NP4–5.
2. Sheen J. Closed versus open rhinoplasty-and the debate goes on. Plast Reconstr Surg. 1997;99(3): 859–62.

Surgical Anatomy of the Nasal Tip

Contents

N. Balaji, *Textbook of Nasal Tip Rhinoplasty*, https://doi.org/10.1007/978-3-030-48157-5_2

Learning Objectives

- To learn the surgical anatomy of the nasal tip and its relationship to the pathology of the nasal deformity.
- To understand the various aesthetic parameters of the nasal tip in relation to cosmesis.

2.1 Introduction

The nasal tip is formed by the two lower lateral cartilages or tip cartilages and is the most projecting part of the nose. Nasal tip defining points are usually considered as the junctional zone between the lateral crus and the intermediate crus. The distance from the nasion to the tip defining points determines the length of the nose. The shape of the nasal tip and function is dependent on the structure and tensile strength of the two lower lateral cartilages, along with caudal septum. Nose is anatomically subdivided into bony upper third made of nasal bones and the frontal process of maxilla, cartilaginous mid third formed by the two upper lateral cartilages and the septum and the lower third made of the tip cartilages, otherwise called lower lateral cartilages. The tip is a floating structure, the entire skeleton being supported by the cartilaginous septum anteriorly and bony septum posteriorly. The lower two thirds of the nose are soft and movable side to side at the cartilaginous and bony junction with rigid upper third. Below is the description of the anatomy of the nasal tip, pertinent to the nasal plastic surgeon.

2.2 Surgical Anatomy of the Nasal Tip

- Nasal tip is formed by the two alar cartilages, also called lower lateral cartilages, both in harmony with each other. They are called so as they are lower and laterally placed to the midline.
- These are incompletely curved semi-lunar pieces of cartilage, soft and pliable situated in the lower third of the nose contributing to the lower third architecture of the nose. They are roughly 2–3 mms with varying thickness.
- The two lower lateral cartilages on both sides along with its fibrous attachments to the caudal septum offer not only structural stability to the tip of the nose but also functional support to the external nasal valve region.
- Anatomically each alar cartilage is composed of three segments, the larger, wider lateral crus, the smaller, narrower medial crus and the narrow transitional intermediate crus, all forming a single curved piece like a "boomerang" with the lateral crus being in a "frontal" plane and the medial crus in a sagittal plane, with fixed points laterally and medially, resulting in both the intermediate crura projecting out from the frontal plane forming the nasal tip [1, 2].
- The size, shape and position of these three segments on each side are quite variable "within" anatomical normality. The two medial crura being smaller and lighter than their lateral counterparts forming a conjoined segment to support the weight of the lateral crus and the tip of the nose. Hence they are attached by fibrous connective tissue to each other and also to the caudal septum to form the "conjoined" medial crus. It is the "conjoining" of the medial crural cartilage (Fig. 2.1) plus the sagittal orientation of the two medial crura which gives support to the tip. Hence any surgical intervention to support the tip should be directed to increasing or strengthening the medial crus and make the two medial crura into a "conjoined" piece in a sagittal plane to offer support. This can be done with sutures or even additional pieces of cartilage secured in between.
- The two medial crura are slightly convexing towards each other at the mid-point and start to diverge away superiorly towards the intermediate crus, the angle of divergence being around 60 degrees [3]. Similarly the two medial crura diverge

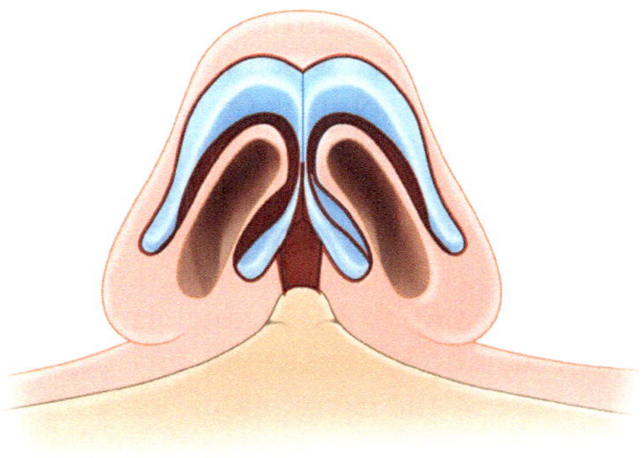

Fig. 2.1 Schematic representation of basal view of the nose showing the "conjoining" of medial crura with diverging footplates inferiorly

from each other inferiorly forming the footplate of the medial crus. This diverging footplate inferiorly (Fig. 2.1) sits on either side of the anterior nasal spine or in some patients on either side of the excess posterior septal angle cartilage. This diverging footplate of the medial crura lifts up the columellar skin causing an elevation called the "sill" just below the columella in the basal view. This space is usually filled with soft tissue and fat.

- The orientation of the lateral crus is usually around 45 degrees [4] from the midline (Fig. 2.2) and oriented towards the lateral canthus. If this angle is reduced and the orientation of the lateral crura is facing towards the medial canthus (Fig. 2.3), then by definition there is a cephalic migration causing a "parenthesis" of the tip. This is seen as a double bracket of the dome cartilages facing each other on the frontal and basal view, with under rotation of the tip and weakness of the lateral alar region on inspiration causing functional issues as well. This is usually genetic or post-traumatic.
- As the two intermediate crura go up and turn laterally to become the lateral crus, they move away from the alar skin margins at the "soft triangle". The cartilage then turns laterally as the "lateral crus" and comes towards the soft triangle skin margin again and then moves back laterally

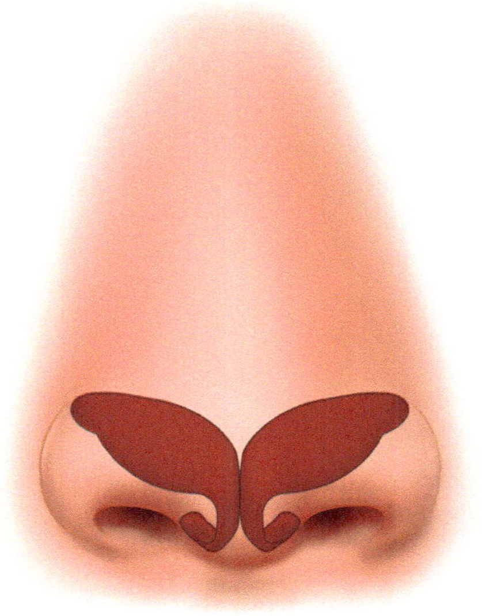

Fig. 2.2 Schematic representation of frontal view of the nasal tip showing the orientation of the lateral crus towards the lateral canthus 45 degrees from the midline

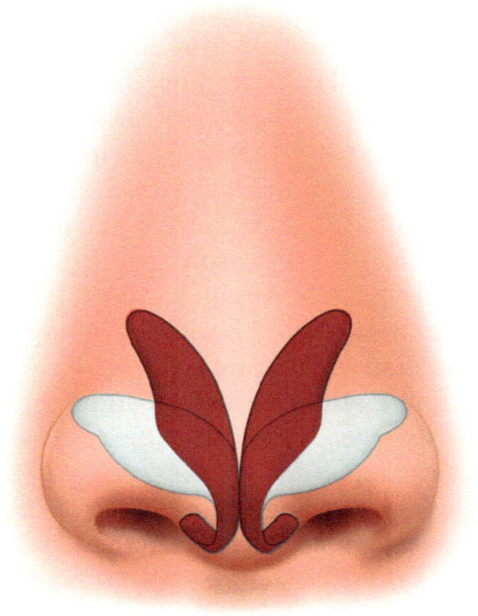

Fig. 2.3 Schematic representation of frontal view of the nasal tip showing the orientation of the lateral crus towards the medial canthus in a parenthesis tip

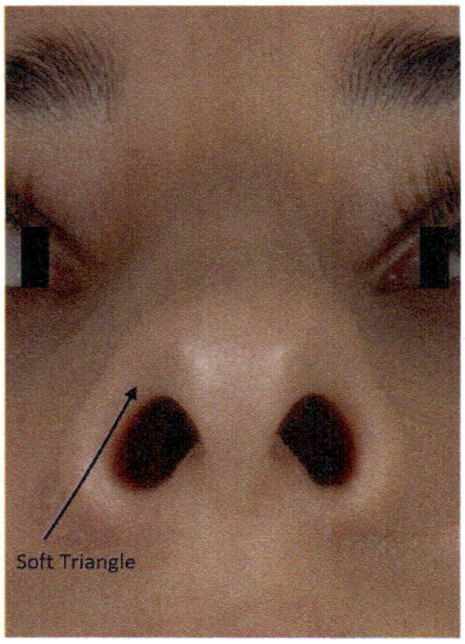

Fig. 2.4 Basal view of the nose showing the location of the soft triangle

going "away" from the alar skin margin. This anatomical orientation creates the so called "soft triangle" at the apex of the alar rim (Fig. 2.4) as seen in the basal view, where there is no alar cartilage and only skin on the outside and the mucosa on the inside.

- This soft triangle at the apex of the alar rim area should not be breached during surgery while elevating the dorsal skin flap as it can cause scarring and contracture. On a similar note, any deformity with scarring involving the soft triangle cannot be satisfactorily repaired either and best left to heal by secondary intention.
- The soft triangle is a misnomer, in that the area is definitely soft due to lack of cartilage in between, but not a triangle even in so called "normal" looking noses. The shape of this area can be a triangle or a square or a rectangle based on the angle of divergence between the medial and lateral crus.
- This soft triangle area deserves special assessment as it denotes the divergence angle between the medial and lateral crus and also helps in the diagnosis of cephalic malposition of the lateral crura, if present.
- The angle formed by the lateral crus and the medial crus at the dome is the dome angle and this is around 45 degrees. If this angle is wider, this can contribute to a wide nasal tip.
- The upper lateral cartilage is a rectangular piece of cartilage which is attached to the cartilaginous septum in the midline (central "K" area). Superiorly they can extend under the nasal bones and the frontal process of the maxilla to a variable distance. Various studies have shown that it can extend up to 12–14 mms. This is called the lateral "K" area, and any depressed fracture of the lateral nasal bones and the frontal process can damage this union.
- Based on the underlying variable attachment of the upper lateral cartilage in the lateral "K" area, following a fracture reduction of the depressed lateral bony complex, the upper lateral cartilage may not come out with the frontal process of the maxilla even after the bony complex is lifted out. In these situations, you may need a spreader graft unilaterally to lift the upper lateral and stabilise this to the dorsal septum in the new position. Failure of upper lateral to lift out is one of the common causes of persistent deviation and depression of the side wall after osteotomy and mobilisation.
- Laterally the upper lateral cartilages are attached to the edges of the frontal process of maxilla by fibrous attachment. Inferiorly as the caudal margin extends downwards towards the alar cartilage, it diverges away from the septal midline forming a floating piece. This junctional zone caudally is the internal nasal valve region, where the space is lined inside by nasal mucosal lining and externally with the continuation of the periosteal and SMAS layer. This is an important anatomical orientation to remember while doing a spreader graft or a spreader flap.
- The most prominent projecting part of the nasal tip lobule is the tip defining point and the part of the tip complex above that is supra tip lobule leading to the mid dorsum and the part below that leading to the columella is the infra tip lobule, altogether forming the tip lobule complex (Fig. 2.5).
- The supra tip lobule width is assessed in the frontal view, but the projection in relation to the dorsal profile line is assessed only in

Fig. 2.5 Schematic representation of the profile view of the nose showing the components of the nasal tip lobule complex

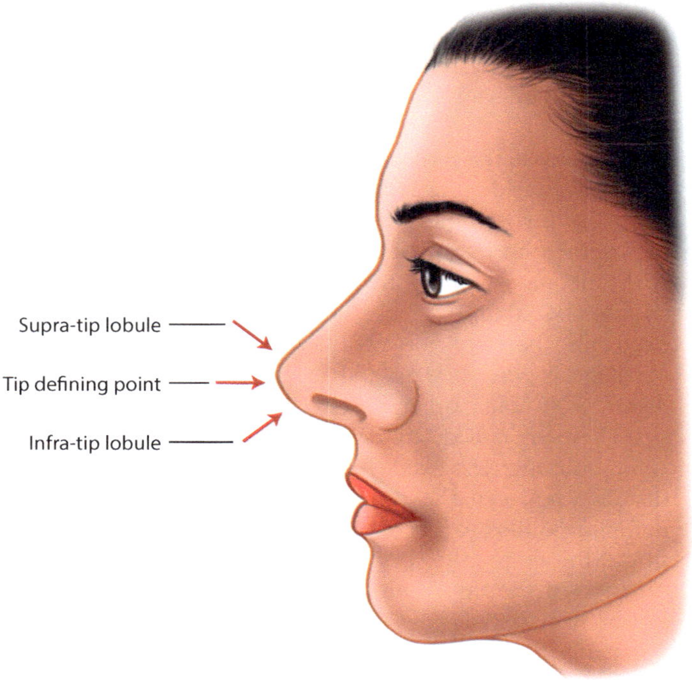

the lateral view. By contrast, the infra tip lobule is seen well in the basal view.

- Anatomically the infra tip lobule is formed by the intermediate crus and the cephalic portion of the medial crura. The supra tip lobule is formed by the medial side of the dome of the two lateral crura.
- Nasal alar base is the terminology used to describe the lateral alar part of the nasal tip complex as seen on the basal view (Fig. 2.6). Alar base surgery is a terminology restricted to surgery of the lateral alar base. This is the point of the ala where it meets the facial sulcus.
- Anatomically alar base is made of skin and soft tissue only and does not have any cartilage, as the lateral crura does not come caudally and as lateral as the alar base. Lack of cartilage makes soft tissue control in the alar base more difficult, and any inadvertent incisions can cause external scarring in the region, which will be very difficult to correct.
- The *nasal tip is defined* as the most projecting part of the nose and represents the junctional zone between the lateral crus and the intermediate crus. This junctional zone not only points slightly laterally but also forwards in the frontal plane away from the face, contributing to the so called "projection" of the tip. This is the most projecting part of the lower lateral cartilages.

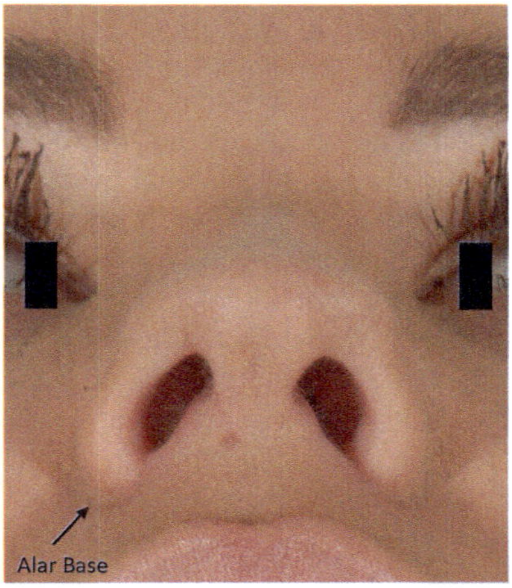

Fig. 2.6 Basal view of the nose showing the location of the alar base

- Also it is important to be aware that the tip is "not" the junction between the medial and intermediate crus, which is medial and inferior to the maximum point of the tip.
- So to increase the projection or define the nasal tip, consider the above two junctional zones as "pivot points" to work on.
- A frontal photograph of the face taken with adequate lighting to avoid shadows should be able to pick up the most projecting parts of the two lower lateral cartilage as two white dots, spaced around 4 mm from each other in a well-defined tip. These are called "tip defining points". In a bulbous, less well-defined tip, this distance between the right and left "tip defining points" can be more than 4 mm, in addition to the asymmetry in the position of the tip defining points or may not be seen at all.
- Normally there are variations in the size, shape and thickness of the alar cartilages between different sexes and races with no dependable expectations in the author's practice.
- Long-standing damage due to trauma or surgery can cause damage to the support mechanisms of the medial crus with loss of tip support. The medial crura are the most damaged part of the nose in a traumatic nose in majority of patients in the author's practice.
- The upper border of the lateral crura is in contact with the upper lateral cartilage laterally at the scroll region and the lower border of the lateral crura starts to follow the alar margin at the soft triangle and slowly slopes laterally away from the cutaneous alar margin. Be aware of this when making incisions in the lateral alar region.
- Each lateral crus is then anchored to the side of the caudal nasal septal cartilage close to the anterior septal angle, so that the tip complex when viewed from the lateral view may be seen to be at, below or above the anterior septal angle based on ethnicity, age and sex. This relationship should be noted before nasal tip surgery, and patient's wish of this anatomical relationship is important in addressing the final outcomes, as the concept of nasal tip surgery involves not only redefining the nasal tip anatomy of the lateral and medial crus, but also to re-establish the relationship of the nasal tip cartilages to the anterior caudal septum and the profile line. Awareness of this concept is important in achieving long-term stability to the position of the nasal tip.
- The nasal tip is a free-floating structure in the lower third of the nose, hence supported by "major" and "minor" tip support mechanisms.
- The major tip support is provided by the "intrinsic" size, shape, thickness and weight of the Lateral and medial crus and the intermediate crus. The surgeon should be aware that there are no specific parameters available regarding the size or shape or weight of the lateral crus or medial crus in any sex, age or race.
- In any particular patient, it is the "relative balance of the weight, strength or power" between three anatomical structures on each sides, namely the medial crus, intermediate crus and the lateral crus, which decides the ultimate tip deformity. Any trauma or deformity to any of these six anatomical variables can introduce a wide variety of tip deformities particularly in a revision surgery patient.
- The caudal septum and the anterior septal angle of the dorsal septum is also a major contributing factor for the tip support. The "minor" tip support mechanisms being the fibrous attachments between the two medial crura which gives "conjoined" strength to the two medial crura to support the tip. The other minor tip support mechanisms are fibrous attachments between the caudal septum and the conjoined medial crus and the position and prominence of the anterior nasal spine and fibrous attachments at the scroll region between the upper lateral and the lower lateral cartilages.

- The relationship between alar margins in the side view with the columella is important anatomically. If there is an excess columellar show, it could be due to an over hanging columella or could be due to upward retraction of the alar margin.
- In the author's experience, this division of major and minor tip supports are an arbitrary one, as even damage to a so called "minor" tip support mechanism may result in a "major" tip deformity and vice versa.

In practice, the following factors affect the tip support [5, 6]:

- The size, shape, and strength of the two lateral crura.
- The width, bulk and thickness of the lateral crura.
- The size, shape, and strength of the two medial crura.
- The separation of the medial crura.
- The position (e.g., cephalic migration) and orientation of lateral and medial crura.
- The structural integrity of the two medial crura and lateral crura (fracture, discontinuity or scarring).
- Complete or incomplete interruption of the medial or lateral crus. In the majority of our patients with nasal trauma, damage to medial crus is invariably just below the dome, while any fracture line in the lateral crus is usually just lateral to the intermediate crus with a deep concavity of the rest of the lateral crus, particularly in deformities causing functional issues in the external valve region.
- Position, strength and integrity of the caudal septal cartilage.
- The effect of the above factors either on one or both sides will lead to various tip deformities, predominantly causing loss of tip support, de-projection and sometimes over rotation or under rotation, with or without functional external valve issues. Primary deformities of the tip are classified as pathologies limited to or intrinsic to lower lateral cartilages and secondary deformities are due to the caudal septal pathology causing secondary tip changes.

2.3 Nasal Tip "Tripod" Concept

- Jack Anderson in 1969 [7] described the "tripod" nasal tip concept, whereby he compares the nasal tip complex to a three-legged (tripod) stool with a base to sit on.
- This concept has stood the test of time. Even after all these years, it is still a very valid tool to understand the tip dynamics.
- Imagine sitting on the nasal tip (analogous to the "base" of the stool) of someone lying supine on the operating table, like sitting on a stool and looking forward towards the patient's feet! The position and strength of the seat is determined by three limbs of the stool, which are the "conjoined" medial crus in the front and the two separate lateral crura in the postero-lateral position. By manipulating the length of the three legs alone or in combination, the projection and rotation of the nasal tip can be altered [6–8].

2.4 Concept of "Big Guy – Small Guy"

- Anatomically the tip complex is not "an ideal" creation of nature.
- The lateral crus is usually bigger, wider and heavier when compared to the medial crus; hence the "conjoining" of medial crura is needed in supporting both the lateral crural weight. This is an important concept to be aware of in nasal tip reconstruction.
- In trauma and revision surgery of the tip, there is always this disparity of worsening relationship between the two lateral crus and the conjoined medial crus. The usual pathology being the weak, fractured or separated medial crus which cannot support the weight of the relatively heavier lateral crus.
- So the author's personal concept of nasal tip surgery is "*to make the big guy (lateral crus) smaller and lighter and the small (medial crus) guy bigger and stronger*". This concept has been published in the past, which has been referenced [9, 10].

2.5 M-Arch Model

- "The M-arch model" was introduced by Prof. Dr. Peter Adamson, from Toronto, in 2006 [7]. He considers this concept as an extension of the simple tripod concept with the inclusion of the intermediate crus which recognises the importance of the length of each medial, intermediate and lateral crura.
- Changes in the length of these subdivisions (particularly any vertical resection of the lateral crus) will affect changes in length, projection and rotation of the nasal tip and can be used as a model to help the thought process in planning the surgical techniques.
- Both the "tripod" concept and the "M"-arch model are helpful in analysing the pathogenesis of the deformities and also in the planning of various surgical steps to correct the deformities. These concepts help in the thought process.

2.6 Skin and Soft Tissue Envelope

- The anatomy of the skin envelope is an important factor in nasal tip surgery, be it a primary or secondary procedure.
- There is a normal variation in the skin thickness over the nose, with thicker skin in the upper and lower third and thinner skin over the mid dorsum.
- The surgical outcomes will not be optimum if the skin envelope is thicker, oedematous or very thin and scarred.
- People with thickened skin of the nasal tip and also bulbous tip should not be given assurances of any surgical technique to narrow the tip [5, 8]. This is akin to a mannequin in a shop window. The skin has to be thin and be able to drape around the tip cartilages; otherwise any clever tip plasty techniques will not be visible to the patient and the surgeon.
- Thin skin has its own disadvantages as well, with even minor irregularities of the dorsum seen or felt easily, hence the need for using crushed cartilages (CATS graft) to camouflage any minor dorsal irregularities in patients with thin skin.

2.7 Aesthetic Sub-units of the Nose

The framework of the nose is divided into nine aesthetic nasal segments externally. This is not based on any specific underlying anatomical structures, but it is based on the way light shadows and contours fall on the nose, so that any scars placed on the margins or borders of these sub-units are less visible to the eye. Although these sub-units are more relevant in excision and reconstruction of cutaneous lesions, rather than rhinoplasty, it is still worthwhile having knowledge of these facial sub-units, as they may be significant in patients needing revision rhinoplasty requiring some unusual incisions to access the nose. The external nasal sub-units are totally nine, with three in the midline and six paired sub-units laterally.

The three midline sub-units from top down are:

- A single dorsal nasal segment
- One tip lobule segment
- Single columellar segment

The three paired lateral sub-units from top down are:

- Two lateral nasal-wall segments
- Two soft-tissue triangle segments
- Two alar segments

2.8 Blood Supply of the Nose

- Majority of the blood supply of the external skin and soft tissue framework of the nose comes from the external carotid artery system through a dorsal artery, lateral artery of the nose and through the angular and facial arteries.
- Nose is very vascular and the distribution and anastomosis of the different arterial systems allows the nose to have a variety of surgical approaches, including external approach and also simultaneous alarotomy to be performed without compromising the vascularity of the overlying skin flap. In my experience, even opening the nose third or fourth time does not jeopardise the blood supply to the flap, until

injudicious use of diathermy to the flap, which if done even the first time, can cause damage to the skin flap.

- The main arterial blood supply to the nose including the nasal cavity and internal mucosa is from both internal and external carotid systems. The percentage distribution of the nose is roughly 30–40% by the internal carotid artery via the anterior and posterior ethmoidal arteries and around 50–60% via the external carotid artery through the sphenoplatine, facial and angular vessels.
- Persistent nasal bleeding in the post-operative period involving the septum is usually from the external carotid system, while intra-nasal bleeding from the nasal cavity is usually from the internal carotid system from the osteotomy sites.
- The external nose is supplied via facial artery, which becomes the angular artery running along the medial side of the nasal external skin at the junction of the lateral nasal sub-unit with the cheek sub-unit ending at the medial canthus. These vessels give branches horizontally across the lateral nasal sub-unit with rich anastomosis with the dorsal nasal artery, which enters the lateral and superior part of the nasal skin with branches of the internal maxillary artery from the external carotid system. Hence majority of the external nose is supplied by the external carotid system.
- This rich blood supply allows us the flexibility of combining the hemi transfixation incision with an open approach trans-columellar incision. We have also combined the above with a unilateral alarotomy incision without any issues with the blood supply. We have not done a double alarotomy with a trans-columellar incision. Tip has slightly less blood supply when compared to the rest of the nose. But in essence, the blood supply to the nose is generally robust even allowing multiple revision procedures to open the nose. Personally, in some patients, We have raised a flap "fourth" time without any issues to the blood supply.
- Every attempt should be made while raising the skin flap to be just under the SMAS layer and above the perichondrial and periosteal layer. It is important to use the bipolar diathermy judiciously on the skin flap. Sometimes a sub-perichondrial or sub-periosteal dissection may be needed.
- Internally, the lateral wall of the nose is supplied by the spheno-palatine artery and posterior ethmoidal artery. The nasal septum is supplied by spheno-palatine artery and also anterior and posterior ethmoidal arteries.
- The venous drainage of the nose is anatomically significant, as they do not have any "valves" in the vessels. Hence they are in direct circulatory communication with the cavernous sinus. This makes the potential intracranial spread of any bacterial infection of the nose a possibility.
- In any revision surgery requiring skin flap elevation, we usually give broad-spectrum single-dose antibiotic on induction.
- The medial canthal veins are usually seen as a blue structure in a Caucasian skin just lateral to the medial canthus of the eye. Care must be taken to avoid injury to this structure while doing the external osteotomies. The area you are more likely to catch this vessel is the junction between the superior and lateral osteotomies. Sometimes this area of the bone of the ascending process of the maxilla is so thin that it can be fractured through finger pressure after the lateral and superior osteotomy, thus avoiding direct trauma with the 2 mm osteotome.
- The lymphatic drainage follows closely the vessels and drains into the retropharyngeal nodes posteriorly and to a smaller extent into the anterior upper deep cervical nodes or into the sub-mandibular glands.
- It is of practical significance to note that the lymphatic drainage of the columella is less compared to the rest of the nose and hence cause minimal post-operative oedema of the columella even in revision procedures.

- A certain degree of finesse and fine movements on the part of the surgeon definitely helps in the healing. The degree of post-operative oedema and bruising of the face is directly related to the degree of damage to the soft tissues and bony structure of the nose and also the age of the patient and the state of soft tissue envelope. Still it is very difficult sometimes to predict who will get more bruising compared to the others.
- Extreme care should be taken while thinning or defatting the skin of the nasal tip as the blood supply to the tip lies above the SMAS layer and just beneath the dermis, and any aggressive thinning of the subcutaneous tissue can end up in skin necrosis.

2.9 Aesthetic Tip Parameters (Definition, Projection and Rotation)

There are three parameters which contribute to the aesthetics of the nasal tip. They are definition, projection and rotation. A patient needing nasal tip surgery may present with any of these parameters being abnormal in any combination. These are described in detail in the ► Chap. 4.

Definition

- Definition of the nasal tip means, "how well defined the tip is?" [5, 11]
- In other words, what does the lay man thinks of the "shape" of the nasal tip? Is it big or small, bulbous or narrow, pointed or blunt, straight or twisted?
- Definition is what most patients talk about during the consultation.
- Very few patients rarely talk about projection and rotation, although they may be aware of them.

2.9.1 Projection

- Projection is defined as: "How much the tip is projecting forward when compared to the face or the rest of the nasal dorsum?"
- Either we can compare the projection of the whole nose with the rest of the face or just only the tip in relation to the rest of the nasal dorsum.
- There are various accepted means of measurement of projection by Goode ratio [12] and Crumley.
- These are rough guidelines which are used generally to assess the aesthetic balance of the so called "normal" nose.
- In practice, we tend to use the "projection line" which is measured from the nasal-alar crease to the nasal tip.
- This projection line is roughly 60% of the nasal dorsal line (a ratio of 3:5) from the nasion to the nasal tip. If this line is more than 60% of the nasal dorsal line, then it is an over projected nose, and if it is less it is an under projected nose (◘ Fig. 2.7).
- There are some issues by reporting these measurements as a ratio, which in fact can be counter-productive to the surgeon. Sometimes the length of both the lines are a perfect ratio of 3:5, *but* the length of both the lines may be equally more than "normal", resulting in an actually larger nose which will concern the patient.
- The angle between the nasal dorsal line and the forehead is the naso-frontal angle (◘ Fig. 2.8).
- Ideally this angle should be around 130 degrees for an aesthetically pleasing nose. Again all these angles and measurements are of no practical significance and should be taken in context with the entire pathological deformity of the nose.

2.9.2 Rotation

- Rotation of the nasal tip is defined as the relationship between the nasal tip and the frontal plane of the face. It is defined as an

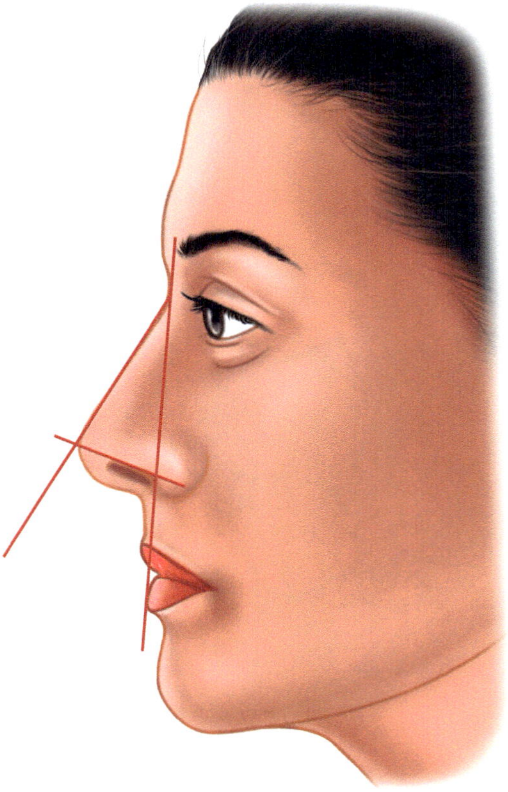

Fig. 2.7 Schematic representation of the profile view of the nose showing the nasal projection line, which is roughly 60% of the nasal dorsal line from the nasion to the tip

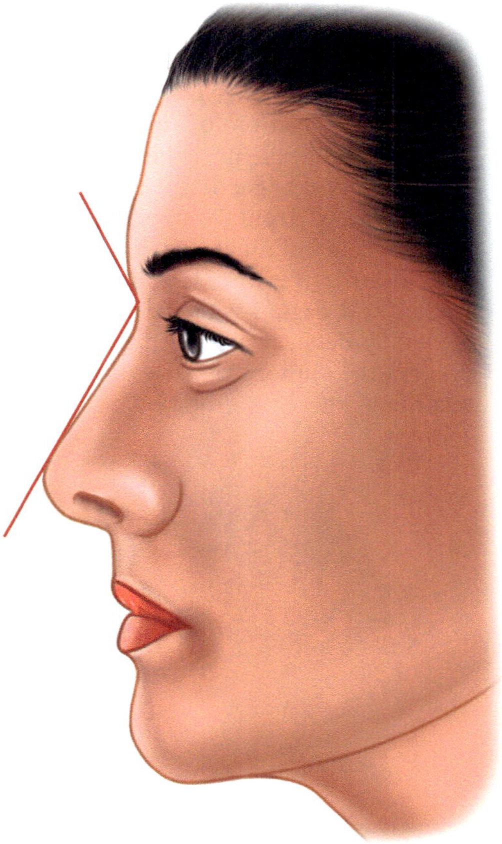

Fig. 2.8 Schematic representation of the profile view of the nose showing the ideal naso-frontal angle of 130 degrees between the nasal dorsal line and the forehead line

arc of rotation in the lateral profile line, an upward movement of the tip resulting in over rotation and a downward movement of the tip resulting in an under rotation or a ptotic tip depending on the severity.

- Rotation of the nasal tip can be divided into two further sub-sets with one between the columella and the upper lip and the second one between the columella and the infra tip lobule.
- Traditional methods of measuring the rotation of the nasal tip based on the angle between the upper lip and the columella can be totally misleading and does not always indicate the position of the infra tip lobule. So for example, the naso-labial angle may be less than 90 degrees suggesting under rotation of the tip, *but* still the infra tip lobule might be over rotated in relation to the columella.
- Although it is easy to look at the naso-labial angle, any abnormalities in the soft tissue or prominent nasal spine can cause spurious judgemental errors regarding rotation of the tip. Hence it is advisable to measure the rotation as an arc cantered on the horizontal projection line of the nasal tip drawn from the alar facial sulcus to the nasal tip. Another vertical line is dropped at the nasal facial sulcus, and the rotation arc is measured as an angle.

- If this tip angle [11] is somewhere between 90 and 100 degrees (less in males than females), then the nasal tip is aesthetically pleasing. Basically rotation defines the position of the two lower lateral cartilages in relation to the anterior septal angle. If the tip is rotated up and "away" from the upper lip, then it is "over rotated"; if it is drooping down and towards the nasal tip, it is "under rotated" (◘ Figs. 2.9 and 2.10).
- Generally detailed measurements are not done in the author's practice, but general recording of over rotation or under rotation is important, so that it tells us about the pathogenesis of the tip deformity and what surgical technique is needed to fix it. The downside of these measurements is that they are made in a 2-D photograph, which does not correlate with a patient in a 3-D orientation. Rotation will also vary when a patient is sitting or lying on the surgical table.
- There is a slight difference in the rotation measured between the two sides as well. We published a study on the effect of caudal septal dislocation on nasal tip rotation, when compared to control group. The results of our study [13] showed that caudal dislocation of the septum causes

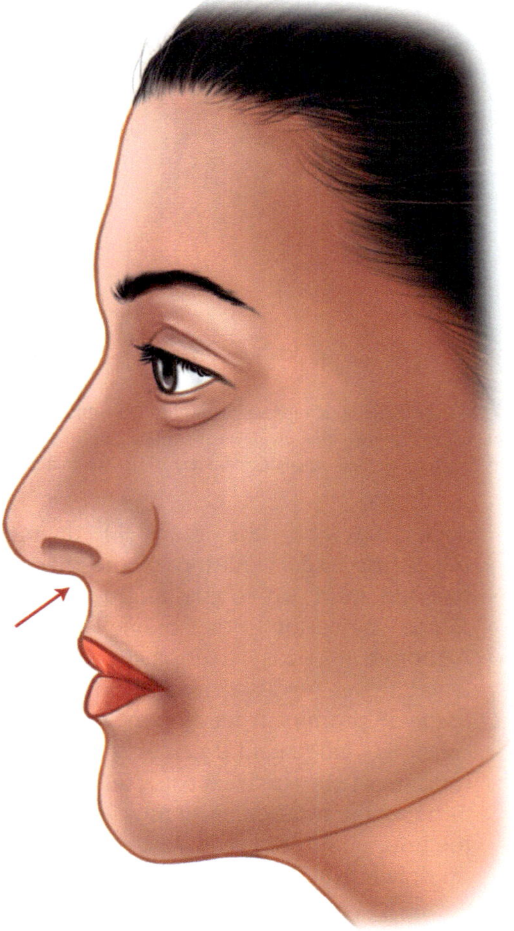

◘ **Fig. 2.9** Schematic representation of the profile view of the nose showing an over rotated nasal tip with the naso-labial angle of more than 100 degrees

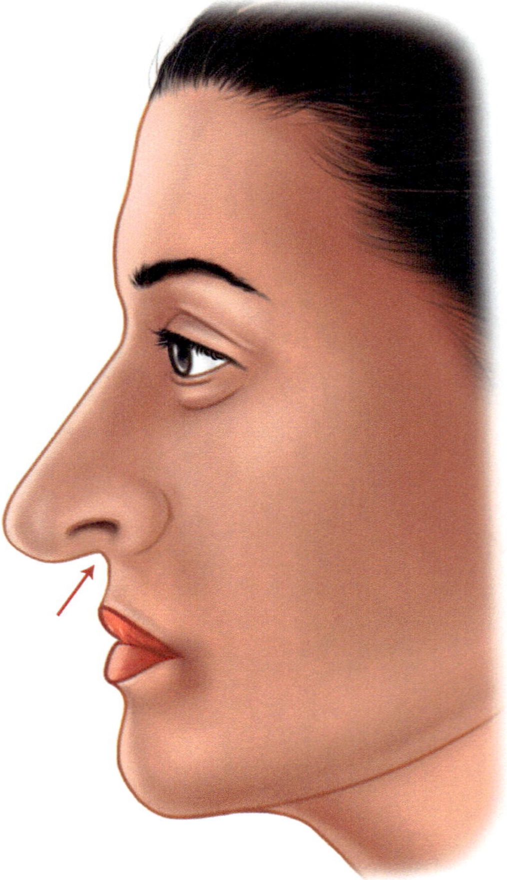

◘ **Fig. 2.10** Schematic representation of the profile view of the nose showing an under rotated nasal tip with the naso-labial angle of less than 90 degrees

significant differences in tip rotation as measured between both sides. There was a correlation between the side of dislocation and rotation with more obtuse angle (over rotation) being demonstrated on the side of the dislocation.

- Thus it is important that while assessing tip rotation, the position of the caudal septum should be taken into consideration. Furthermore, patients should be made aware of this link between the caudal septum and the nasal tip rotation before embarking on septorhinoplasty.
- *The relationship of projection and rotation of the tip to the length of the nose should be looked at here*. There is always a constant relationship between the rotation and the length of the nose. An "under rotated nose is always a long nose" and an "over rotated nose is always a short nose". But the relationship of projection to the length of the nose is variable. An over projected nose is more commonly a short nose but may be a long nose as well. An under projected nose is usually a long nose but may be a short nose as well.
- These concepts are important to bear in mind while planning and executing the surgical techniques particularly when the patient requests are based on these parameters.

Conclusion

In conclusion, the understanding of nasal surgical anatomy is vital for the assessment and surgical management of patients needing nasal tip rhinoplasty. It is important to understand the projection and rotation of the tip in relation to the nasal dorsum by assessing various parameters as mentioned above. But detailed nasal tip measurements, lines and angles may be extremely complex and subjective [5, 11] and, in the author's experience, are of no practical value to the surgeon, apart from teaching and training purposes. Hence clinical examination involving definition, projection and rotation is more significant in arriving at a diagnosis and planning for the surgical treatment [14]. A thorough knowledge of the nasal tip cartilages, along with a clear grasp of the blood supply is necessary before embarking on an open approach nasal tip reconstruction. A clear understanding of the width, position, orientation and angulation of the lateral and medial crura gives you a roadmap for reconstructing a deformed tip. The surgeon needs to be aware of the three-dimensional nature of the lower lateral cartilages and its effect on various aesthetic issues.

Key Points Box

- Detailed nasal tip measurements, lines and angles may be extremely complex and, in the author's experience, are of no practical value to the surgeon.
- The division of major and minor tip supports is an arbitrary one, as damage to even a so called "minor" tip support mechanism may result in a "major" tip deformity and vice versa.
- It is the relative "balance of the strength" between the three structures, namely the medial crus, intermediate crus and the lateral crus, on one side (six in total), which decides the ultimate tip deformity.
- It is the "conjoining" of the medial crural cartilage plus the sagittal orientation of the two medial crura which gives support to the tip. Hence any surgical intervention to support the tip should be directed to increasing or strengthening the medial crus and make the two medial crura into a "conjoined" piece to offer support.
- The degree of post-operative oedema and bruising of the face is directly related to the degree of damage to the soft tissue and bony structure of the nose and also the age of the patient and the state of soft tissue envelope.
- Patients with thickened skin of the nasal tip and also bulbous tip should not be given assurances of any surgical technique to narrow the tip.
- The author's personal concept of nasal tip surgery is "*to make the big guy (lateral crus) smaller and lighter by cephalic trim and the small guy (medial crus) bigger and stronger by grafts or sutures*".

References

1. Daniel RK. The nasal tip: anatomy and aesthetics. Plast Reconstr Surg. 1992;89(2):216–24.
2. Steela NP, Thomas RJ. Surgical anatomy of the nose. In: Stucker FJ, et al., editors. Rhinology and facial plastic surgery. Heidelberg: Springer-Verlag Berlin; 2009. p. 5–13.
3. Sheen JH, Sheen AP. Aesthetic rhinoplasty. Mosby –Year Book Inc: St. Louis; 1987.
4. Sepehr A, Alexander AJ, Chauhan N, Chan H, Adamson PA. Cephalic positioning of the lateral crura: implications for nasal tip-plasty. Arch Facial Plast Surg. 2010;12(6):379–84.
5. Daniel RK. The nasal tip. In: Daniel RK, editor. Aesthetic plastic surgery rhinoplasty. Boston: Little, Brown and Company; 1993. p. 215–81.
6. Tardy ME, et al. Rhinoplasty. In: Cummings CW, editor. Otolaryngology head and neck surgery. St Louis: Mosby–Year Book Inc; 1998. p. 949–99.
7. Anderson JR. A reasoned approach to nasal base surgery. Arch Otolaryngol. 1984;110(6):349–58.
8. Tardy ME, Toriumi DM, Hecht DA. Philosophy and principles of rhinoplasty. In: Papel ID, et al., editors. Facial plastic and reconstructive surgery. New York: Theime Medical Publishers, Inc; 2002. p. 369–89.
9. Balaji N, Ravichandran S. Assessment of nasal valve obstruction: a new nasal "wall" subunit concept. ENT Audiol News. 2012;21(4):111–3.
10. Balaji N, Ravichandran S. Assessment of nasal valve obstruction: a new Glasgow nasal "wall" subunit concept. ENT Audiol News. 2012;21(5):86–7.
11. Daniel RK. Tip. In: Rhinoplasty: an atlas of surgical techniques. New York: Springer-Verlag New York Inc; 2002. p. 59–139.
12. Goode RL. A method of tip projection measurement. In: Powell N, Humphrey B, editors. Proportions of the aesthetic face. New York: Theime-Stratton Inc; 1984. p. 15–39.
13. Smillie I, Sil A, Haddock R, Balaji N. Asymmetrical nostril axis angle in the post traumatic nose. Rhinology. 2013;51(2):176–80.
14. Whitaker EG, Johnson CM Jr. The evolution of open structure rhinoplasty. Arch Facial Plast Surg. 2003;5(4):291–300.

Aetiology, Pathology and Pathogenesis of Nasal Tip Deformities

Contents

N. Balaji, *Textbook of Nasal Tip Rhinoplasty*, https://doi.org/10.1007/978-3-030-48157-5_3

Learning Objectives

- To learn about two types of tip deformities, namely primary and secondary.
- To discuss the aetiology of primary and secondary tip deformities.
- To discuss the pathogenesis of various clinical types of tip deformities including definition, projection and rotation.

3.1 Introduction

Nasal tip deformities can be due to trauma, surgery or genetic in origin and can be complex, requiring many different techniques to correct them. Nasal tip surgery is usually done in association with other rhinoplasty techniques like dorsal or septal work. It is not only important to accurately diagnose the deformities of the lower lateral cartilages before surgery, but also to decide on the "sequence" of the various surgical steps needed to correct the deformity. The peculiarity with this operation is that we rely mainly on the experience of the surgeon rather than relying on any other investigation modalities. Prior to surgery, it is difficult to diagnose accurately the anatomical integrity and pathology of the tip cartilages by any other way. We do not have the advantage of radiological assessment like CT or MRI, which is taken for granted in other specialities in modern day medicine. Hence, an inquisitive mind to acquire the knowledge to understand the aetiology and pathogenesis of the nasal deformity is a prerequisite for developing the optimum rhinoplasty skills.

3.2 Types of Tip Deformities

The tip deformities are classified as *primary* and *secondary*. The primary deformity, meaning that there is an intrinsic structural problem with the two tip cartilages and secondary deformity, meaning issues with the tip secondary to caudal septal issues [1]. Generally most of the deformities, seen in clinical practice, are a combination of both. Usually in familial noses the predominant deformity is primary, where the lower lateral cartilage is deformed, e.g., cleft lip noses. In traumatic noses, it is usually a combination of caudal septal damage and secondary damage to the tip cartilages.

Primary deformities of the tip are due to intrinsic deformities of the lower lateral cartilages involving the following:

- Medial crus, either on one or both sides to varying degrees
- Lateral crus, again either on one or both sides with or without asymmetries
- Intermediate segment or dome
- Varying combinations of all the above giving rise to a myriad of deformities

Secondary deformities of the tip are due to caudal septal issues with no anatomical abnormalities in the tip cartilages. This can involve the following:

- Lack of anterior caudal septal support, causing de-projection and under rotation of the tip
- Caudal septal deviations causing secondary twisting of the tip
- Lack of tip support mechanism due to damaged septal–medial crural fibrous bands causing de-projection and under rotation of the tip.
- Lack of support at the scroll region either due to scarring or weak fibrous support bands (e.g., aging changes) resulting in alar pinching, tip ptosis and functional obstruction

Complex primary and secondary deformities. Most deformities of the nasal tip seen in clinical practice are usually a combination of primary tip cartilage abnormalities and caudal septal defects particularly in traumatic noses. Around 85% of tip deformities in author's practice are patients with a bulbous de-projected nasal tip requesting surgery to narrow the tip and improve the projection.

3.3 Aetiology of Primary Deformities

"Primary deformities" refers to deformities of the nasal tip cartilages per se. This means there could be a deformity in the medial crus, intermediate crus or lateral crus, either on one side or both sides (three on either side and six in total) creating a challenging and complex combination of nasal tip deformities. Weak and deformed cartilages are more common in traumatic patients, whereas strong and over sized cartilages are common in genetic and familial noses. In the majority of the author's patients (around 90% of over 1700) with nasal trauma, it is the medial crura which are damaged and weak and not being able to sustain the weight of the two lateral crura. Surgical aim in these situations would be to strengthen the two medial crura and make it a conjoined segment which then would be able to support the lateral crus. If necessary this is usually combined with a conservative cephalic trim of the lateral crus, which will also help in the tip stability by reducing the weight on the medial crus. Thus increased conjoined strength of the two medial crura will be able to support the less heavy lateral crura. In essence, you are *making the "small (medial crura) guy stronger and the big guy (lateral crura) smaller and weaker". This is an important concept* which will take you through in most nasal tip reconstructions.

The following are a combination of aetiologies in primary tip defects:

- Genetic or familial issues resulting in multiple variations of sizes and shapes involving the lower lateral cartilage
- Congenital deformities – secondary to cleft lip/mid-face abnormalities. Lateral crural abnormalities are common in genetic deformities
- Non-surgical trauma to the nose. Typically, frontal trauma to the nasal tip, like falling over a bike handle. Medial crural damage is more common in traumatic patients. There can be unilateral or bilateral medial crural fractures with loss of tip height and projection. There can be associated concavity of the lateral crus. Medial and lateral crural concavities are usually associated with sharp angulations of the tip with loss of projection. Again these deformities can be unilateral or bilateral (◘ Fig. 3.1a–h)
- Iatrogenic revision rhinoplasty deformities – due to excess cartilage resection, predominantly lateral crus or excess reduction of dorsal cartilage of the septum
- Following surgical tumour excision, most common being inadvertent damage to the alar cartilages during excision of cutaneous tumours
- Aging changes of the elderly with weakness of the tip cartilages and drooping of nasal tip

3.4 Aetiology of Secondary Tip Deformities

These deformities imply that the tip cartilages (lower lateral cartilage) are intrinsically normal but tip abnormality is secondary to other issues predominantly involving the caudal septum, fibrous attachments between medial crus and septum or extensive soft tissue and cutaneous scarring either due to previous surgery or trauma. The aetiologies of secondary tip deformities are as follows:

- The most common aetiology causing secondary tip deformity is trauma to the caudal septum causing moderate or severe caudal septal dislocation, deviation or loss of septal cartilage (◘ Fig. 3.2a–d). This can cause de-projection and upward rotation of the nasal tip.
- Damage to the caudal septum can result in droopy and under rotated tip due to damage to the fibrous attachments to the medial crus.
- Caudal septal retraction or caudal septal loss due to trauma, post-surgery or secondary to septal haematoma and abscess.
- Mid-dorsal septal cartilaginous weakness and collapse causing de-projection and rotating the tip upwards.
- Dorsal bony collapse due to direct severe frontal injury (road traffic accidents), taking "In" the upper lateral cartilages and "K" area along with the dorsal septum and pulling the tip causing de-projection and upward rotation.
- Decrease in the length of the cartilaginous septum due to trauma or surgery.
- Septal perforation due to any trauma, post-surgery or disease.

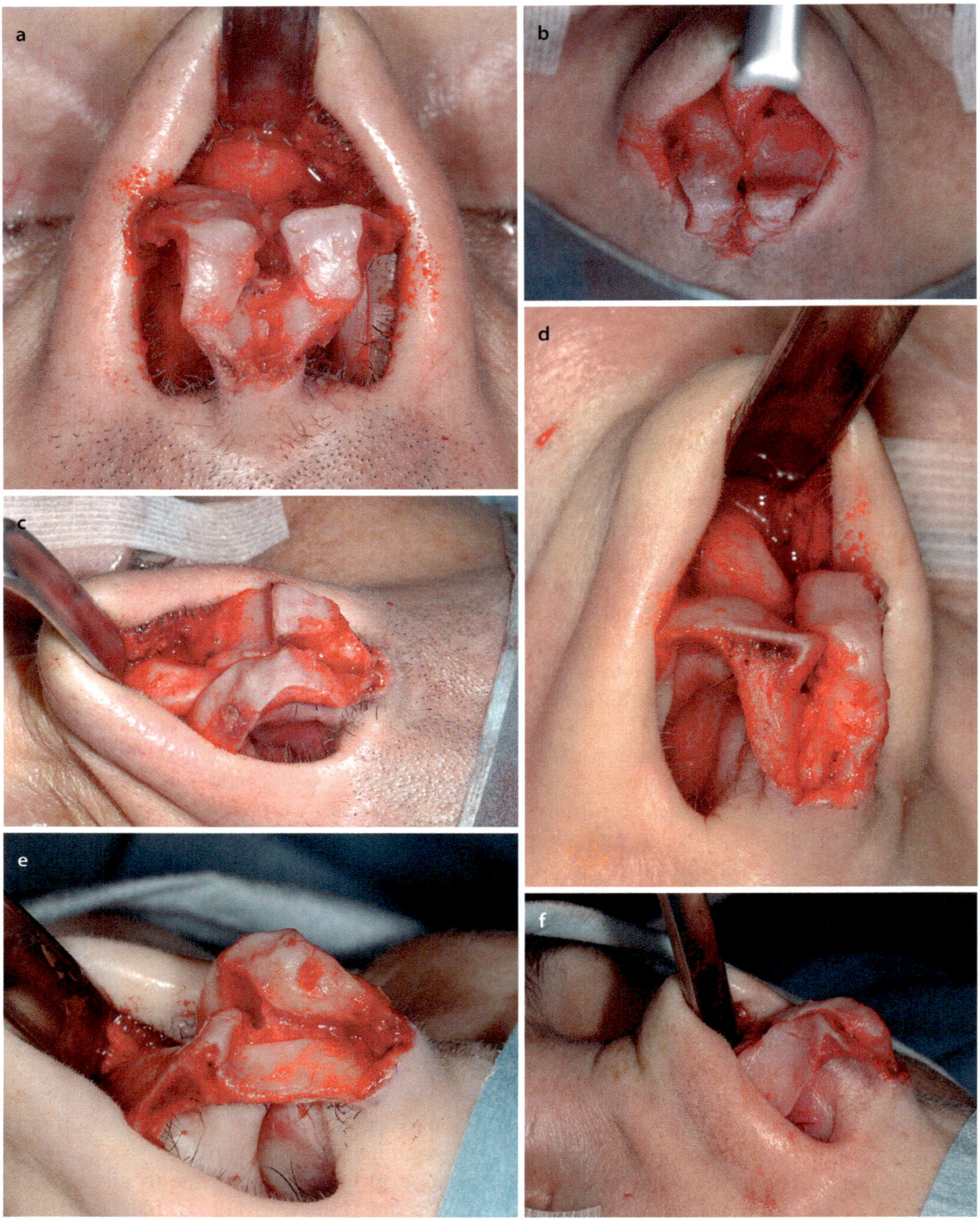

Fig. 3.1 **a–h** Intra-operative pictures showing primary tip deformities. **a** Showing bilateral medial crural fractures. **b** Showing bilateral lateral crural fractures worse on the left side. **c** Showing bilateral lateral crural concavities, both in the horizontal and vertical planes. **d** Showing sharp angulation of the tip cartilage on the right side. **e** Showing sharp angulation of the tip cartilage on the right side and concave medial crura lying in the coronal plane. **f** Showing sharp angulation of the tip cartilage on the right side with smooth concave medial and lateral crus. **g** Showing complex sharp angulations of the tip cartilages due to multiple fractures. **h** Bilateral "volume" loss of the lateral crural cartilage needing a strut graft. ("Reproduced with kind permission from Ref: [1]")

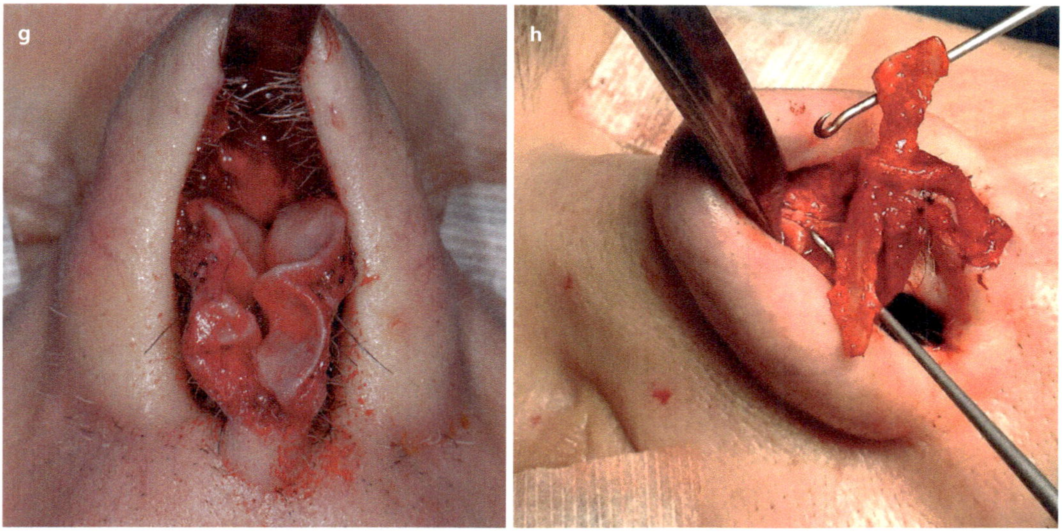

Fig. 3.1 (continued)

- Aging changes resulting in tip ptosis due to weakness of the attachment of the cartilaginous skeleton either to the caudal septum or in the scroll region.
- Columellar soft tissue (skin and subcutaneous) scar contracture with shortening of columella and widening of columella resulting in tip de-projection.
- In patients with nasal trauma, not unusually a combination of septal and lower lateral cartilages abnormalities co-exists.

3.5 Pathogenesis of Primary and Secondary Tip Deformities and Clinical Correlation

A clear understanding of the pathogenesis of the tip deformity is crucial in planning elective surgery. In primary tip abnormalities where tip plasty is indicated, the surgical aim is to address the lower lateral cartilages per se. The principle is to reconstruct and strengthen the lower lateral cartilages predominantly using sutures and avoiding cartilage destructive techniques. In secondary tip abnormalities, it is important to correct the caudal septal support and if necessary anchor the reconstructed and unified tip complex to the rest of the nasal dorsum to achieve a pleasing nasal dorsal profile line. Most of the clinical scenarios due to trauma results in a complex clinical scenarios with both primary and secondary deformities of the tip. Tip assessment should involve history taking, visual examination, palpation, photo documentation and if possible 3D reconstruction. In assessing tip deformities, we need to be aware of this distinction between primary and secondary deformities, as the surgical algorithm should be tailored to individual deformities. Isolated tip plasty procedures are rare in clinical practice, but tip plasty is invariably combined with various other septorhinoplasty techniques involving the nasal dorsum and septum.

3.6 Clinical Types of Tip Deformities

Based on the definition, projection and rotation of the tip, the tip deformities can be classified into various clinical scenarios. The most common tip deformity in Caucasians is a bulbous de-projected nasal tip, with

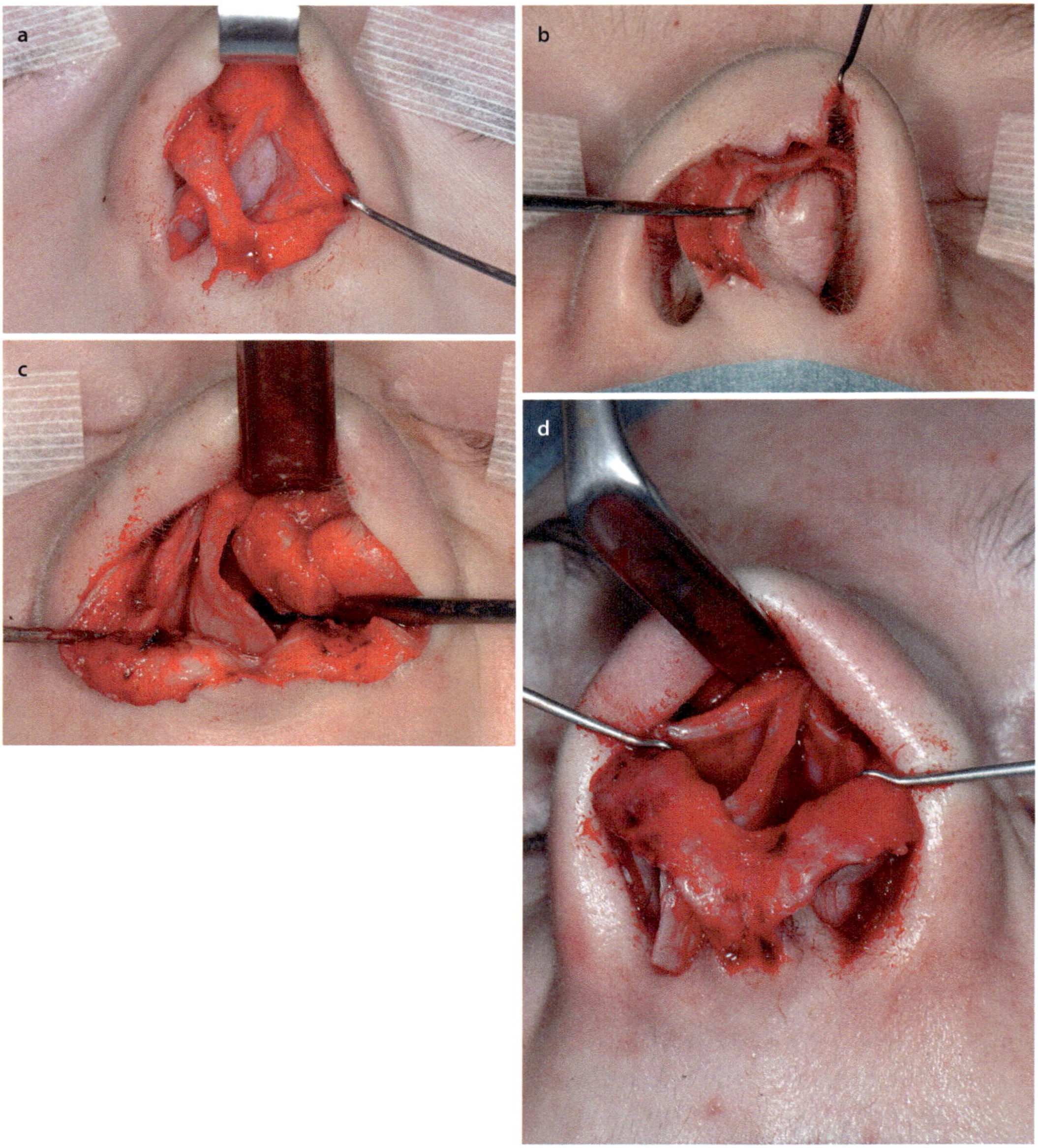

Fig. 3.2 **a–d** Intra-operative pictures showing secondary tip deformities. **a** Open approach view Severe deviation of the septum, including dorsal and caudal septum. **b** Anterior deviation of the septum to the left side. **c** "L" shaped deviation of the septum to the right due to a vertical and horizontal septal fracture. **d** Severe caudal dislocation of the septum to the right side. ("Reproduced with kind permission from Ref: [1]")

patients requesting a more refined and narrower tip. This roughly constitutes majority of the work load with the rest being more rarer combination of defects. Various clinical types of tip deformities will be discussed including the pathogenesis and management algorithms.

3.6.1 Pathogenesis of a Bulbous Nasal Tip

Nasal tip bulbosity may be genetic or secondary to nasal trauma. As mentioned before, the tip defining point is the most projecting part of the nose on the face and is formed by the junction of the intermediate crus with the lateral crus. Normally the tip defining points are about 4 mm wide seen as two dots 4 mm apart in a frontal photograph. A bulbous tip is defined as anything wider than 4 mm between the two tip defining points. In a grossly bulbous tip, they may not be visualised at all. There can be two basic reasons why the tip can be wider. Firstly if the two lower lateral cartilages have moved away from each other, there can be a wider tip with an external depression in between the two lower lateral cartilages almost like a cleft visible on the infra tip lobule segment. Secondly the angle between the medial crura and the lateral crura may be wider either on one side or both sides causing a wider tip, with the angle of divergence being more than 45 degrees. In this situation, the diagnostic clue lies in the width of the soft triangle. The soft triangle area will be a wide open angle rather than a triangle, particularly if there is a cephalic migration of the lateral crus with parenthesis of the tip. Bulbous, wide and trapezoidal, boxy nasal tip could be due to the following factors:

- Genetically large noses due to excess lower lateral crus width and length, resulting in excess bulk of the lateral crus either on one side or both sides, usually seen in Arab, Persian, Punjabi ethnic noses.
- In traumatic noses, there could be a separation of the two lower lateral cartilages (tip cartilages) resulting in a wide tip with more space between the two tip cartilages.
- Separation of the angle between the lateral crus and the medial crus, either on one side causing asymmetric bulbosity or on both sides causing symmetrical bulbosity of the nasal tip.
- A combination of open angle between the medial crus and lateral crus and separation of the two tip cartilages.
- In traumatic noses or revision surgeries, there could be an excess of soft tissue scarring and blubbery tissue with fat in between the two domes which can also contribute to excess width. If so, this should be removed before any tip sutures.

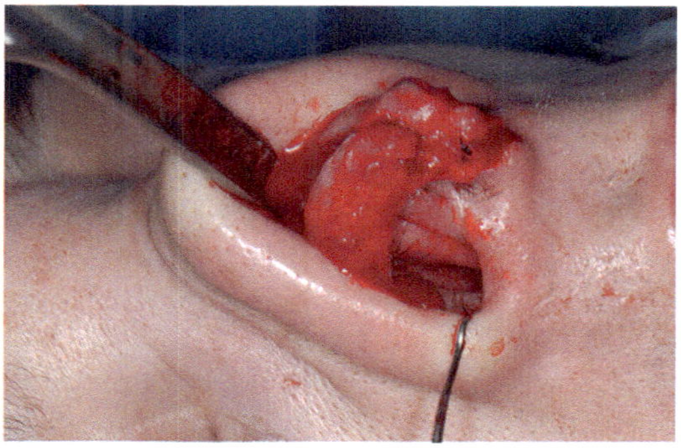

Fig. 3.3 Showing bulbous convex lateral crus on the right side

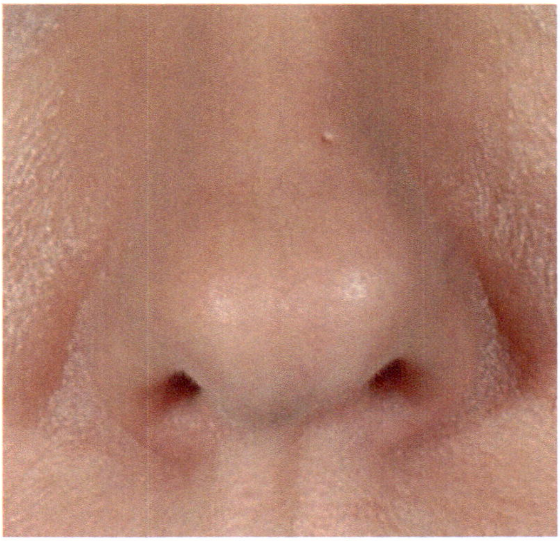

Fig. 3.4 Bulbosity of Tip - Frontal view

- A bulbous tip may also be due to cranial rotation of the domal cartilages on both sides [2].
- Sometimes a unilateral bulbous lateral crus could be due to a weak and fractured medial crus and the weight of the lateral crus pushes down on the dome and causes a bulge of the lateral crus as seen in Figs. 3.3 and 3.4.

3.6.1.1 Clinical Picture

- A bulbous nasal tip is usually the most common deformity of the nasal tip (around 85%) seen in the author's practice over the last 24 years.

- It is usually associated more commonly with an over projected strong nasal tip (▣ Fig. 3.5b).
- It is usually associated with a degree of over rotation (▣ Fig. 3.5b) or normal rotation.
- It can also be associated with under projection (▣ Fig. 3.6) and under rotation (▣ Figs. 3.7 and 3.8).
- There may or may not be a dorsal septal weakness or damage to the dorsal osseo-cartilagenous framework. The dorsal profile line in these noses is usually lower than the tip.
- There is usually an associated supra tip depression due to over projection of the lower lateral cartilages (▣ Fig. 3.5b).
- There can be an associated depression (clefting) in the middle of the tip, either due to strong bulging cartilages imprinting on the skin or due to separation of the two medial crura (▣ Fig. 3.5b) and if present is an indication for a medial crural fixation suture to bring the two

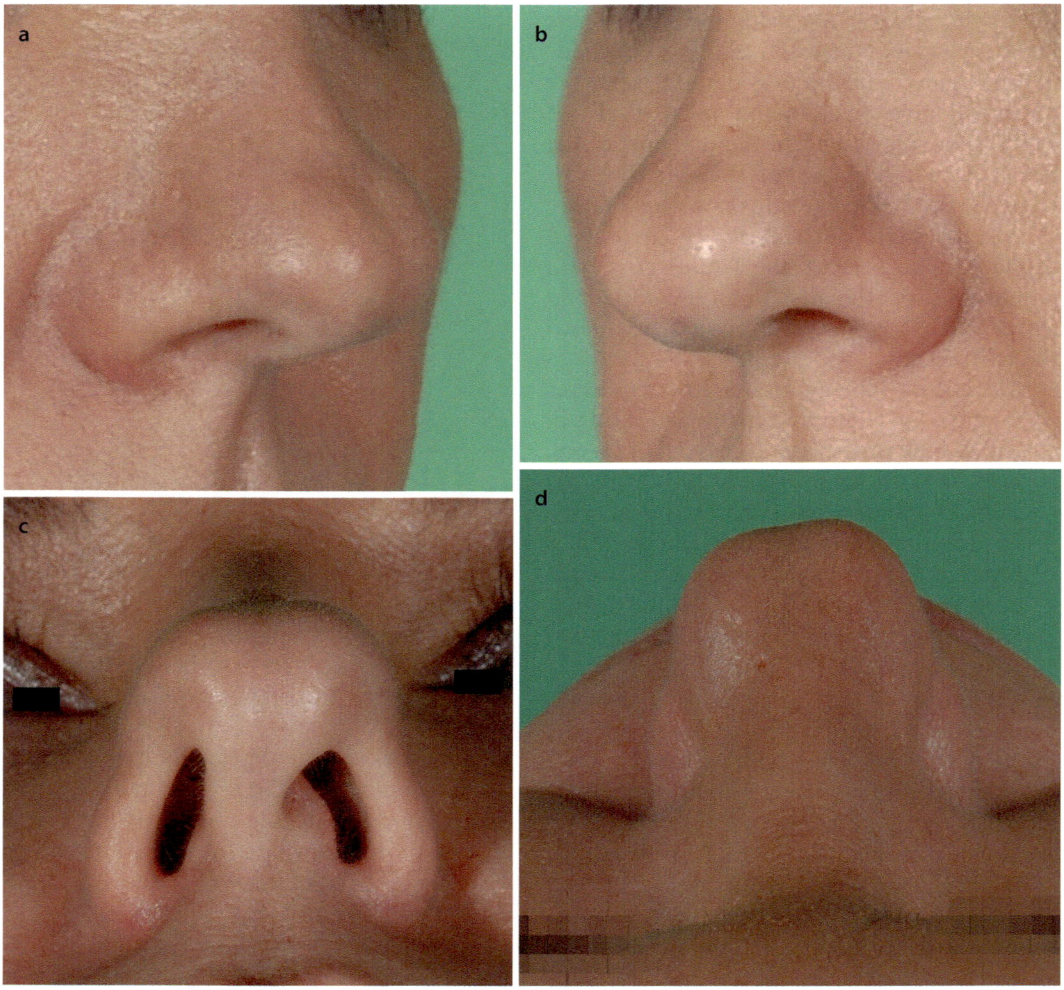

▣ **Fig. 3.5** **a**–**d** Severe bulbosity of the tip with bifidity and over rotation. **a** Right ¾ View. **b** left ¾ view. **c** Basal view. **d** Sky view. ("Reproduced with kind permission from Ref: [1]")

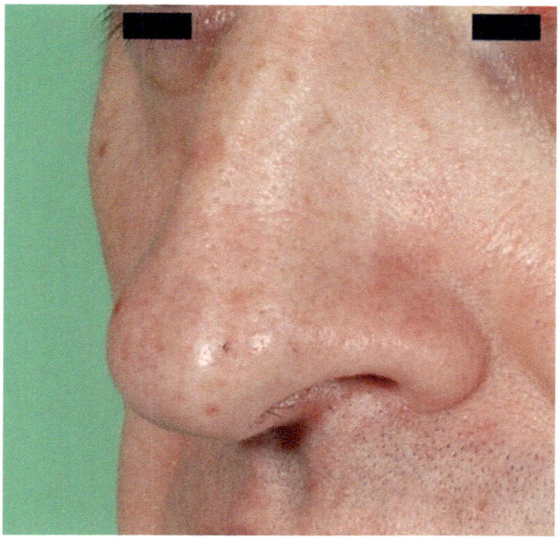

Fig. 3.6 Bulbous tip associated with under projection

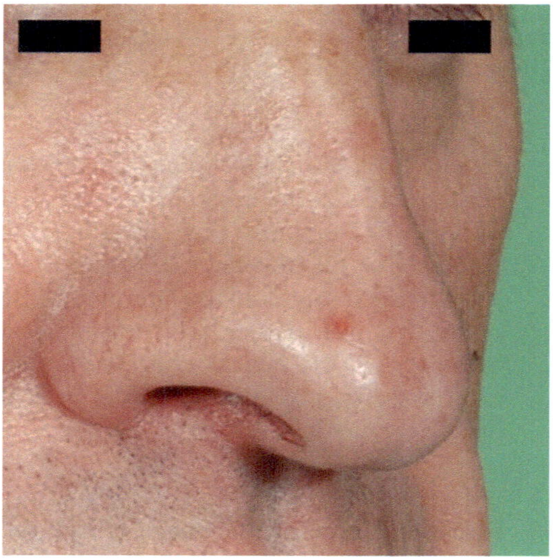

Fig. 3.7 Bulbous tip associated with under rotation

medial crura together (Figs. 3.9 and 3.10).

- Overlying skin in a bulbous strong tip is usually very thin.
- A bulbous tip with a weak tip support can cause medial crural prolapse with excess columellar show (Figs. 3.13 and 3.14). Conversely it can also be associated

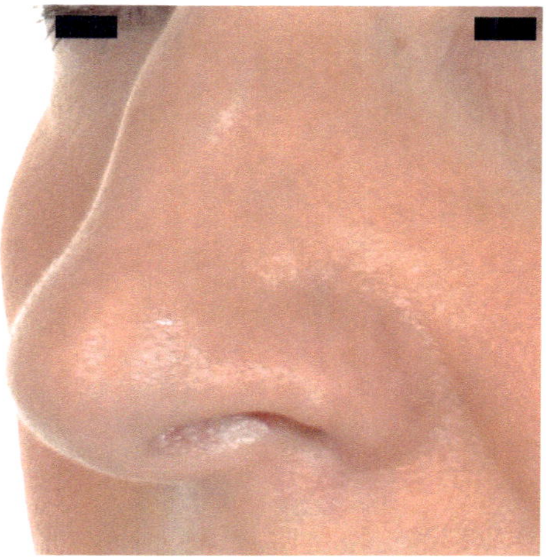

Fig. 3.8 Bulbous tip with over hanging columella

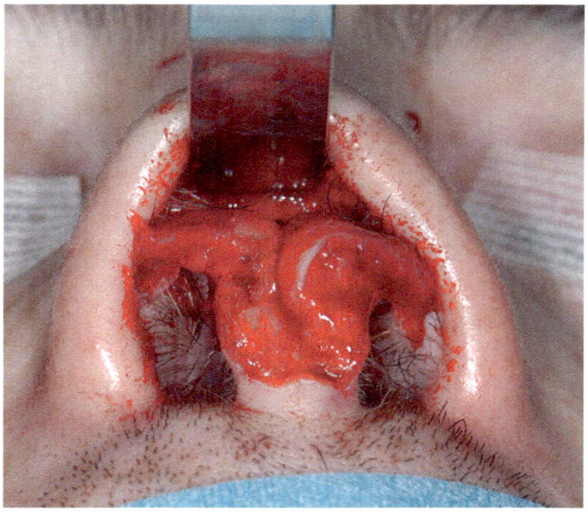

Fig. 3.9 Asymmetric widening of the angle between medial crus and the lateral crus on both sides contributing to widening of the tip

with a retracted columella (Figs. 3.11 and 3.12).

- There could be an asymmetrical bulbosity due to localised weakness of one lateral crus when compared to the other side (Fig. 3.15a).
- Unilateral bulbosity of one lateral crus may be due to the weakness or concavity of the opposite lateral crus with unequal strength. The clinical clue will be a

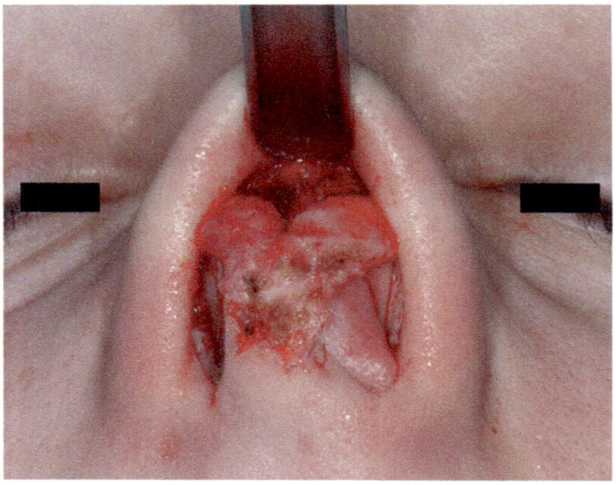

Fig. 3.10 Widening of the angle between medial crus and the lateral crus on the left side contributing to widening of the tip

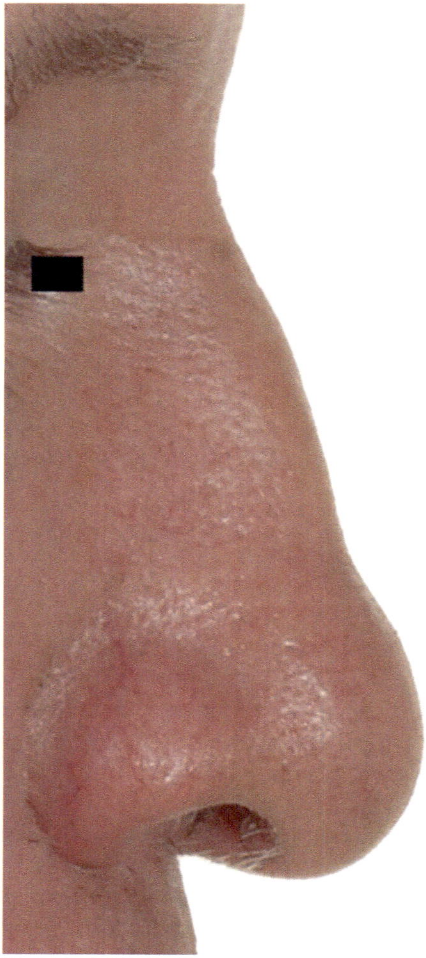

Fig. 3.11 lateral view of bulbous tip with retracted columella with de-projection and under rotation

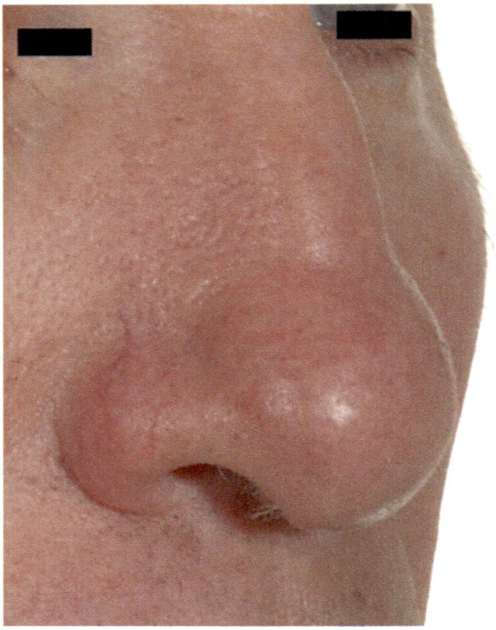

Fig. 3.12 ¾ view of amorphous bulbous tip with retracted columella

deviation of the nasal tip away from the bulbous side to the opposite weaker side (Fig. 3.15a–c). In this situation, the bulbosity of the affected side is due to its unopposed strength of the lateral crus. Be aware that in a patient with a unilateral bulbosity of the lateral crus, the actual issue can be a weaker opposite lateral crus.

3.6.1.2 Target Areas for Surgery

- Essentially targeting the lateral crus of the alar cartilage, particularly de-bulking the lateral crus with bilateral cephalic trim.
- Any excess scar tissue between the domes should be removed before the use of sutures to narrow the tip, particularly in trauma or revision surgery patients.
- Localised bulge can be excised and re secured, but run the risk of shortening the lateral crus and tip asymmetry.
- Plus narrowing the dome with various suture techniques, predominantly trans domal and inter domal sutures [3, 4].
- Localised bulges can also be corrected with mattress sutures.

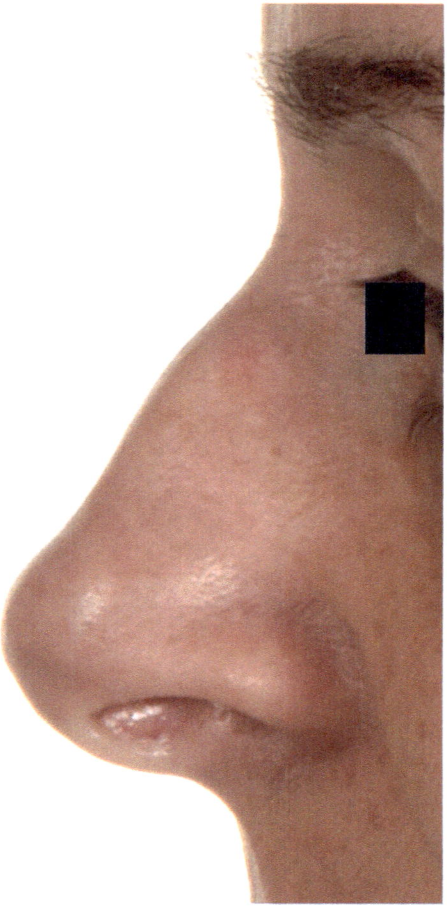

Fig. 3.13 Lateral view of bulbous tip with excess columellar show

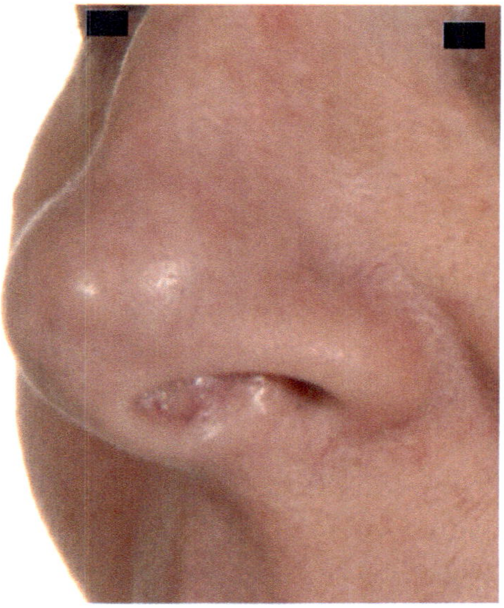

Fig. 3.14 ¾ view of bulbous tip with excess columellar show

3.6.2 Pathogenesis of a Narrow Nasal Tip

A narrow nasal tip may be associated with strong cartilages or weak cartilages. Typically a narrow nasal tip is associated with a strong over projection which may be true or a relative over projection in relation to the rest of the dorsum. It is associated with excess cartilaginous septum in the caudal and the dorsal septum near the anterior septal angle. They may be associated with slight under rotation due to the heaviness of the nasal tip cartilages, particularly if the tip support mechanisms are weak.

Sometimes the tip is very narrow and small in petit noses, particularly secondary to bony and cartilaginous dorsal collapse (Fig. 3.17c), associated with upward rotation with or without tip asymmetry and tip deviation. This is due to retraction and loss of cartilaginous dorsum and caudal septum, causing a bit of inward contraction between the two medial crura. A degree of dorsal de-projection also causes a dead space into which the tip can rotate upwards causing over rotation.

A narrow over projected nasal tip can be genetic, particularly in ethnic middle eastern, Indian, Punjabi, Afghan noses where there is excess length of the lower lateral cartilages associated with a narrow width of the lateral crus. In traumatic noses, there could be a fracture of the lateral crus just lateral to the dome causing an over projection, narrowness and slight upward rotation of the nasal tip. The thickness of the tip cartilages may vary; particularly in the author's experience, majority of over projected thin noses have thinner tip cartilages.

3.6.2.1 Clinical Picture

The following abnormalities are encountered during surgery in a patient with a thin narrow nasal tip:

- Commonly seen with strong tip cartilages and an over projected tip with excess septal

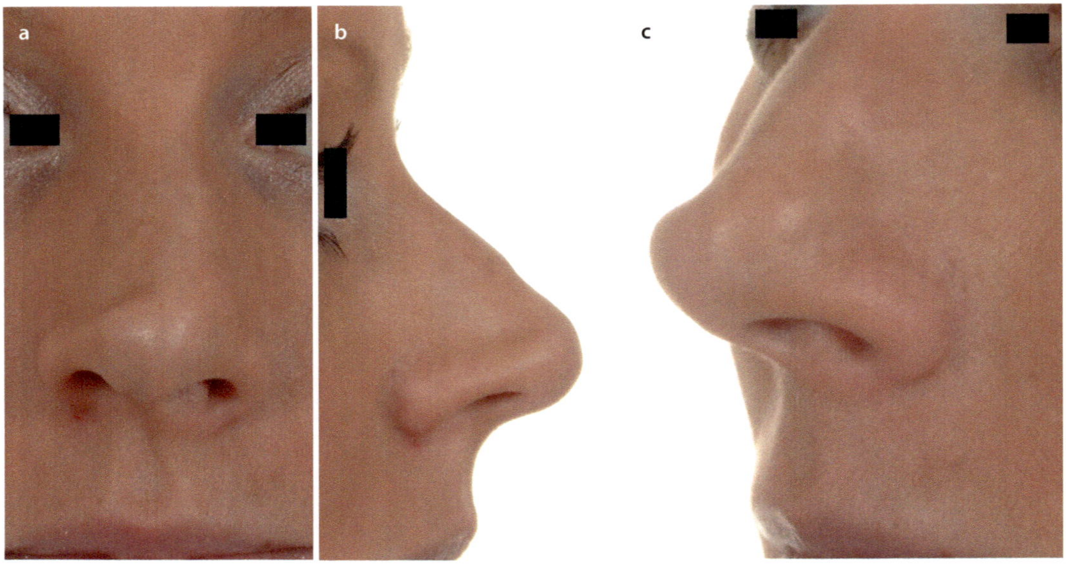

Fig. 3.15 **a–c** Patient with asymmetric bulbosity of the tip with concave lateral crus on the collapsed right side and convex lateral crus on the normal left side and tip deviation to the side of lateral crural weakness. **a** Frontal View. **b** Right lateral view. **c** left ¾ view

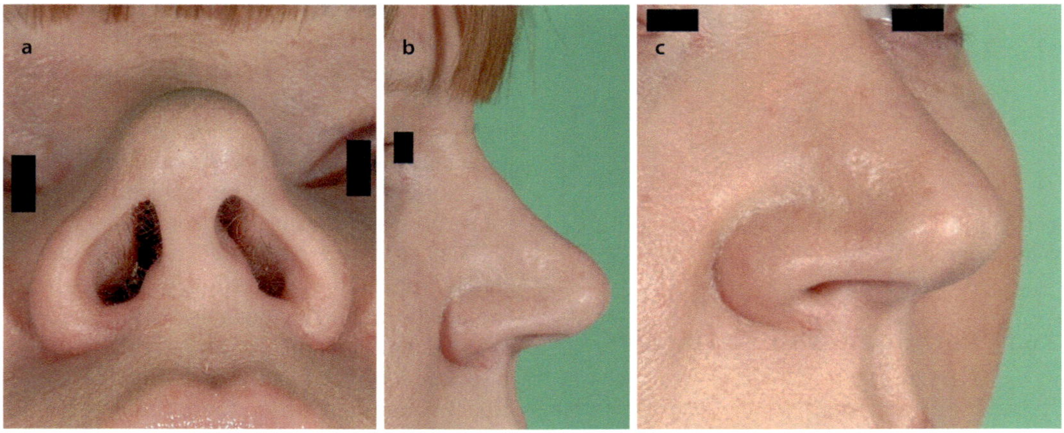

Fig. 3.16 **a–c** Over projecting narrow nasal tip after dorsal hump reduction and failure to address the tip projection. **a** Basal view. **b** Lateral view. **c** Right ¾ View

cartilage in the columella and the anterior septal angle.

- Thin nasal tip can be associated with over projection and over rotation, in a familial nose or after surgery only to reduce the dorsal hump and not addressing the tip (Fig. 3.16a–c).
- Very thin nasal tip can be associated with under rotation and under projection following over resection of the dorsal osseo-cartilagenous framework (Fig. 3.17a–c) or due to a high dorsal septal weakness, absence or perforation.
- Very narrow angle between the medial crus and the lateral crus either due to previous surgery (e.g., VDD or lateral crural steal) or traumatic scarring.
- Sometimes narrow over projected and slightly divergent tip cartilages are due to a fracture of the lateral crus just lateral to

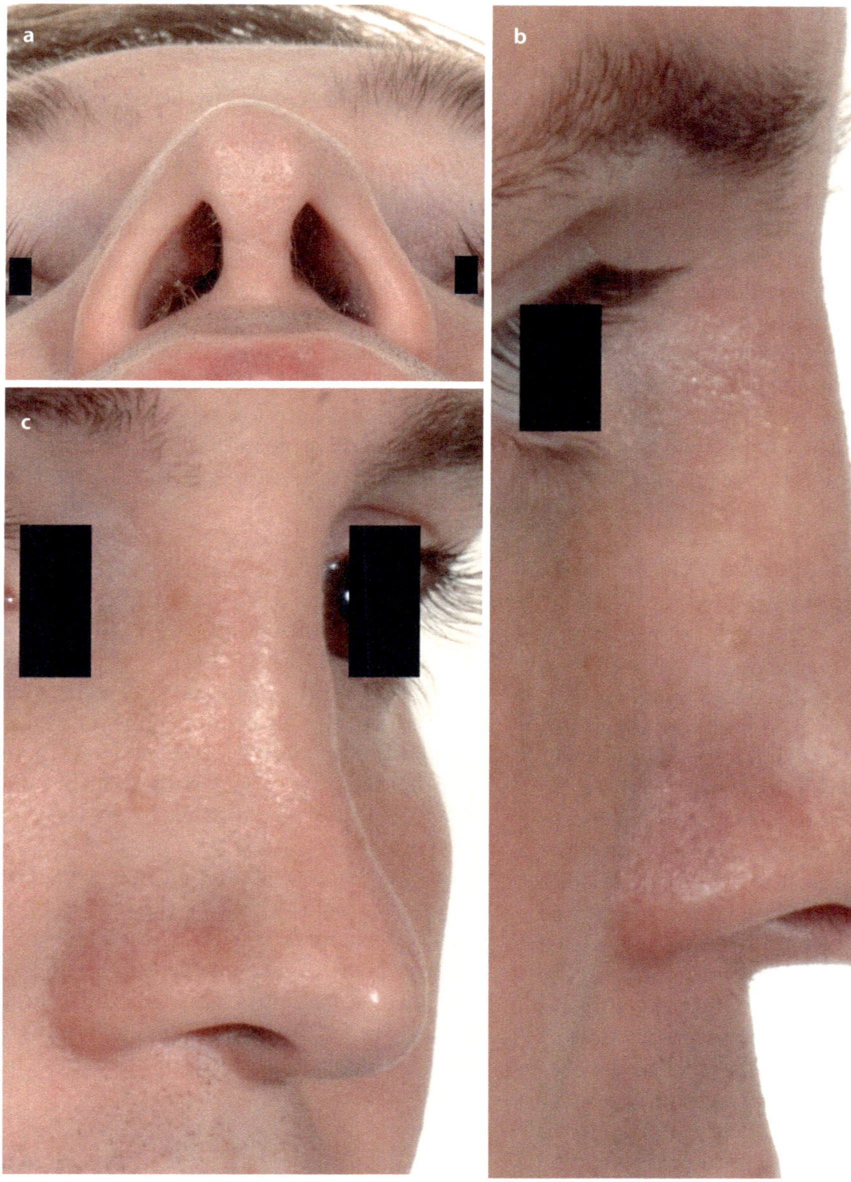

Fig. 3.17 **a–c** Narrow de-projected and under rotated nasal tip after over resected dorsum. **a** Basal view. **b** Lateral View. **c** Right ¾ view

the dome with concavity of the lateral crus caving in and pressing against the medial crus and jacking up the tip (Fig. 3.15a).

- Medial crural weakness with a very narrow space between the medial crus and scarring, usually associated with undue pencil-thin columella in the frontal view. This type of nose might need a strut or a tongue and groove suturing of medial crus to the caudal septum depending on other deformities.

3.6.2.2 Target Areas for Surgery

- A narrow but over projected tip may need reduction of the height of the caudal septum with or without shortening the height of the tip cartilages. By shortening the height of the dome the tip can become wider.

- The reduction of the tip projection can also be achieved by reducing the length of both lateral crus and medial crus, which is time consuming or address the dome directly by a "direct dome technique" of intermediate crural resection and anastomosis of lateral to the medial crus in selective patients with thicker skin. The advantages and disadvantages of this technique are discussed under the surgical techniques.
- A narrow but de-projected petite nasal tip may need additional bulking with either columellar strut plus or minus extra grafting like a shield graft involving the columellar region [5].

3.6.3 Pathogenesis of an Over Projected Nasal Tip

The common pathogenesis of an over projected tip is due to an excess of anterior caudal septum and anterior dorsal septum. It can also be due to an excess length of the lower lateral cartilage. A primary over projected tip is usually familial and associated with excess length of the lower lateral cartilages from the lateral crus in the scroll region to the medial crural footplate in the anterior nasal spine region. An over projected tip is usually also a narrow tip, until otherwise the width of the lateral crus is also wider. Hence any surgical procedure aiming to reduce the projection of the tip should include tools to reduce the dorsal septal cartilage and also caudal septal cartilage, failing which direct techniques to reduce the length of the lateral crus may also be indicated.

3.6.3.1 Clinical Picture

- Usually associated with a strong tip cartilages.
- Associated with under rotation due to weight of the tip cartilages and additional lack of caudal septal support.
- An over projected nose can also be over rotated (◘ Fig. 3.18a–c).
- The length of the nose is usually longer with the patient wishing to reduce the length of the nose along with decreasing the projection of the nasal tip.

3.6.3.2 Target Areas for Surgery

- The dorsal septal cartilage and also caudal septal cartilage, may have to be reduced to decrease the tip projection.
- A parallel shave of the caudal septum will reduce the projection of the tip without altering the rotation (◘ Fig. 3.19a).
- A triangular shave of the caudal septum with the base of the triangle at the posterior septal angle/anterior nasal spine region will cause de projection of the tip and also slight under rotation on the lip (◘ Fig. 3.19b).
- A triangular shave of the caudal septum with the base of the triangle at the anterior septal angle will cause de-projection of the nasal tip and also slight over rotation on the dorsum (◘ Fig. 3.19c).
- May also need direct excision techniques to reduce the projection, like a 4 mm resection (maximum) and or overlap of the lateral crus, along with reducing the height of the medial crus by incision or excision [6].
- Another direct technique that will give an acceptable outcome is to go for an Intermediate crural resection and anastomosis of the medial to lateral crus in selected patients. This is quicker and ideally suited for a slightly older patient with a thicker skin (see case report in ▶ Chap. 19).

3.6.4 Pathogenesis of an Under Projected Nasal Tip

This could be due to a primary tip problem or secondary to caudal septal weakness, absence or a combination of both. Primary tip problems are usually associated with bilateral fractures, scarring and weakness of the medial crus either one side or both sides, with the conjoined medial crus not able to cope with the weight of the two lateral crus, so called "the big guy pressing down on the

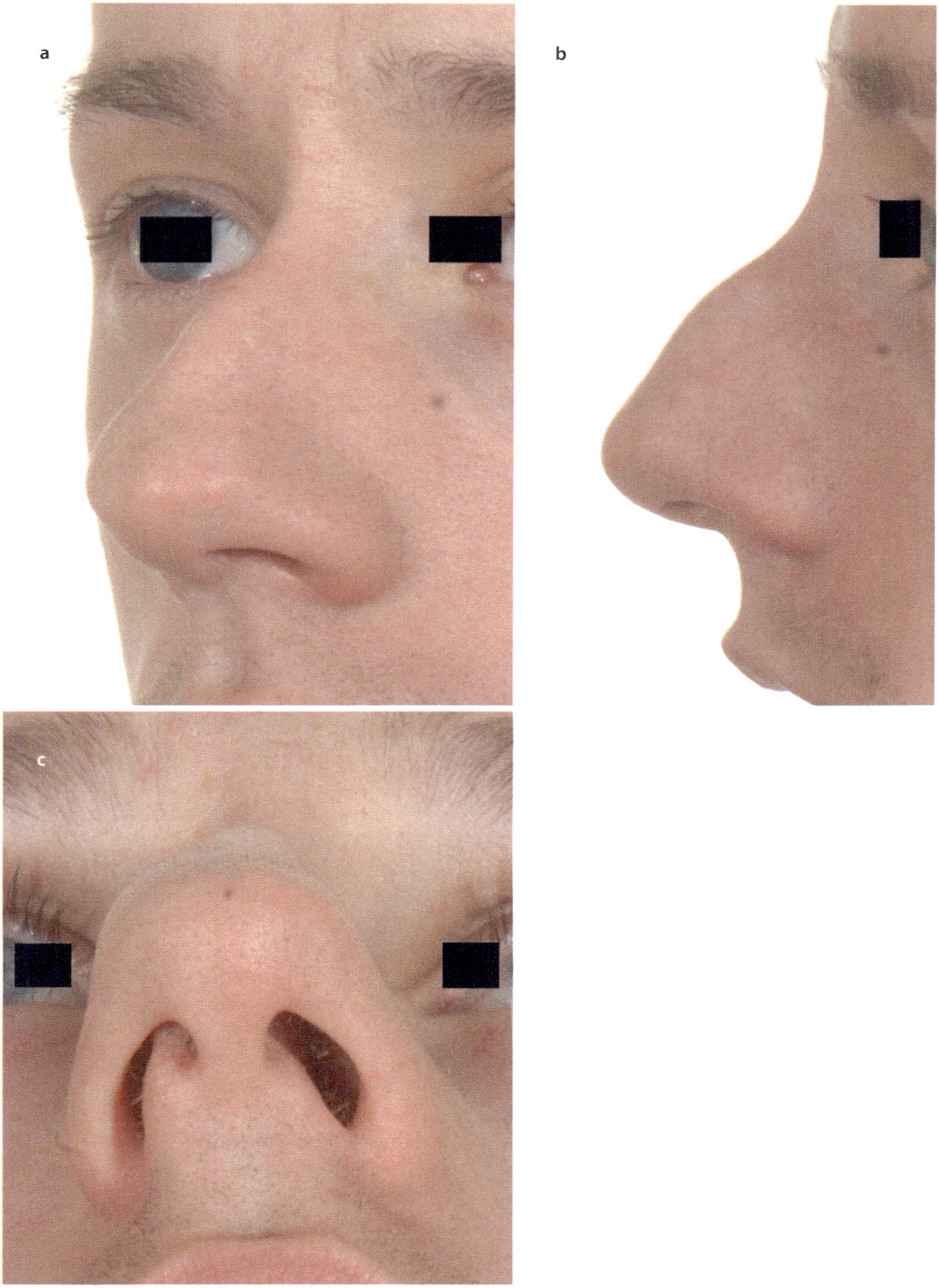

Fig. 3.18 **a–c** Young patient showing over projected and over rotated tip with a short nose and a prominent hump. **a** Left ¾ View. **b** Lateral view. **c** Basal view

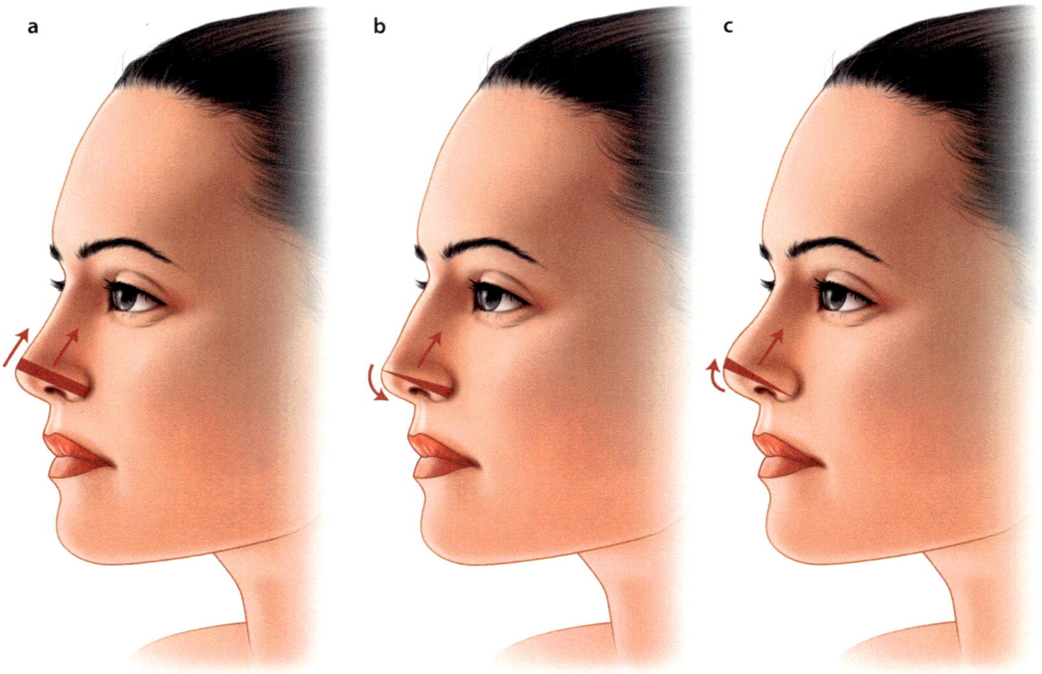

Fig. 3.19 **a–c** Schematic representation of caudal septal shave to reduce projection. **a** Parallel shave reducing the projection. **b** Triangular shave with base of the triangle at the posterior septal angle helps to de-project and under rotate the tip. **c** Triangular shave with base of the triangle at the anterior septal angle helps to de-project and over rotate the tip

small guy". The concept of surgery in these patients would be to make the big guy smaller by cephalic trim and the small guy stronger with either additional columellar grafting with or without medial crural re-enforcement sutures.

3.6.4.1 Clinical Picture

- There is an antero-posterior shortening of the anterior caudal septum (Fig. 3.20a–c).
- Usually, associated with a bulbous, trapezoidal tip. The patient may wish to achieve a narrow tip along with increasing the tip projection.
- Can also be associated with a narrow tip (Fig. 3.21a–c).
- The length of the nose is relatively longer (Fig. 3.21a), as the projection line will be lot lesser than the dorsal length line. Even though the main issue is a de-projected tip, the patients are more likely to complain about the length of the nose. It is up to the surgeon to point out the other deformities, particularly the under projected tip, if any.
- Can be associated with cleft lip noses.
- Can be seen in revision rhinoplasty patients, particularly multiple open revisions with scarring of the columella (Fig. 3.22a).

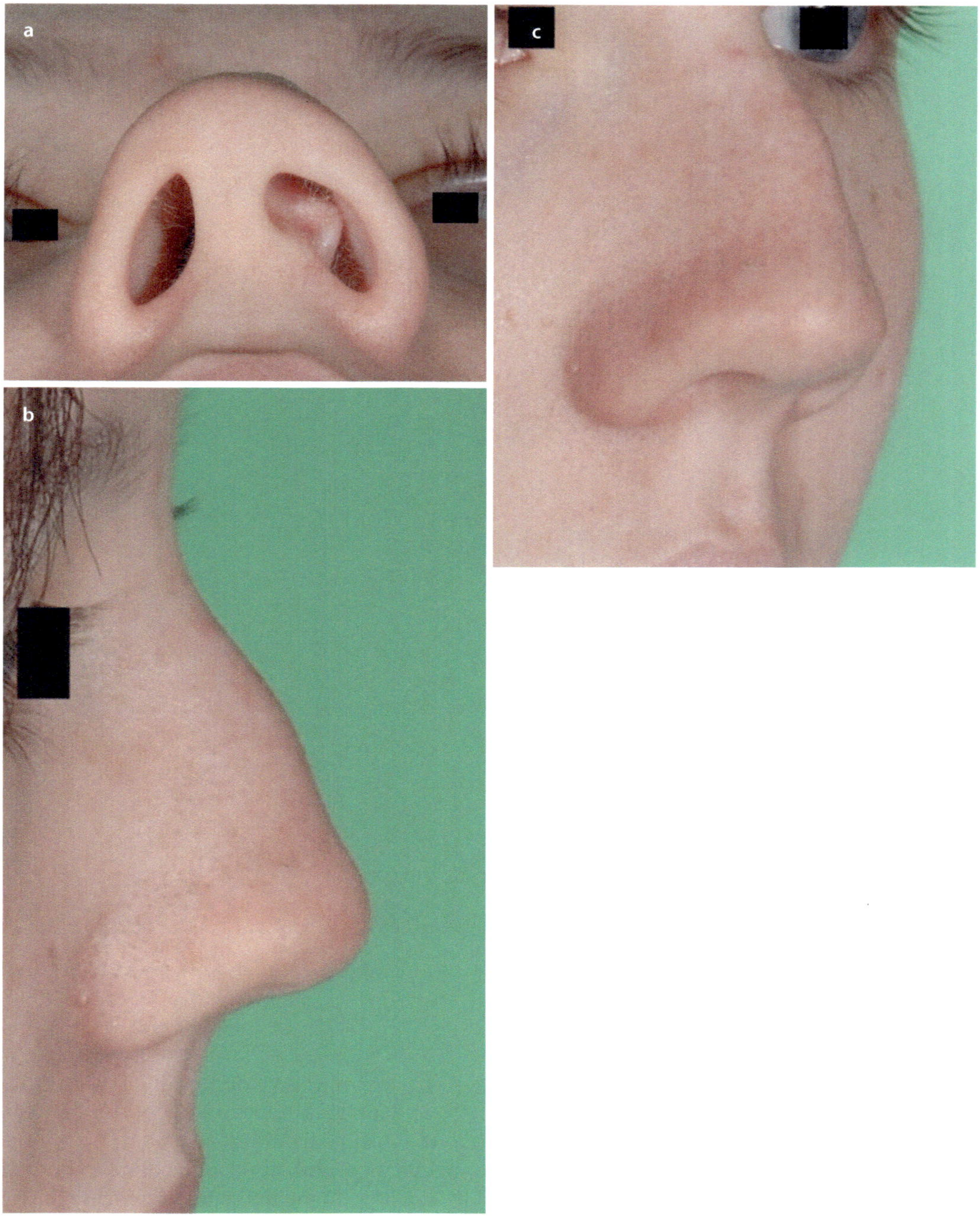

Fig. 3.20 **a–c** Younger patient showing under projected tip due to caudal septal damage. **a** Basal view. **b** Lateral view. **c** ¾ view

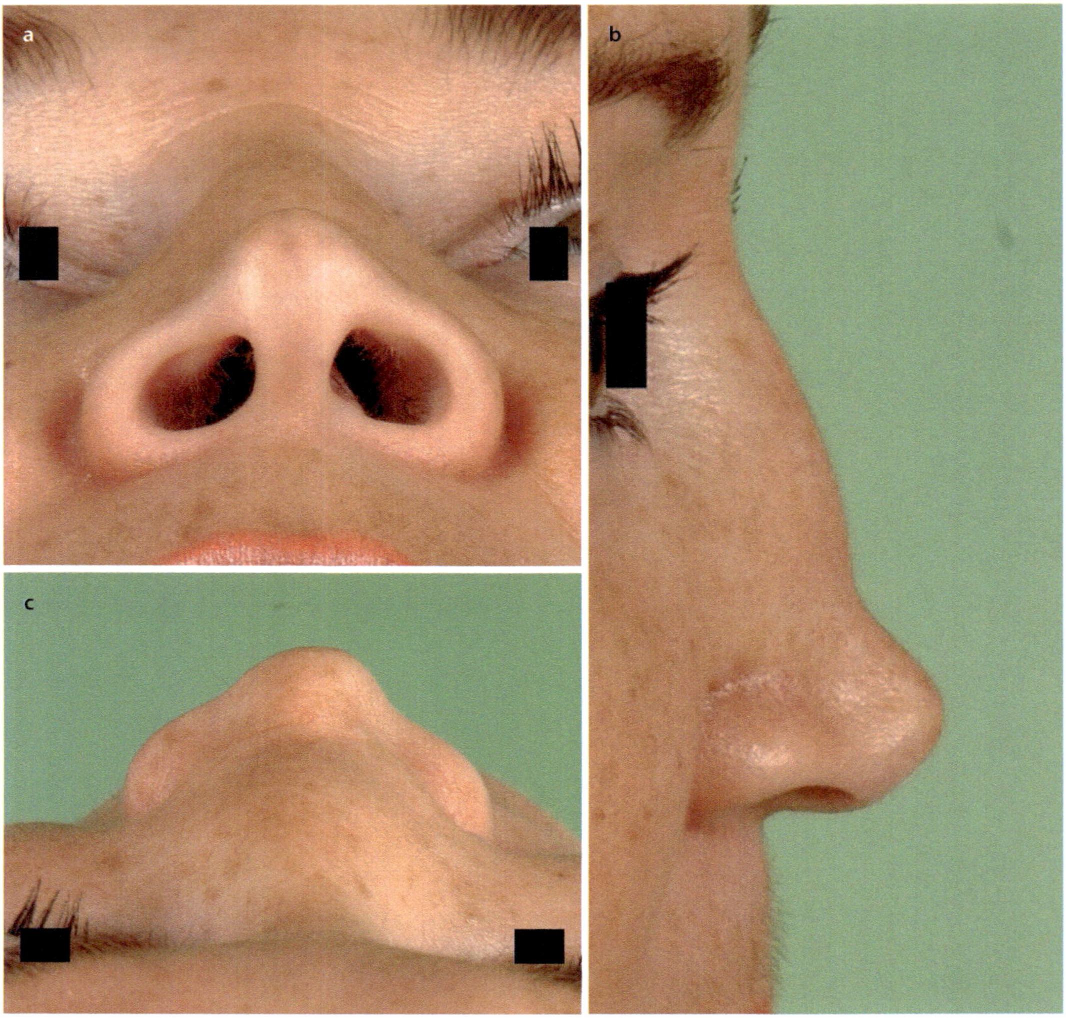

Fig. 3.21 **a–c** Older Patient showing under projected tip due to mid dorsal septal collapse. **a** Basal view. **b** Lateral view. **c** ¾ view

- Can be associated with localised lack of cartilage at the anterior septal angle cartilage, due to trauma or previous over resection.

3.6.4.2 Target Areas for Surgery

- Strengthening the two medial crura creating a "conjoined" force to improve tip projection and give support to the tip.
- The above can be done either with sutures with or without cartilage grafts between the two media crura.
- Lateral crural steel can be done to borrow cartilage to medial crura to increase the tip height [7].
- Additional grafts can be used to increase tip projection like columellar strut grafts, caudal extension grafts or shield grafts.

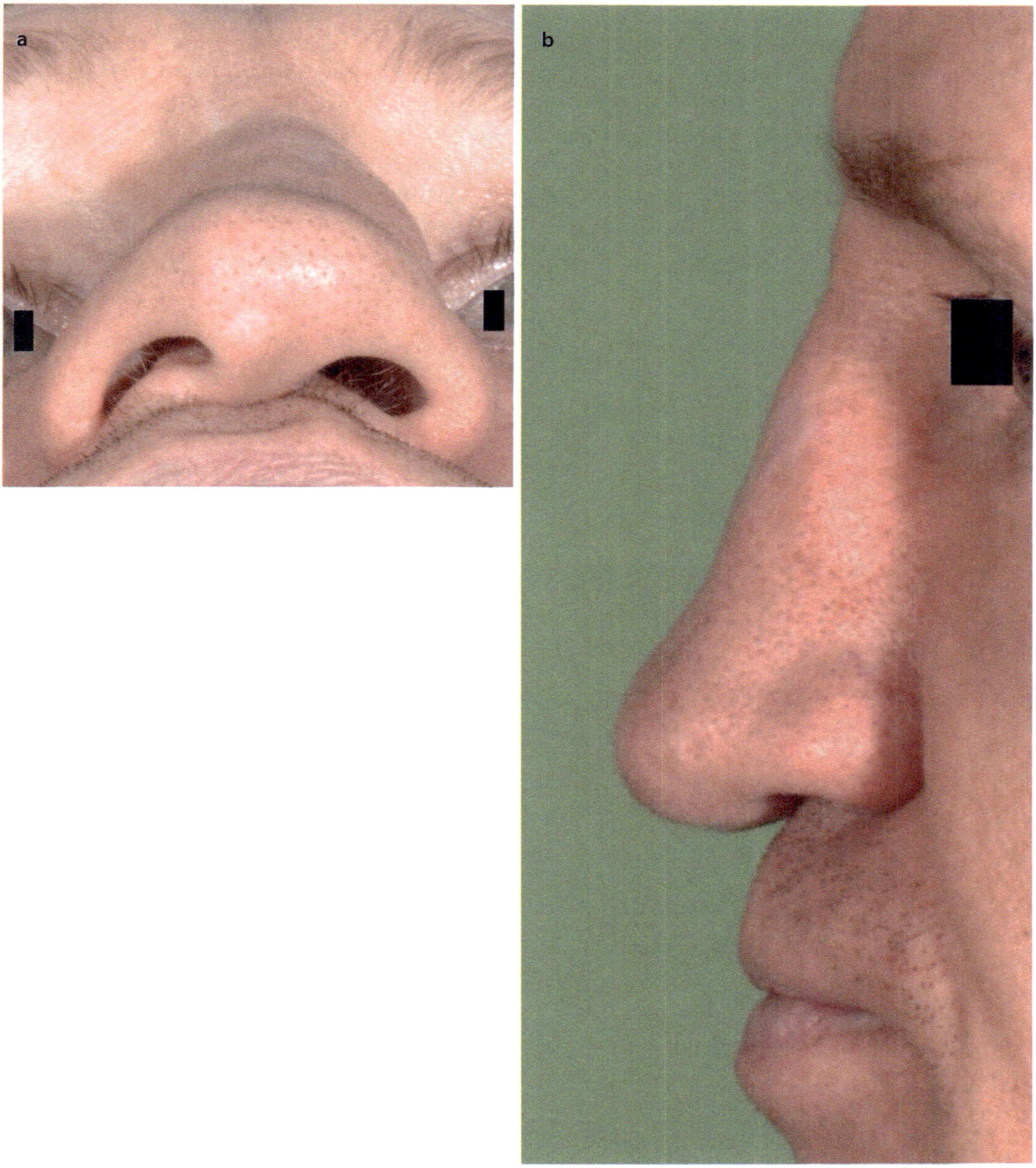

Fig. 3.22 **a**, **b** Older Patient showing under projected and under rotated tip due to caudal septal damage. **a** Basal view. **b** Lateral view

3.6.5 Pathogenesis of an Under Rotated Droopy Nasal Tip

An under rotated droopy tip without tip support is usually due to either a primary issue with the tip cartilages as seen in an aging nose or secondary to lack of caudal septal support and or disconnection from the caudal septum, secondary to trauma or previous surgery. It is associated with under projection as well. This can be associated with columellar shortening along with extensive skin scarring of the columella. The naso-labial angle in a droopy tip is less than 90 degrees with restricted visualisation of the upper lip in the mid line. Sometimes the male patient may have to lift the tip to access shaving the upper lip hair. The aim of correcting the under rotated tip is to strengthen the caudal septum, if necessary with a caudal septal extension graft and strengthening the medial crus with or without lateral crural shortening procedure. The tip has to be anchored to the adequately projected and straightened caudal septum with sutures, for example, the tip anchoring suture.

3.6.5.1 Clinical Picture

- Usually a long nose from the nasion to the tip (◘ Fig. 3.23a).
- Smaller nasal labial angle between the columella and the infra tip lobule.
- Patients don't like their profile side views as it gives an aged look.
- Sometimes male patients complain that they can't see the upper lip clearly in the frontal view and they may have to left the tip to shave (◘ Fig. 3.23b).
- Can be seen in young people after trauma or multiple revision procedures.
- Also seen in elderly patients with weak cartilages with functional nasal obstruction due to change in the direction of airflow.

3.6.5.2 Target Areas for Surgery

- To secure a reconstructed medial crus to the caudal septum with tongue and groove advancement sutures.
- To strengthen caudal septum with either caudal extension grafts.

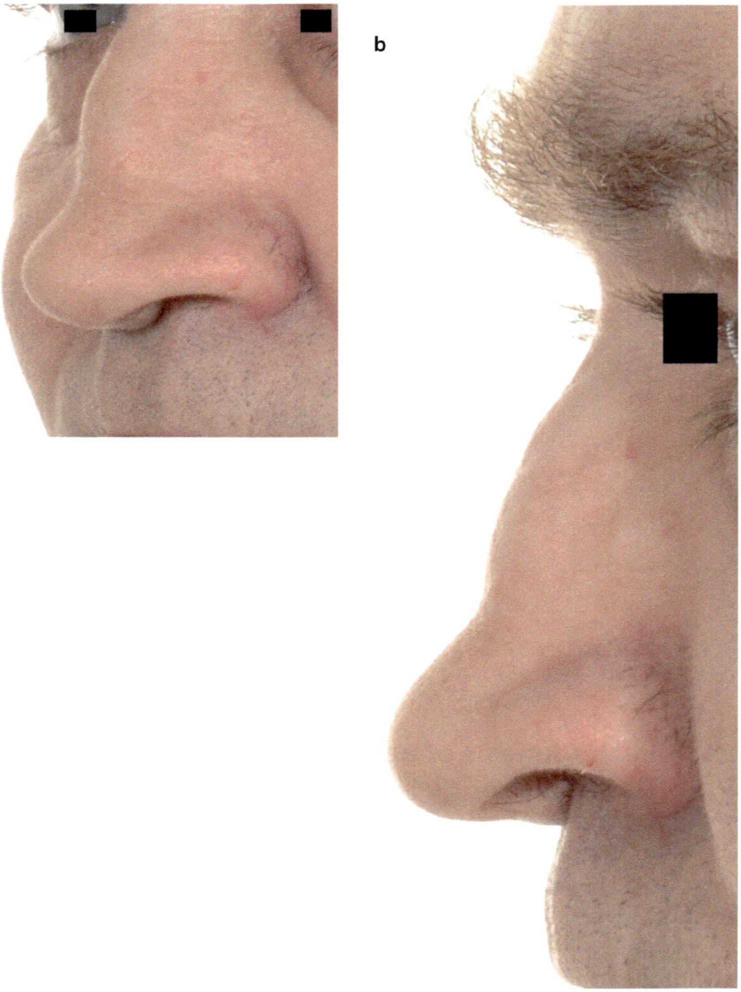

◘ **Fig. 3.23** **a**, **b** Older Patient showing under rotated droopy tip due to caudal and dorsal septal damage. **a** ¾ view. **b** Lateral view

- Medial crural lengthening and strengthening procedure may have to be done along with septal reconstruction.
- Shorten the lateral crus with lateral crural overlap or resection and anastomosis of the lateral crus.
- The dome can also be simply over rotated purely with sutures, namely tip anchoring suture going through the posterior border of both medial crura and the anterior septal angle taking care not to tighten the knot too much.

3.6.6 Pathogenesis of an Over Rotated Nasal Tip with Short Nose

Is usually secondary to lack of dorsal septum either due to disease, perforation, and trauma or over resection. There can also be lack of anterior caudal septum, particularly near the anterior septal angle, where the caudal septum meets the dorsal septum. An over rotated tip usually results in a shorter nose with the dorsal length between the nasion and the tip less than the projection. The angle between the columella and the upper lip is more obtuse with an angle more than 105 degree. There can be an excess frontal show of the two alar nostrils, which the patients may dislike more than the rotation. Can also be associated with supra tip depression and pseudo dorsal hump with wide nasal bones, particularly post traumatic deformities. The novice will quickly understand it is not easy to bring the tip down as opposed to lifting the tip up with any surgical procedure [8].

3.6.6.1 Clinical Picture

- Over rotated tip usually results in a shorter nose, (◘ Fig. 3.24a) with patients wishing to increase the length of the nose.
- The infra tip lobule segment of the tip will be disproportionately larger than the supra

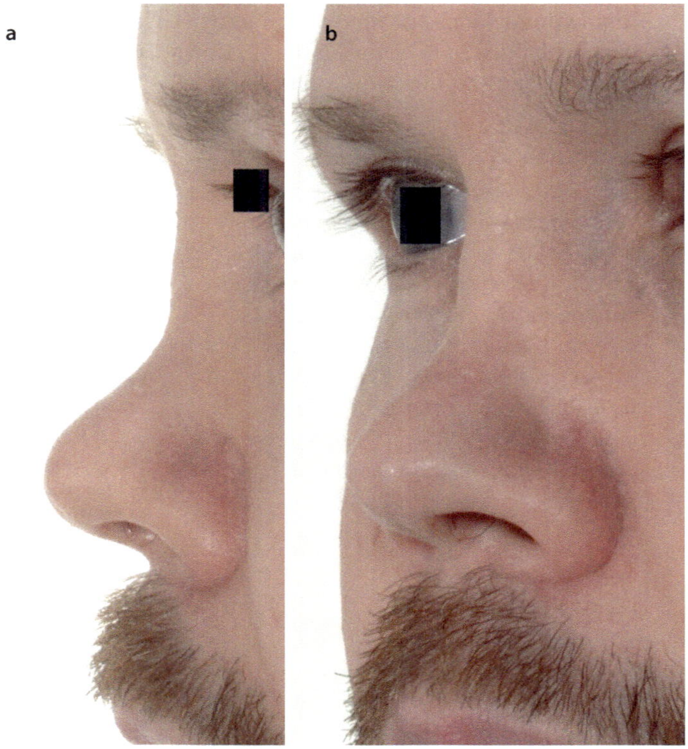

◘ **Fig. 3.24** a, b Younger patient showing collapsed dorsum with over rotated tip and a shorter nose, due to septal perforation caused by granulomatosis. **a** Lateral view. **b** ¾ view tip lobule segment with an exaggeration of the "double break" in the tip. The angle between the columella and the infra tip lobule segment can be more obtuse.

- There could be excess "anterior show" of the alar nostrils when seen in the frontal view.
- Could also be due to excess resection of the lateral crus after secondary rhinoplasty or trauma.
- Can be associated with septal perforation and septal volume loss (Fig. 3.24b).

3.6.6.2 Target Areas for Surgery

- The dorsum and caudal septum may need to be augmented and supported and extended either with a dorsal septal extension or caudal septal extension grafts.
- They may also need lateral crural strut grafts to de rotate and bring down the tip.
- Be aware it is very difficult to surgically bring down the tip (under rotate) than to upwardly rotate a droopy tip.
- Supra tip lobule segment can be augmented by a supra tip or CAP graft to create the illusion of rotating the tip down by increasing the supra tip lobule.

Conclusion

Thus being aware of the aetiology and pathogenesis of the tip deformities are essential before contemplating nasal tip surgery in a deformed nose. A thorough understanding of the knowledge of what is happening under the skin can come only with experience. Being able to understand the pathogenesis and hence able to plan the sequence of surgical steps, helps in the informed consent of the patient and also helps the surgeon to achieve favourable outcomes.

Key Points Box

- Primary tip deformities are due to intrinsic problems with the tip cartilages.
- Secondary tip deformities are due to caudal septal issues.
- Traumatic noses have a combination of primary and secondary tip issues.
- Congenital pathologies like a cleft lip nose is usually due to primary tip deformities involving the lower lateral cartilages rather than septal issues.
- Bulbous tip is the most common tip deformity faced by most rhinoplasty surgeons. There can be two basic reasons for a bulbous tip. Firstly, if the two lower lateral cartilages have moved away from each other with an external depression in between the two lower lateral cartilages almost like a cleft visible on the tip lobule. Secondly the angle between the medial crura and the lateral crura may be wider either on one side or both sides causing a wider tip.
- Any surgical procedure aiming to reduce the projection of the tip should include tools to reduce the caudal septal cartilage, failing which direct tip techniques to reduce the length of the lower lateral cartilage may be needed.

References

1. Balaji N. Top tips in nasal tip surgery, ENT-FPS UK Newsletter— Feb 2018 –Issue 6.
2. Constantian MB. The boxy nasal tip, the ball tip, and alar cartilage malposition: variations on a theme – a study in 200 consecutive primary and secondary rhinoplasty patients. Plast Reconstr Surg.2005; 116(1):268–81.
3. Daniel RK. Surgical techniques for broad, boxy, and ball tips. Op Tech Plast Reconstr Surg. 2000;7(4): 213–23.
4. Rohrich RJ, Adams WP Jr. The boxy nasal tip: classification and management based on alar cartilage suturing techniques. Plast Reconstr Surg. 2001;107(7):1849–63; discussion: 1864–8.
5. Toriumi DM. New concepts in nasal tip contouring. Arch Facial Plast Surg. 2006;8(3):156–85.
6. Foda HM, Kridel RW. Lateral crural steal and lateral crural overlay: an objective evaluation. Arch Otolaryngol Head Neck Surg. 1999;125(12):1365–70.
7. Kridel RW, Konior RJ. Controlled nasal tip rotation via the lateral crural overlay technique. Otolaryngol Head Neck Surg. 1991;117:411–5.
8. Gruber RP. The short nose. Clin Plast Surg. 1996;23(2):297–313.

Assessment of the Nasal Tip

Contents

N. Balaji, *Textbook of Nasal Tip Rhinoplasty*, https://doi.org/10.1007/978-3-030-48157-5_4

Learning Objectives
- How to assess the structural deformity of the nose and the nasal tip.
- How to differentiate primary from secondary tip deformities.
- How to assess the definition, projection and rotation of the nasal tip and come up with a surgical algorithm.

4.1 Introduction

4

Like any aspect of rhinoplasty surgery, assessment of the nasal tip is the "key" in achieving a favourable outcome in nasal tip surgery. The surgeon should develop the art of being able to assess the "aetio-pathology" of the deformity by being able to "look through" the overlying skin. The biggest teacher being the patient. Theoretical knowledge and attending courses helps in the process, but ultimately it is the years of learning experience from the patients which helps the surgeon. Arriving at a diagnosis helps in the informed consent. It is always wiser to cross check the pre-op clinical findings with intra-operative pathology. Also create the habit of going back and looking at the pre-operative pictures to see whether the deformity was visible and whether it was picked up before or during the initial examination. In the author's experience, most of the tip deformities are visible through the skin, but the surgeon fails to "see" them. It is this "art" of diagnosing the deformity under the intact skin which is difficult to learn. It takes years to master this art and still each and every patient can evade the surgeon in this quest for knowledge. The patient should be educated in the counselling stage that there is no radiological or any form of investigation which can aid us in arriving at a correct diagnosis. It is often said that you should envy the "eye" of an excellent rhinoplasty surgeon than his "hands".

What is an "ideal tip" we are trying to achieve? The answer is rather philosophical. In short there is "no ideal tip". Although the beauty is in the eye of the beholder, there are some parameters which make the nose pleasing. One factor is the "symmetry". Leonardo da Vinci, the renaissance painter and sculptor, used the principle of symmetry and proportions, the so-called golden triangle to create aesthetic master pieces like "Vitruvian man", "Last Supper" and "Annunciation". Da Vinci believed in "The Golden Ratio" which is a ratio found in nature and design, also called the "Phi Ratio" and sometimes, also called the divine ratio [1]. This is also seen in other works of art including the Acropolis of Athens, the Parthenon and Mona Lisa. This ratio measures 1:1.618, which is a 3:5 ratio. For example, in an aesthetically pleasing nose, the ratio between the projection line of the nose and the dorsal length should be 3:5. This golden ratio of 3:5 correlates with the Fibonacci sequence in mathematics and hence sometimes also called Fibonacci ratio [2]. Fibonacci numbers are a set of numbers that starts with zero or one and goes up based on the rule that each number is equal to the number of the preceding two numbers. Da Vinci believed the Golden Ratio represented perfect harmony in nature and in design. Whether this is true or not is questionable, but there is a constant relationship between symmetry and beauty, particularly in the nose. "Symmetry" is a key factor between two sides of the face or nose. An asymmetric small twisted nose is more obvious to the observer as "abnormal" than a large over projected but symmetrical nose. An aesthetic looking tip should be narrow with the "two tip defining points" (junction of the intermediate crus with the lateral crus on right and left) closely together with an optimum distance of 4mm between them. The projection of the tip from the face (from the alar facial sulcus to the tip) should be 60% of the length of the nose from the nasion to the tip. In Caucasian noses, an aesthetic looking tip in females slightly over rides the dorsum by roughly 2 mm with a "supra tip break point". Be aware that these ideals can keep changing with the time, fashion, race and culture. So, in essence there is no ideal nose to make the patient happy. The surgeon should be able to offer what the patient is looking for. You do not want to be in a situation where the operation did show an objective change in the shape of the nose for the better, but the patient is still unhappy with the outcome. To understand what changes the patient is looking for is the ultimate quest of the successful surgeon and hence the need for repeated consultations before surgery.

4.2 Assessment of the Patient

Assessing the patent's suitability for the surgery is an important key consideration before going on to clinically assess the patient's deformity of the nose. The assessment of patient's suitability for surgery starts as soon as the patient walks in. More often, just by inspecting the nose, an experienced surgeon can plan the surgical treatment when the patient walks in. This surgery does not need expensive and complex investigations to arrive at a diagnosis. The issue here is not about the nasal diagnosis and management plan alone, but to effectively "manage" the patient and to some extent the close family's expectations. Making sure that the patient's expectations are realistic is the key factor in a successful rhinoplasty. Adequate communication skills in simple vocabulary which the patient can understand are vital. It is often decided by the patient within the first few minutes of consultation whether you are the ideal surgeon they are looking for. The same applies to the surgeon too. Both physical and mental health of the patients should be considered. Aging rhinoplasty is on the ascend particularly for functional reasons. Be aware of highly demanding patients with unrealistic expectations and probably avoid surgery in them. Be aware of the pneumonic SIMON (single, introspective, male, obsessive and narcissistic). Extreme care is needed in counselling these patients, and preferably surgery should be avoided [3]. These issues cannot be explained in words, but only practical experience can help the surgeon to deal with particular circumstances. The surgeon should also be aware of body dysmorphic syndrome (BDS) in patients, which is estimated to affect 1–3% of western population. But the incidence is more (5%) among patients who present for aesthetic medical and surgical treatments [4]. The surgeon needs to be aware that these patients with obvious psychological issues are not the only ones to be concerned about. Often it is the so called "normal" looking and behaving patients who get the surgeon into trouble with unrealistic expectations. It is not easy to consistently fool an experienced surgeon; hence the way to avoid these issues would be to have multiple consultations with the patients before surgery. Of course, the best way to avoid an unrealistic patient is, not to do the surgery at all. It has to be remembered that as we get more experienced, we should not let our ego take on challenging patients, as the surgical skills are not the only criteria in this type of surgery to make a patient happy!

4.3 Assessment of the Tip

Assessment of the structural and functional nasal deformity is the initial step in the surgical planning. It can be a steep learning curve. Functional assessment is covered in the section on nasal valve surgery. If the surgeon is able to correctly assess the deformity and understand the pathogenesis, then it is easier to arrive at a logical sensible management algorithm. The nasal tip should be assessed along with the rest of the nasal dorsum and the nasal septum. The key doctrine in rhinoplasty surgery is, *"if the mind does not know, the eyes don't see the deformity and the surgical algorithm will be flawed."*

4.3.1 Is It a Primary or a Secondary Tip Problem or a Combination of Deformities?

In assessing tip deformities, we need to be aware of this distinction between primary and secondary deformities, as the surgical algorithm can be tailored to individual deformities.

- Primary deformities (true deformities of the tip) involve the lower lateral cartilages with intrinsic deformities of medial crus, lateral crus and intermediate crus on either one or both sides resulting in varying combinations of all the above, particularly in traumatic and revision noses giving rise to complex nasal tip deformities.
- Secondary deformities (pseudo deformities of the tip) are due to caudal septal issues,

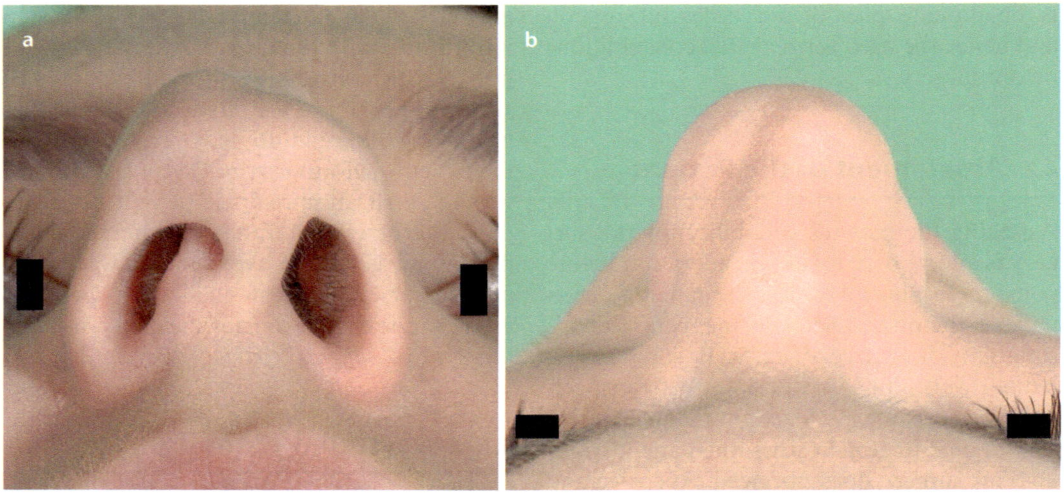

Fig. 4.1 **a**, **b** Patient showing complex tip deformity due to both primary tip cartilage and secondary caudal septal issues. **a** Basal view. **b** Sky view. (Reproduced with permission from Ref: [5])

like caudal septal deviations or lack of caudal septal support, causing secondary tip issues like tip de-projection or under rotation of the tip, with actual structure of the tip cartilages being intact. Thus caudal septum is a significant factor in causing a variety of tip deformities, particularly in a traumatic nose.

- A combination of primary and secondary deformities requires complex reconstructive algorithms. Around 85% of traumatic tip deformities which we encounter in our clinical practice have both primary and secondary tip issues (Fig. 4.1a, b).

4.3.2 How Can You Say on Inspection a Tip Deformity Is Primary or Secondary?

On inspection, one should be able to assess whether the tip deformity is either primary or secondary or a combination of both. Clues for primary deformity (Fig. 4.2a–c), include localised tip bulbosity, localised sharpness or lateral crural concavity with deviation and asymmetry of the tip with distortion of the soft triangle. Clues for secondary deformity include distortion and deformity of the caudal septum, causing secondary asymmetry in the tip regarding its position on both sides (Fig. 4.2c) with or without alar nostril asymmetries as seen in Fig. 4.1a. In practice, in the majority of patients, there is always a combination of primary and secondary deformities, particularly in a traumatic nose.

If the surgeon is aware that a tip deformity is primary or a complex deformity and expect lot of issues with the medial crura, soft triangle or the lateral crura, surgical elevation of the flap through an open approach is advisable and the incisions can be better planned and executed.

4.3.3 Clinical Assessment

It begins with history, particularly the pathogenesis and duration of the trauma, including previous surgical treatment and if possible getting access to the previous operative notes. In a traumatic nasal deformity, it will be worthwhile to know the nature of injury and mode of trauma, etc. If it is a revision rhinoplasty requiring tip surgery, any information regarding previous surgical findings and any techniques carried out before can be vital in the assessment of the tip deformity. Communicating with the previous surgeon is an effective option. Clinical assessment should

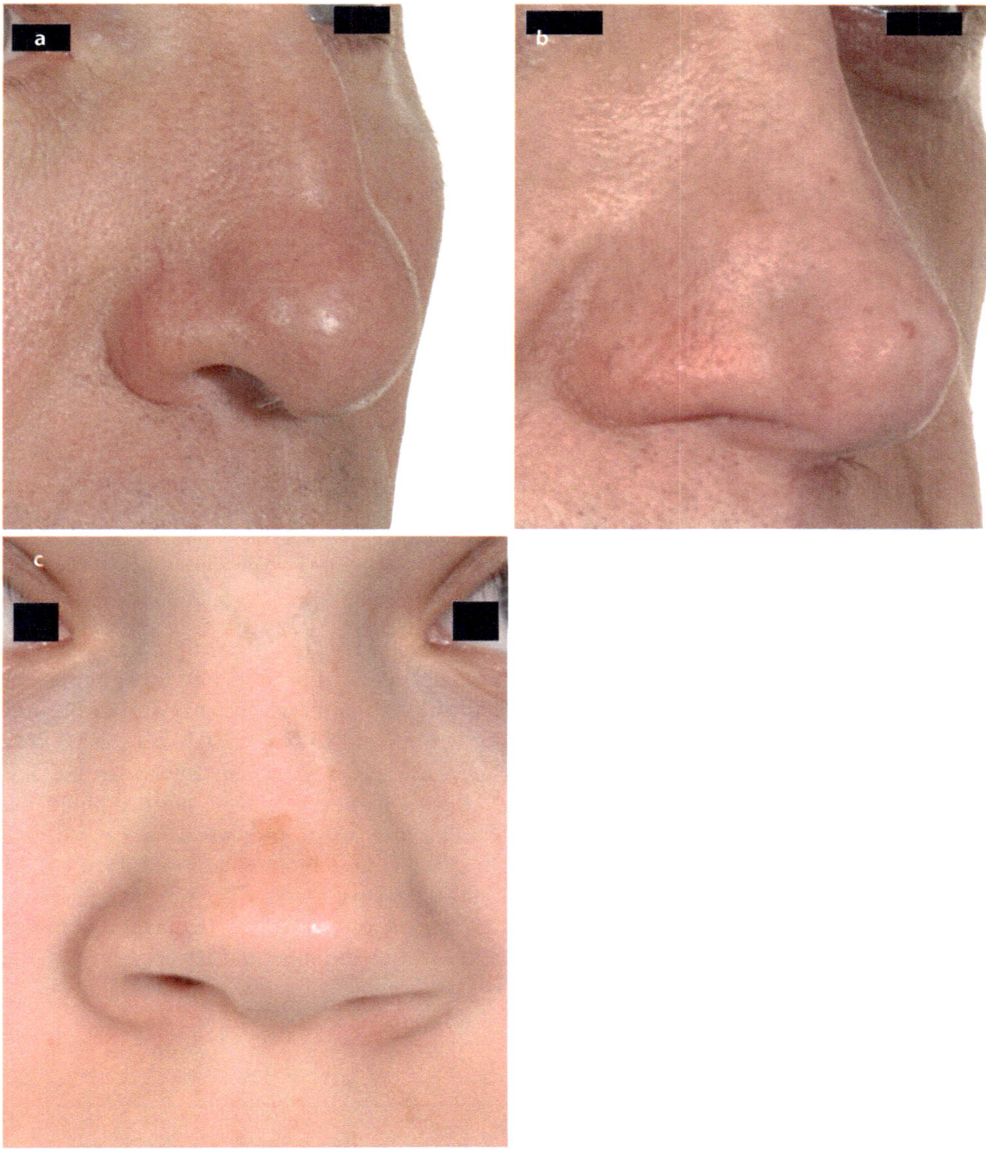

Fig. 4.2 **a–c** Primary tip deformity. **a** ¾ View showing localised tip bulbosity. **b** Isolated concavity of lateral crus. **c** Asymmetry of the tip with distortion of the soft triangle

involve visual examination and clinical palpation. This should be supplemented with 2-D or 3-D photography. Adequate documentation of the examination findings is a must. The aim of the assessment is to diagnose the underlying pathology, understand the pathophysiology of the deformity and then decide on an "Ideal" surgical plan. In my practice, most tip work is done as an adjunctive to other rhinoplasty procedures, with isolated tip work being rare. There are several tools in helping and aiding in the diagnosis of the individual deformities of the nose. *Definition, projection, rotation and dorsal aesthetic lines* are the key tools in the diagnosis of structural and functional traumatic nasal deformities [5]. An accurate diagnosis of the exact pathology of the deformity helps in the management plan.

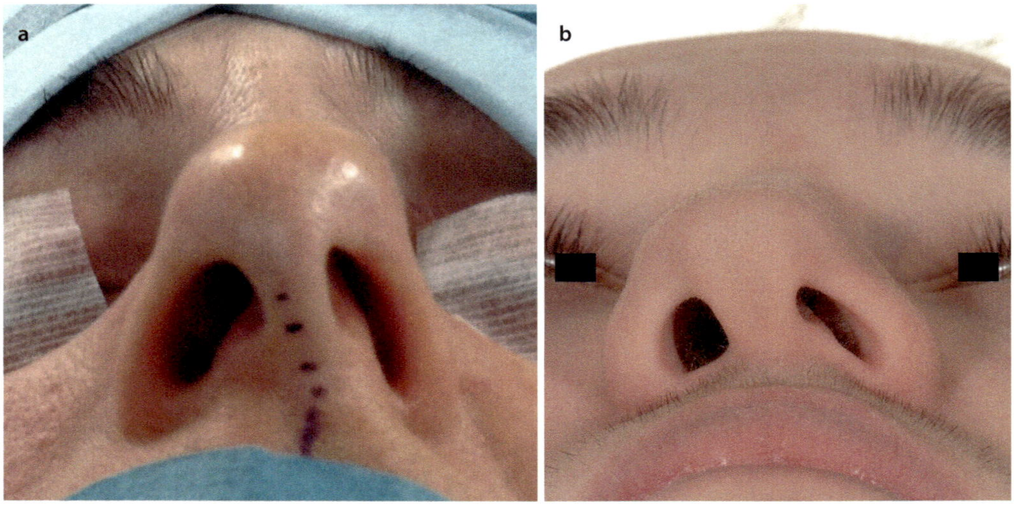

Fig. 4.3 **a**, **b** Patients showing angulation and tilting of the nasal tip away from the midline due to caudal septal deviations. **a** Basal view showing the tilting of the mid-columellar line with over projection. **b** Basal view showing the tilting of the mid-columellar line with under projection

Nasal base is the best view to assess the anatomy of the nasal tip. It has to be an aesthetically pleasing triangle with adequate projection, rather than a boxy or trapezoidal tip. The triangle of the nasal base should be roughly divisible into three equal parts, anteriorly the nasal infra tip lobule, mid and posterior third being the columella. Some surgeons consider the posterior third as a separate "sill" region. Ideally all these three parts visible in the "basal" view should be in symmetrical thirds to make a nasal tip aesthetically pleasing. Apart from being symmetrical in the basal view, the nasal tip should be oriented in the sagittal plane and any angulation or tilting of the nasal tip away from the midline is important (Fig. 4.3a). In our experience, any gross tilt of the nasal tip beyond 15 degrees from the midline sagittal plane is a negative prognostic predictive factor (unpublished data) in achieving successful outcomes in nasal tip surgery (Fig. 4.3b).

Clinical assessment of the nasal tip should include "four dimensions" namely:

- *Definition, projection, rotation and dorsal aesthetic lines*

Definition

- Definition is "what the patient generally thinks of the nasal tip". It represents a lay person's view of the "structure" of the nasal tip. Assessment of definition should be focussed on the size and the shape of the nasal tip, whether it is large or small, bulbous or narrow, pointed or blunted. Is there an abnormal shape to it? Definition also includes assessment of the shape of the nostrils, symmetry between two sides, soft triangle anatomy and columellar show, comparing both sides looking for symmetric and asymmetric tip deformities. Is the basal view an aesthetic pyramid? (Fig. 4.6)
- Most patients talk only about definition during the consultation. Few patients rarely talk about projection, rotation or dorsal aesthetic lines, although they may be aware of them.
- The aim of clinical assessment is to understand the pathogenesis of the damage to the intrinsic size, shape and strength of the lower lateral cartilages (alar cartilages), which ultimately is a major tip support mechanism.

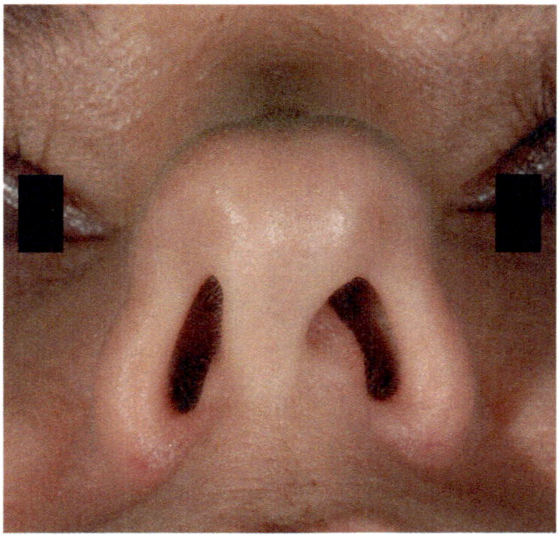

Fig. 4.4 Basal view showing a wide tip due to a wider soft triangle

- The most common tip deformity in Caucasians is a wide, bulbous trapezoidal nasal tip (Fig. 4.4). Bulbosity of the tip could be due to deformity of one alar cartilage or both. It is usually symmetrical due to excess width and length of the lateral crus of the alar cartilages in familial patients or could be asymmetric following trauma. The bulbosity could either be due to widening of the angle between the medial crus and the lateral crus and or due to separation of the two medial crura as evidenced by a skin cleft in the middle (Fig. 4.5). If the deformity is bilateral and familial, it is also usually symmetrical. If it is a localised weakness in the lateral crus causing a bulge secondary to trauma or revision surgery, it is usually asymmetrical. It may or may not be associated with cephalic migration of the lateral crus. A minor but asymmetric deformity will cause more distress to the patients than a severe but symmetric deformity.
- Assessing the skin thickness is a key factor in achieving outcomes. A very prominent bulbosity of the tip also suggests that the tip cartilages are strong and forceful on overlying skin envelope which may be thin. In a bulbous strong tip, if the overlying skin is thin, this can be a favourable scenario to the surgeon as any changes made in the tip cartilages would be visible outside as the skin will drape around the restructured cartilages. At the same time, there are downsides when using destructive techniques and sutures in patients with thin skin. On the other hand, if the skin envelope is thick, any tip technique to narrow the bulbosity may not be obvious enough to please the patient [6].
- A bulbous nasal tip is usually associated with over projected tip due to intrinsically large size of the lower lateral cartilage and

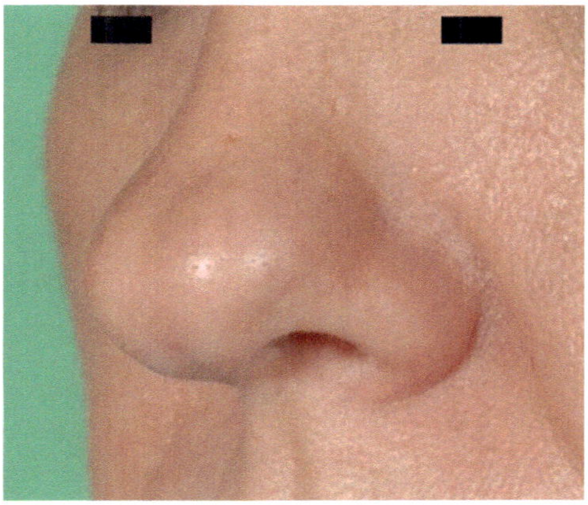

Fig. 4.5 Basal view showing a primary bulbous tip with bifidity

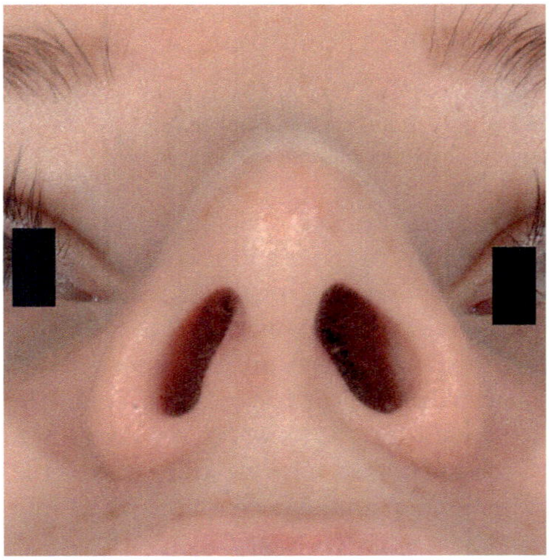

Fig. 4.6 Basal view showing an aesthetic basal triangular pyramid

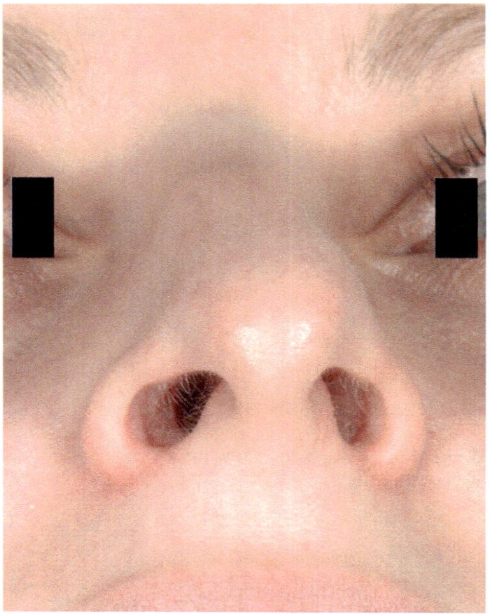

Fig. 4.7 Basal view showing asymmetric soft triangle being wider on right side

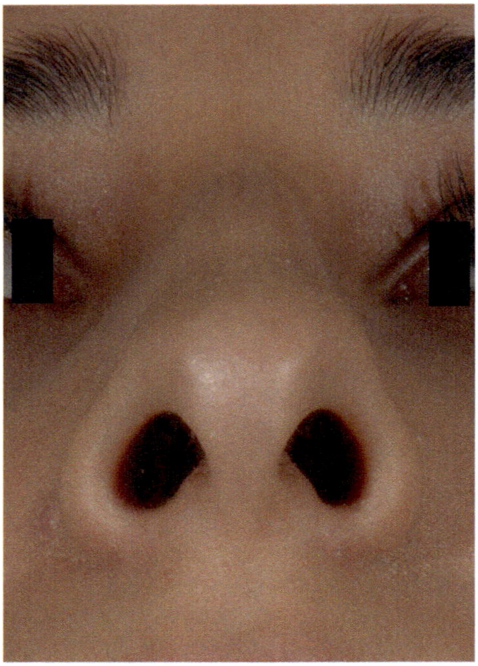

Fig. 4.8 Basal view showing symmetrical soft triangle on both sides.

or due to excess dorsal and caudal septum. If the tip cartilages are genetically large, the tip will over ride, or at least be at the same level as the nasal dorsum in the profile view. If the tip cartilages are large but associated with deficient caudal septum at the anterior septal angle, the tip will be "clinging on" to the anterior septal angle with a nasal tip deprojection and may be a little under rotation as well.

- Assess the soft triangle. This is the area seen at the junction between the columella and the lateral ala at the supero-lateral margin of the alar nostril region. This represents an area where there is no underlying cartilage and has only the skin and mucosa. The soft triangle may be seen or felt (Figs. 4.7 and 4.8). The overlying skin should be thin enough for the margins of the cartilage to be seen through. The soft triangle is visible if the overlying skin is very thin. But if the skin is thicker, it can only be felt and not seen. The soft triangle is due to the angulation of the lower lateral cartilage at the apex of the nostril where the lateral crus diverges away from the medial crus supero-laterally. The angle between the medial and the lateral crus as measured at the inferior border of the lower lateral cartilage is the "dome angle". This angulation between the medial crus and the lateral crus decides the shape of the soft triangle. In the author's view, the soft triangle is always "soft", since there is no cartilage, but not always a "triangle" even in the so called "normal" noses, as the angulation between the medial crus and the lateral crus is not always consistent and has a wider range of normality.
- Always examine both soft triangles and compare each side to assess any asymmetry. Both sides should be symmetric (Fig. 4.8). In patients with cleft lip noses or in traumatic noses, the soft triangle may be asymmetric between two sides (Fig. 4.7). Normally the apex of the soft

triangle is facing up and slightly medially towards 2'O clock position on the right side (▫ Fig. 4.8) and 10'O clock position on the left side. The base of the triangle is inferior abutting on the superior alar skin margin. Check both the base and apex of the soft triangle which can give a lot of clinical clues to the underlying deformity of the tip cartilages. If the apex of the triangle is sharp with a "sharp angulation" of the soft triangle, this is due to a very narrow angle between the lateral crus and the medial crus as seen in an over projected nasal tips. Contrary to this, if the angle is wider, then this leads to blunting of the soft triangle. In an over projected tip, the vertical length of the soft triangle is longer than normal (▫ Fig. 4.9a, b).

- If the base of the triangle is wider and the angle is more obtuse than it suggests, the lateral crus and medial crus have moved away from each other causing bulbosity. The soft triangle may also become a wide rectangular space (as seen in ▫ Fig. 4.10 on the right side), due to cephalic migration of the lateral crus.
- If changes are present only on one side, then it will introduce an asymmetry; a good example would be lateral crural issues in cleft lip patients.
- If the soft triangle is scarred (▫ Fig. 4.11) or retracted or collapsed (▫ Fig. 4.12), it could be either due to surgical trauma of previously misplaced marginal incisions or non-surgical trauma. This examination of soft triangle also helps us to plan the internal marginal incisions and hence avoid any damage caused by misplaced alar incisions.
- Look for sharp domes on one side or other which are due to trauma and asymmetric strength between two alar cartilages with the so called normal lateral crus pushing the tip to the opposite weaker side.
- Columellar show should be assessed in the lateral view. Excess columellar show can be a true deformity due to sagging of medial

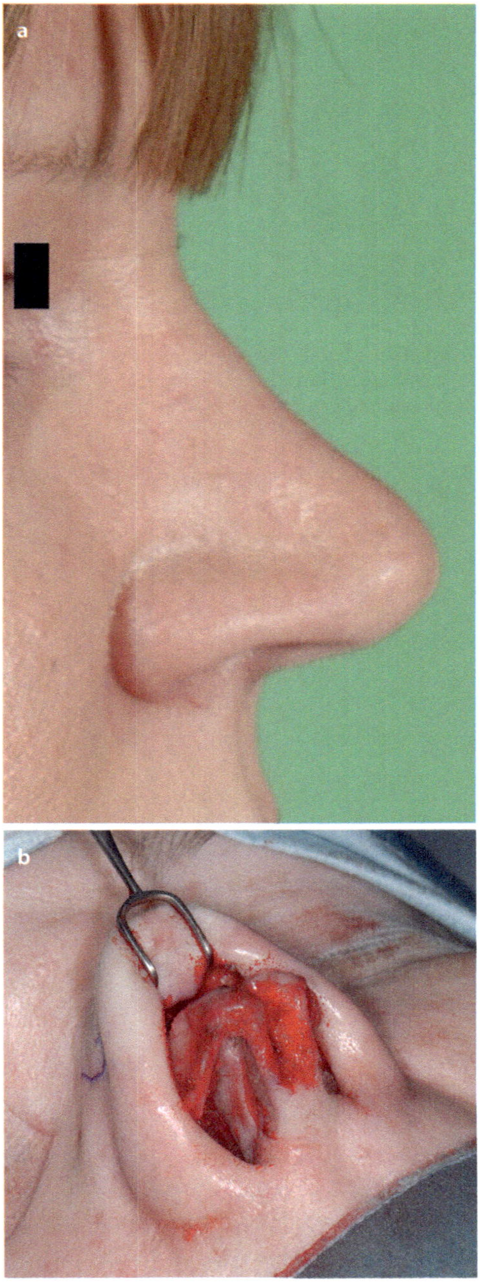

▫ **Fig. 4.9** **a**, **b** Over projected tip with vertical length of soft triangle being longer. **a** Basal view of over projected tip. **b** Open view of over projected tip with vertical orientation of soft triangle between the medial and lateral crura

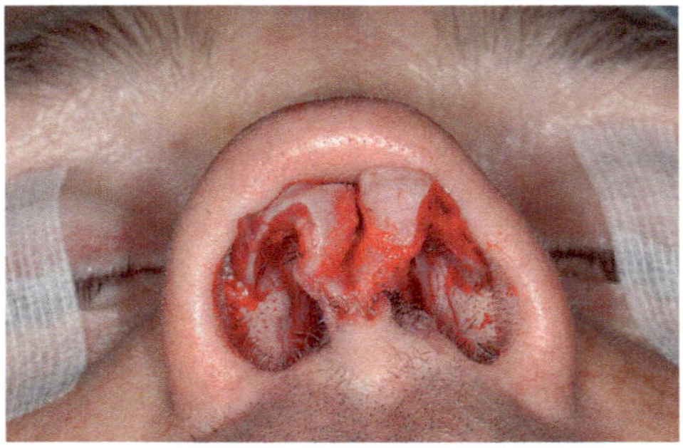

Fig. 4.10 Basal view of under projected tip on the right side with vertical shortening of soft triangle length and widening of soft triangle base

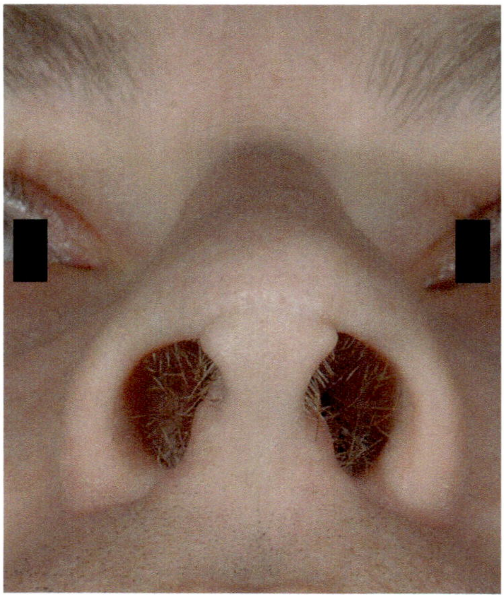

Fig. 4.11 Basal view showing bilateral soft triangle scarring

crus (Fig. 4.13a) causing prolapse of the medial crus or could be a pseudo deformity due to retraction of the lateral alar margin

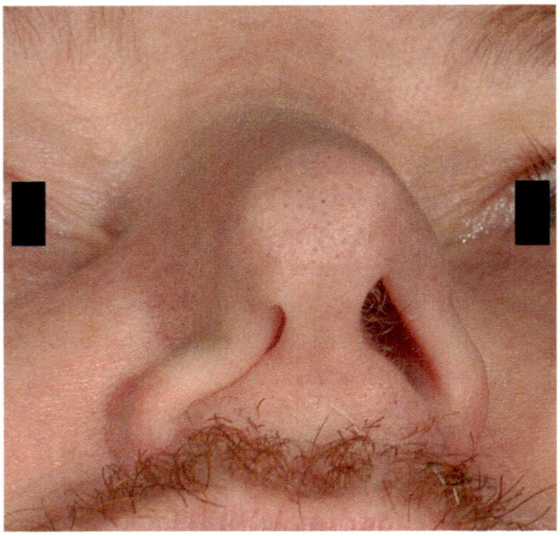

Fig. 4.12 Basal view showing collapsed soft triangle due to lateral alar weakness

(Fig. 4.13b). Although there are various measurements and angles, in practice clinical examination of the lateral view alone will suffice to distinguish between true and pseudo columellar excess show. Contrary to this, a "no-show" columella could again be a true deformity (Fig. 4.14a, b) due to lack of caudal septum and caudal septal retraction or a pseudo deformity due to a weak and thickened downwardly migrated lateral alar margin over riding the columella (Fig. 4.14c).

- Finally, assessment of "nasal tip definition" is not complete without assessment of nostril size and shape in the basal view. Generally they are symmetrical and shaped like a vertical "Tear-drop" angled slightly medially. The caudal septum, medial crural footplate and the skin and soft tissue envelope decide the anatomy of the nostril shape (Figs. 4.15, 4.16, 4.17, and 4.18).

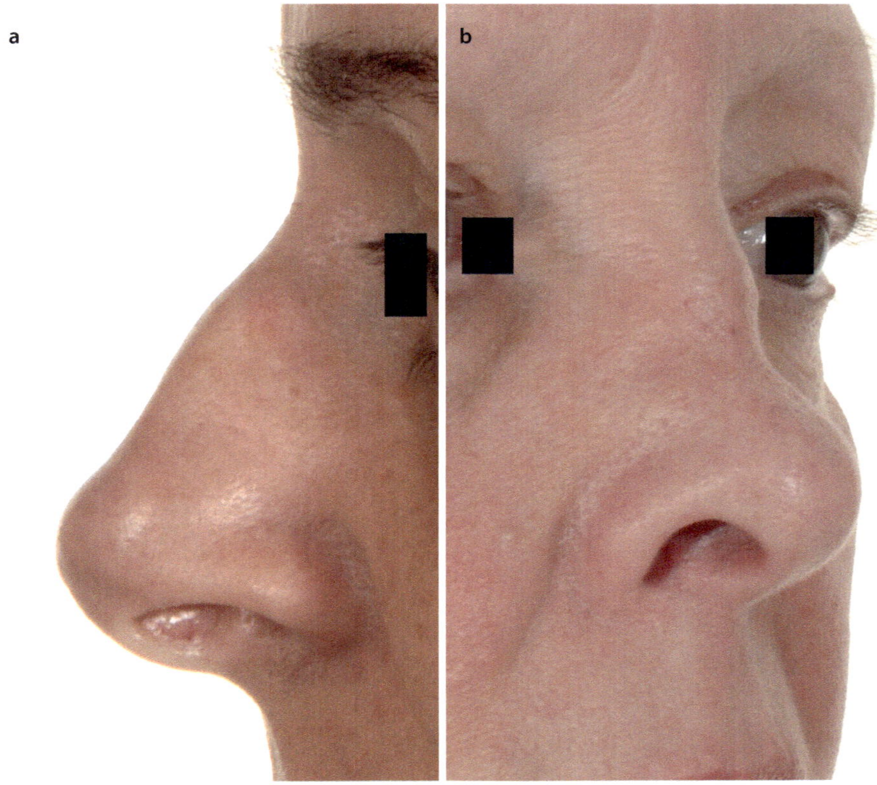

Fig. 4.13 **a**, **b** Excess columellar show. **a** True deformity due to sagging of medial crus. **b** Pseudo deformity due to retraction of the lateral alar margin

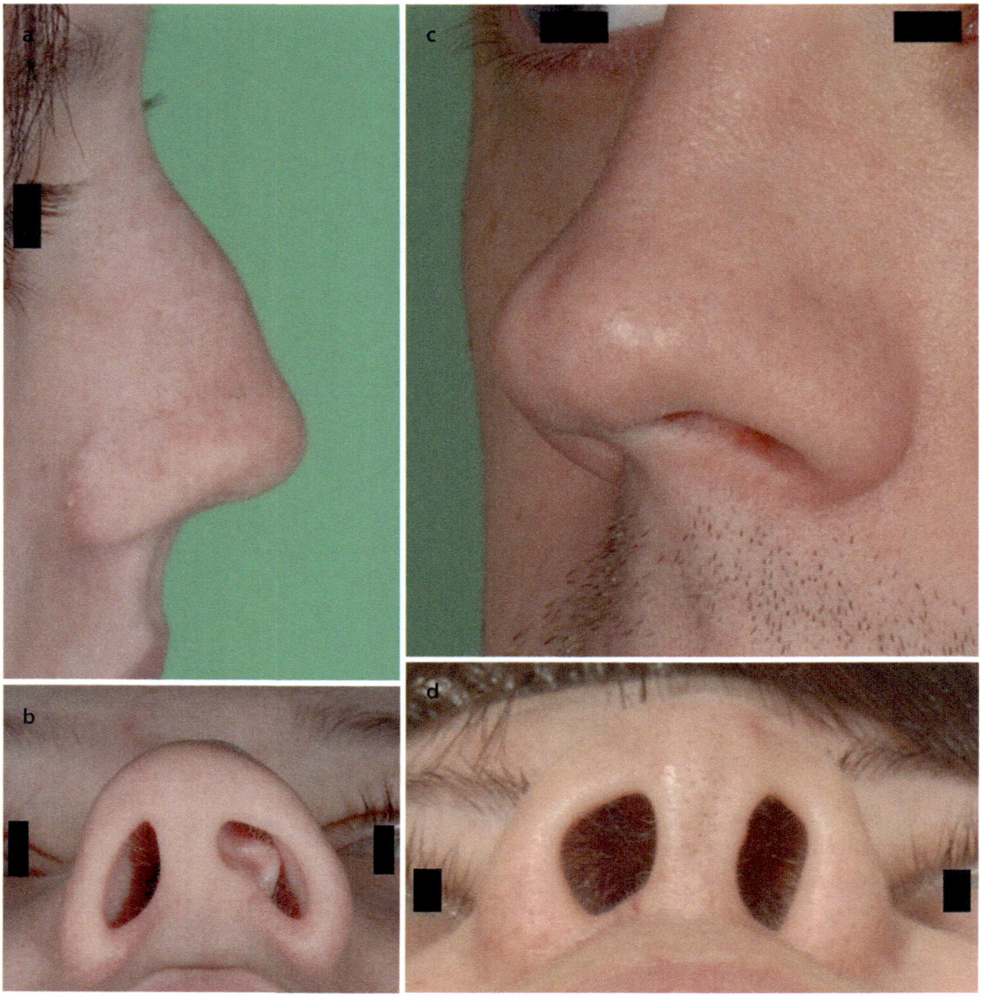

Fig. 4.14 **a–d** "No-show" columella. **a**, **b** True deformity due to retracted columella. **c**, **d** Pseudo deformity due to hooding of the lateral alar margin

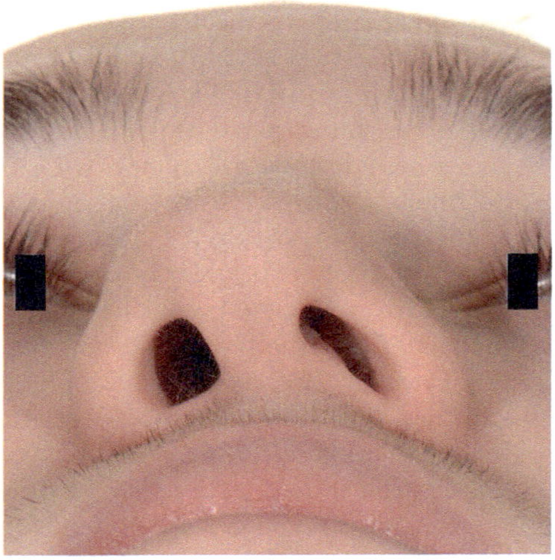

Fig. 4.15 Basal view showing asymmetric nostril size

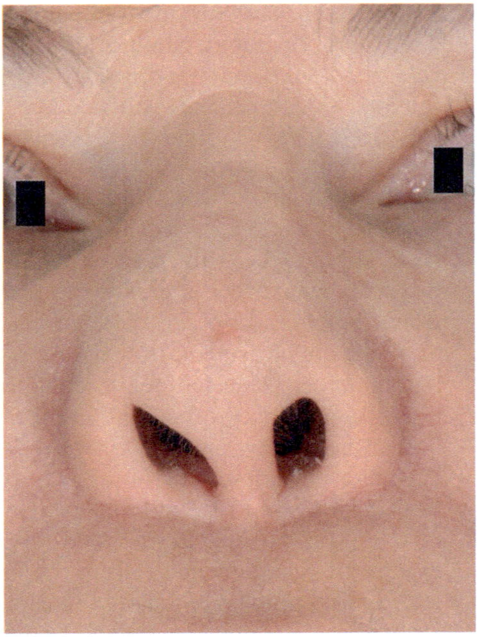

Fig. 4.16 Basal view showing sharp angulation of nostrils due to soft triangle and alar margin scarring

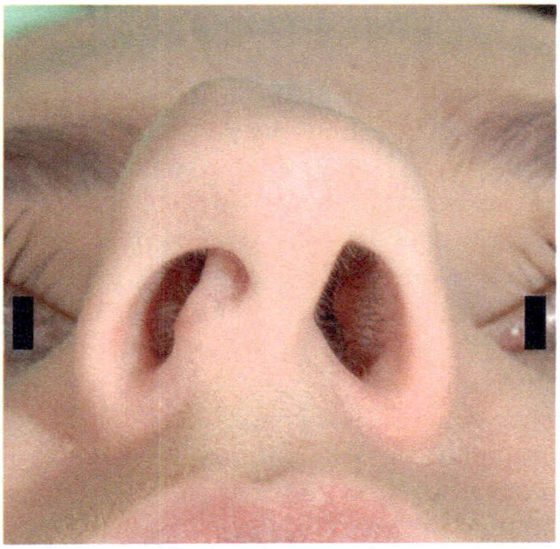

Fig. 4.17 Basal view showing "doughnut"-shaped right nostril due to caudal septal dislocation

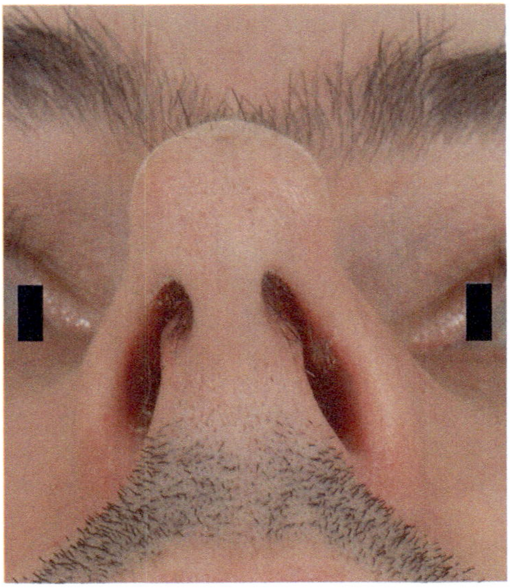

Fig. 4.18 Basal view showing bilateral vertical slit like nostrils due to over projection

4.3.4 Projection

- The term projection of the nasal tip indicates how much it is projecting forward from the face and the rest of the nose. Thus, projection of the nose is measured in two scenarios, namely:
  1. Projection of the *nose in relation to the face* as seen in ¾ view and lateral profile.
  2. Projection of the *nasal tip to the rest of the nasal dorsum* as seen in the lateral profile.
- The commonest abnormality in post-traumatic nasal deformity is a loss of projection of the nose, with deviation or tilting of the nasal tip and nasal base axis to one side usually associated with loss of projection.
- The nasal tip projection is best assessed in the lateral profile view and the basal view. In the profile view, the projection of the nose on the face is measured in various ways. Although several methods are described in literature, in practice clinical examination alone can say whether it is an over or under projected tip. Various methods of assessing tip projection have been described, including those of Goode, Crumley, and Simons, etc. Each of these methods has its own limitations. We generally tend to follow Goode's method, in which a horizontal line is drawn from the naso-facial sulcus to the most projecting part of the nasal tip called the projection line. This line should be roughly less than 60% of the length of the nose as measured by a line from the nasion to the nasal tip [7, 8].
- Be aware that these measurements are relative and not absolute. Beware of situations where the length of the nose is small and hence the projection line looks relatively longer. To compensate for variable clinical scenarios, more than one measuring tool is important. The naso-facial angle and fronto-nasal angle also help in deciding the projection of the nose. An ideal naso-facial angle should be around 35 degrees and an ideal naso-frontal angle between the frontal bone and the nasal dorsum should be 120 degrees average. These angles determine the relative position of the nasal bridge in line with the face, suggesting either over projection or under projection.
- An adequately projected nasal tip in the "basal" view should be an aesthetic triangle with tip lobule, columella and the sill forming equal thirds. Some surgeons include the "Sil" region within the columella, with the result the columella-to-lobule ratio should be approximately 2:1. In the basal view, the infra tip lobule should form a single point at the apex of the triangle. If the tip is de-projected, the basal view may be boxy or trapezoidal. The width of the nasal base should be within the inter-canthal distance. The long axis of the nostrils should be roughly 55 degrees slant with the midline of the columella. On lateral view, the columellar show should be 2–3 mm.
- An ideal nasal base should have a double break of the columella with the Infra tip lobule gently curving into the columella. The supra tip lobule should gently over ride the nasal dorsum by roughly 2mm in females to give a supra tip break point. But these ideals can vary with time, race and culture.
- A trapezoidal boxy nasal tip on basal view is usually an under projected tip. The surgeon should be aware that narrowing a boxy tip would also increase the projection of the nasal tip. On the contrary, an aesthetically pleasing narrow nasal tip can still be under projected due to columellar retraction and lack of caudal septal cartilage, although it is unusual to be so.
- Preoperative assessment of nasal projection is not complete without evaluation of chin projection. Retrognathism may exaggerate the appearance of an over projected nasal tip or give the false illusion of an over projection in a normally projected tip. Chin projection can be evaluated by dropping a vertical line from the vermilion cutaneous border of the lower lip perpendicular to the Frankfort horizontal plane in the lateral view. The pogonion should be in the same plane as the sub-nasal or vermilion border of the lower lip.
- *Relationship of "projection" to the "length" of the nose:* The projection of the nasal tip

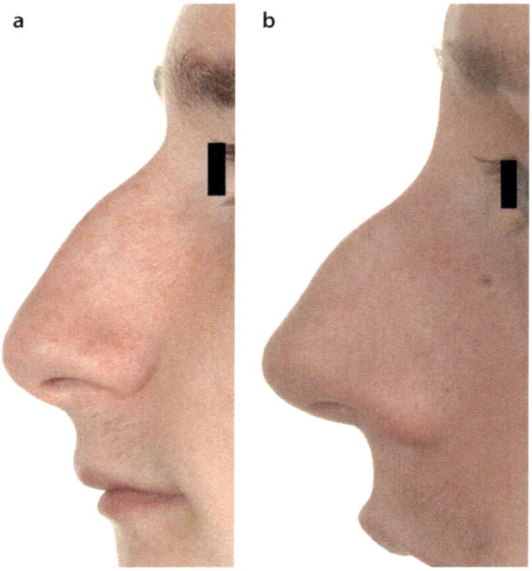

■ **Fig. 4.19** **a**, **b** Over projected tip. **a** Long nose. **b** Short nose

bears no "constant" relationship to the length of the nose. One can have an over projected nasal tip, but the length of the nose can be short or long (■ Fig. 4.19a, b). One can also have an under projected nose and the length of the nose can be long (■ Fig. 4.20a, b) or short. But rotation of the tip bears a direct relationship to the length of the nose as mentioned below.

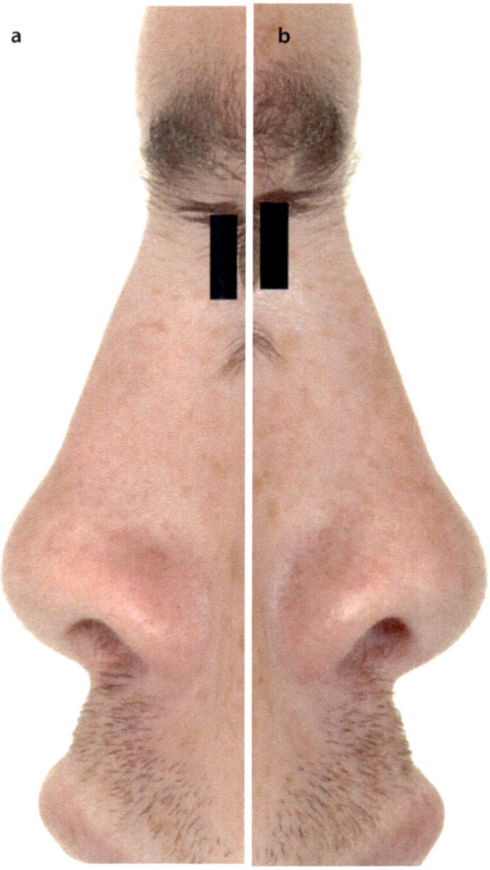

■ **Fig. 4.20** **a**, **b** Under projected tip with a long nose. **a**, **b** Lateral view

4.3.5 Rotation

- Accurate assessment of nasal tip rotation is essential in pre- and post-operative evaluation of patients needing septorhinoplasty. The rotation of the nasal tip can alter the appearance of the nose dramatically with variations depending on sex and ethnic background. Surgical planning and technique is dependent on tip rotation analysis, and it can be used as a quantitative assessment tool for measuring outcomes in rhinoplasty.
- Rotation of the nose by definition is analysed in the lateral profile plane. There are two types (■ Fig. 4.21b) of rotation:
  1. *Rotation of the columella of the nasal tip to the upper lip*
  2. *Rotation of the infra tip lobule segment of the tip complex to the columellar segment*
- Both of these components are important, but in practice the patient's concern is more towards the rotation of the entire columellar tip complex in relation to the upper lip and dorsal profile line, rather than the rotation of the infra tip lobule on the columella which is more of a concern to the surgeon. ■ Fig. 4.21a, b, shows more rotation of the Infra tip lobule segment to the columella when compared to the rotation of the columella to the upper lip (■ Fig. 4.22).
- There are numerous methods described to measure tip rotation prior to septorhinoplasty. Rotation of the nasal tip complex to the dorsal profile line is his-

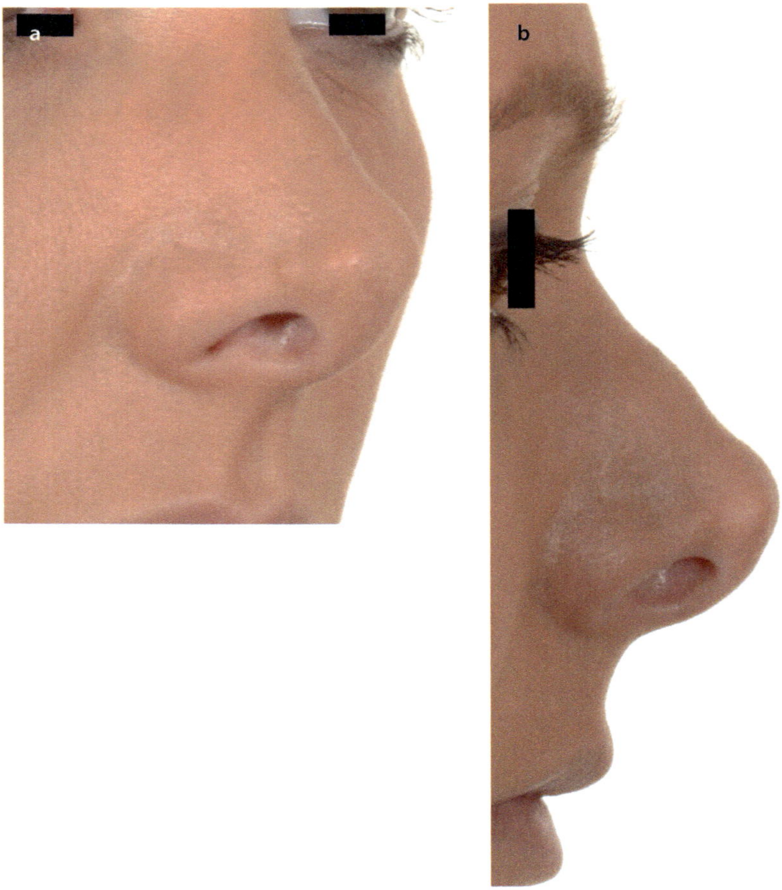

Fig. 4.21 **a**, **b** Over rotated tip with excess angulation of columella and infra tip lobule. **a** ¾ View, **b** Lateral view

torically measured by analysing the nasolabial angle. This angle (NLA) is measured as the angle between the columella of the nose and the upper lip. The aesthetically attractive range in a Caucasian population for tip rotation is described as being an angle between 90° and 100° in men and 105° and 110° in women. This means Caucasian men prefer a neutral rotation and women prefer a slightly upturned nasal tip on the dorsal line. An angle of over 90 degrees in men and over 110 degrees in women is defined as over rotation and a lesser angle is defined as under rotation [9]. Again these measurements are relative depending on ethnicity, age, sex, etc. Individual wishes should be discussed with the patients before surgery.

- It is also important to understand what it means when we use the words like "over" rotation or "under" rotation. Over rotation suggests the tip is rotated up on to the dorsum of the nose and under rotation means the nasal tip is turned down towards the upper lip (Figs. 4.23, 4.24, and 4.25). Because the arc of tip rotation is measured in the dorsal profile line, it contributes to the so called "length" of the nose. The length of the nose extends from the fixed nasion to the mobile nasal tip. Since the nasal tip is mobile and can be in any position of rotation arc in relation to the dorsal profile line, the length of the nose is related to the nasal tip rotation. This relationship of rotation to the nasal tip is "constant" when compared to the

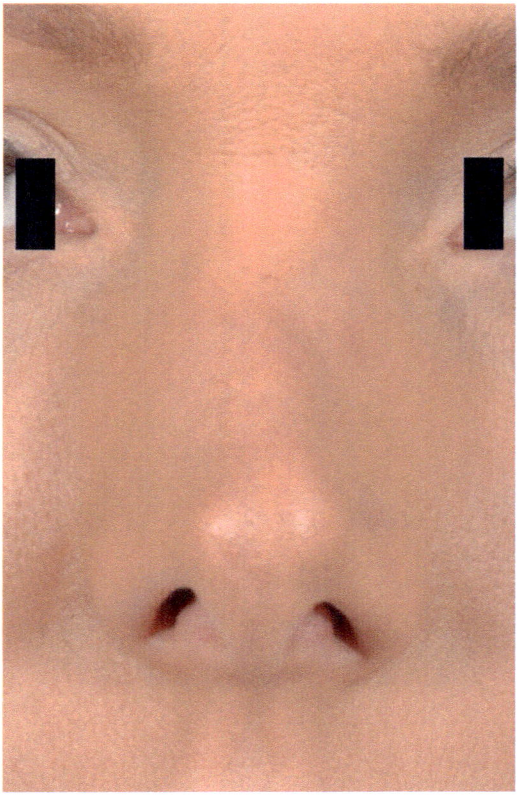

Fig. 4.22 Frontal view showing over rotated tip with infra tip lobule show

relationship of projection to the length of the nose.

- Measuring tip rotation is often inconsistent due to lot of variables. The ranges of angles and measurements are only a reference baseline and must be used in the context of patient's height, facial features, sex and ethnicity. However, variations in anatomical landmarks including upper lip and soft tissue columella and facial expression can make this measurement inconsistent. In addition, a large nasal spine, a tension nose deformity or an over projected tip may cause a larger more obtuse naso-labial angle. In contrast, a hypoplastic mid-face may cause a more acute naso-labial angle. In the post-traumatic nose, a common potential variable in tip rotation analysis is "dislocation of caudal septum into a nostril" causing secondary tip deformity. Studies have shown that vertical malposition of the columella (hanging or retracted columella) may affect the position of the reference line for quantitative analysis (using naso-labial angle measurement) and therefore affect the assessment of tip rotation.

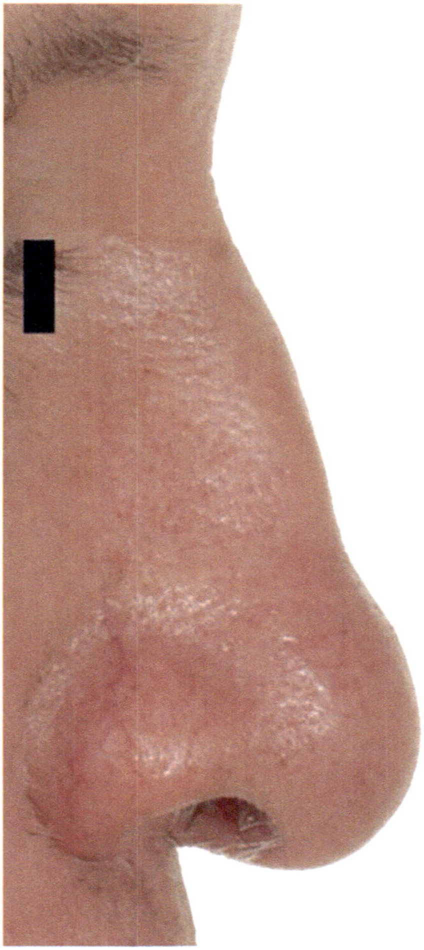

Fig. 4.23 Lateral view showing under rotated tip

- In posttraumatic noses, malposition of caudal septum is more common than malposition of columellar soft tissue. Be aware in the post-traumatic noses with caudal dislocation of the nasal septum, the tip rotation can look different in the same patient when viewed from right and left side. Nostril axis line is a line drawn along the longest nostril axis in the profile view. The "nasal

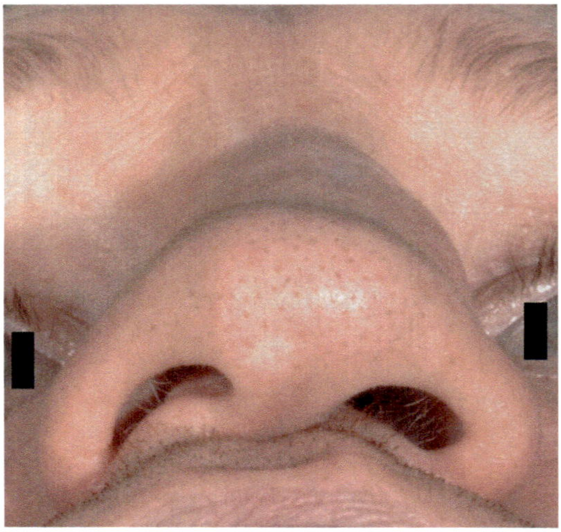

Fig. 4.24 Frontal view showing collapsed tip causing under rotation

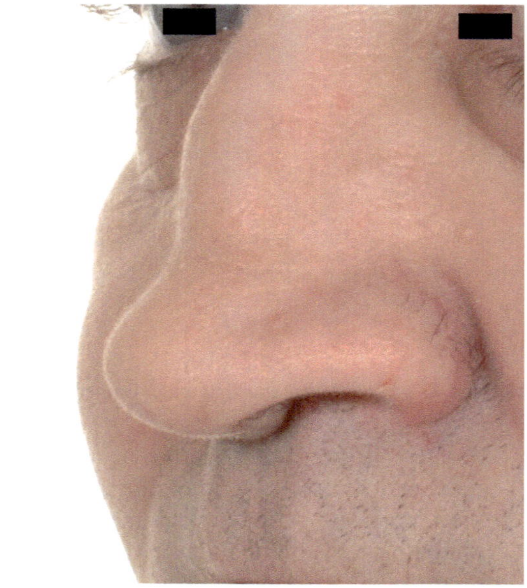

Fig. 4.25 ¾ View showing under rotated droopy tip

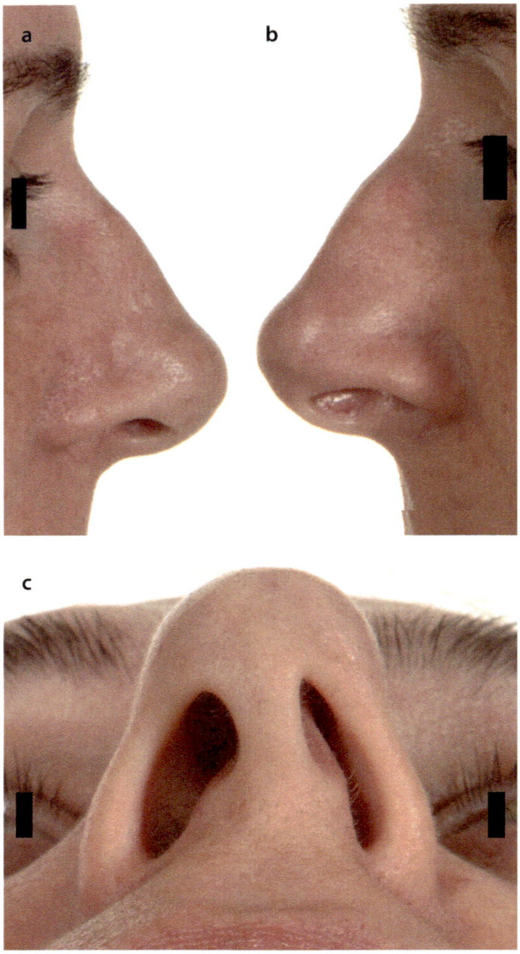

Fig. 4.26 **a–c** Variable columellar show due to septal dislocation in the same patient. **a** Right lateral view. **b** Left lateral view. **c** Basal view

axis angle", formed by the angle between the nostril axis line and the vertical perpendicular drawn to the Frankfort horizontal plane can be used to measure rotation of the nasal tip between the two sides in patients with caudal septal dislocation. The main advantage of this method is that it is not subjected to variability due to columella or upper lip position. We used this method to assess the difference in tip rotation between ipsilateral and contralateral side in relation to caudal septal dislocation in the same patient. The results of our study [10] have shown that caudal dislocation of the septum causes significant differences in nostril axis angle and tip rotation as measured between both sides (Fig. 4.26a–c). There was a correlation with the side of the caudal dislocation with more obtuse angle (over rotation) being demonstrated on the side of the dislocation. Our study emphasised that while assessing and planning surgery for nasal tip rotation, the surgeon should be aware of the fallacy that caudal

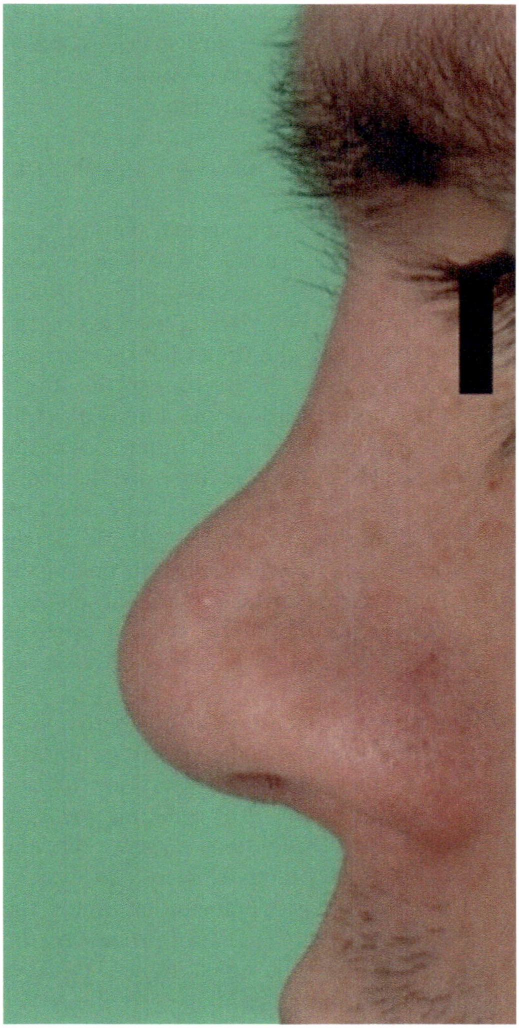

Fig. 4.27 Lateral view showing "short" nose with over rotated tip

septal issues can result in differences in tip rotation when measured from both sides.

- *Relationship of "rotation" to the "length" of the nose:* Rotation of the nasal tip has a direct and constant relationship to the length of the nose. An over rotated nasal tip is *always a short nose* (Fig. 4.27) and under rotated nasal tip will *always be a longer nose* (Fig. 4.28). This is an important concept to remember when compared to projection, particularly when the patient complains about the length of the nose.
- Thus rotation is a measurement analysed in the profile line (straight lateral view) which

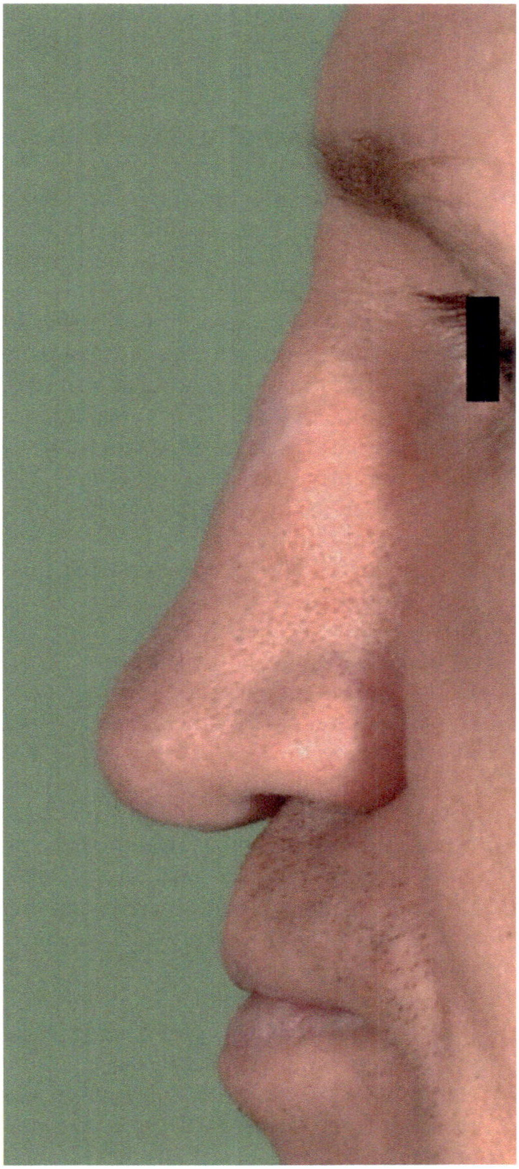

Fig. 4.28 Lateral view showing "long" nose with under rotated tip

sometimes is not an ideal view to measure the "3-D depth" of the under rotation of the nasal tip. This so called "depth" is best seen in a three quarters view when compared to the straight lateral view, although both being two dimensional.
- Be aware that any technique to alter the projection will also affect the rotation as both the factors are inter-related. This

concept is important before embarking on tip surgery [11].

4.3.6 Dorsal Aesthetic Lines (D-A-L)

- To be aesthetically pleasing, the paired dorsal aesthetic lines should be seen as a smooth "gull-wing" appearance. Any alterations in the "anatomy" of this line helps as a good diagnostic tool to accurately arrive at the pathogenesis and the pathology of the various nasal deformities. They are one of the several tools in helping in the nasal assessment, apart from the definition, projection and rotation. It can also be used as an outcome measure after a successful rhinoplasty.
- It is a pair of cosmetically pleasing lines seen on the frontal view and is a gentle smooth flowing line starting from the medial end of both the eyebrows superiorly with a slight superior convexity towards each other and then coming down and following the side of the nasal bones and upper lateral cartilages. As the line comes down, it widens gently from each other and depending on where they are going it can be divided into an "eyebrow tip line", going towards the tip defining points, or called an "eyebrow facial sulcus line", if they are traced laterally towards the naso-facial sulcus. These lines on both sides, if uniform, give a very pleasing smooth "gull-wing" appearance to the shape of the nose, when viewed on the frontal plane. The D-A-L on both sides, although best visualised in the "frontal view", is also seen from the cranial view by tilting the face backwards and viewing down on the nose.
- This line has three components, starting from above downwards (◘ Fig. 4.29a):
  1. The upper one third is a smooth convexity starting on the medial edge of the eye brow, gently coming down towards the medial canthus in a smooth convexity facing each other (concave towards the eyeball). Predominantly the shape of the nasal bones and the nasal process of the frontal bone contribute to the contour.
  2. The middle third is parallel to each other and extends from the medial canthus to the cephalic border of the lateral crus. The frontal process of the maxilla and the upper lateral cartilage contribute to the contour of this line.
  3. The lower third of this line is a gentle divergent from each other extending towards either the naso-facial sulcus or straight down towards the nasal tip defining points. The shape of the tip cartilages contributes to this line. If the line extends to the nasal facial sulcus, it represents the lateral crus as opposed to the line extending only towards the nasal tip.
- The smooth appearance of the paired lines gives an aesthetically pleasing appearance to the nose, and restoration of this line would be an ideal outcome measure after a septo-rhinoplasty surgery. This line also helps as a diagnostic tool to localise the various nasal deformities. Since the line extends from the nasal process of the frontal bones, the nasal bones, through the upper lateral cartilages to the lower lateral cartilages, any deformity along this line, involving the nasal skeleton, will compromise the integrity of this line and helps to focus on the specific area of discontinuity or distortion of this line. Any assymetrical distortion of this line helps in the comparison of the deformity between two sides of the face. The "eyebrow facial sulcus line" (◘ Fig. 4.29b) is more of a diagnostic help than "eyebrow tip line" (◘ Fig. 4.29c), as it takes into account the lateral crural pathology. Be aware that

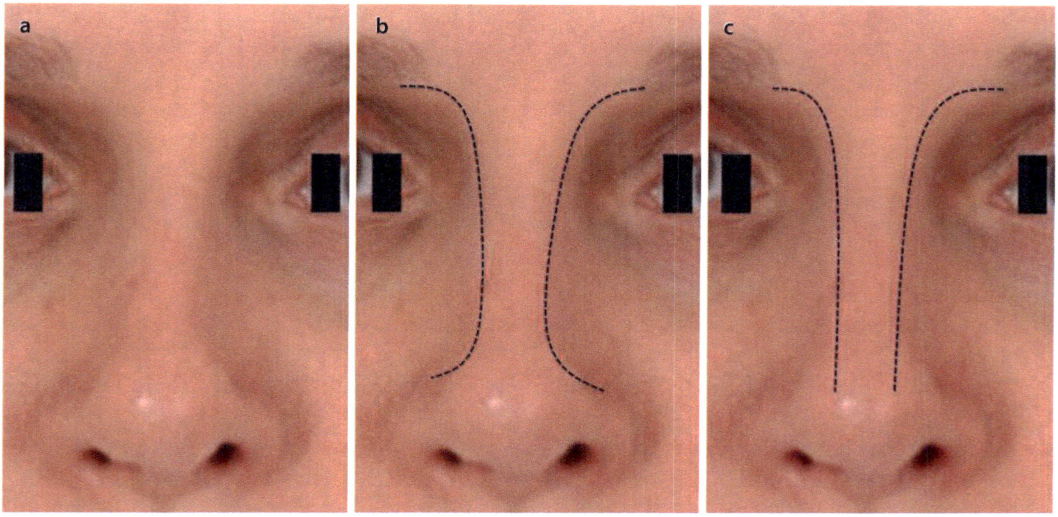

Fig. 4.29 a–c Dorsal aesthetic lines. **a** Frontal view. **b** Frontal view showing "eyebrow facial sulcus line". **c** Frontal view showing "eyebrow tip line"

the eyebrow tip line may look aesthetically pleasing even in patients with excess width of lateral crus with lateral crural ballooning or malposition.

4.4 Assessment of Skin and Subcutaneous Tissue

- Assessing the skin of the patient's nose is vital in predicting good outcomes. The thickness of the skin should be noted with any overlying seborrhoea or rhinophyma changes which can affect any tip narrowing procedure.
- Patients with thick skin, particularly of the tip should never be guaranteed to give a narrow tip. If the skin and subcutaneous tissues are thickened, it will not drape around the sculpted cartilages and hence the outcome of the surgical procedure might not be obvious to the patient, much like dressing a mannequin in a shop window. This is significant in the nasal tip than the rest of the nose [12].
- Similarly, if the skin envelope is very thin, it can show through small dorsal irregularities and any cartilage grafts used can be visible. Any non-absorbable tip sutures also run the risk of extrusion through the thin skin.
- Overlying scar should also be noted as any localised scar should be released during the flap elevation, so that the skin envelope can re-drape nicely without any tethering. Patients should be pre-warned that any depressed dorsal scar may be more obvious soon after the procedure, before it gets better looking. Always any depressed scars should be plumped up with crushed cartilage at the end of the procedure.
- Any pigmentation, vascular changes should be noted, particularly in multiple revision procedures. If so it is an indication to increase the vascularity and thickness of the flap with either temporalis fascia, temporo-parietal fascia or fascia lata. These factors should be taken into account in the assessment and planning stages of the surgery.

4.5 Assessment Checklist

On inspection the tip should be assessed in conjunction with the nasal dorsum and the lateral profile line. As mentioned above, definition of the nasal tip, projection, rotation and eyebrow tip line should be assessed. All the deformities which the surgeon encounters during surgery are invariably seen on external examination. The surgeon should adequately train themselves to "see" these deformities, so that a *realistic* surgical plan can be formulated and the patient can have an informed choice about the outcomes of the surgery.

What the eyes "should see" in the "frontal" view

1. Width of the nasal dorsum
2. Orientation and asymmetry of the dorsal profile lines
3. Localised depressions of the nasal dorsum or the upper lateral cartilages
4. Deviations of the nasal bones with or without upper lateral cartilage "K" Area deviations cartilaginous structures
5. If there is an "open" book deformity, is it parallel, or diamond shaped
6. Localised scarring, pigmentation, vascular changes in the skin

What the eyes "should see" in the "profile" view

- Dorsal profile line/relationship of upper third, middle third and the lower third tip region
- Any dorsal hump or depression
- Length of the nose
- Projection of the nose in relation to the face and the projection of the tip in relation to the rest of the nasal dorsum

What the eyes "should see" in the "three quarters" view

- This view particularly is useful in assessing the depth of the nose, particularly an over projected or under projected nose.
- Most important view to document.
- More useful in accurately recording the under rotation or over rotation of the nasal tip.
- Accurate assessment of the length of the nose.

What the eyes "should see" in the "basal" view

- Aesthetic triangle of the nasal tip.
- Symmetry of the sill, columellar and infra tip lobule section of the nasal tip.
- Dislocation of the caudal nasal septum
- Dislocation or fracture of the medial crural footplates of the lower lateral crus.
- Shape of the nostrils.
- Shape and angulation of the soft triangle.
- Any additional soft tissue scarring and functional collapse of the alar margins should be noted as well.

4.5.1 Palpation

- Tip recoil and strength should be assessed on palpation.
- A springy recoil suggests the integrity of the length of the medial crura. Lack of tip recoil suggests issues with medial crus and a surgical plan should include medial crural sutures to strengthen both the crura.
- Always remember to feel the septal cartilage, particularly in patients needing septal cartilage harvest leaving an "L" strut. Also it helps to plan whether the patient needs caudal strengthening.

4.6 Functional Assessment

Functional assessment of the nasal tip is slightly more difficult than structural assessment which can be confusing and not easily understood and not easily reproducible. Generally nasal tip structural issues involving the lateral crura cause functional external nasal valve dysfunction. Apart from this, middle vault collapse or an upper lateral collapse can also cause functional internal nasal valve obstruction. Lack of lateral crural support due to misplaced lateral crus or a deformity of lateral crus can cause functional obstruction with an alar collapse in the lateral alar sidewalls. Examination in quiet breathing and forced inspiration may show the degree of obstruction (◘ Fig. 4.30a, b). Even experienced rhinoplasty surgeons may not agree with each other in diagnosing internal nasal valve deformities from external nasal valve deformities and hence management options can vary widely even within experienced consultants, leave alone surgical trainees. Lack

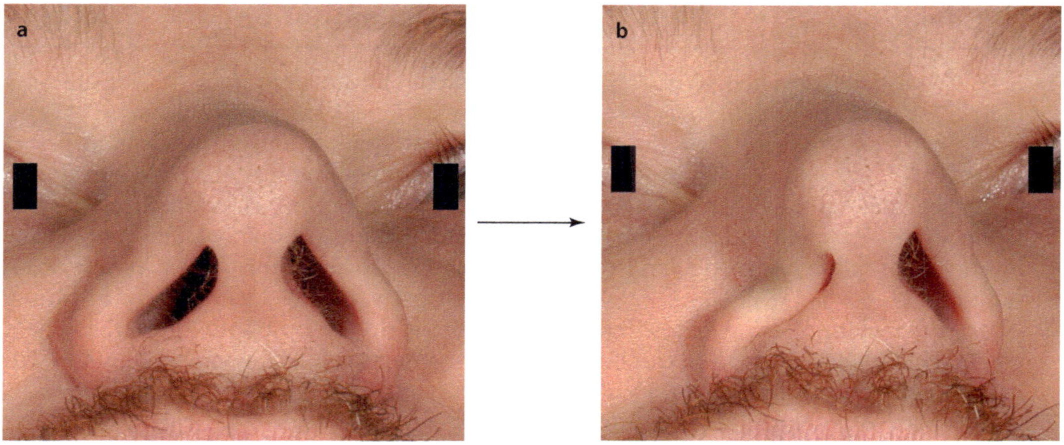

Fig. 4.30 **a**, **b** Lateral alar weakness on the right side with concavity. **a** Quiet inspiration. **b** Forced inspiration

of consistency between trained surgeons also leads to inconsistency in diagnosis and confusion regarding management, unable to tailor individual surgery to the patient's needs. This also leads to confusion in teaching and training junior surgeons. Over the last 13 years, the author has been using a nasal "wall" sub-unit assessment system [13, 14] concentrating on individual anatomical sites in the medial wall of the nose and the lateral wall of the nose, rather than external and internal valve areas. Various concepts have also been put forward by other surgeons [15–19]. Functional assessment should concentrate on individual anatomical components inside the nose rather than on the traditional internal and external nasal valve regions. This will help in the understanding of the pathology, introduce consistency in the management plan and improve teaching and training.

4.7 Pathology Checklist

4.7.1 Septum

1. Is there a caudal deviation?
2. Is there a mid-septum/posterior septal deviation?
3. Is there a dorsal septal deviation?
4. Is there a combination of deformities requiring an extra-corporeal septoplasty?

4.7.2 Hump

5. Bony or cartilaginous or both.
6. True or pseudo.
7. Is there an "open" book deformity, or the bony dorsum is smooth and rounded?
8. If there is open book, is the deformity parallel or diamond shaped?
9. If it is diamond shaped, is there a lateral "K" area collapse?
10. Is it associated with over projected strong tip or under rotated tip?
11. Do they need composite reduction or component reduction?
12. Do they need dorsal crushed cartilage?
13. Depth of nasion.

4.7.3 Depression

1. Is it bony, cartilaginous or both?
2. Is there upper lateral collapse?
3. Is there an inverted "v" deformity?
4. Is there an over rotation of the tip?
5. Do they need spreader grafts?
6. Do they need caudal septal grafts?
7. Assess the width of the nasal base.

4.7.4 Deviation

1. Is it "C" shaped – deviated nose?
2. Is it "S" shaped – squinted nose?
3. Is the problem at the roof of the nose – nasion?
4. Is the problem in the "K" area as well?
5. Is the septum deviated and how is it affecting the external shape particularly dorsal septum?
6. What is the width of nasal bones – so that you need to know whether you can borrow nasal bone from other side?
7. Have a plan for a sequential osteotomy.
8. Is it associated with unilateral depressed fracture?

4.7.5 Tip

1. Shape – bulbous, wide, narrow, any clefting.
2. Strong or weak LLC.
3. Projection.
4. Rotation.
5. Soft triangle.
6. Infra tip lobule blunting.
7. Naso-labial angle blunting.
8. Any other issues in the naso-labial sulcus?
9. Columellar retraction or hanging columella.
10. Tip ptosis.
11. Loss of medial crural height.
12. Columellar scar.

4.7.6 Palpation

1. Palpate the caudal septum.
2. Palpate the width and orientation of nasal bones.
3. Palpate the lower marginal edge of lateral crus and soft triangle.
4. Assess the tip recoil.

4.7.7 Skin and Subcutaneous Tissue

1. Localised scar.
2. Pigmentation.
3. Increased vascularity.
4. Thickness of the skin.

4.8 Documentation

Adequate documentation of the consultation process, clinical assessment findings, 2-D or 3-D photographic documentation and surgical operative findings are all important in the entire process of rhinoplasty surgery to achieve a successful outcome and protect the surgeon from litigation. Pre-op photo documentation is a legal document. In litigation, if there is no pre-op photograph, the benefit of judgement will be favourable only towards the patient.

Conclusion

Knowledge gained by "clinical assessment" is the key for a successful rhinoplasty and a positive outcome. Getting the thought process right is key for a successful tip work. It is based on the surgeons' knowledge of what the author refers to as *"conscious thinking"*, the so called *what and why* of the deformity. This knowledge can be acquired not only by clinical examination but also by direct observation during surgery, particularly when done through an open approach. Clinical assessment of the nose should include both structure and function. Do not approach structure without considering the function as they are both interrelated. Structural assessment includes definition, projection, rotation and assessment of dorsal aesthetic lines. In conclusion, the key to a successful rhinoplasty ultimately depends on the accurate assessment and planning of the surgical treatment.

Key Points Box

- There is no "ideal" nose which will make the patient happy. Be aware that these ideals can keep changing with the time, fashion, race and culture.
- One should develop the art of being able to assess the "aetio-pathology" of the deformity by being able to "look through" the overlying skin. We do not have the luxury of any other tools like MRI or a CT scan to make the right diagnosis.

- To understand what changes will make the patient happy is the ultimate quest of the successful surgeon and hence the need for repeated consultations before surgery.
- Assessing the patent's suitability for the surgery is an important key consideration. Making sure that the patient's expectations are realistic is the key factor in a successful rhinoplasty.
- The soft triangle is always "soft", since there is no cartilage, but not always a "triangle" even in so called normal tips.
- *Definition, projection, rotation and dorsal aesthetic lines are* the key tools in the assessment and diagnosis of structural and functional traumatic nasal deformities.

References

1. Hemenway P. Divine proportion: phi in art, nature, and science. New York: Sterling; 2005. p. 20–1.
2. Dunlap RA. The golden ratio and fibonacci numbers. Singapore: World Scientific Publishing; 1997.
3. Bulstrode NW, Waterhouse N, Forrester P. Male aesthetic patients to avoid, slap-simon. Plast Reconstr Surg. 2007;119(1):452.
4. Veale D, De Haro L, Lambrou C. Cosmetic rhinoplasty in body dysmorphic disorder. Br J Plast Surg. 2003;56(6):546–51.
5. Balaji N. Top tips in nasal tip surgery, ENT-FPS UK Newsletter— Feb 2018 –Issue 6.
6. Tardy ME, Hendrick D, Alex J. Refinement of the nasal tip. In: Bailey BJ, editor. Head and neck surgery – otolaryngology. 2nd ed. Philadelphia: Lippincott-Raven; 1998.
7. Robinson S, Thornton M. Nasal tip projection: nuances in understanding, assessment and modification. Facial Plast Surg. 2012;28(2):158–65.
8. Goode RL. A method of tip projection measurement. In: Powell N, Humphrey B, editors. Proportions of the aesthetic face. New York: Thieme-Stratton; 1984. p. 15–39.
9. Tasman AJ, Lohuis PJ. Control of tip rotation. Facial Plast Surg. 2012;28(2):243–50.
10. Smillie I, Sil A, Haddock R, Balaji N. Asymmetrical nostril axis angle in the post traumatic nose. Rhinology. 2013;51(2):176–80.
11. Soliemanzadeh P, Kridel RWH. Nasal tip over projection: Algorithm of surgical deprojection techniques and introduction of medial crural overlay. Arch Facial Plast Surg. 2005;7:374–80.
12. Tasman AJ, Helbig M. Sonography of nasal tip anatomy and surgical tip refinement. Plast Reconstr Surg. 2000;105(7):2573–9.
13. Balaji N, Ravichandran S. Assessment of nasal Valve obstruction: a new nasal "wall" subunit concept. ENT Audiol News. 2012;21(4):111–3.
14. Balaji N, Ravichandran S. Assessment of nasal Valve obstruction: a new Glasgow nasal "wall" subunit concept. ENT Audiol News. 2012;21(5):86–7.
15. Tsao GJ, Fijalkowski N, Most SP. Validation of a grading system for lateral nasal wall insufficiency. Allergy Rhinol (Providence). 2013;4(2):e66–8.
16. Vaezeafshar R, Moubayed SP, Most SP. Repair of lateral wall insufficiency. JAMA Facial Plast Surg. 2018;20(2):111–5.
17. Ziai H, Bonaparte JP. Reliability and construct validity of the Ottawa valve collapse scale when assessing external nasal valve collapse. J Otolaryngol Head Neck Surg. 2018;47:15.
18. Spielmann PM, White PS, Hussain SS. Surgical techniques for the treatment of nasal valve collapse: a systematic review. Laryngoscope. 2009;119(7):1281–90.
19. Goudakos JK, Fishman JM, Patel K. A systematic review of the surgical techniques for the treatment of internal nasal valve collapse: where do we stand? Clin Otolaryngol. 2017;42(1):60–70.

Nasal Tip Rhinoplasty: Consultation Process

Contents

N. Balaji, *Textbook of Nasal Tip Rhinoplasty*, https://doi.org/10.1007/978-3-030-48157-5_5

Learning Objectives
- To understand the nuances of the consultation process.
- To understand the need for effective communication with the patient.
- To deal with individual patients and their families.

5.1 Introduction

Consultation for a rhinoplasty is tedious both to the surgeon and the patient and approached by both parties with lot of apprehension. The key to the process is "effective communication". This is one particular art for the surgeon which cannot be taught in a book or attending a course. Consultation phase is important and patients should feel well supported. This is the time most surgeons should concentrate to avoid future issues. There are lot of things which will be learnt not in the initial stages of the practice, but may be only after few years.

Assessing a patient for rhinoplasty often starts at the time the patient "walks in" for the first consultation. The patient usually comes alone or with just one of their closest relative or a friend during the first consultation. There should be adequate time allocated for the consultation process. Often examination of the nose and clinical assessment is a shorter period for an experienced surgeon. It is more often talking about the whole process and finding what the patient wants takes time. The aim of the initial consultation is to figure out:
- What exactly the patient wants from the surgical procedure?
- How realistic is the patient's expectations?

The issues can be functional, structural or both. Unfortunately the word "cosmetic" is used synonymously with structural changes in the nose when compared to any other organ in the body. Beware functional outcomes are more difficult to achieve when compared to structural improvements. The patient should be encouraged to describe "all" their deformities and prioritise the top three things which bother them the most. If there are deformities the patient has not noticed particularly alar margins and alar size asymmetry, this should by default discussed with the patient and documented before proceeding with surgery. Always encourage the patients (and not the relatives or friends) to talk. The role of the relatives or friends is "to listen" to what the surgeon has to say and perhaps re-enforce the patient later on. Do not allow relatives to make decisions. Sometimes there are patients who turn towards the relative to ask for their approval. Encourage them to make their own decisions.

The patients should be seen two or three times before proceeding with surgery, the so called "cool off" period. This not only allows the patient to understand what you discussed, but also for medico-legal reasons. Also the "cool-off" period gives the vital time needed for the surgeon to know what the patient actually wants from the operation and also helps the surgeon to understand how realistic the patient is. Seeing the patient few times also helps the surgeon to understand the mental framework of these patients and may be not to go ahead with the procedure if the surgeon is not satisfied. This "cool off" time is an important consideration in favour of the surgeon if a medico legal situation arises.

5.2 Following Are the 'Top" Tips of the Clinical Consultation Process

1. *Handling the patient's and the family's expectations* is an important aspect and peculiar aspect of this surgery. Patients demanding aesthetic or cosmetic rhinoplasty without any functional issues are more difficult to please and their expectations can be unrealistic. Be on-guard all the time for patients with unrealistic expectations. It is not always easy to pick these patients up before surgery. Every rhinoplasty surgeon with years of experience will be in this scenario where he or she has repented doing surgery in the wrong patient. Numerous studies have highlighted these issues [1, 2]. Even after

years, it is not surprising to be caught out. These are patients to be avoided or counselled properly before surgery. Even after years of experience the surgeon is likely to miss a difficult patient if not on guard all the time. Always listen to the third sense which may alert the surgeon about a difficult patient with unrealistic expectations. Beware of a "lone" patient coming in for consultation. Patient usually comes alone or with just one relative during the first appointment, but invariably comes with the two or three close relatives or friends when the nasal splints come off in a week's time. This can be a recipe for disaster for the surgeon. It is always wiser to see a patient with his relatives during the pre-operative discussion so that everyone is aware of the identified goals and outcomes. In the first postop week, when the splints comes off, a relative or a friend, who has come for the first time and not aware of the agreed outcomes, can pass a judgemental negative comment for example, "oh the tip is very swollen" or "I thought the nose will be much smaller". This can set off a chain of negative thoughts in the patient's mind and can lead to an unhappy patient, which invariably be projected to the surgeon during the subsequent visits as "being not happy with the surgery". Some patients complain about very obvious deformities like deviation or a large hump, but may not notice or concentrate on minor deformities. The surgeon should point out the other deformities particularly nostril asymmetries prior to surgery although patient is concentrating on only a few. This should also be recorded in the patient's files. Always deal with patient's expectations genuinely and sincerely as the surgeon can only improve the deformity by moving the grade of deformity better by a point or two, but will never make a nose 100% better.

2. *Always have a "cool off" period before surgery*. Seeing patients twice or even thrice is important. This gives them enough time at least 4–8 weeks before proceeding with surgery. *"Patients have to be sure of what they want from the surgeon and the surgeon also needs to be sure of what he or she can offer the patient."* Look for consistency in the patient's demands when they come second time. Be careful not to operate before you are convinced that the patient is fully aware of what you can offer or you are convinced that the patient's expectations are realistic. Having said that, most patients have decided whether they like the surgeon or not at the very first appointment.
3. *Agree a set of goals or outcomes which are practical and easy to quantify* before proceeding for surgery. Few appointments may be needed to figure out the key objectives. The patient should be able to see these outcomes when the plaster comes off, bearing in mind some of the outcomes may not be obvious for few months.
4. *Providing written material and leaflets are important*. This should be sent to the patient and the referring doctor along with printed leaflets well ahead of the surgery. On the day of surgery, this should be included in the "informed consent".
5. *Adequate record keeping is vital*. Key objectives should be recorded. Also the gist of the consultation process including the pros and cons of the surgery should be recorded, including the expected outcomes and results. Adequate record keeping saves lot of hassle particularly when there is a litigation. Written material is better than verbal advice. Do not alter or amend the operation notes or clinic notes without prior consultation with the patient. This results in loss of faith and a major source of litigation and falling foul with the peers.
6. *In patients undergoing functional septo rhinoplasty*, you need to emphasise that the functional improvement in breathing will take time and may not be better for 6 weeks. In septoplasty surgery, it will also be worthwhile pointing out that the sep-

tum is a midline structure and can be accessed through the right or the left nostril and whichever side you access it, there will be sutures on that side. This prevents patients to assume quickly in the immediate post-op period that the lack of improvement in the nasal function is because you have done the "wrong" side, simply because they saw the sutures on the opposite side of the nasal obstruction! If trying to explain this after surgery, it will be difficult to win their trust.

7. *Beware of patients with bipolar disorders*, psychological issues and body dysmorphic syndrome. Beware of the acronym single, introspective, male with obsessive neurosis (SIMON). On the contrary, the acronym SYLVIA (secure, young, listener, verbal, intelligent and attractive) is supposed to indicate a favourable candidacy for surgery [3, 4, 5]. These guidelines does not always help the surgeon, as often it is the so called "normal" looking people who lands the surgeon in trouble.
8. Be aware of over patronising patients. "I have been referred to you because you are the best" – Statements like this may be a trap that surgeon should avoid falling in.
9. *Be aware of cocaine and recreational drug users*, which is getting more common these days. They are powerful vasoconstrictors causing damage to septal mucosa and cartilage preventing flap elevation. Cocaine is often contaminated with anti-helminthic drug Levamisole, which can cause agranulocytosis and make them more prone for post-operative infection and the risk of septal perforation [6, 7, 8].
10. *Handling revision surgery patients needs a lot of skill.* Remember, the surgeon who undertakes revision procedure, will be held responsible for all the previous issues. Although the previous surgeon may have created some of the deformities, only the last surgeon will be in the patients' mind and hence technically responsible for everything which has happened before! It may not be possible to correct all the deformities or even if you correct them it may not be to the patient's satisfaction. It is not about technically correcting a deformity that matters, but what matters most is whether the surgeon will make the patient happy after the revision procedure.
11. *Use of computer morphing*: There has been an increasing use of computer software to morph patient's images from pre-op situation to show the post-operative changes. It will be nice for the patients to appreciate what the nose "may" (but not "will") look like after the surgery and more importantly gives the surgeon a rough guidance of what exactly the patient is looking for. The downside being the patients may expect miracles looking at the morphed images and runs the risk of raising patient's expectations, although this is generally found to be untrue in literature [9, 10]. The author personally do not use computer morphing as it can raise patient's expectations and be counterproductive, as small incremental changes possible in the computer may not be possible in real life, taking into consideration the healing process.
12. *Post-operative period and visit* is very important – Expect issues in the post-op period. All post op concerns should be addressed very quickly and reassured. Unhappy patients are usually due to wrong selection of patients with emotional instability rather than surgeon related factors [11, 12]. There should always be a system where patient can contact you with queries. Repeated consultations allay anxiety and reassure the patient. Surgeon being readily accessible to the patient is an important positive factor in the post-operative period. Sometimes the offer of a second opinion from a peer is a gesture which is liked by the patients. Most medico-legal issues are due to inadequate and poor communication skills.

5.3 Consultation Scenarios

We have put forward following clinical scenarios encountered in our practice of 24 years, which a beginner should be familiar with, when doing this type of surgery. We would like to share our views on these and hope the reader will find some nuggets, which will help them to avoid difficult patients and not get caught out with unrealistic patients.

5.3.1 Scenario 1: The Over Flattering, "Ego" Flaming Talkative Patient

There are some patients who come in and say "I heard that you are the best in this and I am sure you will know what is wrong with my nose and you will fix it for me." Be aware of this type of over flattering personality where they try to flame the surgeon's ego to try and shift the entire burden of responsibility to the surgeon, instead of taking responsibility themselves. In this scenario, it is easy to fall in the trap as the patient is playing with the ego of the surgeon, either deliberately or not. These patients should be counselled right from the outset that apart from the surgeon, there are many equally important factors, including patient related factors in the healing process, to achieve a favourable outcome. At the initial consultation itself, it is important to point out that complication do happen in your hands and be honest and tell your revision rate and keep the conversation very clear and make sure you back it up with your own personal information leaflet and a "cool off" period.

5.3.2 Scenario 2: The Young Patient Who Comes in with a Relative but Remains Silent During the Consultation

This scenario can be difficult to handle as any question you put to the patient is usually answered by the relative, even themselves pointing the fingers to the part of the patient's nose that need correction. It is best for the surgeon to be assertive and make sure the patient talks and not the relative or the mother, if the patient is in his or her teens. This should be done fairly bluntly at this stage, by looking towards the relative and telling them that the conversation will be better if you have with the patient as they are the ones who will be having the surgery. The patient should be encouraged to have the conversation. If you do this at this stage, the patient also feels empowered. This will encourage the patient to tell what the concerns are about the surgery. This also helps the surgeon to decide whether the patient is having the surgery to please someone else.

5.3.3 Scenario 3: "Beware of Young Lone Males" with Psycho-social Issues and on Anti-depressants

Beware of the pneumonic, SIMON-single, introvert, male, with obsessive narcissistic views. Patients obsessive about their noses may not be limited to one sex. Sometimes patients are not easy to detect until otherwise you see them few times. It is very important not to operate on someone who is obsessed with his or her nose, particularly when there is not much of a deformity. The reason being even if you have an objectively better outcome, subjectively it will not be possible to satisfy the patient.

5.3.4 Scenario 4: Guilt, Low Self-Esteem and Wants to Justify the Money Spent

Beware of patients who turn towards the relative every few minutes during the discussion, as if they are looking for approval before they proceed. This may be for many reasons, either they are financially dependable on their relatives or psychologically labile with a low self-esteem, guilt and not able to come to terms with spending money to justify the surgery.

5.3.5 Scenario 5: Patients Who Came Alone for the Initial Consultation but Comes with Three People in the Post-op Period – Dealing with the Family

The author has come across situations where patients come for the pre-op consultation few times *alone*, but in the immediate post-op they bring few of their relatives and look at them for their comments as soon as the plaster comes off. This is a recipe for disaster. Even a small comment by the relative saying the tip is swollen (which it will be for few months!) will set a chain of negative thoughts in the patient's mind that will make them unhappy. It is important right from the very first consultation that the patient comes with a closest relative and make sure the same person comes with the patient when the plaster comes off, so that all concerned are aware of the planned outcomes and pros and cons of the surgery and also helps the surgeon to see if either of them are unrealistic in their expectations.

5.3.6 Scenario 6: Dealing with Expectations of Revision Surgery

Multiple revision rhinoplasty procedures are a totally different issue. Technically it can be difficult to execute any corrective surgery third or the fourth time. There may not be enough cartilage to harvest. They may have extensive scarring. The surgeon is also dealing with a very upset patient who is looking to correct all the previous issues by revision surgery. The surgeon should be honest with the patient about the results. Sometimes it is not possible to execute the surgery skilfully and the tissues may not heal, despite the best efforts of the surgeon. Adequate communication is a must. Record keeping should be accurate.

5.4 Patient Information Leaflet for Septo-Rhinoplasty

The term rhinoplasty means reshaping the structure and function of the nose. It is the most commonly performed facial plastic surgery procedure. The term "rhinoplasty" means changing the shape of the nose. The term "septoplasty" means straightening the nasal septum to improve the nasal breathing. The term "septo-rhinoplasty" means correcting the breathing (septoplasty) and the shape of the nose (rhinoplasty). Most people need septo-rhinoplasty for post-traumatic nasal obstruction and deformity. Septo-rhinoplasty surgery is also indicated in elderly patients when aging changes cause functional nasal valve obstructions and tip droop due to lax tissues. Septo-rhinoplasty is also performed for deformed nasal tissues in people born with cleft lip. The word "Primary" rhinoplasty means first time surgery. Persistent or new problems after a primary rhinoplasty requiring revision surgery are called "secondary" rhinoplasty. Rhinoplasty is also done for functional reasons when for example over resection of tissues resulting in scarring causing narrowing at the valve regions of the nose. This might need complex surgical procedures, including cartilage grafting to help breath better. This is called "functional" rhinoplasty. Sometimes cartilage grafts have to be taken from ears or rib cartilage in the chest.

There is no ideal age for this surgery, although young people recover quickly with less oedema. The older a person is, the longer the recovery, particularly tissue oedema and tip swelling take longer to clear. The techniques for correcting traumatic noses are more complex and the outcomes are difficult to judge. The favourable age is any time after 16–18 years when the development of the mid face is complete.

Most operations like tonsillectomy or appendectomy have fixed outcomes, but in septo-rhinoplasty there are usually a variety of outcomes possible. Patient might want different outcomes which may be realistic or unrealistic. Even if it is realistic, sometimes, the outcomes are not achievable without having some other negative effect on the nose. I proceed with surgery only when patients understand the outcomes and be realistic about the outcomes. I usually see my patients twice or even thrice before proceeding for surgery.

5.4.1 How Is This Operation Performed?

In the UK, this operation is usually performed under general anaesthetic. Septoplasty operation is done through incisions inside the nose to straighten the septum. The incision is made either on the right or left side of the septum depending on the surgeon's preference to correct the deviation which may be to one side or other. The sutures used are absorbable sutures and they may take 6–8 weeks to absorb and disappear. Sometimes the sutures may be needed to be taken out on the follow-up visit.

Rhinoplasty is done either through inside or through outside "open approach". Inside approach is suitable for limited deformities and I prefer outside approach open approach, as this has more advantages to deal with all the eventualities we may encounter. Open approach is needed in revision procedures and in primary procedures needing complex procedures, including tip work. Open approach will leave a small scar across the columellar region of nose, which is usually less obvious in 6 weeks, but still can be seen if you are looking for it. In my practise scarring has never been a major issue, when compared to the benefits achieved in correcting the deformities. Extra-cartilage usually taken from the ears might be needed to reconstruct some noses.

5.4.2 What to Expect After the Operation?

The operation for septoplasty as mentioned above is a much smaller procedure which may require nasal packing for up to 5–6 hrs. The patient can be discharged either the same day or next day. The nasal breathing will take 3 months to recover fully as there will be tissue oedema. There will not be any facial bruising or change in the shape of the nose with this procedure. Avoid lifting weights or heavy exercise for 2 weeks as there may be some bleeding on and off.

On the contrary septo-rhinoplasty or rhinoplasty is a bigger procedure, sometimes complex reconstructions taking up to 2 hrs. There will be swelling and bruising around the eyes as often the skin has to be lifted and bones had to be broken and reset in new positions. Patient has to wear an external nasal splint for 7 days. Any external stitches will come out the same time as the plaster in 7 days. It is advisable to be off work for about 10 days and rest at home. Avoid heavy exercise or trauma for about 3 months. Stopping smoking certainly helps in the healing process.

5.4.3 What Are the Possible Complications?

Bruising and swelling are expected for few days after surgery. Nasal bleeding, blood clots around the suture sites, may be annoying sometimes. Nasal tip swelling may be present for up to 3 months or even up to a year in patients having tip plasty. Septal haematoma, infection, septal abscess, loss of septal cartilage, septal perforation and loss of dorsal height are all rare, but significant complications. Some of the outcomes agreed may not be achieved and may need revision procedure to achieve them. In the author's practice, around 5% of patients need revision surgery. Antibiotics are usually given single dose intravenously during the procedure and simple pain killers like paracetamol would suffice.

5.5 Informed Consent

The term "informed consent" strictly speaking does not apply to the nasal tip work particularly as it is difficult to predict what exactly is happening under the skin, contrary to any other surgical speciality where there are investigatory tools like radiography. If it is difficult for the surgeon to predict the diagnosis strictly speaking, it is not possible to give an "informed" consent to the patient. Nevertheless the surgeon should discuss all the facts of the surgery based on the surgeon's experience. The patient should be seen few times and the information backed up by written leaflets. The timing of the consent must be at least few weeks before the surgery and preferably not on the day of the procedure.

Conclusion

Consultation process can be tedious both for the surgeon, and the patient and can cause anxiety for both patients and the surgeon. The whole process is about effective communication skills and some surgeons are better at it than others and most surgeons get better with time based on their personal experience.

Key Points Box

- Patients should be encouraged to talk about "all" their deformities and then prioritise the top three deformities which bother them the most.
- Dealing with patient's expectations is vital and initial time spent will be quite rewarding later.
- If there are deformities, the patient has not noticed particularly alar margins and alar size asymmetry; this should by default discussed with the patient and documented before proceeding with surgery.
- Always have a "cool off" period before surgery, seeing the patient at least twice before surgery.
- Beware of patients with bipolar disorders, psychological issues and body dysmorphic syndrome.
- Agree a set of goals or outcomes which are practical and easy to quantify before you proceed for surgery.
- Adequate record keeping is vital.

References

1. Slator R, Harris DL. Are rhinoplasty patients potentially mad? Br J Plast Surg. 1992;45:301.
2. Macgregor FC. Social, psychological and cultural dimensions of cosmetic and reconstructive plastic surgery. Aesthet Plast Surg. 1989;13:1.
3. Gorney M, Martello J. Patient selection criteria. Medical-legal issues in plastic surgery. Clin plast surg. 1999;26:37.
4. Tardy ME Jr. Rhinoplasty: the art and the science. Philadelphia: W.B. Saunders Company; 1997.
5. Rohrich RI. Streamlining cosmetic surgery patient selection – just say no. Plast Reconstr Surg. 1999;104:220.
6. Thompson JS, Herbick JM, Klassen LW, et al. Studies on levamisole-induced agranulocytosis. Blood. 1980;56(3):388–96.
7. Kopp SA, High WA, Green JJ. Levamisole-induced Wegener's granulomatosis following contaminated cocaine abuse. Skinmed. 2012;10(4):254–6.
8. Nolan AL, Jen KY. Pathologic manifestations of levamisole-adultered cocaine exposure. Diagn Pathol. 2015;10:48.
9. Sheen JH, Sheen AP, editors. Aesthetic rhinoplasty. 2nd ed. St. Louis: Quality Medical Publishing; 1998.
10. Gruber RP. Computer imaging and surgical reality in aesthetic rhinoplasty. Plast Reconstr Surg. 2005;116(3):922–3.
11. Moses S, Mahler D. After aesthetic rhinoplasty: new looks and psychological outlooks on post-surgical satisfaction. Aesthet Plast Surg. 1984;8:213.
12. Goin MK, Rees TD. A prospective study of patients' psychological reactions to rhinoplasty. Ann Plast Surg. 1991;27:210.

"Surgical Principles" in Nasal Tip Rhinoplasty

Contents

N. Balaji, *Textbook of Nasal Tip Rhinoplasty*, https://doi.org/10.1007/978-3-030-48157-5_6

Learning Objectives
- The role of "tripod" concept and its significance in arriving at an algorithm to correct the lower lateral cartilage deformities.
- To understand the role of overlying skin and soft tissue envelope.
- To understand the role of surgical planning and tissue handling.

6.1 Introduction

Nasal tip rhinoplasty is one of the most demanding and complex surgical procedures with in the gamut of rhinoplasty surgery. The two lower lateral cartilages, otherwise called alar cartilages, form the nasal tip. Each lower lateral cartilage has three components namely medial crus, lateral crus and intermediate crus. Hence damage to any of the three components on each side (6 in total) can create a myriad of complex deformities. It is more complex than upper third or middle third deformities of the nose due to the multiple variations it can present. Tip plasty is an essential and indispensable part of rhinoplasty. It is important to realise that every nose is different and the attention to finer details is important and defines the good rhinoplasty surgeon. Nasal tip reconstruction is complex, particularly in post-traumatic noses and compliments the surgery on nasal dorsum.

6.2 The Aims of Nasal Tip Plasty

The aim of nasal tip reconstruction is to achieve patient satisfaction with both structure and function. The aims are:
- To achieve good definition and symmetry of the nasal tip
- To achieve adequate projection of the nasal tip
- To achieve adequate rotation of the tip in relation to the dorsum

Following a pre-op assessment, the surgeon aims to reconstruct the tip by changing either/or the definition, projection and rotation. Due consideration should be given to the final outcome and position of the tip in relation to the nasal dorsum, taking into account the skin thickness, race and ethnic variations.

6.3 Knowledge and Understanding of the Pathogenesis of Tip Deformities

In assessing the pathogenesis of the tip deformities, the surgeon needs to make a distinction between *primary and secondary deformities.*

Primary deformities (■ Fig. 6.1) refer to deformities intrinsic to the tip cartilages, which can involve the lateral crus, medial crus or the intermediate crus on one or both sides. Thus six variables, three on either side can create a multitude of tip deformities, which makes nasal tip surgery more complex.

Secondary deformities (■ Fig. 6.2) are due to the caudal septal deformities causing poor tip support and secondary tip changes.

But in practice, there is always a combination of primary and secondary tip deformities (■ Fig. 6.3), particularly in traumatic and revision noses.

In the author's experience, in most of the traumatic patients (over 90%), complete or near complete interruption of the medial crura with loss of medial crural support is the cause of primary tip deformity. In a smaller percentage, there are issues with lateral crus. In the medial crus the interruption is invariably just below the dome, while the fracture

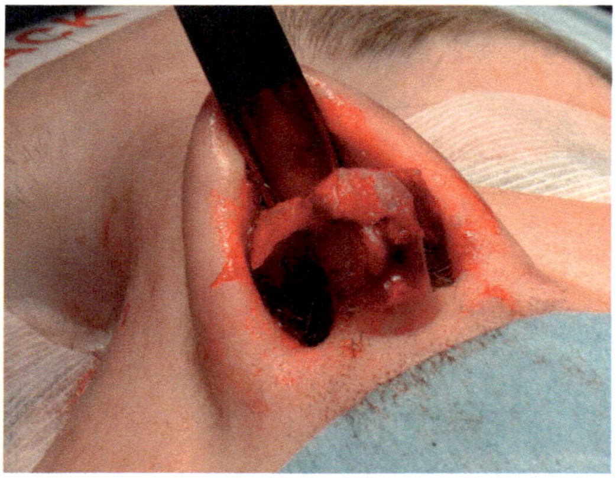

■ **Fig. 6.1** Primary tip deformity due to lateral crural fracture

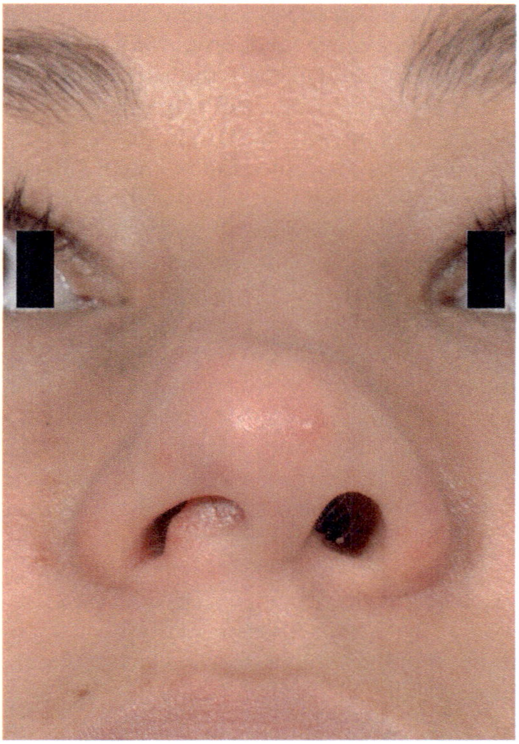

Fig. 6.2 Secondary tip deformity due to caudal septal issues

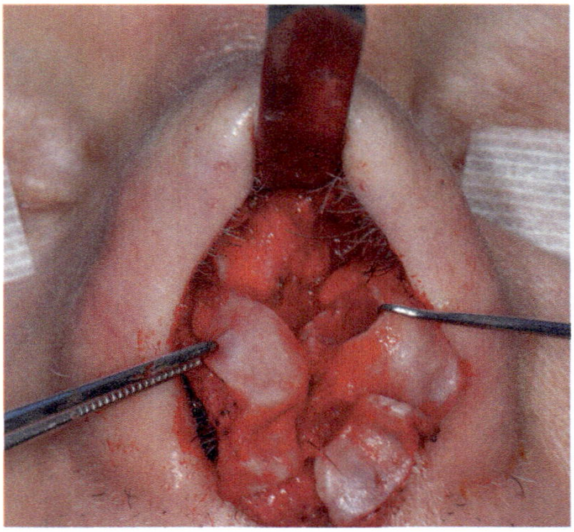

Fig. 6.3 Complex tip deformity due to both primary tip cartilage and secondary septal cartilage damage

line in the lateral crus is usually just lateral to the dome with a deep concavity of the rest of the lateral crus (Fig. 6.3), caused by constant "in drawing" on inspiration and resulting restriction of airflow in the external valve region.

The effect of the above factors can lead to a *variety* of tip deformities, predominantly causing loss of tip support, de-projection and sometimes over-rotation, with or without functional external valve issues.

The key to achieving optimum outcomes in nasal tip surgery lies in the following *"three pillars of learning"*, namely:

- Knowledge derived from *"Accurate assessment"*
- Knowledge in using the *"Right tools and techniques"*
- Knowledge in executing the techniques in the right *"Sequence"*

6.4 Knowledge and Understanding of the Nasal Tip "Tripod" Concept

A clear understanding of the following factors affecting the nasal tip support is a prerequisite before doing tip surgery. Although described as "major" and "minor" tip support mechanisms, in practice this distinction is arbitrary. Damage to a minor tip support structure can become a major issue, particularly in a traumatic nasal tip deformity. Hence all the factors mentioned below should be given *"equal"* importance.

- The size, shape and integrity of the two medial crura
- The size, shape and strength of the lateral crura
- The conjoined strength of the medial crura
- The position, angle and orientation of lateral and medial crura
- The position and strength of the caudal septum and its attachments to the medial crura

Any pathology involving the above tip support mechanisms can cause a nasal tip deformity, in terms of definition, projection and rotation.

Although not a rule, an understanding of the tripod concept gives us an *"insight into the algorithms"* for correcting tip deformities. The nasal tip has been compared to a tripod where the two lateral crura form the lateral legs of the tripod and the conjoined medial crura forms the medial leg of the tripod. As per Anderson's *"tripod" concept* [1], the tip is analogous to a tripod stool. The position of the tip (base of the stool) is determined by the length and strength of the three legs of the stool, namely the two lateral crura and the third conjoined medial crura in the front. Note the front leg is the "conjoined" medial crus, emphasising the fact that the strength of the front pod of the tripod depends on the combined strength of the medial crus rather than a single healthy medial crus, which alone is not enough to give adequate support. The other two latero-posterior pods of the tripod being the length and strength of the two lateral crura. The projection and rotation of the tip can be adjusted by manipulating the three legs of the stool. By shortening the lateral crura (lateral crural excision or incision and overlap), the tip can be de-projected and over rotated up and similarly increasing the medial crural strength and height can increase the tip projection. Various techniques that lengthen or shorten the legs of the tripod, can affect the projection, definition and rotation of the tip. Although *not as simple as this*, being aware of these concepts helps in the understanding of tip dynamics and helps in the management algorithm.

Anatomically the weight of the individual lateral crus is more than that of the individual medial crus. Hence the "conjoined" strength of the two medial crus put together is needed to counter balance the weight of the two heavier lateral crus. Anatomically this is not a favourable arrangement as even a minor damage to the integrity of the medial crura is enough to cause a major tip deformity. Thus the aetio-pathology of any tip deformity is directly related to the poor support of the medial crus and the aim of nasal tip reconstruction should be focussed first on strengthening the medial crus and also may be to decrease the weight of the lateral crus to counter balance the tip. Reducing the length of the conjoined medial crus (either by surgical or non-surgical trauma) alone will not only bring the seat post (which is the tip) down towards the face (de projection) but also turn in towards the face (under rotation). Reducing the two posterior legs of the tripod, namely the two lateral crura, will take the tip back on the dorsum with over rotation of the tip and reducing the projection of the tip. To de-project the tip without altering the rotation, it is advisable to reduce all three limbs of the tripod, namely the conjoined medial crus and the two lateral crus. If performed individually, the tip rotation can be altered. The credit for developing advanced concepts in nasal tip dynamics goes to Dr. Adamson from Toronto, who had proposed the "M-arch" model for a further understanding of tip dynamics [2]. This model not only allows us to delineate the contribution of each medial and lateral crus but also emphasises the importance of the "intermediate" crus. "M"-arch model is an extension of the tripod concept with the inclusion of the intermediate segment which angles away from the conjoined medial crus, creating an aesthetic "M"-arch model.

6.5 Knowledge Gained by "Clinical Assessment"

Getting the thought process right is the key for a successful tip work. It is based on the surgeons' knowledge, of what the author calls *"conscious thinking"*, the so called *"what and why"* of the deformity. This knowledge can be acquired by not only clinical examination, but also by direct observation during surgery, particularly when done through an open approach. Clinical assessment of the nose should include both structure and function. Do not approach structure without considering the function. Both these are interrelated. Structural assessment includes definition, projection, rotation and assessment of the dorsal aesthetic lines. Functional assessment should concentrate on individual anatomical components inside the nose rather than on the traditional internal and external nasal valve regions [6, 7]. An assessment checklist should be able to mentally trigger an algorithm for managing the deformities.

6.6 Concept of "Big Guy – Small Guy"

As mentioned before, anatomically the tip complex is not "an ideal" creation of nature. The lateral crus is usually bigger and wider and heavier when compared to the medial crus, hence the "conjoining" of medial crus in supporting both the lateral crura. This is an *important concept* to be aware of in nasal tip reconstruction. In trauma and revision surgery of the tip, there is always this disparity of worsening relationship between the two lateral crura and the conjoined medial crus. The usual pathology being the weak, fractured or separated medial crus (◘ Figs. 6.4, 6.5, and 6.6) being not able to support the weight of the relatively heavier lateral crura. So the author's concept of nasal tip surgery is "*to make the big guy (lateral crus) smaller and lighter and the small (medial crus) guy bigger and stronger*" [3].

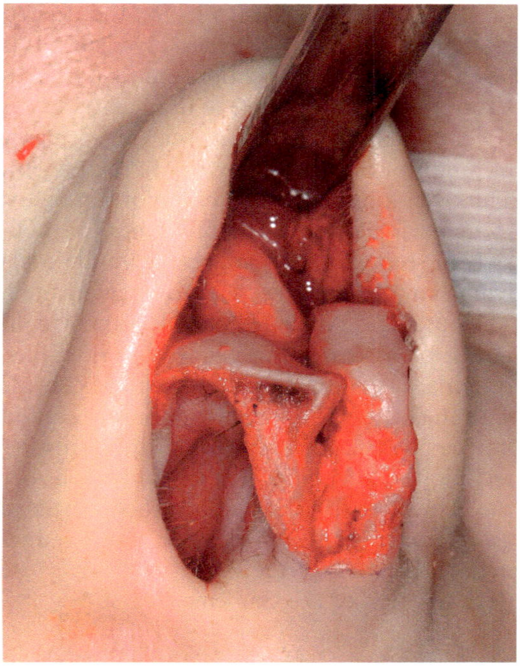

◘ **Fig. 6.5** Showing a fracture of right medial crus below the dome and the weight of lateral crus "jack-knifing" the lower lateral cartilage on the right side. ("Reproduced with permission from Ref: [3]")

6.7 Understanding the Importance of Skin and Soft Tissue Envelope

The nasal tip reconstruction not only demands creating ideal structural changes in the cartilaginous skeleton of the nasal tip, but the overlying soft tissues should also re-drape

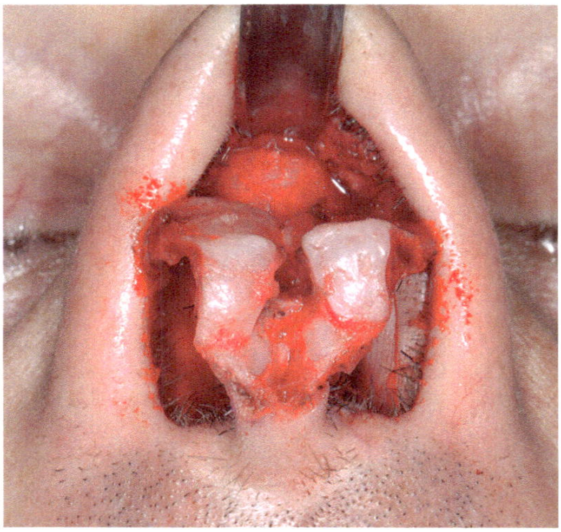

◘ **Fig. 6.4** Showing bilateral medial crural fracture with de-projection of tip due to the weight of lateral crus not being supported. ("Reproduced with permission from Ref: [3]")

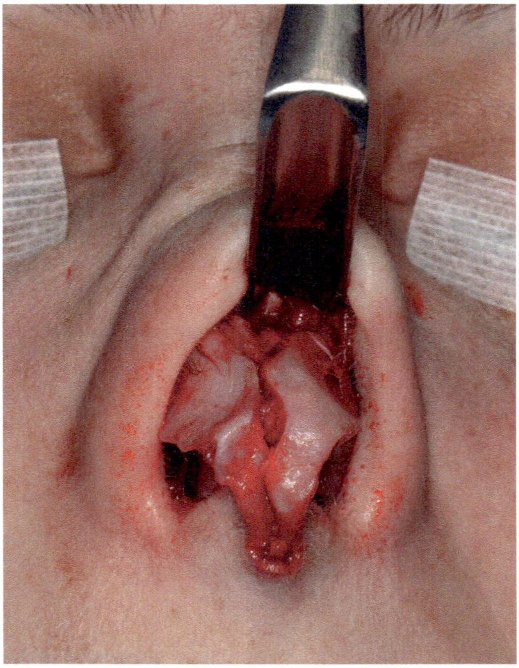

◘ **Fig. 6.6** Bilateral weak and damaged medial crus causing caudal prolapse due to the weight of unsupported bilateral wide lateral crura. ("Reproduced with permission from Ref: [3]")

on the cartilaginous skeleton for the desired aesthetic outcome to be externally visible. It is like a mannequin in a shop window. The skin has to be thin and be able to drape around the tip cartilages, otherwise any clever tip plasty techniques will not be obvious to the patient. Thus the skin envelope is an important factor in achieving the desired outcomes, particularly in secondary procedures where the overlying skin may be thin, scarred or pigmented. The outcomes, which the patient wants, might not be possible if the skin envelope is thicker, oedematous or very thin and scarred. People with thickened skin with a bulbous tip should not be given assurances of the tip narrowing techniques. If thin skin is an issue, consider the use of fascia lata or crushed cartilage grafts under the skin. Be aware of not reducing the thickness of the skin as this may cause devitalisation of the skin envelope.

6.8 Selecting the Surgical Approach and Tissue Handling

Nasal tip surgery can be performed by both "open" and "closed delivery" techniques. Open approach gives an excellent access to the tip cartilages and also the entire nasal septal cartilage (Figs. 6.8 and 6.9). Open approach can be combined with hemi-transfixation incisions of a closed approach (Fig. 6.7). Open approach also helps to execute various tip techniques with ease, which may be difficult through a closed approach. Again to reiterate, the surgical approach does not matter in the hands of the surgeon who is good at what he is doing. Fine tissue handling dur-

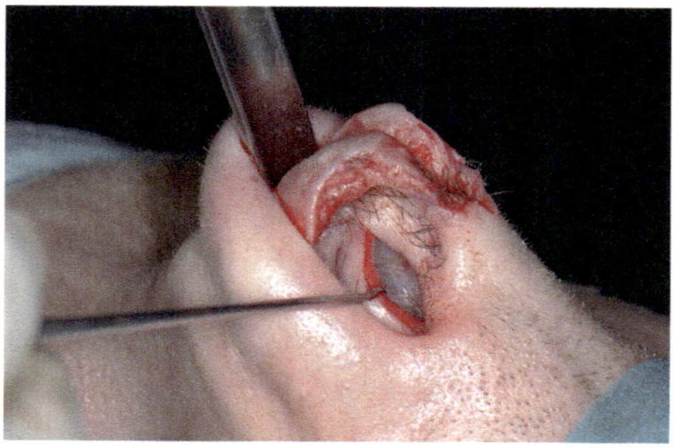

Fig. 6.7 Combination of "open" approach and hemi-transfixation approach. ("Reproduced with permission from Ref: [3]")

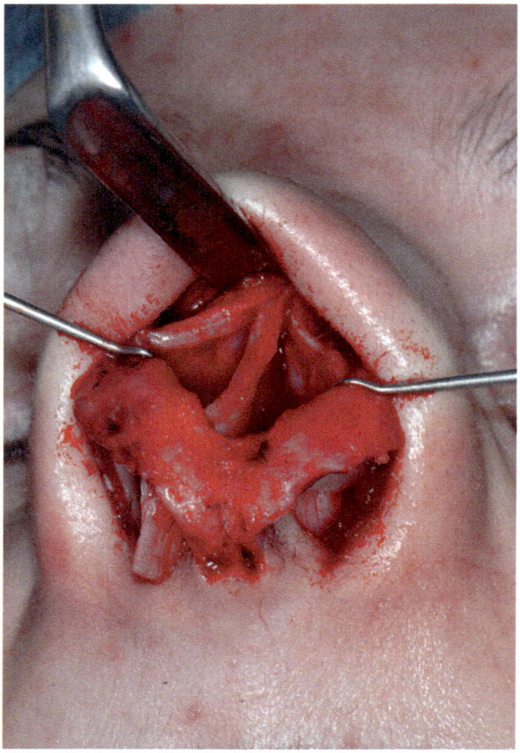

Fig. 6.8 Open approach showing excellent access to dorsal septum. ("Reproduced with permission from Ref: [3]")

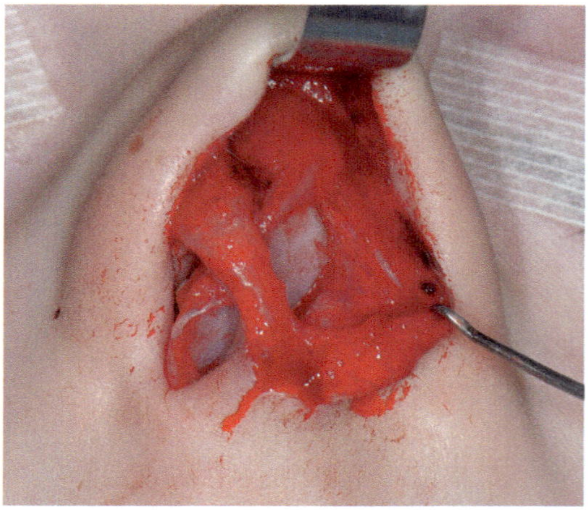

Fig. 6.9 Open approach showing excellent access to the entire septum and tip cartilages. ("Reproduced with permission from Ref: [3]")

ing the procedure helps to keep the morbidity less. Instrumentation and finger control of the two-pronged retractors add to the ease and elegance of the procedure. Traction and counter-traction helps in fine dissection.

6.9 Selecting the "Right" Tools and Techniques

The *"Contents"* of the tool box should include:

- Suture techniques [4]
- Grafting techniques [5]
- A combination of sutures and grafts
- Non-suture/non-grafting techniques

Sutures are predominantly used for primary surgery. We use 5 O′ ethilon sutures. One can also use PDS. In secondary rhinoplasty, a combination of sutures and grafts are used. Avoid destructive techniques in primary surgery. Sutures are versatile in achieving definition and projection of the nasal tip cartilages. The author has been using 5–0 ethilon non-absorbable sutures for tip plasty not only in primary rhinoplasty, but also in secondary rhinoplasty as an adjunct to grafting techniques for over 24 years without any major problems – just four patients with suture granuloma and extrusion in over 1700 patients). The surgeon can use 5 O′ PDS or any absorbable suture with less chances of extrusion.

Sutures have the following advantages:

- They are non-destructive.
- They are reversible.
- Non-absorbable sutures are less susceptible to fibrosis induced remodelling of cartilage as the suture material generates less of an inflammatory reaction compared to absorbable sutures.

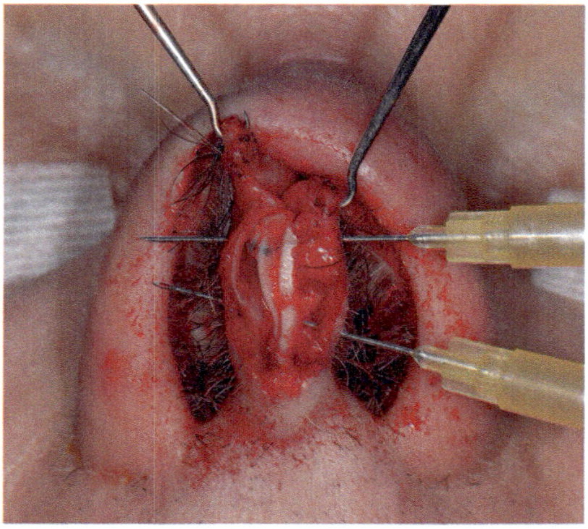

Fig. 6.10 Open approach showing the use of hypodermic needles as a "tool" for stabilisation before the use of sutures. ("Reproduced with permission from Ref: [3]")

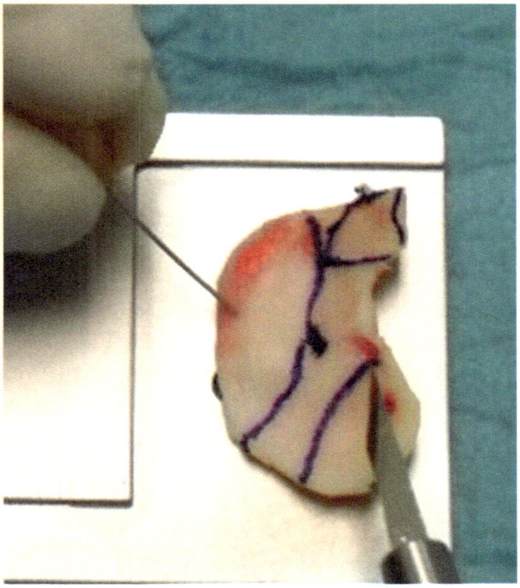

Fig. 6.11 Showing the use of hypodermic needle and a cutting plate for measurement and marking of conchal cartilage as a "tool" before incising. ("Reproduced with permission from Ref: [3]")

Grafting techniques (Fig. 6.12) are valuable when there is loss of structural integrity or functional issues or a combination of both structural and functional issues. Generally revision procedures require structural grafting. The toolbox should also have fine hypodermic needles, cartilage crusher, licensed tissue glue, crushed cartilages, etc. Practice the use of fine hypodermic needles (Figs. 6.10 and 6.11), whenever there is a need for stabilisation. Try and use crushed autologous cartilage grafts (CATS) to smoothen the dorsum and cover the suture knots, where and when possible (Figs. 6.13 and 6.14). This will prevent suture exposure and ensures a smooth dorsum, thereby preventing any revision pro-

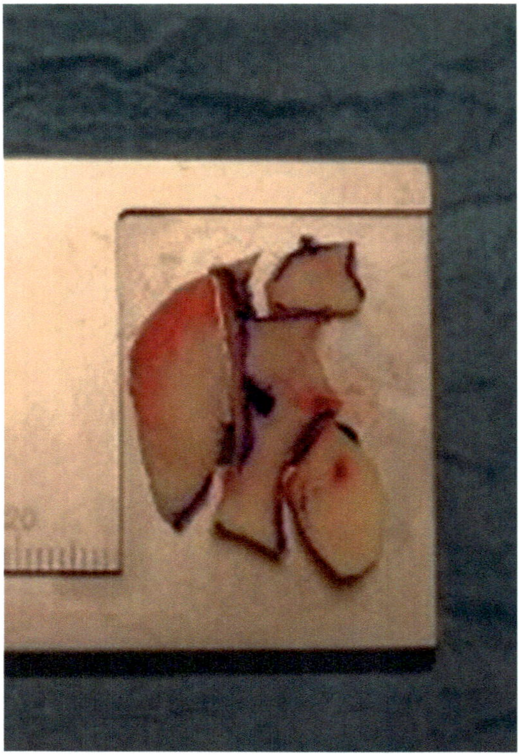

Fig. 6.12 Showing the "optimum" utilisation of conchal graft for dorsal augmentation, columellar strut and a shield graft

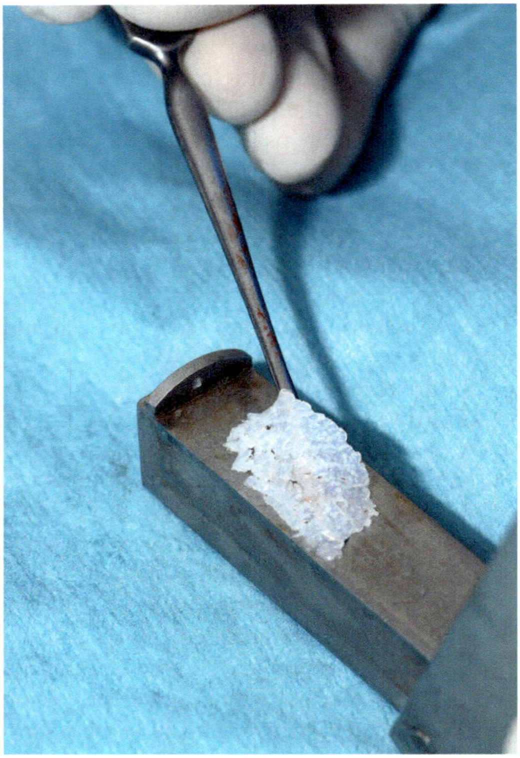

Fig. 6.13 Showing autologous crushed septal cartilage. ("Reproduced with permission from Ref: [3]")

cedures. If possible try and use biological acceptable licensed tissue glue (Fig. 6.15) instead of sutures for stabilisation as sutures can make the cartilage split or friable. Check with local guidelines before using tissue glue.

6.10 Selecting the "Right Sequence" to Reconstruct the Nasal Tip

"Surgical sequence" is an important concept in nasal tip reconstruction. Surgical sequence is vital to optimise the outcomes in nasal tip surgery [8], particularly when there are multiple deformities involving the caudal septum and also the medial and lateral crura on one or both sides, making the situation very challenging. It is better to have some starting

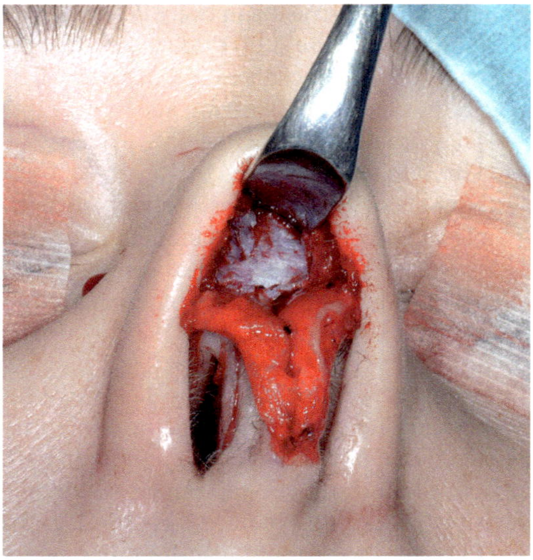

Fig. 6.14 Showing autologous crushed septal cartilage to smoothen the dorsum, after hump removal

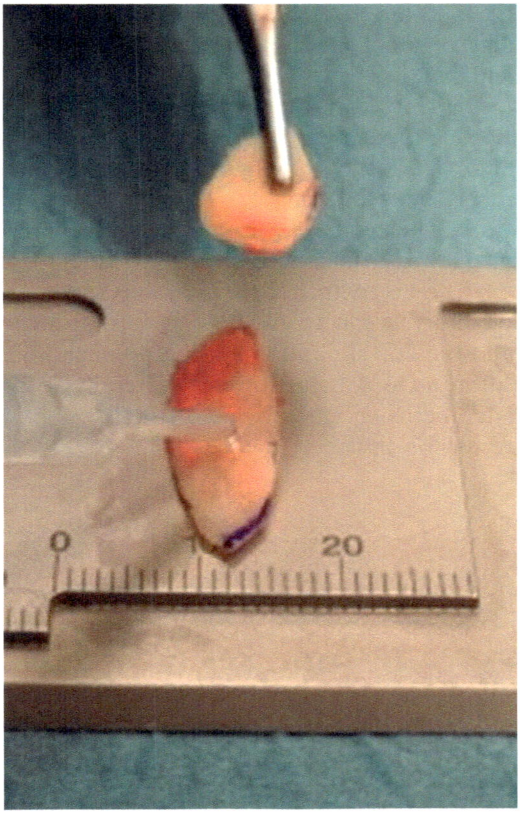

Fig. 6.15 Showing the use of tissue glue in securing layers of conchal cartilage

point in nasal tip surgery and we find starting from medial and working laterally offers the best outcomes as there is only limited space medially to accommodate the changes when compared to the lateral alar region.

Once a decision is made to do nasal tip reconstruction, the important thing to consider is "*the surgical sequence of reconstruction algorithm*". The author prefers to do the dorsal work like hump reduction and osteotomies first before doing tip work. The tip work is more finesse and should be kept last. One of the tools we use in our training programme is to ask the residents prior to the surgery to come up with three columns in a black board. The first column is to write down all the deformities which need to be corrected. The second column should include all the available techniques and procedures to correct the deformities mentioned in the first column and the third column is to "sequence" the various techniques or steps shown in the second column. The third process of "sequencing" all the necessary techniques needed to correct the deformity is the most important step which will be acquired by the surgeon only after a long learning curve. The sequencing of techniques helps the surgeon to understand the pros and cons of various techniques and helps to optimise the surgical time, preventing repetition and avoiding unnecessary steps. In our experience this is the most important factor which makes the surgeon stand out from the rest, and good surgical sequence does reflect in good patient outcomes.

The following are the sequential steps of tip work:

- *Step 1:* Caudal septal correction and strengthening
- *Step 2:* Shaping and unification of the medial crura and creation of basic dome height and symmetry (cephalic trim and medial crural fixation and flare control sutures)
- *Step 3:* Shaping of lateral crura and domes (inter-domal and trans-domal sutures)
- *Step 4:* Positioning the unified tip complex in relation to the rest of the nose and face (tip anchoring sutures)

6.10.1 Reconstructing the Caudal Septal Support

Adequate planning of the surgical steps should be followed by a clear thought process of "why" and "how" to sequence the steps. Before considering tip work, the position, strength and integrity of the caudal nasal septum should be reconstructed if necessary. The caudal septum should be of adequate strength, length and in the midline with adequate projection before considering the tip work. This means the dislocated or bent caudal septum needs to be straightened. This may require a proper septoplasty, a posterior SMR or dorsal spreaders. Patients who lack the caudal septal support may need a columellar strut or septal extension grafts. In most situations, the source of graft for dorsal and caudal reconstruction of the septum can come from the posterior septum leaving behind an "L" strut. Costal cartilage is a good alternative for dorsal and caudal septal correction.

Once the caudal septum is reconstructed, then the attention is given to the actual tip cartilages. Tip reconstruction can be achieved in the majority of patients with sutures, grafts and a combination of both. Generally sutures are reserved for primary surgery and grafts for revision procedures. Planned sequential tip work should start from *"medial to lateral"*. If there is a complex deformity of the tip cartilages (▪ Fig. 6.16a–c), a clear sequence of surgical intervention starting medially from medial crus and then working towards the Intermediate and then lateral crus should be followed, as there is more space in the alar region laterally to accommodate extra lengths and changes, when compared to medially near the anterior nasal spine region. Reconstructing the medial crus on both sides and securing the strength of the conjoined medial crus and height is the first step in tip work. Then consider reconstructing the intermediate and lateral crus on both sides. The final step is to anchor the conjoined tip complex in relation to the anterior septal angle and the dorsal nasal line using tip anchoring sutures. Do not start tip work laterally at the lateral crus and move medially. This will be a recipe for disaster.

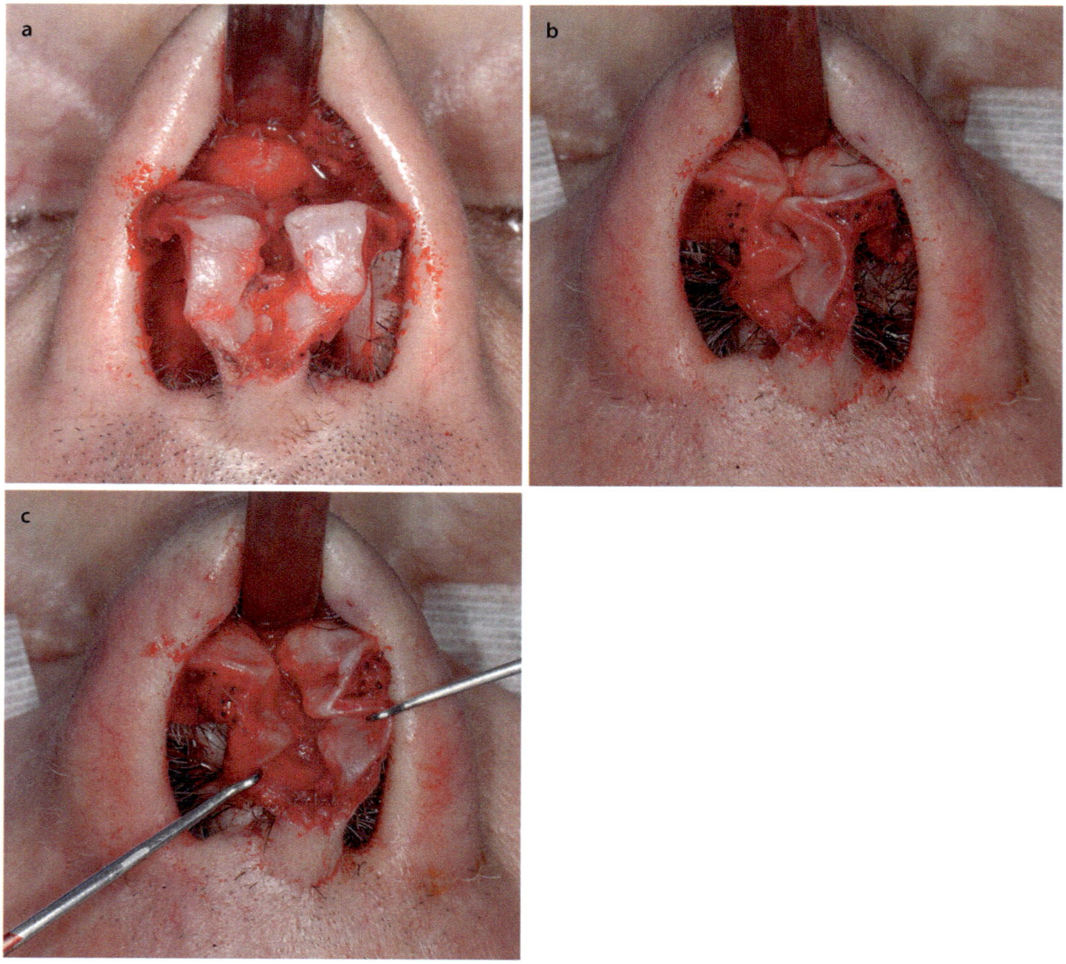

▪ **Fig. 6.16** **a**–**c** Showing complex tip deformities involving medial and lateral crura

Conclusion

Nasal tip surgery is complex and the key to achieving good outcomes lays in three pillars of learning namely, accurate assessment, selecting the right tools and techniques and using them in the right sequence. Every patient should be given due importance despite your level of expertise. Even then be prepared for unpleasant surprises in your entire career.

Key Points Box

- The most important factor in the success of nasal tip surgery is the surgical sequence of "where to start the reconstruction". The surgical steps should follow a specific "sequence" with caudal septal reconstruction being done first, followed by tip work. In the tip, the sequence should be from the medial and inferior part of the nose working on the medial crura first, followed by the domal work and at last lateral crural work in that sequence. Starting the surgical sequence from lateral to medial is a recipe for disaster.
- The distinction between "major" and "minor" tip support mechanisms is arbitrary. A minor tip support structure can become a major issue in a particular patient, particularly post trauma. Hence all the factors should be given "*equal*" importance.
- Anatomically the weight of the individual lateral crura is more than the individual medial crus can cope. Hence the "conjoined" strength of the medial crus put together is needed to counterbalance the weight of the two heavier lateral crus. This fact should be appreciated before nasal tip reconstruction.
- The concept of nasal tip surgery should be "to make the big guy (lateral crus) smaller and lighter and the small (medial crus) guy bigger and stronger".
- The surgical "tools" being used are generally sutures for primary surgery and grafts for secondary revision procedures or a combination of both in revision surgery.

References

1. Anderson JR. A reasoned approach to nasal base surgery. Arch Otolaryngol. 1984;110(6):349–58.
2. Adamson PA, Litner JA, Dahiya R. The M-Arch model a new concept of nasal tip dynamics. Arch Facial Plast Surg. 2006;8(1):16–25.
3. Balaji N. Top tips in nasal tip surgery, ENT-FPS UK Newsletter—Feb 2018 –Issue 6.
4. Sil A, Ravichandran S, Balaji N. Suture Techniques in posttraumatic nasal tip reconstruction. ENT Audiol News. 2009;18(5):98–102.
5. Sil A, Ravichandran S, Balaji N. Non- suture techniques in posttraumatic nasal tip reconstruction. ENT Audiol News. 2010;19(2):109–12.
6. Balaji N, Ravichandran S. Assessment of nasal valve obstruction: a new nasal "wall" subunit concept. ENT Audiol News. 2012;21(4):111–3.
7. Balaji N, Ravichandran S. Assessment of nasal valve obstruction: a new Glasgow nasal "wall" subunit concept. ENT Audiol News. 2012;21(5):86–7.
8. Paul S. White, Pater D. Ross. Open structure rhinoplasty. 2nd ed. Tuttlingen: Endo Press GmbH; 2012.

Open (External) Approach: Incision and Flap Elevation

Contents

N. Balaji, *Textbook of Nasal Tip Rhinoplasty*, https://doi.org/10.1007/978-3-030-48157-5_7

Learning Objectives

- To learn the placement of various incisions in an "open" approach technique.
- To learn to raise the skin flap in the correct plane without causing any unwanted side effects.
- To learn the surgical technique stepwise as described below with clinical photographs.

7.1 Introduction

The tip plasty surgery can be performed through various approaches to the osseo-cartilaginous skeleton of the nose. This can be either via internal cartilage delivery techniques or via an open external approach, raising the skin flap and having a direct access [1]. Open approach was first described by Rethi and was later modified by Sercer and Padovan [2, 3]. But modern-day systematic approach to open rhinoplasty owes its beginnings to the work of Goodman [4]. A survey conducted in the USA among facial plastic surgeons showed that more than 25% of the surgeons use open approach almost always [5]. There are pros and cons of open and closed approaches. Open approach gives excellent access for better diagnosis of the pathology and helps in the correct placement of sutures and grafts [6, 7, 8]. The downside of this procedure is the columellar scar, although generally negligible issues if closed with care [9]. Prolonged tip oedema and loss of projection have also been accepted downsides of the open approach. As mentioned before, the discussion about what approach does not matter as long as the final outcome is acceptable to the patient.

The emphasis in this book, will be only on "open" approach techniques. In this chapter, we will be describing the author's way of raising the skin flap in an open approach rhinoplasty showing the various steps with intraoperative photos and relevant tips. The role of antibiotics is questionable. But there is a general agreement that a single shot of broad-spectrum antibiotic given during induction is far better than a week's course of antibiotic [10]. Most surgeons tend to use the antibiotic prophylaxis during induction particularly when grafts are used. The role of systemic steroids to reduce oedema is not routinely recommended in rhinoplasty surgery, although studies have shown marginal improvement on eyelid oedema for a short time [11].

The following are the *primary indications* for an open approach rhinoplasty:

1. Primary rhinoplasty needing nasal tip reconstruction
2. Severe caudal septal deformities associated with tip deformities
3. Multiple revision rhinoplasty
4. Complex nasal tip deformities requiring various grafting techniques

7.2 Surgical Technique

The surgical techniques of raising the skin flap vary between surgeons, but the technique described below is that of the author.

The "external or open" approach rhinoplasty involves lifting the skin and soft tissues "off" the osseo-cartilagenous skeleton of the nose starting from the columella in a sub-SMAS plane to have a direct access to the chondro-osseous skeleton of the nose. *To achieve this, three incisions are made, two of them being in the columella and one in the alar region.* The first incision is a horizontal trans-columellar incision, second is a vertical medial marginal columellar incision and the third is a horizontal alar marginal incision. The trans-columellar incision is visible, and hence getting it right is important to avoid an unsightly scar and a poorer outcome. Also, of equal importance is the junction between the horizontal columellar incision with the vertical marginal columellar incision. Extreme care should be taken at this junction to prevent tissue loss, which can cause notching.

7.3 Instruments Required

Number 15 blade knife, (Beavers' knife preferable) two small skin hooks, one double hook, Q-tips, sharp curved scissors, Aufricht's elevator and small fine Adson's bipolar cautery. Be extremely cautious in using the diathermy on the flap.

7.4 Planning the Incision

Planning and making the incisions in the right place is of paramount importance in raising the skin flap in an open rhinoplasty to prevent any unsightly scars. This can be easy and simple in primary rhinoplasty, but in secondary revision procedures with extensive scarring of the columella, fore-shortened columella and deformed columella due to septal dislocation, as shown in the Figs. 7.1, 7.2 and 7.3, raising the flap can be challenging.

In the UK, we do this procedure under general anaesthetic with topical vasoconstriction. The surgery is done in the head up position with preferably hypotensive anaesthesia, the eyes being taped with steristrips.

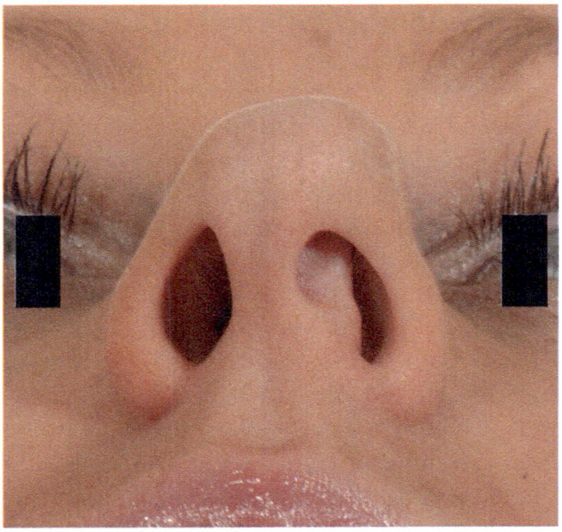

Fig. 7.1 Basal view showing distorted columella due to septal dislocation

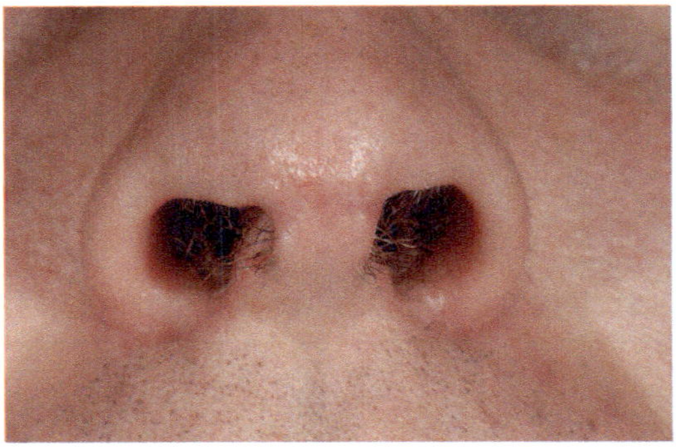

Fig. 7.2 Basal view showing extensive scarring and fore shortened columella

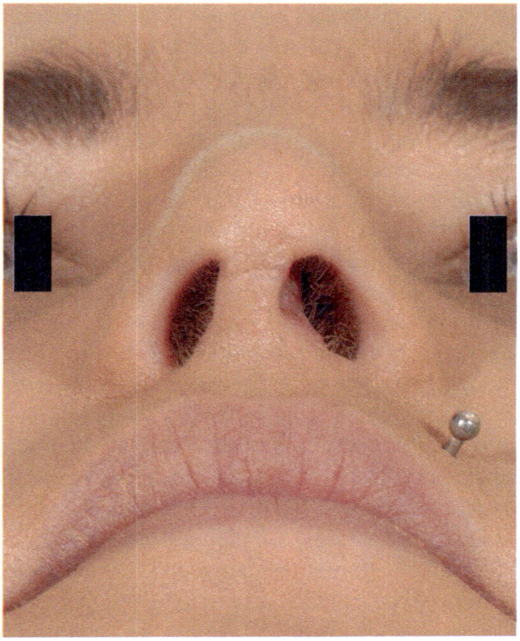

Fig. 7.3 Basal view showing scarred and distorted columella

7.5 Planning/Marking the Trans-columellar Incision

Always mark out the incision first before injecting the local anaesthetic, so that there is no tissue distortion.

First mark the trans-columellar incision which can be an inverted "V" or "W". The incision should be roughly at the middle of the columella. The author's preference is a "W" incision in primary rhinoplasty as it offers a wider area to redistribute the forces of contraction. However, in revision procedures, the author prefers an inverted "V" incision. If the columella is of adequate width and height with no distortion, the ideal location of this incision is at the midpoint of the columella, overlying the medial crura. There are pros and cons of going too far high or too far low on the columella depending on the pathology. Do not make the incision too far up close to the tip, as this restricts access to the columella and medial crus. At the same time, do not go too low down towards the sill where there is no underlying cartilage. Based on the author's experience, the most deciding factor is the presence of underlying medial crural cartilage under the skin incision to prevent soft tissue notching. If the incision is placed too far down towards the sill, where there is no underlying medial crural cartilage to support due to divergence of the footplates, then there is a possibility of soft tissue notching at the edges of the wound.

Sometimes, the columella is so much distorted that you need to imagine the final shape of the columella and plan your incision accordingly. Do not hold the columella with fingers, particularly in a fore shortened columella. *There should be adequate "traction and counter traction" with double hooks* (Fig. 7.4) to stretch and lengthen the columella and plan the incision accordingly. If the columella is extremely short and retracted, you can lengthen the columella at the expense of the width by a vertical "z- plasty". Remember a longer, thinner well-projected columella is aesthetically pleasing than a short, wide and de-projected columella.

In revision surgeries, there can be horizontal scars and vertical scars in the columella. Vertical scars are modified as a "Z" incision. If unsightly horizontal scars of previous rhinoplasty are present, avoid going through them again, as it increases the chance of notching. If there is adequate space above it, make a separate incision about 2 mm above the old one in an "inverted V" fashion. When a "W" incision is made, make sure that all three key points in the top of the "W" and all the two key points in the bottom of the "W" are roughly in a staright horizontal line. Make sure the lateral limb of the "W" does not go up obtusely to meet the vertical marginal incision, if this happens the healed scar will be asymmetric and cause asymmetric hourglass narrowing of columella.

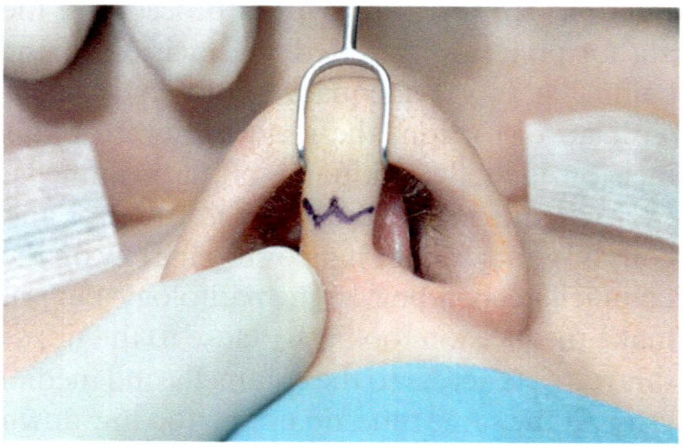

Fig. 7.4 Basal view showing the use of fingers for traction and counter traction

7.6 Planning/Marking the Medial Marginal Incision

Then *mark the second part of the incision* which is a medial marginal columellar incision. Start from the edge of the trans-columellar incision and stop at the angle of the nostril. Make sure this incision is really marginal and strictly vertical. Avoid extending gently posterior into the membranous septum, as this may cause flaring and webbing of columella.

7.7 Planning/Marking the Lateral Alar Incision

Then *mark the third part of the incision* in the lateral alar margin following the margin of the lateral crus cartilage and NOT following the alar cutaneous margin. Then, connect this incision under vision to the medial marginal columellar incision at the soft triangle. Clinical palpation of the inferior margins of the lateral crus of the lower lateral cartilage to assess its proximity to the alar skin margin is very important. This helps you to plan the incision and follow the lower margin of the lateral crus without damaging the cartilage. Again, following the alar lateral crus margin is not without any issues. If you are very close to the cartilage with no soft tissue to take a bite while closing, you may end up taking a bite in the cartilage which will cause alar thickening on the incision site. Being pedantic and being aware of the pros and cons of every move and altering your practice based on your results are important than being dogmatic about each technique.

7.8 Injecting Local Anaesthetic

This step is performed *ONLY* after the incision is planned and marked; otherwise, there will be tissue distortion. How much to inject is also debatable. The author believes in small volume injection to avoid distortion of tissues. Some surgeons inject a lot using the local anaesthetic for hydro dissection. It is an individual choice. Once the skin incision is marked, traction is applied to the tip superiorly with a double hook to stretch the columellar skin and a local anaesthetic with a vasoconstrictor (we use 0.5% xylocaine with 1 in 80,000 adrenaline) is injected in the following sequence (Fig. 7.5a–h).

- Inject 0.5 ml just under the skin of the columella anteriorly with a gentle pierce with the needle and gently withdrawing the needle and then injecting (Fig. 7.5a).
- Then with a twist of the double hook, inject 0.5 ml at the vertical marginal incision on both sides (Fig. 7.5b, c).
- Then inject 0.5 ml into the lateral alar marginal incision site (Fig. 7.5d, e).
- Then 0.5 ml is injected at the bony lateral osteotomy sites by going through the muco-cutaneous junction at the lateral ala (Fig. 7.5f–g).

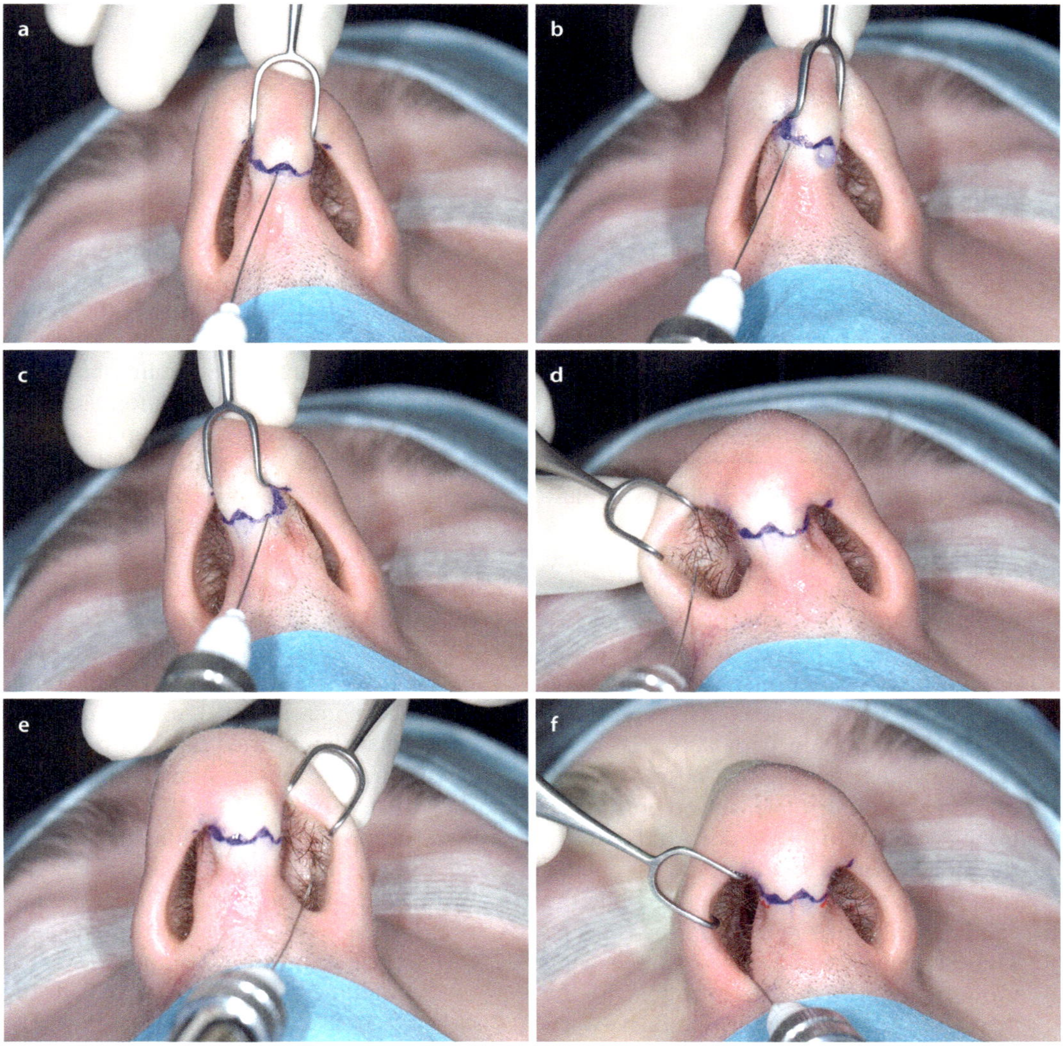

Fig. 7.5 **a–h** Technique of infiltrating local anaesthetic and vasoconstrictor agent. **a** Trans-columellar injection. **b** Right lateral columellar marginal injection. **c** Left lateral columellar marginal injection. **d** Right lateral alar marginal injection. **e** Left lateral alar marginal injection. **f–h** Pyriform aperture infiltration

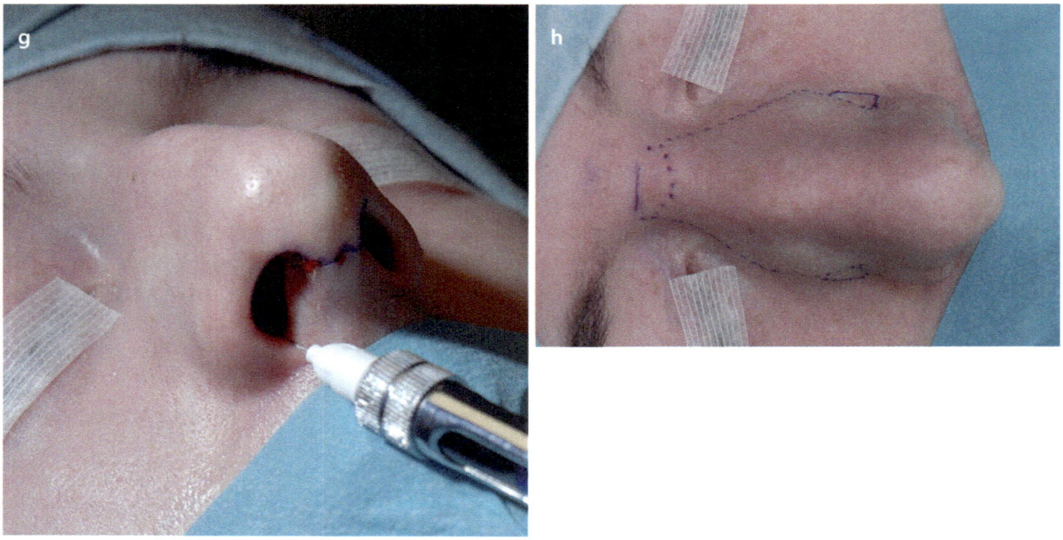

Fig. 7.5 (continued)

- Then 0.5 ml is injected at the anterior columellar septum.
- Then 0.5 ml is injected at the dorsal septal bony cartilaginous junction.

7.9 Surgical Steps

- Make the *first part of the incision* namely the "W" shaped horizontal trans-columellar incision applying traction and counter traction. With a double hook, apply traction at the infra tip lobule as shown in the Fig. 7.6b. With a finger apply counter traction at the alar base. Now with the columella stretched, start making the incision with a No 11 blade starting at the apex of the "W" in the middle and extending it laterally on both sides, taking care not to go too deep and damage the medial crus. Remember the columellar skin flap is in the coronal plane, while the caudal border of the medial crus is in the sagittal plane. Avoid stabbing or sawing motions to prevent direct trauma to the medial crus. Also avoid dissecting between the two medial crura.
- Then make the *second part of the incision* namely the medial marginal columellar incision (Fig. 7.6c) extending strictly vertical from the edge of the trans-columellar incision inferiorly to the apex of the nostril superiorly keeping along the caudal border of the medial crus of the lower lateral cartilage and not extending beyond a millimetre into the membranous septum. The key to this incision is keeping it *truly marginal and truly vertical*. Avoid swaying posteriorly into the membranous septum, as this will cause widening and gull winging of columella and it will be difficult to bring it out again to connect with the lateral alar marginal incision. *After this STOP, before you proceed to the third part of the incision.* It is better not to make the lateral alar incision at this stage until the columellar flap is lifted till the tip as making all the incisions together can be messy due to bleeding.
- Now deepen the trans-columellar incision (Fig. 7.7a) [12] and start raising the columellar flap by applying superior traction with an alar double hook on the columellar skin. The trans-columellar vessels in the midline should be coagulated and cut to release the tension in the flap. The rest of the columellar flap is raised with fine scissors using the technique of "*small snips and big spreads*", staying just deep to the SMAS layer and superficial to the

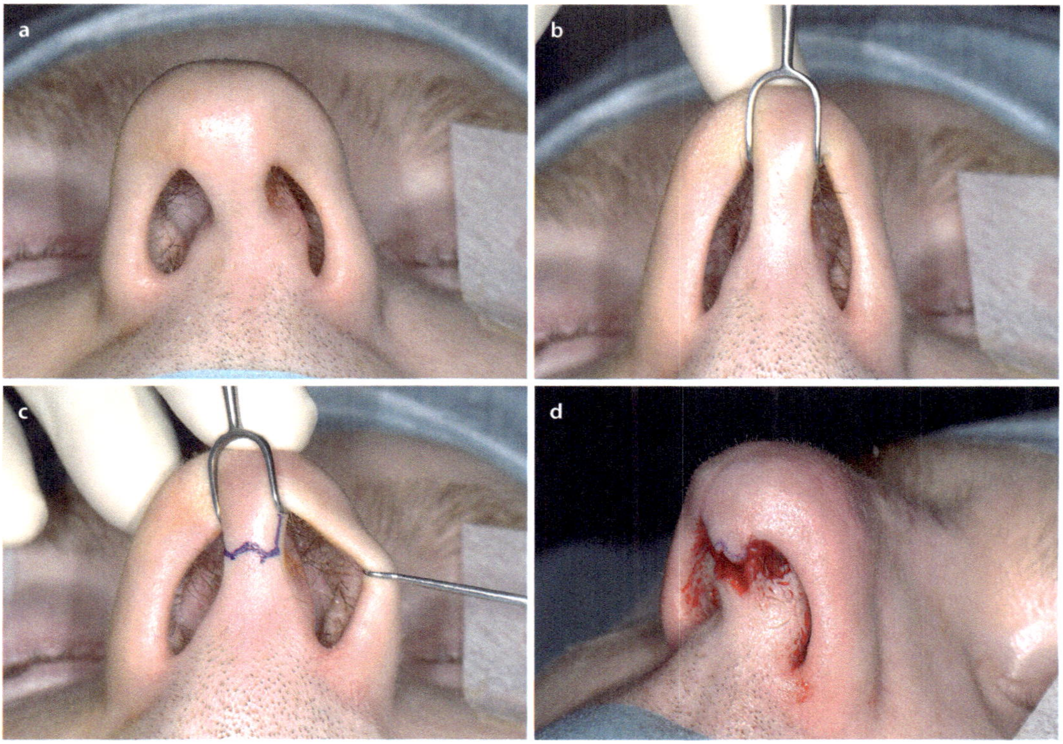

Fig. 7.6 **a–d** Traction and counter traction before marking and making the horizontal columellar skin incision. ("Reproduced with kind permission from Ref: [12]")

perichondrium of the cartilage. Try not to dissect between the two crura and damage them.

- Once the flap is raised up to the infra tip lobule (Fig. 7.7b), then make the *third part of the incision* along the lateral alar margin (Fig. 7.7c) [12] to join the medial marginal incision at the angle of the nostril using a double alar hook for traction. Care must be taken to avoid damage to the soft triangle and the alar cartilages as this may result in alar notching. This part of the incision should be made under direct vision with adequate traction and counter traction.
- Elevate the flap further to expose the cephalic border of the lower lateral cartilage (Fig. 7.7a, b) [12]. Finally, release the tension on the flap by releasing the soft tissues along the cephalic border of the lateral crus. This can be done with bipolar cautery dissection. Once the soft tissues over the cephalic border of the lateral crus are released, then the tension on the flap is released and you can continue the dissection superiorly towards the nasal dorsum and the nasion.
- Now with an Aufricht's elevator under the flap continue elevating the flap deep to the SMAS plane. Then continue the dissection along the dorsum of the nose till the nasion staying just above the perichondrium [13] and either above (Fig. 7.8b) or below the periosteum of the nasal bones and the frontal process of maxilla. It is preferable to lift the periosteum over the nasal bones and frontal process, as it can be used to cover minor dorsal irregularities, particularly after hump reduction. While dissecting at the nasion region, vestigial nasal dorsal muscles can bleed at this point, hence sharp dissection is favoured. Dissecting deeper to the SMAS layer is important to reduce bleeding and also keeping the muscles and facial layer on the flap makes the flap thicker and helps to

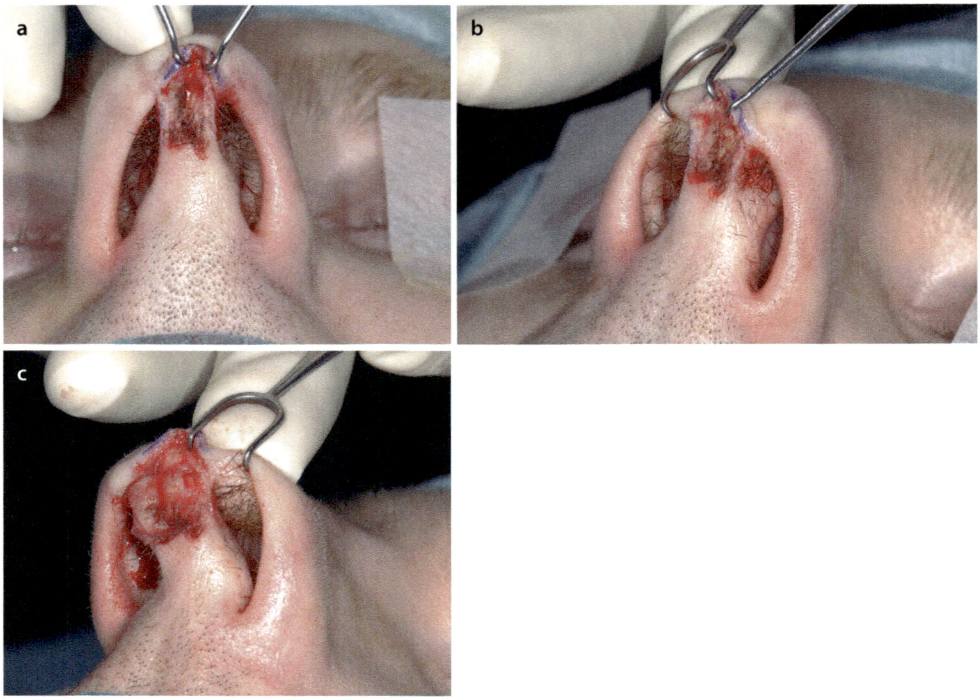

Fig. 7.7 **a–c** Raising the columellar flap with skin hooks and three-point traction. ("Reproduced with kind permission from Ref: [12]")

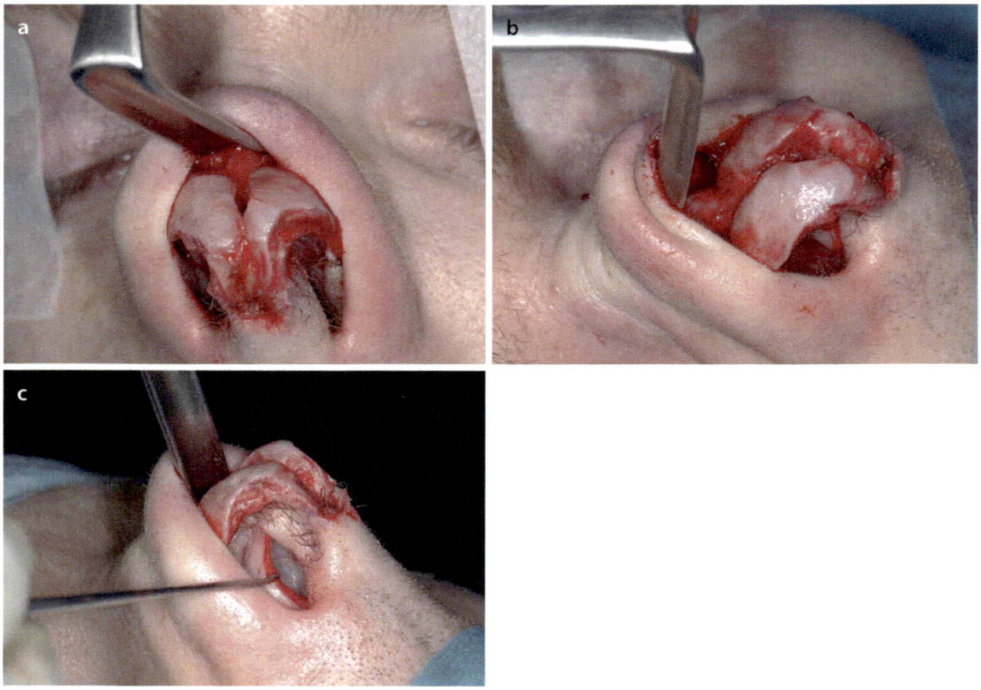

Fig. 7.8 **a–c** Raising the dorsal flap by releasing the soft tissues along the cephalic border of the lateral crus. ("Reproduced with kind permission from Ref: [12]")

smoothen small irregularities. The extent of skin elevation in the dorsum depends on the extent of surgery and re-draping needed. Tardy advocates elevation of muco-perichondrium endonasally while removing a large hump [14].

- If access to the septum is needed, this can be done sub-perichondrially either through a separate hemi-transfixation incision (◘ Fig. 7.8c) or can dissect between the two medial crus going through the inter domal ligaments and identifying the anterior septal angle. Then dissection can be carried along the caudal border of the septum going inferiorly towards the nasal spine area and create muco-perichondrial tunnels on both sides.
- At the end of the procedure, the transcolumellar incision is closed with two to three 5-0 ethilon sutures and marginal incisions closed with 5-0 ethilon or vicryl sutures. Final scar should be aesthetically pleasing.
- If needed, the entire septum can be accessed through open approach (◘ Figs. 7.9 and 7.10), by approaching either from the caudal septum "anteriorly" or coming from above downwards through a "Sky View" approach. The entire septum can be accessed and reconstructed through an open approach if necessary.

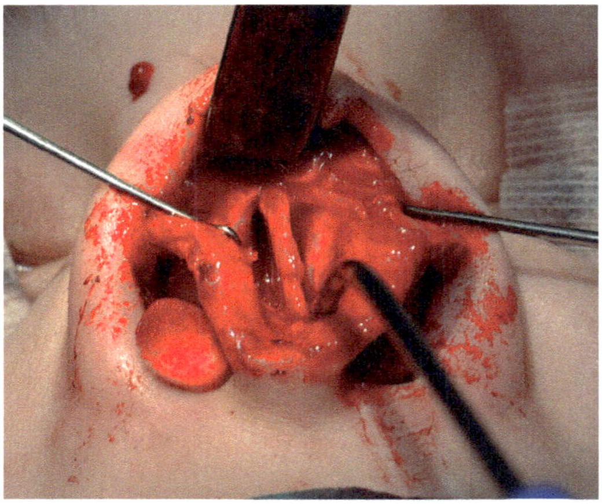

◘ **Fig. 7.9** Open approach exposing the dorsal septum

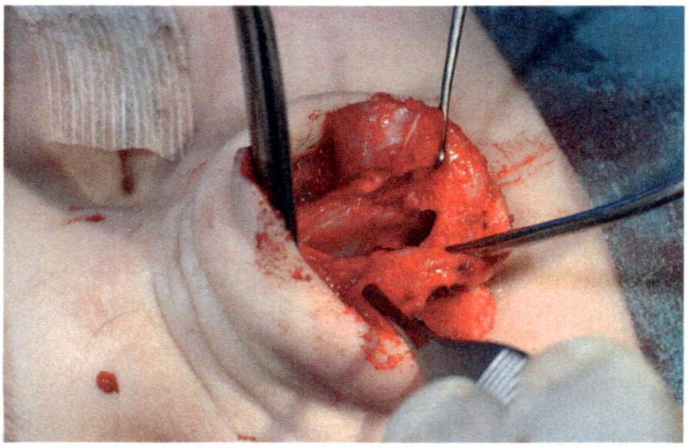

◘ **Fig. 7.10** "Sky-View" exposing the septal cartilage on both sides through an open approach

Conclusion

Open approach tip surgery will leave a scar in the columella. Hence making the incision in the right place with fine tissue handling and good approximation in closing the skin is paramount in preventing unwanted scarring in the alar columellar region.

Key Points Box

- Nasal tip surgery can be performed through various approaches to the osseo-cartilaginous skeleton of the nose.
- The approach does not matter, as long as the surgeon is able to execute the techniques. There are more important factors than approach to achieve a satisfactory outcome.
- Always mark out the incision first before injecting the local anaesthetic, so that there is no tissue distortion.
- There should be adequate traction and counter traction with skin hooks and fingers.
- Use small curved scissors in a sequence of "small" snips and "big" spreads.
- Take care to not to damage the free border of the medial crus while making the horizontal columellar incision.

- Take care to keep the vertical marginal incision exactly vertical at the margin of the columella and not sway into the columellar mucosa.
- Take care to keep the lateral marginal alar incision at the margin of the lower lateral cartilage and not at the margin of the soft tissue ala.
- Take care not to dissect between the medial crura while raising the columellar skin.
- Take care to perform flap elevation in the correct sub-SMAS plane without the need to have too much diathermy or damage to the overlying skin.

References

1. Adamson PA, Doud Galli SK. Rhinoplasty approaches. Arch Facial Plast Surg. 2005;7:32–7.
2. Sercer A, Mundinhc K. Plastiche Operationen an der nase un an der Ohrmuschel. Stuttgart: Georg Thierne; 1962.
3. Padovan LF. Combination of extra nasal and intranasal approach in surgery of the nasal pyramid and nasal septum (decortication). Can J. Otolaryngol. 1975;4:522–8.
4. Goodman WS, Charbonneau PA. External approach to rhinoplasty. Laryngoscope. 1974;84(12):2195–201.
5. Adamson PA, Galli SK. Rhinoplasty approaches: current state of the art. Arch Facial Plast Surg. 2005;7(1):32–7.
6. Rohrich RJ, Griffin JR. Correction of intrinsic nasal tip asymmetries in primary rhinoplasty. Plast Reconstr Surg. 2003;112(6):1699–712.
7. Smith O, Goodman W. Open rhinoplasty: its past and future. J Otolaryngol. 1993;22:21–5.
8. Gruber RP, Friedman GD. Suture algorithm for the broad or bulbous nasal tip. Plast Reconstr Surg. 2002;110:1752–64.
9. Adamson PA. Incision and scar analysis in open (external) rhinoplasty. Arch Otolaryngol Head Neck Surg. 1990;116:671–5.
10. Rajan GP, Fergie N, Fischer U, Romer M, Radivojevic V, Hee GK. Antibiotic prophylaxis in septorhinoplasty? A prospective, randomized study. Plast Reconstr Surg. 2005;116(7):1995–8.
11. Kara CO, Gokalan I. Effects of single-dose steroid usage on edema, ecchymosis, and intraoperative bleeding in rhinoplasty. Plast Reconstr Surg. 1999;104(7):2213–8.
12. Paul S. White, Pater D. Ross. Open structure rhinoplasty. 2nd ed. Tuttlingen: Endo Press GmbH; 2012.
13. Huizing EH, de Groot JAM, editors. Functional reconstructive nasal surgery. Stuttgart, New York: Thieme; 2003.
14. Tardy ME Jr. Rhinoplasty: the art and the science. Philadelphia: W.B. Saunders Company; 1997.

Suture Techniques in Nasal Tip Rhinoplasty

Contents

N. Balaji, *Textbook of Nasal Tip Rhinoplasty*, https://doi.org/10.1007/978-3-030-48157-5_8

Learning Objectives

- To learn the indications, contra-indications, actual surgical steps and key learning points of various suture techniques used in nasal tip reconstruction, which will help the surgeon navigate most of the nasal tip deformities.

8.1 Introduction

Nasal tip sutures are an important tool to define, project and alter the position of the tip cartilages, either on one side or both. The credit for using sutures as a versatile tool to modify the nasal tip goes to the visionary surgeons, mainly Dr.Tardy [1], Dr.Tebbetts [2] and Dr.Daniel [3] from North America. They had the "thought process" to look into various ways of modifying the tip anatomy with reversible means. The sutures preserve the structural integrity and anatomy of the tip cartilages without the need for any destructive manoeuvres. Generally, they are versatile tools in primary rhinoplasty and also used as an adjunctive to grafting in secondary or revision procedures. Generally non-absorbable sutures like 5-0 ethilon or prolene are preferable. Absorbable PDS sutures or coated vicryl sutures can also be used with equally good results. It is advisable to use a particular suture material which works best in your hands based on your clinical practice. If a suture goes through a mucosal surface then it has to be an absorbable suture. Sutures are used predominantly in the lower lateral tip cartilages to correct the structure anatomy and position, whereas sutures in the upper lateral cartilages are used more for functional reasons (e.g. ULC flare sutures). Dr. Tardy [1] introduced the concept of narrowing a wide dome with sutures using a trans-domal-spanning suture going through both domes performed through a cartilage delivery technique. Daniel [3] later on used open approach to describe individual suture techniques to create an aesthetic dome. But the current concepts of using sutures is largely attributed to the conceptual thinking of Tebbetts [4] and no doubt the credit for the development of modern suture techniques goes to Tebbetts, who introduced more formalised and systematic approach to complex tip suturing techniques with algorithms to modify the tip cartilages through an open approach using permanent sutures. There has been a steady increase in the use of sutures recently in view of the versatility, simplicity and non-destructive nature of the sutures as compared to the use of grafts [5]. Most of the publications since then by various surgeons around the world have been a further refinement of concepts put forward by Tebbetts [6, 7].

8.1.1 Advantages of Tip Sutures

- The suture helps to bring the tip cartilages which are soft and pliable to a particular shape and position keeping it in place for 6 weeks, till the healing process helps to stabilise the cartilages in the "new" position.
- Either absorbable or non-absorbable sutures can be used. It is an individual choice based on the personal experience of the surgeon. The author prefers to use 5-0 ethilon non-absorbable sutures for nasal tip work. Although these are considered as non-absorbable sutures, they do not have any stabilising function after 6 weeks, so has the potential to be removed later on if there are any issues with infection or extrusion without causing much change to the tip structures. There are always pros and cons of using absorbable over non-absorbable sutures. The common alternative being an absorbable PDS suture [8]. Both absorbable and non-absorbable sutures work equally well to achieve the desired outcomes [9].
- Sutures are non-destructive and they preserve the structural integrity of the tip cartilages.
- They are reversible and achieve long-term reliable outcomes.
- Suture techniques are easier to execute.
- Non-absorbable sutures are less susceptible to fibrosis-induced remodelling of cartilage as the suture material generates less of an inflammatory reaction compared to absorbable sutures.

8.1.2 Disadvantages of Non-absorbable Sutures

Although using non-absorbable sutures gives consistent long-term results with less tissue response, sometimes there can be issues, particularly if the knots are not buried or not trimmed very short. Suture extrusion has been extremely rare. In the author's practice, only five patients in over 1700 needed sutures to be removed. This can happen if the cut edges are left long and if the knot is not hidden or camouflaged with crushed cartilage.

If non-absorbable sutures like ethilon is used, the following tips are useful:

- Cut the sutures yourself and not the assistant!
- Always use a fine curved scissors, like iris scissors.
- Cut the knots very close by angling the scissors sideways.
- If possible get the knots buried from outside skeleton.
- If possible put crushed cartilages to cover the knots.

8.1.3 Planning and Preparation of the Site

Adequate exposure of the lower lateral cartilages either through open or closed approach is important. The cartilages are dissected free in the SMAS plane. Any scar tissue over the cartilages and between the medial crura are removed (◘ Fig. 8.1).Use of surface bipolar diathermy leaves black scars of damaged and dead tissue over the cartilages which needs to be removed with Adson's forceps and curved iris scissors. Removing the scar over the convex dorsum of the lateral crus is easy to do, but care is needed to remove the scar tissue on the medial surface of the medial crus taking care not to buttonhole the mucosa of the caudal septum. The way to avoid is to apply gentle traction to the free caudal border of the medial crus and dissect the soft tissues off at an angle working towards the cartilage and not towards the midline. The sequence of tip sutures should be always from medial to lateral, starting with the medial crus and bringing the two medial crura together, restoring the height and symmetry of the tip. Then the intermediate and lateral crus are addressed.

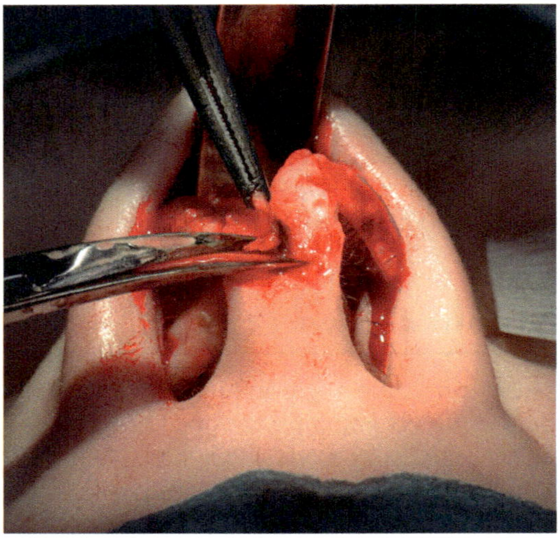

◘ **Fig. 8.1** Open approach view showing the technique to remove scar tissue (held on the forceps) over the medial crura

8.1.4 Sequential Steps in the Use of Sutures

Once the skin flap is raised over the nasal tip, sometimes the tip deformities may be so confusing (◘ Figs. 8.2 and 8.3) that you are in a dilemma where to start. Always resist the idea of starting with easy options. Stabilisation of tip should "always" begin from the medial crural area going towards the tip and then fanning out laterally, ironing out any loss of height or projection issues of the medial crus. There is more space in the lateral alar region than the medial nasal spine region to accommodate any extra changes in the definition and projection.

Once a decision is made to do nasal tip sutures, the important thing is to consider in *What sequence to use the sutures?* After the septal support is re-established and secured in the midline, then the attention should be directed towards primary reconstruction of the tip [10]. This can be achieved in the majority of patients with sutures, grafts and a combination of both.

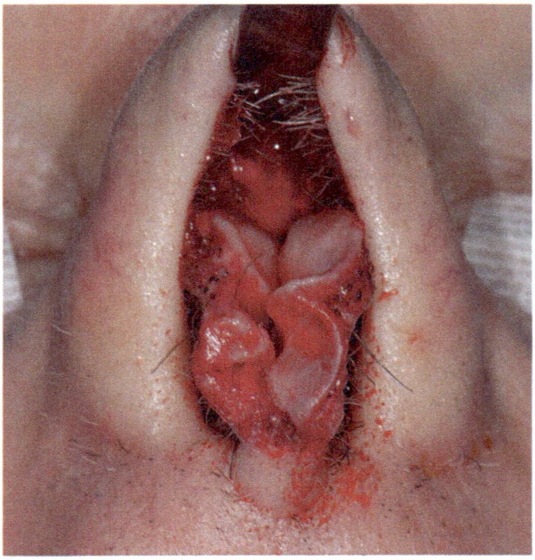

■ **Fig. 8.2** Open approach view showing complex deformity of the lower lateral cartilage

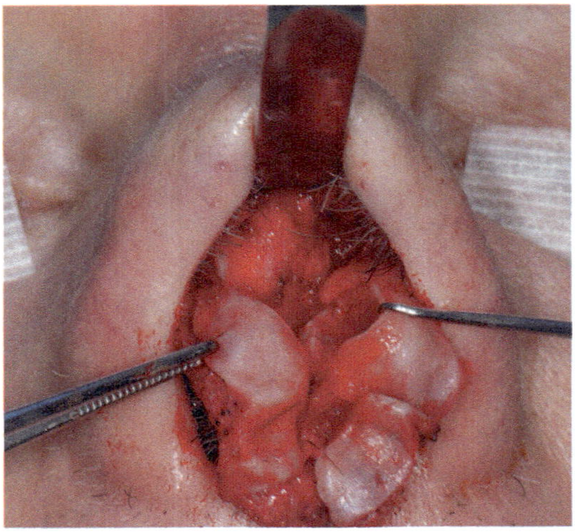

■ **Fig. 8.3** Open approach view showing complex deformity of the lower lateral cartilage and dorsal septal damage

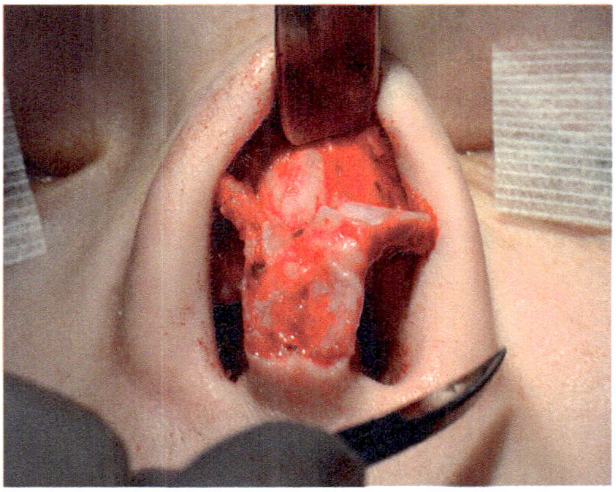

■ **Fig. 8.4** Open approach view showing scar tissue over the medial crura which are in a frontal plane

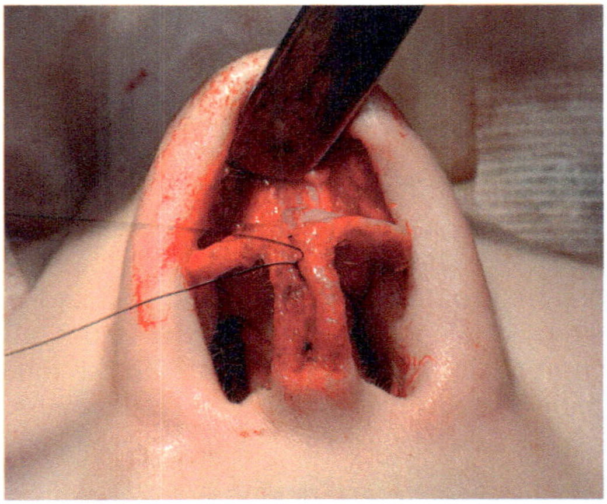

■ **Fig. 8.5** Open approach view showing the two medial crura being turned "in" to a sagittal plane with medial crural flare control suture (MCFS), thus increasing the "conjoined" medial crural support

The sequential steps in tip suturing are as follows:

- Reconstructing the medial crus on both sides and creating a "conjoined" medial crura. The orientation of the medial crus may need to be changed from a frontal plane to a sagittal plane (■ Figs. 8.4 and 8.5). The medial crural height may need to be increased, equalised and any weak area be supported with grafts thereby increasing the strength of the conjoined medial crus and re-establishing the symmetry between the two alar cartilages. This is usually achieved with medial crural fixations sutures (MCFS), medial crural flare control sutures (MCFCS) and if necessary medial crural ironing out sutures. Collectively they are referred to as medial crural stabilising sutures. These sutures are often considered as "basement" sutures before doing any domal work.
- Then reconstruct the intermediate crus and the domes of the tips with trans-domal (TDS) and inter-domal sutures (IDS).

- This is followed by lateral crural flare control sutures (LCFCS) to correct any lateral crural flare or convexity caused by the trans-domal sutures.
- The final step is to anchor the unified symmetrical tip complex in relation to the anterior septal angle and the dorsal profile line using tip anchoring sutures (TAS).

Sutures should be used at the right place and with the right tension. Be aware all suture techniques have more than one effect and is important to ascertain what is the most wanted outcome with each suture. For example, a trans-domal suture will not only narrow the tip, but also increase the projection in the dorsal profile line. This factor of additional effect should be *"factored in"* while using the tip sutures in the surgical algorithm [11, 12]. We will be describing the following suture techniques, which the author has been using in his practice over the last 24 years. Be aware that different type of suture nomenclatures are described in literature resulting in lot of confusion. In practice, the nomenclature should be based on exactly what the sutures achieves. Please note that not all sutures are used in all patients. In any one patient the surgeon may need a maximum of 4–5 sutures only to achieve desirable outcomes [13–15].

8.2 Medial Crural Fixation Suture (MCFS)

8.2.1 Introduction

Medial crural fixation suture (MCFS) as the name suggests brings together (more importantly prevent the two crura from moving away from each other) and fixes the two medial crura to create a unified tip complex and gives structural support and integrity to the medial crura [16, 17]. This suture is often the first suture performed in tip plasty. The author considers this suture as a "basement" suture before re-building the rest of the nasal tip. It can also be used to adjust the heights of both the domes to establish the tip projection and tip symmetry.

8.2.2 Indications

- This suture is used to secure the two medial crura to each other (◘ Fig. 8.6a–d) and/or to secure the two medial crura with a columellar cartilage strut (◘ Fig. 8.7a–c).
- This suture helps to prevent the two medial crura moving away from each other.
- To adjust an asymmetric tip height due to malpositioned medial crural height, by adjusting the point of entry and exit of the sutures.
- It helps to prevent posterior migration of the columellar strut cartilage.
- To narrow a wide nasal tip, as a "basement" suture before using the trans-domal suture to narrow the tip.
- To correct a bifid tip with a depression in the middle of the tip lobule complex.
- To achieve structural stability to the tip by creating a conjoined medial crural segment.

8.2.3 Contra-indications

There are virtually no contra-indications to this suture, except perhaps when there is no need for tip work.

8.2.4 Surgical Technique

- Open approach offers a direct view of the surgical site.
- Once the skin flap is raised, both lower lateral cartilages are exposed.
- Overlying scar tissues should be removed and the cartilage skeletonised.
- If no cartilage strut is required and only two medial crura need to be brought together, then the two domes are aligned at the desired height symmetrically with a skin hook placed under the dome one on either side.
- The posterior superior free border of the two medial crura are exposed (◘ Fig. 8.6a) and sutured together by a simple 5-0 ethilon suture.
- This suture goes "outside in" starting at the posterior-superior margin of the lat-

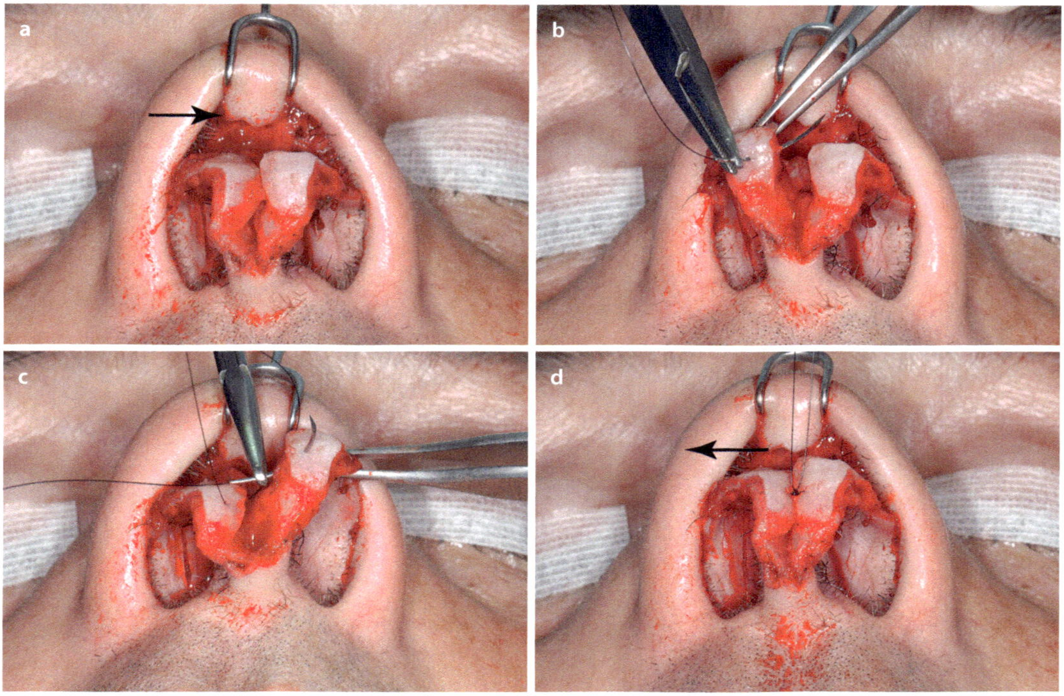

Fig. 8.6 **a–d** Open approach view showing the medal crural fixation suture (MCFS) between the poster-superior border of each medial crura. ("Reproduced with kind permission from Refs: [18–20]")

eral crus (Fig. 8.6b) on the right side staying just below the intermediate segment and going through the other side from "inside out" at the posterior-superior margin of the medial crus (Fig. 8.6c). You can also start "outside in" from the patient's left medial crura and entering the right medial crura "inside out" [18–20].

- A single knot is tied and is buried between the two crura (Fig. 8.6d). The knot brings the two medial crura together and stabilises the complex.
- This suture helps to pulls up the height of the dome, thus increasing the tip projection.
- If used with a piece of caudal cartilage strut to reinforce the medial crura, then the strut can be sutured to the medial crus going through the mucosa with an absorbable 5-0 vicryl (Fig. 8.7a–c). If non-absorbable ethilon is used, then make sure the suture does not go through the mucosa.

8.2.5 Surgical Sequence

- Surgical sequence of the individual steps for tip plasty should be always from medial to lateral direction starting from medial crus and working towards the lateral crus.
- MCFS should always be the first suture before starting any tip sutures. It is considered as the basement suture.
- Should be followed by medial crural flare control suture and then trans-domal and lateral crural sutures if needed. Otherwise, there is always a risk of two tip cartilages moving away from each other causing unwanted residual deformities.
- It is usually proceeded by cephalic trim of the lateral crus to reduce the bulk and the width of the lateral crus.
- It is preferable to do the tip work after dorsal bony work.

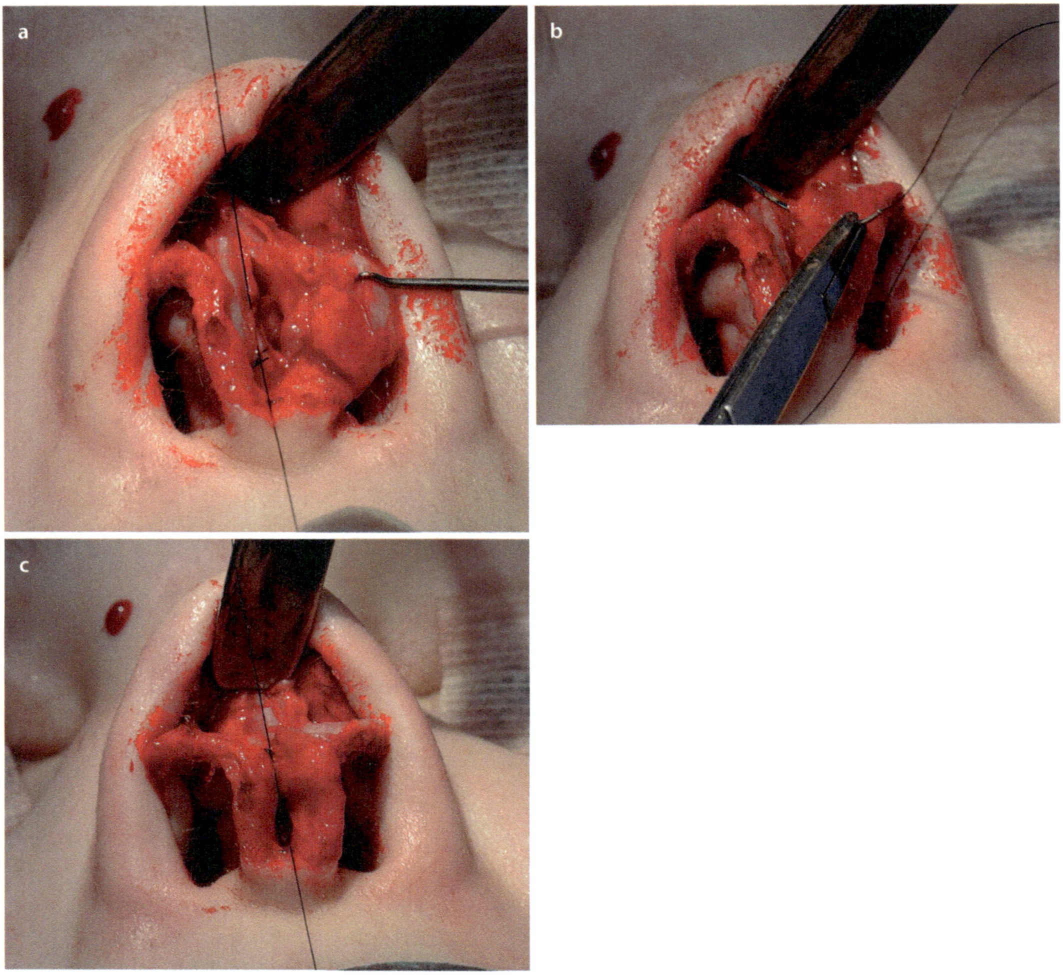

Fig. 8.7 **a–c** Open approach view showing the medal crural fixation suture (MCFS) going through the caudal septal strut for added support

Key Points

- Always start with medial crus before moving to dome or lateral crus.
- Make sure the suture bite in the medial crus is taken at the posterior border of the medial crus leaving a considerable width of the medial crus anteriorly to accommodate columellar strut if needed.
- Make sure the tip height between the two lateral crus is achieved before you proceed to further suturing.
- Make sure the knot is buried between the two medial crus and cut the knot very close.

Conclusion

- Medial crural fixation suture (MCFS), as the name suggests, brings together and fixes the two medial crura to create a unified tip complex and gives structural support and integrity to the nasal tip.
- Medical crural fixation suture is considered as the "basement suture" before commencing any primary tip work. It is often the first suture performed in tip plasty helping to prevent the two medial crura from moving away from each other.
- By bringing together the two medial crus it also helps in narrowing the width of a bulbous tip.

- It also corrects the cleft in the nasal tip due to separation of the two lower lateral cartilages.
- It can be used to address the asymmetric tip height by adjusting the point of entry and exit of the sutures.

8.3 Medial Crural Flare Control Suture (MCFCS)

8.3.1 Introduction

Medial crural flare control suture (MCFCS) brings together the two medial crus along the entire height of the medial crus and helps to control any flare or widening of the medial crura. Thus it creates a unified medial crural complex which is one of the major arms of the nasal tip tripod concept. This suture as the name suggests helps to control the medial crural flare, by approximating the two medial crura along its entire vertical length, helping to strengthen the medial crus and making it a conjoined force which will support the nasal tip better.

8.3.2 Indications

- De-projected nasal tip and loss of tip height due to damaged or fractured medial crus, secondary to trauma or revision surgery.
- To correct an "S" shaped kink in the medial crura with loss of tip height.
- Excess widening of the columella due to scar tissue and fat between the two medial crus. This suture helps to narrow the width of the columella after removal of scar tissue.
- To correct a wide columella due to abnormal orientation of the medial crura in a coronal plane. This suture helps to change the direction of the medial crura from this abnormal "coronal plane" to an anatomically normal "sagittal plane" (◘ Fig. 8.8a–c), thus controlling the flare of the columella.

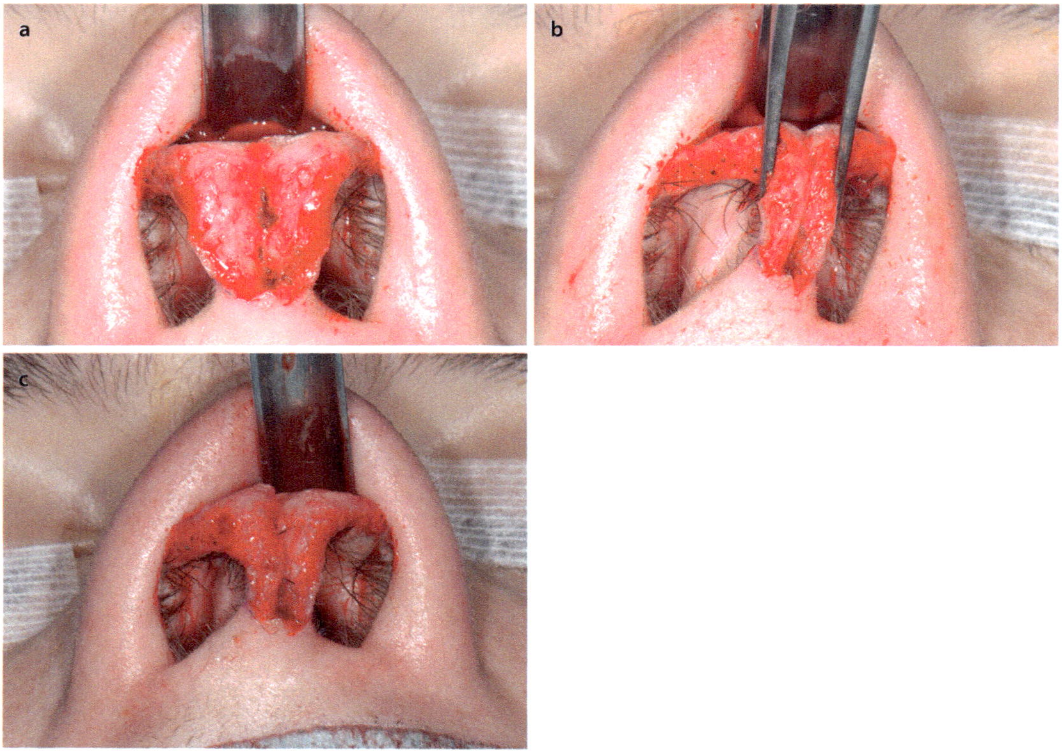

◘ **Fig. 8.8** **a**–**c** Open approach view. **a** Both medial crura in a frontal plane. **b**, **c** Change in the direction of medial crus to a sagittal plane with medial crural flare control suture

- To increase tip support by strengthening the “front” leg of the nasal tripod. By bringing together both the medial crus, it helps to create a “conjoined” medial crura which is stronger than a single medial crus in offering tip support.
- It helps in reducing and controlling an asymmetrical unilateral or a symmetrical bilateral medial crural footplate “flare”, thereby narrowing the columella and helping to open the external nasal valve vestibular region.

8.3.3 Contra-indications

- MCFCS is not necessary, if a caudal septal strut is used.
- MCFCS is not necessary, if planning a septal extension graft.
- If there is multiple level fractures of the medial crus.
- Extremely weak medial crus.
- Extremely short vertical height of the medial crus.

8.3.4 Surgical Technique

- This is a vertical mattress suture that is placed along the vertical length of the medial crus to control the flare of the medial crus (◘ Fig. 8.9a), thus narrowing the width of the columella.
- The suture can be a single suture extending along the entire length of the medial crus

8

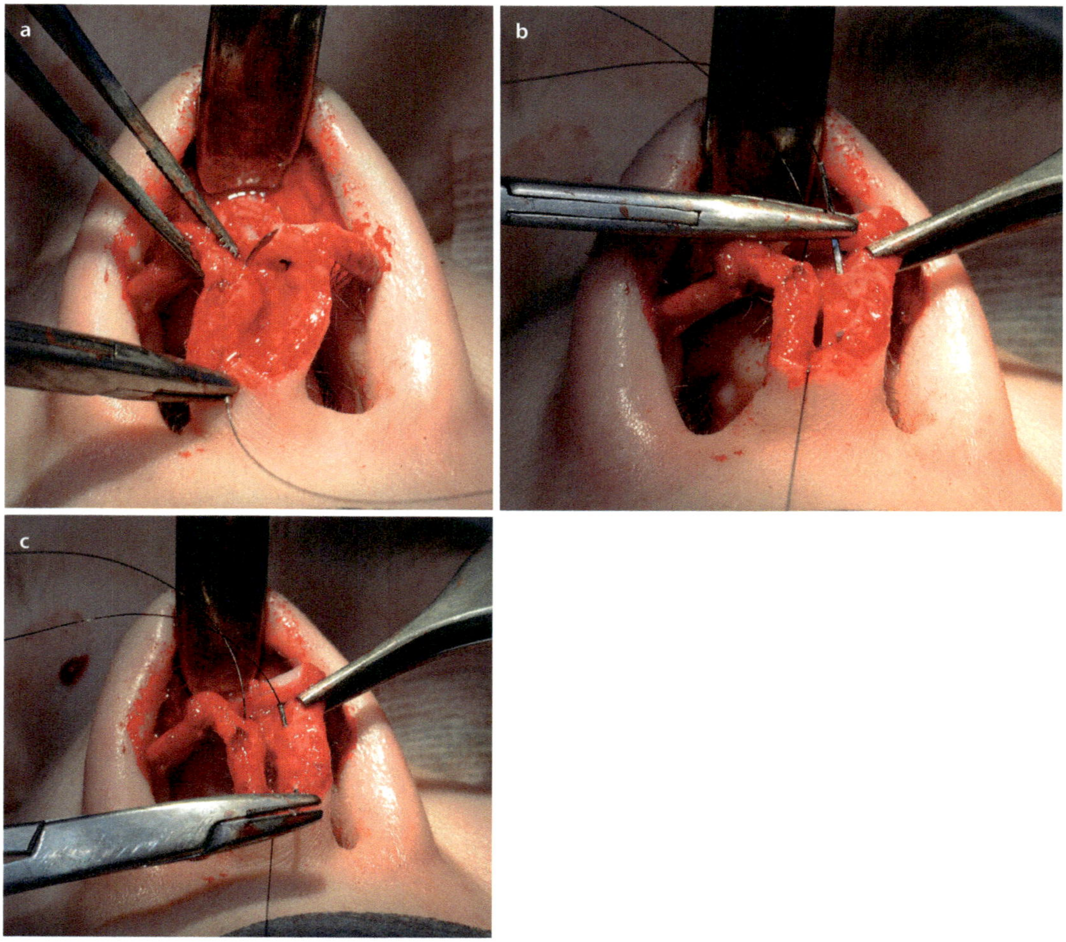

◘ **Fig. 8.9** **a–c** Open approach view showing the sequence of medial crural flare control suture (MCFCS)

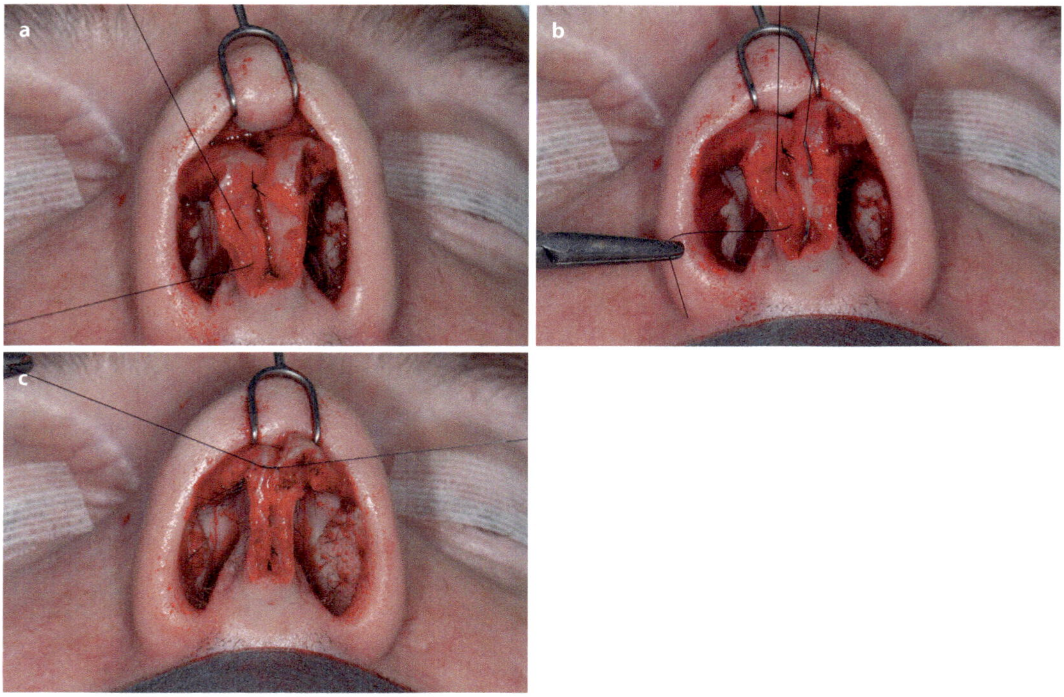

Fig. 8.10 **a–c** Open approach view showing the sequence of medial crural flare control suture (MCFCS) in another patient. ("Reproduced with kind permission from Refs: [18–20]")

or multiple short segment vertical mattress sutures of the medial crura.

- Start the suture at the lower end of the medial crural footplate on the medial surface of the right medial crus and take it out superiorly staying within the cartilage thickness. (Fig. 8.9a–c). Make sure this suture does not come through the mucosa particularly when using non-absorbable sutures like ethilon.
- The suture is then taken through the other medial crus, starting superiorly (Fig. 8.9b) and exiting inferiorly (Fig. 8.9c) [18–20].
- Then using a long non-toothed forceps gently squeeze the two media crura (Fig. 8.8b) to achieve the desired thickness before the knot is tied.
- Be aware that, position and tightness of the suture determines the width of the columella (Fig. 8.10a–c).
- The suturing can be done with or without a columellar strut.
- A variant of the above technique which is quicker and easier to execute is to use multiple vertical mattress sutures going through the nasal mucosa with an absorbable material (Fig. 8.11a–c). Suturing the cartilage together with non-absorbable suture without the mucosa is more effective in the long run to give predictable outcomes.

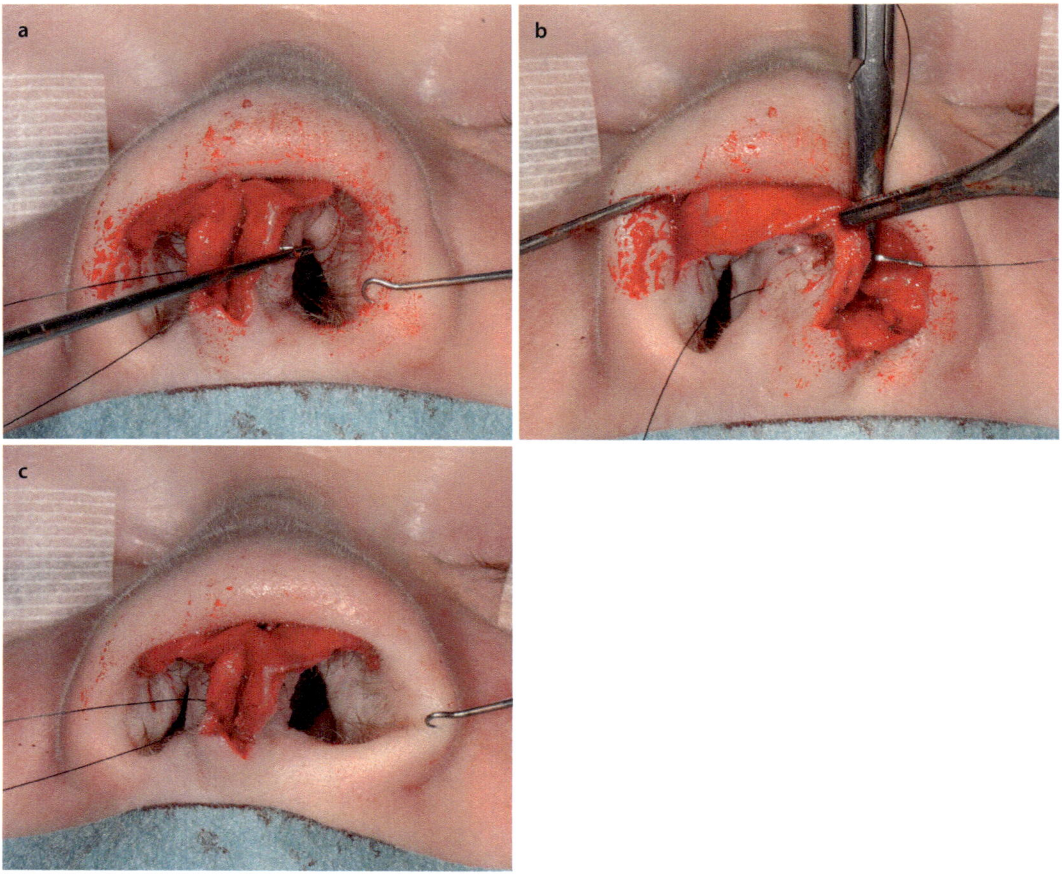

Fig. 8.11 **a–c** Open approach view showing the sequence of medial crural flare control suture (MCFCS) going through the septal mucosa with an absorbable suture.

8.3.5 Surgical Sequence

- It is advisable to precede this suture by the medial crural fixation suture to stabilise the medial crus.
- If needed, follow by trans-domal and inter-domal suture to achieve the desired outcome of increasing the definition and bringing the tip together.
- Does not need to use this suture if a decision is made to use a columellar strut.

Key Points

- Make sure the suture is not too close to the caudal border of the medial crus, as this will cause a pencil-thin narrow columella with cosmetic issues.
- Make sure the superior point of the suture is few millimetres below the intermediate crus, otherwise there will be distortion of the intermediate crus, which can pull the two intermediate crura and cause unnecessary alteration in tip projection due to change in the inter-domal angles.
- If the medial crus is too long in a large over projected nose, it will be better to do two or three MCFCS one below the other, than to use a single long vertical mattress suture which may be counterproductive in causing crimpling and loss of medial crural height.
- If there is a horizontal fracture in the medial crus, either on one side or both, make sure the sutures are tightened

"just enough" to approximate and give strength and not to over tighten, as it will cause buckling and vertical shortening at the fracture site.

Conclusion

- Medial crural flare control suture (MCFCS), as the name suggests, brings together any flare in the medial crus and fixes the two medial crura to create a unified tip complex and gives structural support and integrity to the medial crura.
- It also helps in narrowing the width of the columella by bringing together the two medial crus.
- It also helps to change the direction of the medial crura from an abnormal "coronal plane" to an anatomically normal "sagittal plane" and thus creates a "conjoined" medial crus which is stronger than a single medial crus in offering tip support, thus offering structural support to the tip complex.

8.4 Medial Crural Ironing out Suture

8.4.1 Introduction

Medial crural ironing out sutures brings together the two medial crus along the entire height of the medial crus by a series of individual horizontal mattress sutures to control any flare, irregularity, concavity or convexity or widening of the medial crura. When compared to single vertical medial crural fixation suture described above, the medial crural ironing out sutures are a series of multiple horizontally placed sutures to correct various asymmetric deformities of medial crus. It is aimed to create a unified medial crural complex which is one of the major arms of the nasal tip tripod concept. These are a series of individual (but multiple) simple or horizontal mattress between the two medial crural footplates inserted from below upwards, working to "Iron-Out" the crinkled medial crus by straightening and strengthening the medial crus and creating a stronger conjoined medial crura. The "sequence" of using these multiple sutures should always be from near the anterior nasal spine region at the base of the columella and slowly worked up towards the tip thereby "ironing out" and straightening the deformed medial crura, as you work your way up. This gives conjoined strength to the columella region and also increases the projection and gives a good tip support in a deprojected unsupported tip.

8.4.2 Indications

- This suture helps to iron out either bilateral or unilateral buckled medial crura (Fig. 8.12a), thereby helping to increase the height of the columella and the tip complex.
- Can be used with or without a columellar strut cartilage.
- Ideally indicated in multiple asymmetric deformities of the medial crura.
- Vertically buckled medial crus, unilateral or bilateral causing loss of tip height.
- The medial crural length should be intact and not unduly short.
- The medial crus should not be weak at its midpoint due to scar tissue, fracture or discontinuity.
- Basically indicated when there is multiple medial crural buckling, to create a conjoined crus which will give strength and create enough support for the tip projection.

8.4.3 Contra-indications

- Multiple fracture segments of the medial crus.
- Very thin and weak medial crus.
- Replacement of the medial crural cartilage by scar tissue.

8.4.4 Surgical Technique

- The ideal indication for these type of sutures should be a vertically buckled, but long and wide medial crus either on one

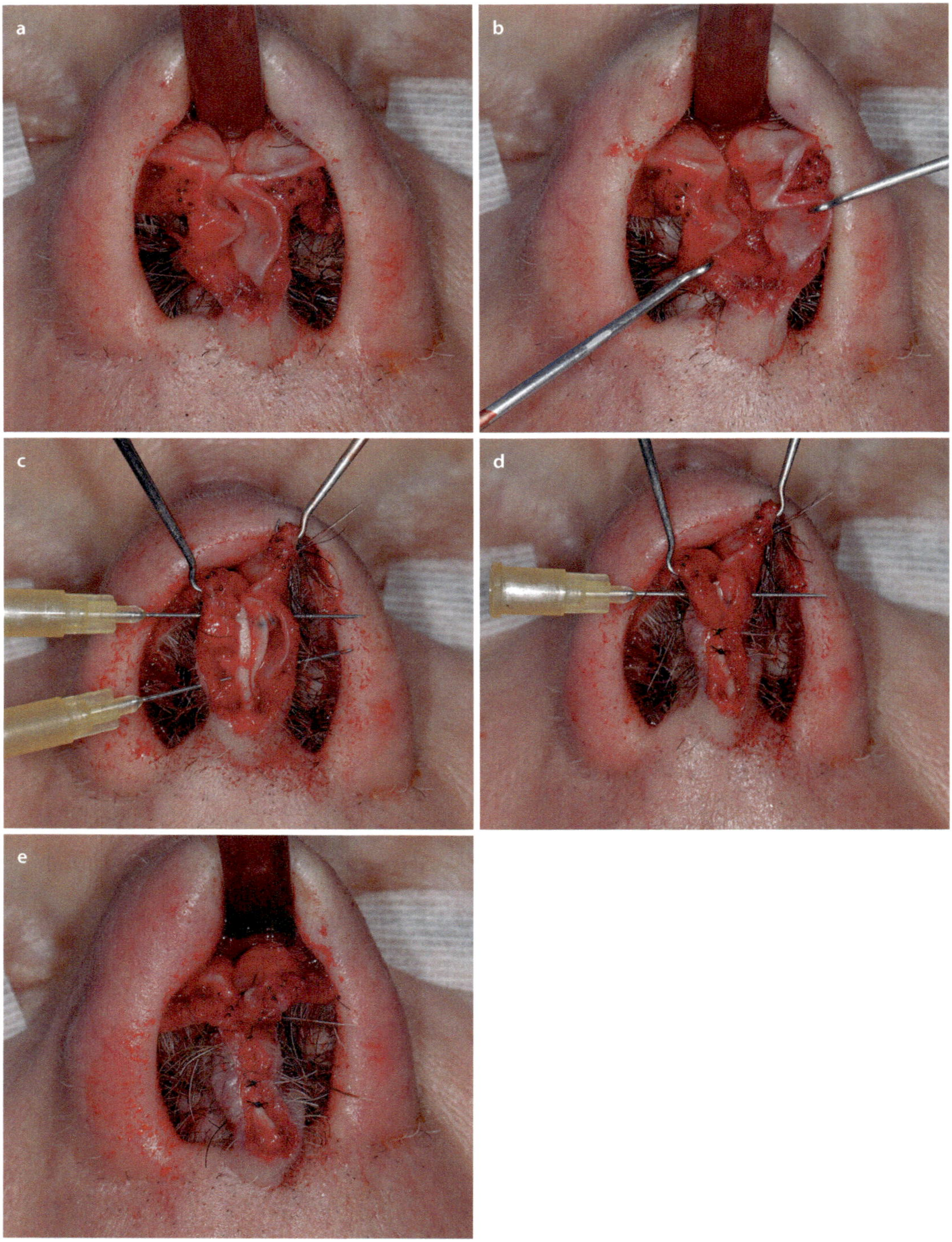

Fig. 8.12 **a–e** Open approach view showing the sequence of medial crural horizontal "ironing out" sutures going through the septal mucosa and a strut with an absorbable suture. ("Reproduced with kind permission from Refs: [18–20]")

side or both sides, but with quite a good strength intrinsically. These are rare group of patients who do not need a columellar strut to support the tip, since the width of the medial crus is quite good and by suturing the two medial crura, the conjoined crus is strong enough to hold the tip.

- If the two medial crus is buckled and lost vertical height and if the medial crural fixation suture is not able to adjust the vertical height without introducing an asymmetry, then consider using this suture.
- First assess the intrinsic width and strength of the medial crus. Simple buckling without fracture is an indication to do this suture. In the presence of any fracture of the medial crus or replacement with scar tissue, we may need to use a columellar strut (◘ Fig. 8.12c).
- Once a decision is made to use this suture, the first step would be to start with simple sutures between the two medial crus starting from the base of the ala and working towards the tip.
- Start the sutures from the medial crural footplate to footplate and slowly iron out the buckling from below upwards ironing them out and securing them together as you go upwards [18–20].

8.4.5 Surgical Sequence

Should always be preceded by the medial crural fixation suture to stabilise the medial crus and then if needed followed by trans-domal and inter-domal suture to achieve the desired outcome of increasing the stability to the tip.

Key Points

- It takes between 2 and 3 simple horizontal sutures to iron out the medial crus, depending upon the length of the medial crura.
- The bites in the medial crus should be 2–3 mm away from the free border (◘ Fig. 8.12c) and not at the edge. Otherwise the columella will become pencil thin.
- Make sure "ALL" the bites should be at the same level in a vertical orientation.
- There should roughly be the same tension in all the knots.
- Make sure the knots are not too tight in some places as these can cause some columellar retraction in the frontal view.

Conclusion

- Medial crural ironing out sutures, as name suggests, are used to "iron out" any crinkling in the medial crus resulting in loss of medial crural height.
- These are versatile and "tailor made" for each patient and can be used as individual horizontal mattress between the two medial crura.
- They should always be "ironed out" from below upwards starting low in the columella and NOT from above downwards.
- Thus, this suture helps to gain height and as well as strength to the medial crural complex.

8.5 Trans-domal Suture (TDS) or Dome-Spanning Suture (DSS)

8.5.1 Introduction

As the name suggests, trans-domal sutures involve going "through" the dome (trans dome) starting medially from the medial crus entering the lateral crus and coming back again as a horizontal mattress from the lateral crus back to the medial crus basically to pinch the dome and help to narrow the dome. By doing so, it slightly changes the direction of the dome and also helps to increase the projection. They are also called domespanning sutures. Since the height of the medial crus is increased, they may need a high medial crural flare control suture to narrow the top end of the columella. Thus these sutures help to control the width of the dome of the lateral crural cartilage. The sutures can go through each dome separately or through both the domes, as a single suture helping to narrow the width of the nasal tip. When used a single suture, they can also be used to bring the two domes together thus narrowing the gap or cleft between the tip cartilages.

8.5.2 Indications

- Wide symmetrical bulbous tip.
- Asymmetrical unilateral bulbous tip.
- Bulbosity and excess width of the nasal tip due to widening angle between the medial crus and the lateral crus.
- De-projected and wider tip – as a means to increase the definition, and increase the projection.
- This suture helps to bring together medial and lateral crura *only on ONE side*, thus ultimately helping to narrow the width of the lower lateral cartilage on that side.
- This suture can be done on both sides, helping to narrow the width of the entire tip complex.
- This suture by narrowing the tip also increases the projection of the tip.
- Also helps to narrow the dorsal aesthetic tip line at the level of the tip lobule complex.

8.5.3 Contra-indications

- If an intermediate crural resection and anastomosis has been performed.
- If a lateral crural excision or incision and overlap has been performed.
- If the integrity of lateral crus is re-established with sutures, say after lateral crural excision, doing a domal suture may put extra tension and disrupt the suture line with alar collapse with functional issues.
- Beware of doing this in a patient with very thin skin, as it can cause a sharp tip.

8.5.4 Surgical Technique

This technique was initially described by Tardy through a closed approach, although later refined by Tebbetts through an open approach [21].

- Ideally an open technique offers the versatility of putting this suture at various levels, although can be done through tip delivery techniques as well.
- A unilateral dome suture helps to increase the projection of the nasal tip without altering the tip support mechanics.
- This is a horizontal mattress suture in the axial plane starting from the medial crus just below the dome and entering the lateral crus about 2–3 mm below the intermediate crus and coming back medially and securing the knot between the two domes (◻ Fig. 8.13a–c) [18–20].
- Make sure the entry and exit points of the suture is in the middle of the dome and not too far anteriorly placed to prevent a unicorn nasal tip.
- There should be a slight angle of divergence of the domes both anteriorly and posteriorly.
- Usually there is no need to elevate the underlying mucosa, but may have to do so, if the dome is quite wide and if using non-absorbable sutures [22].
- The suture entry should be medial so that the knot lies medial to the two domes.
- The knot should be trimmed very close and buried between the tip cartilages deep in the dome.
- Instead of using separate suture on the two domes, a single suture can be used going through both the domes together, as popularised by Dr.Tardy who executed this technique through a "closed" approach and I have seen him doing this technique with a degree of ease and perfection [1, 23].
- There are variants of this technique described by Gruber like a hemi suture to prevent lateral crural concavity [24, 25].

8.5.5 Surgical Sequence

- The sequence of these sutures should be *after* the medial crural re-modelling and just *before* lateral crural re-modelling.
- Should always be preceded by the medial crural fixation suture and followed by inter-domal suture to achieve the desired outcome of increasing the definition and bringing the tip together.

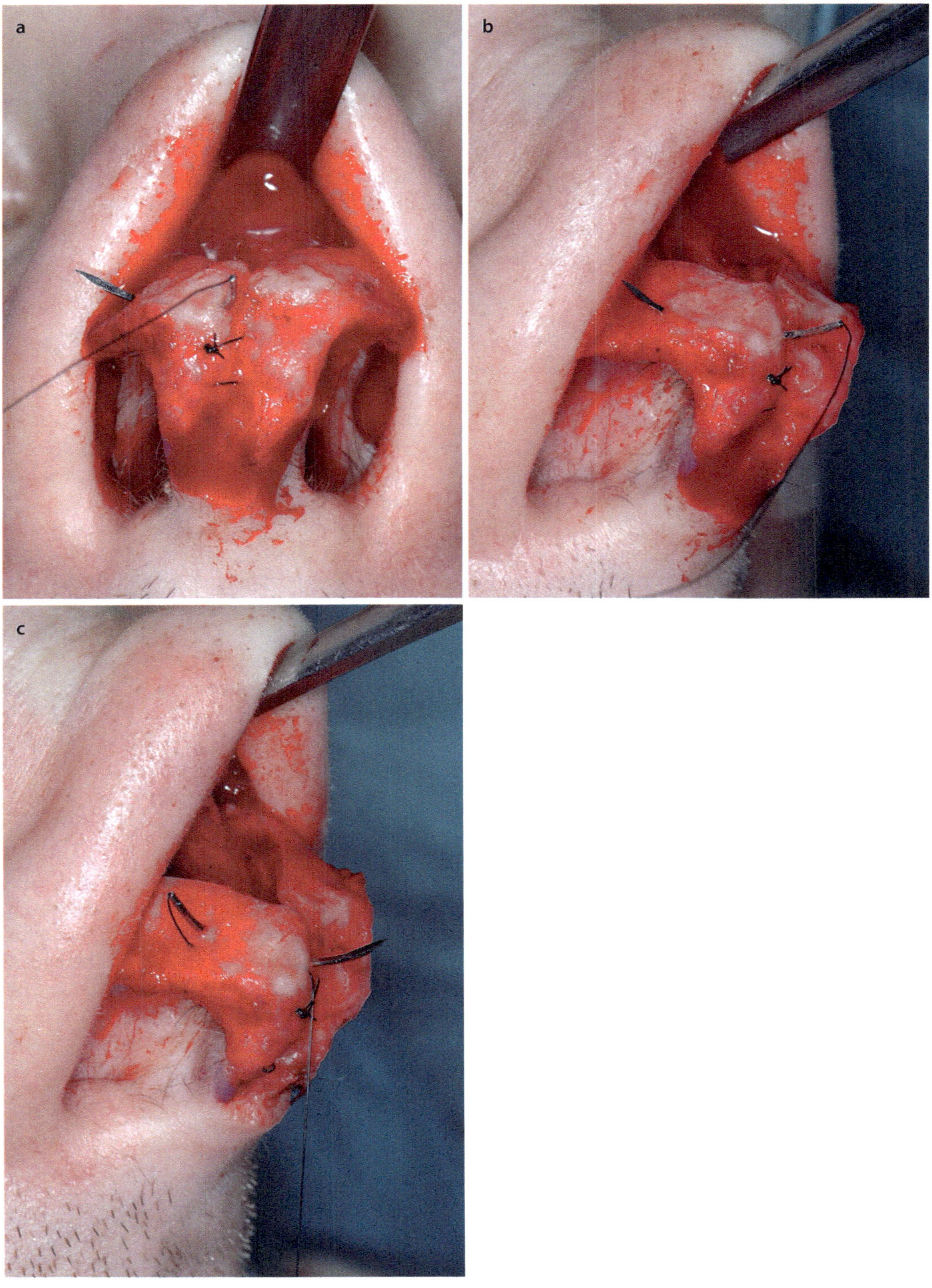

Fig. 8.13 **a–c** Open approach view showing the sequence of trans-domal suture (TDS). ("Reproduced with kind permission from Refs: [18–20]")

Key Points
- Not to tie the knot too tight, otherwise may end up with a very narrow unicorn nose.
- Burry the knot between the two domes securely and cover the knots with crushed cartilage.
- When done on both sides maintain the symmetry of the height of the two domes by keeping the sutures in the same horizontal axis.
- Too tight sutures may narrow the dorsal aesthetic lines too much with resulting asymmetry of the line from above downwards.
- Beware pinching the domes together with this suture will cause lateral alar ballooning due to flaring of the lateral crura on both sides, akin to the use of a clip on a paper board. If you pinch the clip at the top, it will flare the lower part. Hence a lateral crural flare control suture to compensate the lateral flare may also be needed. Be aware that trans-domal suture will increase the projection as well as narrowing the tip.

Conclusion
- As the name suggests the trans-domal suture passes through the domes narrowing either one dome or both the domes, thus helping to narrow the width of the entire tip complex.
- When used as a through and through suture, it helps to bring the two domes together thus narrowing the gap or cleft between the tip cartilages.
- This suture also helps to increase the projection of the tip and strengthens the tip complex.

8.6 Inter-domal Suture (IDS)

8.6.1 Introduction

Inter-domal sutures (IDS), as the name suggests, involve going "between (inter)" the two domes starting from one dome and going through the other dome by a simple suture at the middle of the dome with the knot under the skin or alternatively through a horizontal mattress suture hidden on the inner medial surface of the two domes with the knot being hidden between the two domes. Inter-domal suture (IDS), as the name suggests, helps to bring the two domes together, by placing the suture in the inter-domal region of the two tip cartilages.

8.6.2 Indications

- This suture helps to narrow a wide, trapezoidal and symmetrical bulbous tip.
- This suture helps to narrow the angle of divergence between two domes.
- This suture helps to unify and efface the cleft seen in a bifid tip due to increased distance between the two domes.
- As an adjunct technique along with trans-domal suture to improve the definition in a wide trapezoidal tip as seen in the basal view.
- As an adjunct technique along with trans-domal suture to increase the projection in a wide de-projected tip.
- Increases the firmness and strength of the tip lobule complex.

8.6.3 Contra-indications

- If an intermediate crural resection has been performed.
- After lateral crural excision or overlapping technique has been done, doing a domal suture can cause disruption of the suture site in the lateral crus and can cause collapse of the lateral alar region.
- Beware of doing this in a patient with very thin skin.

8.6.4 Surgical Technique

- This suture can be done in two ways.
- One way of doing this is a simple suture passing through both the domes centred around the middle of the dome (◘ Fig. 8.14) avoiding too close to the caudal edge of the intermediate crus, thus helping to bring the domes together. This

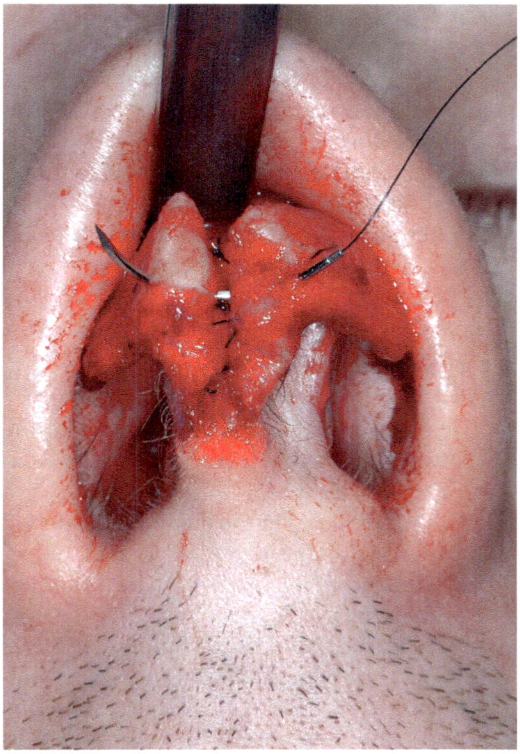

Fig. 8.14 Open approach view showing the inter-domal suture (IDS). ("Reproduced with kind permission from Refs: [18–20]")

simple suture is advisable if the dome width is narrow [18–20].

- Measure the antero-posterior (Caudal-dorsal) distance on the maximum projecting part of the dome and place the suture in the middle of it, taking care not to come too close to the caudal or dorsal border of the intermediate crus.
- Throw a double knot and a single knot and cut the suture very close and slightly bevelling the edges of the suture by tilting the edge of the scissors.
- Since the edges of the suture are just underneath the skin, it will be advisable to use absorbable PDS suture and then put some crushed septal cartilage or a small piece of the excised cephalic portion of the lateral crus between the suture and the dorsal skin.
- Another way of doing this suture is through a horizontal mattress suture on the "inside" of the dome going through one side and coming out on the inside of the opposite dome so that the knot is buried between the two domes. This suture is advisable if the domes are very wide [26].

8.6.5 Surgical Sequence

Should always be preceded by the medial crural fixation suture and trans-domal suture to achieve the desired outcome of increasing the definition and bringing the tip together.

Key Points

- Make sure that the suture placement on the dome cartilages is somewhere midway between the caudal and dorsal part of the intermediate crus and not too far anteriorly, as this will cause a "unicorn" nasal tip which will give an unsightly pointed "single" tip. This will result in dorsal aesthetic line converging towards the tip rather than gently diverging from each other, something akin to the proboscis of a simian.
- If the knot is too tight, can cause tip rotation and thus affect the dorsal profile line.
- If the knot is too tight, can cause very "rigid tip".
- Note that this suture is very superficial under the skin. So take care to cut the knot very close and if possible cover the knot with some crushed cartilage, so that there is no issue of suture extruding through thin skin.

Conclusion

- Inter-domal suture (IDS), as the name suggests, helps to bring the two dome together, by locating the suture in the inter-domal region of the two tip cartilages. The suture can be placed over the dorsum of the dome or on the inside (medial surface) of the tip cartilage.
- This suture helps to narrow a boxy tip and helps to unify and efface the cleft seen in bifid tips.
- It also helps to increase the tip definition and tip projection.

8.7 Lateral Crural Flare Control Suture (LCFCS)

8.7.1 Introduction

A lateral crural flare control suture (LCFCS) first described by Tebbetts, as the name suggests, helps to bring "in" a bulging lateral crus, controlling the lateral crural flare and thus defining the nasal tip. It is a single horizontal mattress suture passing between the two lateral crural arches and best done under vision through an open approach. This is commonly done following an iatrogenic alar flare caused by a trans-domal suture used to narrow a dome. Care must be taken not to tighten the knot too much as it may cause over narrowing and "pinched in" lateral crus ending in both structural and functional external nasal valve issues [2, 27].

8.7.2 Indications

- Wide lateral alar region with symmetrical or asymmetrical alar ballooning of the lateral crus.
- This suture helps to narrow the lateral alar flare and lateral alar ballooning. Hence they are also called "alar-spanning sutures".
- Also helps to narrow the dorsal aesthetic tip lines near the alar lobule.
- Adds definition to the nasal tip.
- This suture should be considered in patients who undergo trans-domal sutures to counteract the lateral alar flare caused by pinching the dome. This is analogous to a using clip on a board. If you pinch the top part of the clip, the lower half will open. Similarly when the domes are pinched together with a trans-domal suture, usually there is a flare in the lateral alar region, which may need to be controlled with the lateral crural flare control suture.

8.7.3 Contra-indications

- If the lateral crus is weak or damaged.
- If an intermediate crural resection has been performed.
- If lateral crus is strengthened with sutures, after lateral crural excision.
- Functional nasal obstruction due to weakness of the lateral alar region.

8.7.4 Surgical Technique

- This suture is a horizontal mattress suture between the two lateral crura to reduce lateral alar ballooning.
- This suture helps in the medial and upward movement of the lateral crus, thus reducing the lateral alar ballooning and under-rotating the tip.
- The suture should be placed in the lateral crus at the maximum point of the alar ballooning as far laterally as it allows starting from "inside out and then going back outside in" on "the right side" and then going "inside out and outside in" on "the opposite side" (◘ Fig. 8.15a–d) [18–20].
- With Aufrichts' elevator in place, the suture is placed under vision.
- Once the knot is tied, the skin flap is replaced and the tightness of the knot is checked and adjusted with optimum pressure internally in the middle between the two domes taking great care *not to tighten the knot very much*, as this may cause internal lateral alar wall narrowing and also unwanted under rotation of the tip with de-projection.
- If the knot is tied too much or if the bites in the cartilage is placed too caudally in the lateral crus, then there is a risk of upward retraction of the alar margin and medial migration of lateral crus with functional external nasal valve issues. Extreme care is needed to execute the desired effects of this suture, without any unwanted side effects [28].

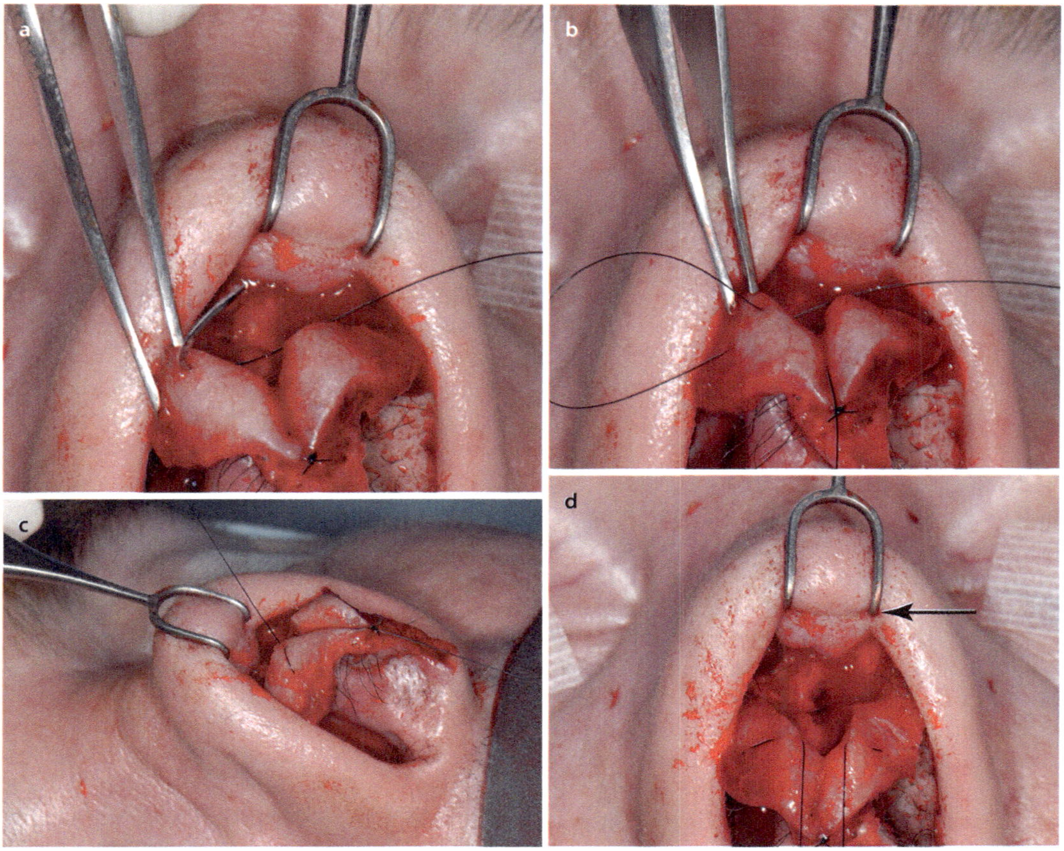

Fig. 8.15 **a–d** Open approach view showing the sequence of lateral crural flare control suture (LCFCS) in helping to control the lateral crural flare. ("Reproduced with kind permission from Refs: [18–20]")

8.7.5 Surgical Sequence

In a patient with a bulbous tip requesting narrowing of the tip, this suture may need to follow the trans-domal suture, particularly if there is an unwanted lateral alar flare. If you stop at the trans-domal suture in a patient with an already bulbous tip, then you may end up like a unicorn narrow tip with a wide lateral ala, which can distort the dorsal aesthtic tip lines.

Key Points

- Do not tie the knot too tight, otherwise may end up with a very narrow external nasal valve with functional obstruction.
- Too tight suture may end up in a pinched up dome giving rise to a unicorn nose.
- Burry the knot between the domes properly.
- When done on both sides, maintain the symmetry of the height of the two domes by keeping the sutures in the same horizontal axis.
- Too tight sutures may narrow the dorsal aesthetic lines too much with resulting asymmetry of the line from above downwards.
- Sometimes an alar spreader may be needed to stabilise a medial migration of the lateral crus after a lateral crural flare suture.

Conclusion

- Lateral crural flare control suture (LCFCS), as the name suggests, helps to control the lateral crural flare on both sides and helps in the lateral alar ballooning.
- It also helps in narrowing the width of the lateral tip and re-establish the dorsal aesthetic tip lines.

8.8 Tip Anchoring Suture (TAS)

8.8.1 Introduction

Tip anchoring suture (TAS), as the name suggests, helps to anchor the tip to the anterior septal angle to achieve a favourable overriding of the tip (2–3 mm) on the dorsum. As the name suggests, this suture is invaluable for achieving the final position of the unified tip complex. This suture helps in aligning the tip in line with the dorsum of the nose, particularly in patients wanting a slight over ride of the tip complex with reference to the dorsal profile line. This suture also helps in preventing "tip ptosis" after correction of a ptotic tip. Extreme care is taken not to tighten the knot too much as it may cause over rotation of the tip with frontal nostril show. Also if the caudal septum is not straight, the tip can be held rigid in one particular direction with a twisted tip complex.

8

8.8.2 Indications

- TAS is indicated when there is an obvious tip droop or ptosis of the tip in relation to the dorsum. This suture helps in preventing undue tip drop after open surgery and also positively to increase the tip rotation [29, 30].
- In an under projected tip, it can marginally increase the degree of tip projection.
- If the tip columellar complex is made heavier due to the use of columellar struts, there is a chance the nasal tip can droop over time. In these patients, the TAS can be used as a prophylactic suture to prevent future ptosis. Hence the name tip anchoring suture.
- This suture helps in securing the final position of the unified tip complex slightly higher in relation to the dorsal profile line to create a slight ski-slope. Depending on the entry points of the suture, the actual location of the unified tip complex can be varied to achieve a favourable position in relation to the dorsum particularly in women to create a slightly overriding tip which can be aesthetically pleasing.
- Also helps in improving the nasal tip support.
- This simple suture can be used as a sole procedure for lifting a droopy tip in an elderly rhinoplasty with functional obstruction.
- It can be used prophylactically in any patient who may be expected to develop tip under rotation due to surgical intervention.

8.8.3 Contra-indications

- In over resected anterior septal angles and over resected dorsal septal cartilage following revision rhinoplasty, when there is not enough dorsal height to secure the tip. In this situation, if the TAS is used it will result in extreme over rotation of the tip and shortening of the length off the nose with excess nostril show.
- Not advisable to use when extended spreader grafts or septal extension grafts are used, as this suture may result in excess width of the nasal tip.
- Even if there is a small chance that tip can become rigid or shift to one side, avoid this suture.
- If the caudal septum and the anterior septal angle are not exactly in the midline even after reconstruction, then it is advisable NOT to suture the tip complex to the anterior septal angle due to the risk of tip deviation.

8.8.4 Surgical Technique

- Open approach is preferable.
- Like in a dome-spanning suture, the surgeon takes a bite from one dome, going from "inside out" but also goes through

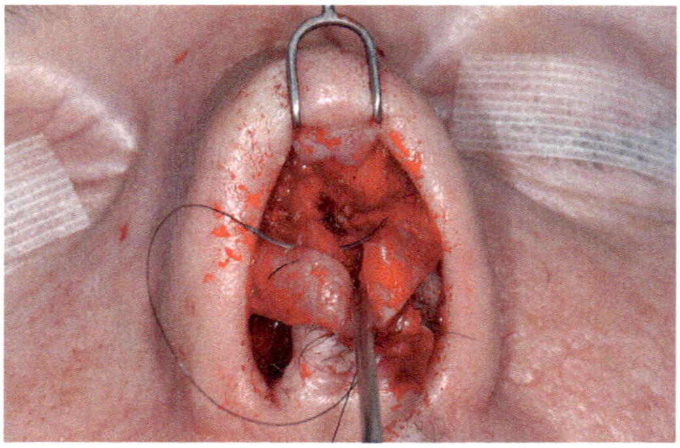

Fig. 8.16 Open approach view showing the tip anchoring suture (TAS), with the tip cartilage being anchored to the anterior septal angle of the septal cartilage. ("Reproduced with kind permission from Ref: [18]")

the "anterior septal angle" of the septal cartilage (Fig. 8.16) at the very tip of the most prominent projection point and comes out through the other dome from "inside out" and secures the knot on the dorsum, thus "anchoring" and "positioning" the tip in relation to the dorsum of the nose.

- This can be a simple suture or a mattress suture.
- The knot should *not be too tight*, but just enough to achieve the desired position without undue over rotation of the tip.

8.8.5 Surgical Sequence

- Should be done as a final step after refining the tip complex and narrowing the tip.
- This suture should be the last one to be used after the medial crural, tip and lateral crural sutures.

Key Points

- Too tight suture will over rotate the tip and cause an excess nostril show in the frontal plane.
- Tip can become very rigid and interfere with smile and can give an operated look.
- If the caudal septum is not exactly in the midline, it can cause asymmetrical rotation and turning of the tip to one side.
- Remember, this suture helps to secure the tip at a higher position in relation to the dorsum and prevent it from drooping down and hence used to prevent tip drop and not to effectively lift the tip up.

Conclusion

- Tip anchoring suture (TAS), as the name suggests, helps to hold the tip at a higher position when compared to the dorsum, so that the tip overrides the dorsum for an aesthetically pleasing nose in female patients.
- This should be done last, always looking not to tighten the suture to avoid over rotation of the tip.

8.9 Upper Lateral Flaring Sutures (ULFS)

8.9.1 Introduction

As the name suggests, this suture helps in "flaring" the caudal portion of the upper lateral cartilages to open the internal nasal valve region. This suture was described by Park to open a narrow and dysfunctional internal valve [31]. In essence, this is a functional suture aiming to improve the internal nasal valve function and not a structural suture. It also helps to widen the mid dorsum. This is best done through an open approach. This is a mattress suture at the caudal border of the upper lateral cartilage creating a flare to open the internal nasal valve region, not a commonly used procedure in the author's practice. Please note there are other more reliable techniques like spreader grafts or spreader flaps to open the internal valve, than these sutures which can be difficult to execute and difficult to achieve meaningful and consistent results in improving the nasal airway.

8.9.2 Indications

- This suture is indicated when there is an obvious narrowing of the middle vault and internal nasal valve narrowing, particu-

larly isolated narrowing of the caudal border of upper lateral cartilage at its junction with the septum. So basically described as a functional operation and not a structural suturing.
- The suture is intended to open a narrow and dysfunctional internal valve [31].
- Can be done through open or closed approach but best done through an open approach.

8.9.3 Contra-indications

- If there is an associated deformity involving the dorsal septum, doing this suture alone will not give long-term results.
- Weak upper lateral cartilage, on one or both sides.
- Parts of upper lateral cartilage fractured or missing.

8.9.4 Surgical Technique

It is a horizontal mattress suture, starting from the lateral caudal border of one ULC and involving the caudal border of the opposite upper lateral and the knot is tightened over the dorsum. The tighter the knot, the more the flare.

8.9.5 Surgical Sequence

Should be done as a final step after refining the tip complex and narrowing the tip. Preferably done before closing the flap in an open approach.

Key Points
- Too tight suture will over rotate the ULC and cause very wide mid dorsum.
- Difficult to execute through an internal approach.

Conclusion

This suture is not a very commonly performed suture and we need to be aware of various alternatives including spreader grafts and spreader flaps, before we attempt this technique.

Key Points Box
- Nasal tip sutures are an important tool to define, project and alter the position of the tip cartilages, either on one side or both.
- They offer a safe, reliable and reversible tool in the reconstruction of nasal tip cartilages.
- The sutures are predominantly advisable in primary rhinoplasty, although also used in combination with grafts in secondary revision rhinoplasty.
- Generally non-absorbable sutures like 5-0 ethilon or prolene are preferable. Absorbable PDS sutures or coated vicryl sutures are used if the sutures go through the mucosa or when the knots are near the surface skin.
- Sutures are used predominantly in the lower lateral tip cartilages to correct the structure anatomy and position, whereas sutures in the upper lateral cartilages are used more for functional reasons.
- Nasal tip sutures preserve the structural integrity and anatomy of the tip cartilages and are non-destructive and hence the long-term outcomes are predictable.

References

1. Tardy ME, JrChen E. Transdomal suture refinement of the nasal tip. Fac Plast Surg. 1987;4:317–26.
2. Tebbetts JB. Primary tip assessment and modification. In: Primary rhinoplasty a new approach to the logic and the techniques. St. Louis: Mosby-year Book Inc; 1998. p. 99–133.

3. Daniel RK. Rhinoplasty: creating an aesthetic tip. A preliminary report. Plast Reconstr Surg. 1987;80:775–83.
4. Tebbetts JB. Secondary tip modification: shaping and positioning in the nasal tip using non destructive techniques. In: Tebbetts JB, editor. Primary rhinoplasty: a new approach to the logic and the techniques. St Louis: Mosby; 1998. p. 261–440.
5. Guyuron B. Discussion: changing the convexity and concavity of nasal cartilages and cartilage grafts with horizontal mattress sutures; part I. experimental results and part II. Clinical results. Plast Reconstr Surg. 2005;115(2):607–8.
6. Tebbetts JB. Shaping and position the nasal tip without structural disruption: a new, systematic approach. Plast Reconstr Surg. 1994;94:61–77.
7. Tebbetts JB. Open rhinoplasty: more than an incisional approach. In: Ked DR, editor. Aesthetic plastic surgery rhinoplasty. Boston: Mass Little Brown & Co Inc; 1993. p. 525–53.
8. Rohrich RJ, Adams WP. The boxy nasal tip: classification and management based on alar cartilage suturing techniques. Plast Reconstr Surg. 2001;107:1849.
9. Gruber RP, Weintraub J, Pomerantz J. Suture techniques for the nasal tip. Aesthetic Surg J. 2008;28(1):92–100.
10. Balaji N. Top tips in nasal tip surgery, ENT-FPS UK Newsletter— Feb 2018 –Issue 6.
11. Daniel RK. Rhinoplasty: a simplified three-stitch, open tip suture technique. Part I: primary rhinoplasty. Plast Reconstr Surg. 1999;103:1491–502.
12. Baker SR. Suture contouring of the nasal tip. Arch Facial Plast Surg. 2000;2:34–42.
13. Behmand RA, Ghavami A, Guyuron B. Nasal tip sutures part I: the evolution. Plast Reconstr Surg. 2003;112:1125–9.
14. Lee KC, Kwon YS, Park JM, Kim SK, Park SH, Kim JH. Nasal tip plasty using various techniques in rhinoplasty. Aesthet Plast Surg. 2004;28:445–55.
15. Toriumi DM. New concepts in nasal tip contouring. Arch Facial Plast Surg. 2006;8:156–85.
16. Guyuron B, Behman RA. Nasal tip sutures part II: the interplays. Plast Reconstr Surg. 2003;112:1130–45.
17. Gruber RP, Friedman GD. Suture algorithm for the broad or bulbous nasal tip. Plast Reconstr Surg. 2002;110:1752–64.
18. Balaji N. Suture techniques in nasal tip reconstruction. Romanian J Rhinol. 2014;4(14):105–10.
19. Sil A, Ravichandran S, Balaji N. Suture Techniques in posttraumatic nasal tip reconstruction. ENT Audiol News. 2009;18(5):98–102.
20. Paul S. White, Pater D. Ross, Open Structure rhinoplasty. 2nd ed. Tuttlingen: Endo Press GmbH; 2012.
21. Tebbetts JB. Shaping and position the nasal tip without structural disruption: a new, systematic approach. Plast Reconstr Surg. 1994;94:61–77.
22. Akkuzu G, Cakmak O. Primary tip rhinoplasty and suture techniques, in rhinoplasty. Archives.com.
23. Tardy ME Jr, Patt BS, Walter MA. Transdomal suture refinement of the nasal tip: long-term outcomes. Facial Plast Surg. 1993;9:275–84.
24. Gruber RP, Chang E, Buchanan E. Suture techniques in rhinoplasty. Clin Plast Surg. 2010;37(2):231–43.
25. Gruber RP, Weintraub J, Pomerantz J. Suture techniques for the nasal tip. Aesthet Surg J. 2008 Jan-Feb;28(1):92–100.
26. Lo S, Rowe-Jones J. Suture techniques in nasal tip sculpture: current concepts. Laryngol Otol. 2007;121:e10.
27. Gruber RP, Friedman GD. Suture algorithm for the broad and bulbous nasal tip. Plast Reconstr Surg. 2002;110(7):1752–64; discussion: 1765–68.
28. Gunter JP. Secondary rhinoplasty: the open approach. In: Aesthetic plastic surgery rhinoplasty: Boston, Mass Little Brown & Co Inc; 1993. p. 833–47.
29. Gruber RP, Friedman GD. Suture algorithm for the broad or bulbous nasal tip. Plast Reconstr Surg. 2002;110:1752–64.
30. Cardenas JC, Carvajal J, Ruiz A. Securing nasal tip rotation through suspension suture technique. Plast Reconstr Surg. 2006;117(6):1750–5.
31. Park SS. The flaring suture to augment the repair of the dysfunctional nasal valve. Plast Reconst Surg. 1998;101:1120–2.

Grafting Techniques in Nasal Tip Rhinoplasty

Contents

N. Balaji, *Textbook of Nasal Tip Rhinoplasty*, https://doi.org/10.1007/978-3-030-48157-5_9

Learning Objectives
- To overview different grafts and implants available for nasal reconstruction.
- To understand the pros and cons of using different graft materials.
- To learn the indications and surgical techniques of using different grafts both for structural and functional rhinoplasty.

9.1 Introduction

Grafts are used in either primary rhinoplasty or more frequently in secondary rhinoplasty to reconstruct structural defects of the nose and to restore function. Dr. Jack Sheen [1] has been credited as one of the early proponents of the use of various grafts in rhinoplasty. They are an important tool either used alone or in conjunction with sutures [2]. They are also used to camouflage defects which cannot be reconstructed. The purpose of using grafts in the nasal tip region is slightly different from using grafts in the internal nasal valve region or in the mid dorsum or in the septum. Tip grafts are used predominantly for structure than function. Be aware tip is a stable, but mobile structure and any grafting in the tip runs the risk of increasing the stiffness of the nasal tip and causing rigidity to the nasal tip region.

9.1.1 Types of Grafts

There are three major categories of grafts used in structural and reconstructive rhinoplasty.

1. *Structural grafts* – These are used to give structural support and stability to the region.
2. *Functional grafts* – These are used for functional reconstruction to improve nasal valve function, often at the expense of some cosmetic issues, particularly when used in the external valve region.
3. *Camouflage grafts* – These are non-structural and non-functional grafts used to mask or camouflage the defects, which cannot be reconstructed.

9.1.2 Sources of Graft Materials

There are an array of graft materials available, both alloplastic and autologous but in practice, We prefer autologous grafts (patient's own tissues), either fascia (temporalis fascia, fascia lata), cartilage (conchal bowl [3], helical rim, scaphoid fossa of the pinna, or costal cartilage grafts from 6th rib) [4]. The advantages of autologous grafts outweigh the use of alloplastic graft materials (e.g. silastic, gortex, medpore, proplast) in our experience [5, 6]. An array of alloplastic materials are available and used by surgeons as per their preference and outcomes in their own population group with varying success. The author feels that it is outside the scope of this book to discuss the pros and cons of various alloplastic materials, as patients' own tissue is safer as there is no risk of rejection or transmissible infections. But there is a risk of morbidity in harvesting the grafts. Donor site morbidity can cause issues of scarring and donor site deformity. It also adds to the surgical time. The advantages of the alloplastic materials are that they are easily available from the shelf with no donor site morbidity and quicker surgical time. The biggest disadvantage of alloplastic materials is the risk of infection, which in turn can result in scarring, sinus and fistula formation in the overlying skin and can lead to a situation where reconstructive surgery is impossible to achieve any reasonable outcomes, even after removal of the implants [7]. There are also irradiated homologous rib cartilage available and also porcine collagen material which are available "off the shelf" and avoid donor site morbidity and surgical down time of harvesting the grafts. These choices should be discussed with individual patients based on the deformity and the experience of the surgeon and even religious beliefs.

At present, the main sources of grafts in the vast majority of the author's patients are from the ears and to a lesser extent from the costal cartilage. The author rarely considers the use of alloplastic material grafts for the septal reconstruction using thin perforated PDS sheets [8], as long as there is no tear in the septal mucosa. Ear cartilages are pliable and softer than rib cartilages and can conform to the shape of the nose, particularly the dorsum of the nose and can easily integrate with tissues. Costal cartilages are more firmer, may undergo warping and if used in the dorsum may not integrate and may keep moving under the skin, particularly annoying to someone who wears glasses. Costal cartilage grafts are good for septal reconstruction, lateral crural struts, spreader grafts and extended spreader grafts. Conchal bowl ear cartilage grafts are good for soft tissue augmentation for the de-projected dorsum, where it conforms to the convex shape of the nasal dorsum. Fascia lata and temporalis grafts are used in revision surgeries to strengthen a very thin dorsal skin, to help resolve pigmentation of the skin and also helps in wrapping up diced cartilages to give some vascularity and protection. In choosing a graft material, the patient should have an informed choice of all the pros and cons of the materials and the surgeon should choose graft materials which he or she is familiar, with the least risk of complications. The surgeon should also take into account the clinical needs, texture of the overlying skin envelope, previous surgery, ethnic background, religious beliefs, etc.

9.2 Harvesting Conchal Bowl Cartilage

9.2.1 Introduction

Auricular cartilage of the pinna offers a good and reliable source of pliable, yet strong cartilage for augmentation of the nasal defects [9, 10]. Conchal bowl cartilage harvesting from one or both sides is a good and easy source of cartilage harvest for nasal reconstruction in the majority of our patients. Conchal bowl cartilage is our work horse for autologous cartilage grafting in the nose. Structurally it is a versatile graft in most nasal reconstructions involving either a primary or secondary surgery. Generally grafts are used more in secondary revision rhinoplasties than primary procedures.

9.2.2 Indications

- Double-layered conchal graft to camouflage a de-projected nasal dorsum.
- Single-layered conchal graft for reconstructing alar region weakness as a structural batten and also as a functional rim graft. These two grafts can be combined as a single graft unit as well. The graft is usually harvested from the opposite conchal bowl to reconstruct the contralateral ala.
- For replacing or strengthening of the damaged lateral crus as a strut grafts. These are for structural reconstruction to support the lateral nasal valve region and also to rotate the tip down and increase the length of the nose in an over rotated short nose. Again it is advisable to harvest the cartilage from the opposite concha.
- For reconstruction of the columellar sil region to strengthen the medial crus done as a hay stack.
- Pieces of conchal bowl cartilage from the central part of the concha can be used for strengthening the columellar region as well.

9.2.3 Contra-indications

- Patients who do not wish to have conchal graft due to a combination of factors involving anxiety of either scarring or the possibility of change in the shape or position of pinna or the possibility of a floppy pinna. Pre-operative consultation can allay the anxiety.
- Previous use of conchal cartilages with inadequate availability of required amount for grafting.
- Extensive scarring of the pinna either due to trauma.
- Previous pinnaplasty.

9.2.4 Surgical Technique

- Conchal bowl is the deep concave area of the pinna just lateral to the cartilaginous part of the external auditory canal. The root of the helix (crus of the helix) starts at the concha abutting into the conchal bowl dividing them into a slightly larger concave "cavum" concha inferiorly and a smaller concave "cymba" concha superiorly.

- It is advisable to harvest the entire conchal cartilage as a single unit including cavum concha and cymba concha, as partial resection can cause the overlying skin to stick around the cut edges of the cartilage making it visible in the conchal bowl in the post-operative period.
- If however, only a small sliver of conchal cartilage is needed care must be taken to bevel the remaining edges to prevent overlying skin getting stuck to the cut edges of the cartilage, causing a puckered scar.
- The cartilage can be harvested via *anterior approach or posterior approach*.
- Anterior approach is easier for the surgeon, and cartilage area of excision can be precise without the risk of damage to the helical fold and also there is less risk of bleeding through anterior approach [11].
- The anterior approach also offers much better visualisation and hence a larger piece of cartilage can be harvested without the risk of damaging the anatomical structure of the pinna cartilage [12].
- The downside of the anterior approach being the visible scar, although this can be camouflaged in the conchal bowl shadow.
- Posterior approach is slightly more difficult, can bleed more and difficult to identify the margins of cartilage excision from the back. There is a risk of some cosmetic deformity if the anti-helical cartilage fold is breached. The main advantage of posterior approach being the scar hidden behind the pinna.

9.2.5 Surgical (Anterior) Approach (◘ Fig. 9.1a–o)

- Place a cotton wool soaked in Vaseline in the ear canal and tie the hair if it is long.
- Mark the lateral extent of the cartilage excision keeping it just few millimetres medial to the anti-helical fold, so that the scar is camouflaged under the shadow of the anti-helical fold.
- Inject the overlying skin with local anaesthetic of choice, to elevate the skin off the cartilage. We use Xylotox, which is lignocaine with adrenaline.
- Then the skin incision is made along the marked area.
- The skin edges are lifted with two skin hooks and a curved iris dissection scissors used to elevate the skin keeping on the cartilage. Once the skin is lifted a little, the rest of the skin elevation can be done with a wet pledget on an Allis forceps and peel the skin off the conchal cartilage as shown in the ◘ Fig. 9.1j.
- Then the cartilage is incised at the same level using a single deep incision (avoid multiple scores in cartilage) with the edge of the blade angled to bevel the edges of the cut cartilage. Always the cartilage is more thicker than you think. Try to be bold and make a single deeper cut than multiple irregular cuts.
- Once the cartilage is incised, then the posterior skin is elevated with sharp dissection with controlled haemostasis using wide, non-toothed forceps to gently hold the cartilage. Do not hold the cartilage at the margins or use skin hook at the cartilage margins as both of these will frail the cartilage edges.
- Once the posterior skin is free, lift the anterior skin with skin hooks and cut the cartilage starting from the superior end and working down with scissors, being aware that at the root of the helix the cartilage is thicker and triangular and not flat. At this point you may have to use a knife rather than the scissors.
- Take care to bevel the edges of the cartilage margin left behind.
- After excising the cartilage, the anterior skin is rolled back laterally with a Q tip and sutured in place taking care to suture the medial edge of the skin to the skin and cartilage laterally. This is called "differential suturing", as you are suturing one structure on one side (skin flap medially) to more than one structure on the other side (skin and cartilage laterally). We close the skin with absorbable 5-0 Biosyn, so that sutures need not be taken out, as

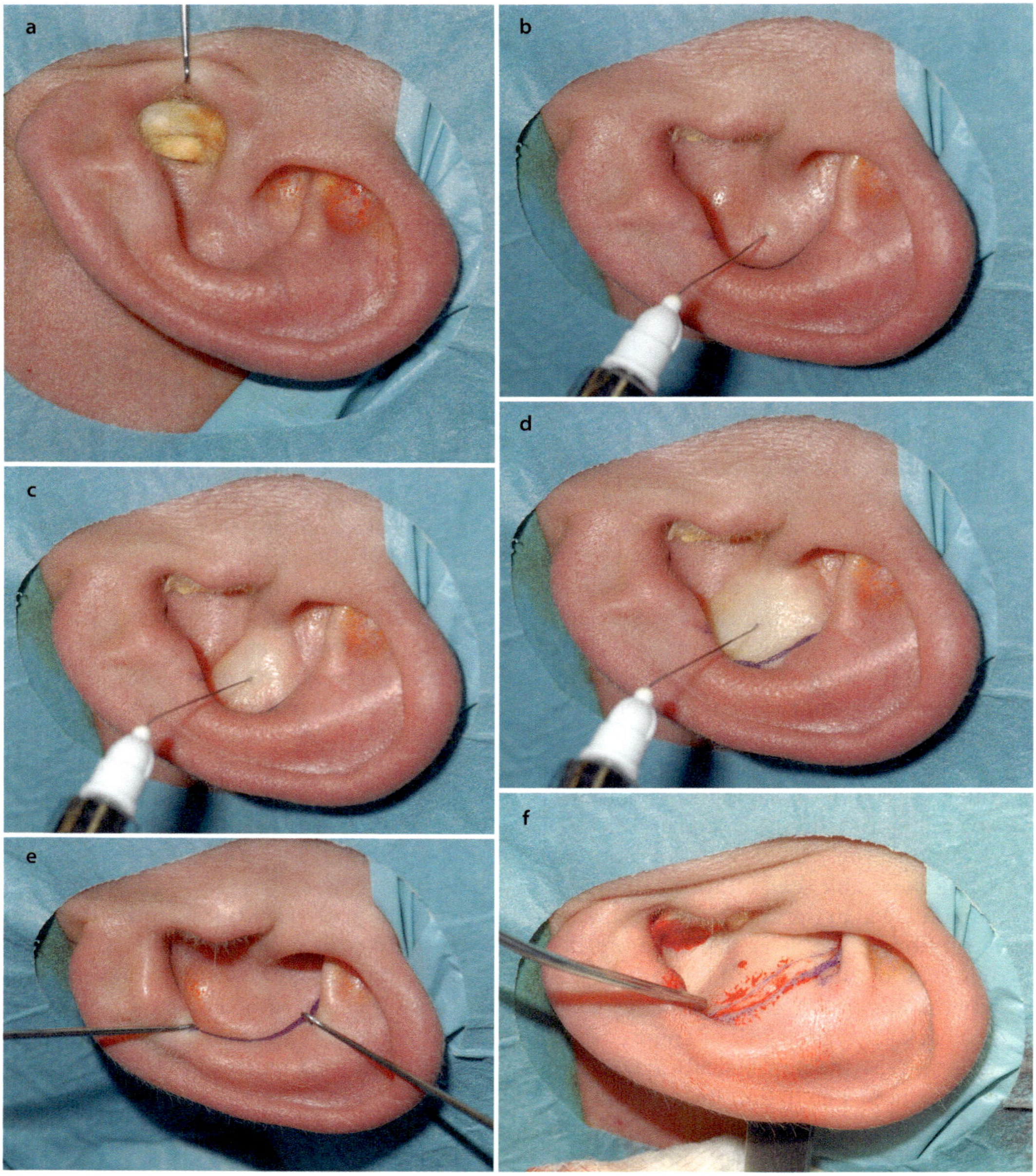

Fig. 9.1 **a–o** Sequential steps in harvesting conchal bowl cartilage from the left pinna by "anterior" approach. **a** Cotton wool in canal. **b–d** Injection technique to lift the skin. **e** Skin incision. **f–i** Skin elevation. **j–m** Dissecting the conchal cartilage out. N-O Replacing the skin flap

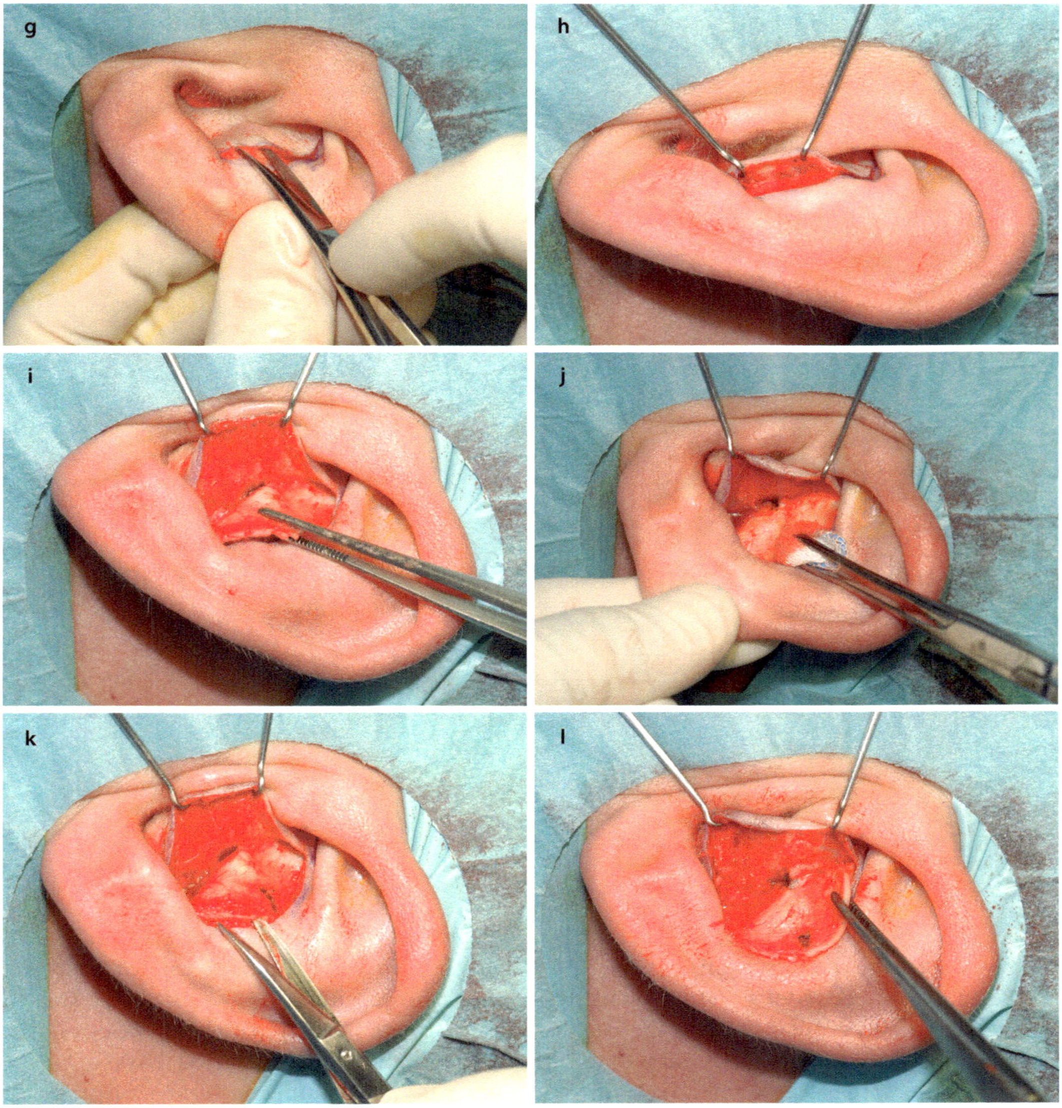

Fig. 9.1 (continued)

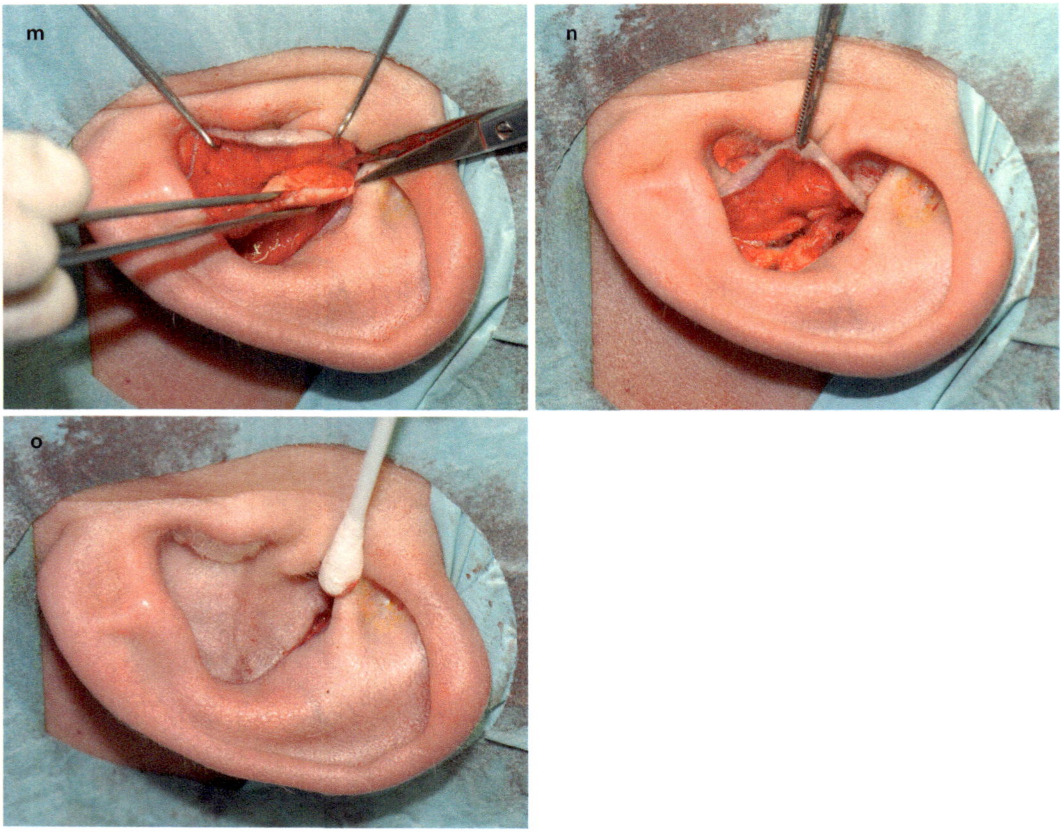

Fig. 9.1 (continued)

removal of sutures in the pinna can be very traumatic to the patient.

- Be aware the vector of pull of the cutaneous scar contracture is towards the meatus and hence by securing the skin to both skin and cartilage composite laterally, it will resist the forces of contraction and will avoid scar migration to the centre of the conchal bowl, which may be a major issue in the post-operative healing stages.
- There is no need to make stabs in the anterior skin for drainage as long as the haemostasis is secured and a pressure dressing is applied. These stabs can result in multiple pigmentations and scarring. Proflavin-soaked cotton ball and pressure dressing is applied to the pinna for 12 hours. By following this regime, we have had only one pinna haematoma done through anterior approach in over 500 patients needing conchal grafting.

The *posterior approach* involves the same technique, except the margins of cartilage excision are identified anteriorly with a needle soaked in methylene blue so that the markings in the cartilage are visible from the back once the skin is lifted. The only advantage of posterior approach is the absence of a scar anteriorly, but it runs the risk of damaging the anti-helical fold, if not careful.

9.2.6 Shaping and Designing the Grafts

- Once the full conchal bowl graft is removed, the dimensions of the graft in an adult Caucasian male would be around 3 cm in vertical direction (length) and just less than 2 cm at the widest point. Remember, if this graft is going to be used to augment the dorsum of the nose, the average length in an adult Caucasian nose needed to be augmented will be around 4 cm, so may have to stagger two layers of cartilage lengthwise and secure them together. Hence a two-layered cartilage graft is preferable. In an Asian nose, the length needed may be less, but at the same time the size of the conchal bowl is also less, hence the same principle applies in an Asian nose as well.

- The graft may be shaped in many ways depending on the requirements. We tend to shape it in two ways which fulfil most of our requirements.
- One way is to split the conchal graft into three segments along lengthwise, without wasting any pieces of cartilage. The central as bit shown in ◘ Fig. 9.2b is used for columellar strut or shield graft, and the other two pieces are used, smaller one below the bigger larger piece for dorsal boat graft augmentation.
- Another way of shaping the conchal graft is shown above (◘ Fig. 9.2c) where again the superior and inferior portion is used for double-layered dorsal grafts and the middle bit used for the columella and infra-tip lobule for a columellar strut and a shield graft.
- In patients needing reconstruction of smooth nasal sil region to establish the slant of the sil region, we can use the natural curvature of the conchal bowl cartilage to re-establish the sil region as shown in (◘ Fig. 9.3a–f). The root of the helix creates a convex elevation anteriorly in the conchal bowl (◘ Fig. 9.1a), separating the conchal bowl cartilage into a smaller concave superior cavum concha and a larger concave inferior cymbha concha. The whole conchal bowl cartilage is harvested and split horizontally at the convexity caused by the origin of the root of the helix into two separate concave units (◘ Fig. 9.3b). These units of concave cartilage are then reduced in width to the required measurements (◘ Fig. 9.3f) usually 4–5 mm width and up to 8 mm height and sutured to the remains of the medial crural footplate and to each other, leaving the other end to spring naturally away from each other, looking like a haystack (◘ Fig. 9.3e). This wider area can be anchored on either side of the anterior nasal spine, thus recreating and reconstructing the sil region and also supporting the columella and increasing the length of the columella. This technique provides an alternative tool for increasing tip projection, apart from strengthening the medial crus with a septal extension graft or a free columellar strut. The *main advantage of this technique* is that it not only increases the columellar length and provides tip support, but also establishes a pleasing smooth, concave nasal sil region with preservation of the anatomical thirds of the nasal base. The only downside being a slightly wider columella. The natural curvature of the conchal bowl cartilage is used to re-establish the sil region.
- Thus, there are many ways of designing the conchal bowl grafts without wastage and used for various reconstructions. Hence forward planning is necessary.
- If used as double-layered grafts, always take care while securing two pieces of cartilage graft together. Two graft pieces can be secured with sutures or using tissue glue (always check the local guidelines before using any tissue glue). If tissue glue is used always wash away the excess in saline and the graft dipped in a broad-spectrum antibiotic solution.
- If sutures are used to secure two layers, be careful not to shatter or fray the cartilage and not tighten the sutures very much. The advantage of the suture is to thread it through the overlying skin and help to stabilise the graft in the required position.
- Also make sure the edges of the graft and also the edges of cartilage left behind in the patient must be bevelled to avoid sharp edges of the graft showing through the overlying skin. The cartilage is subject to slipping and some mobility, hence should be secured in a tight pocket.

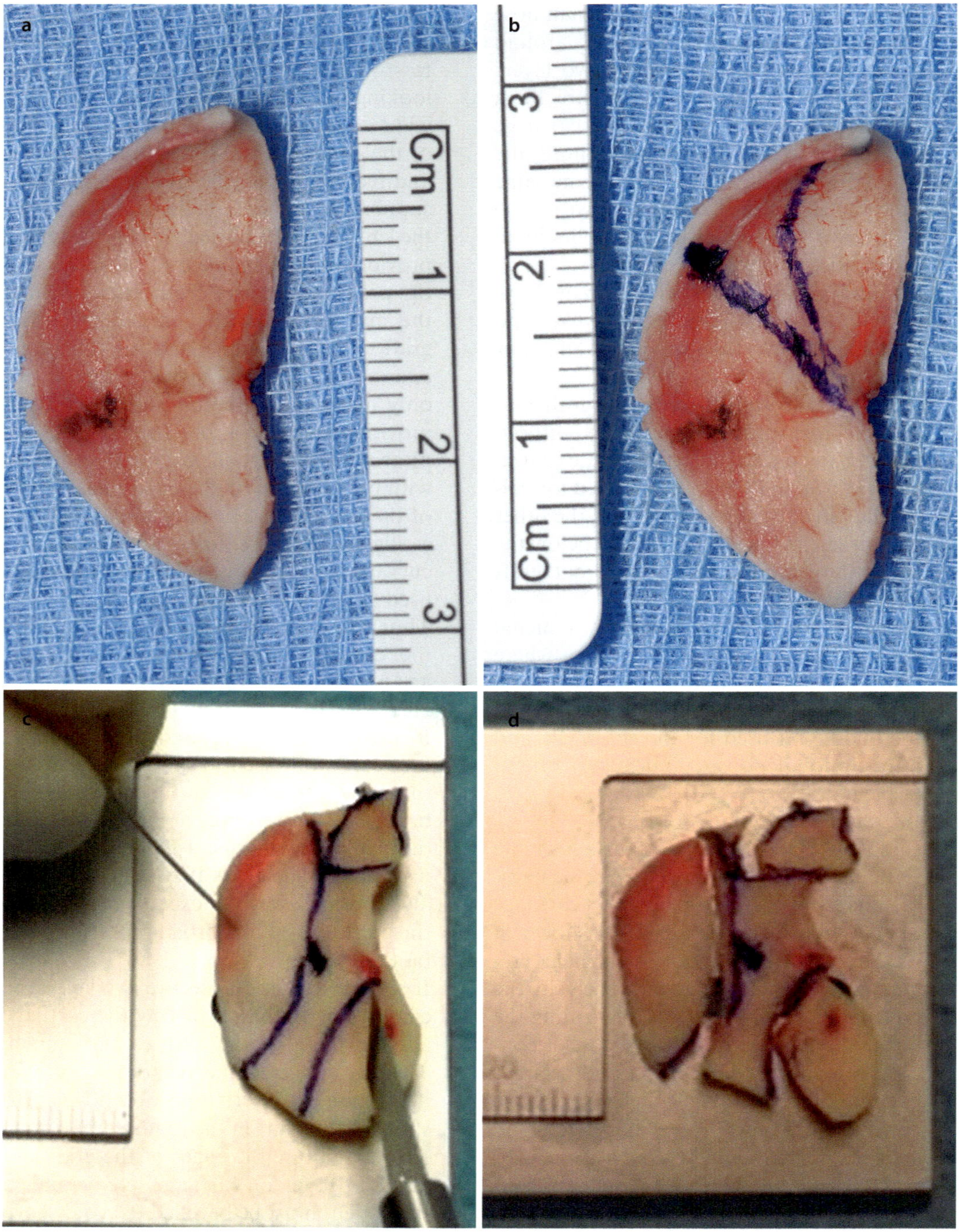

Fig. 9.2 **a–d** Designing the harvested conchal bowl cartilage. **a** The dimensions of the conchal bowl cartilage. **b** Splitting the conchal graft into three segments. **c, d** Splitting the conchal graft into four segments

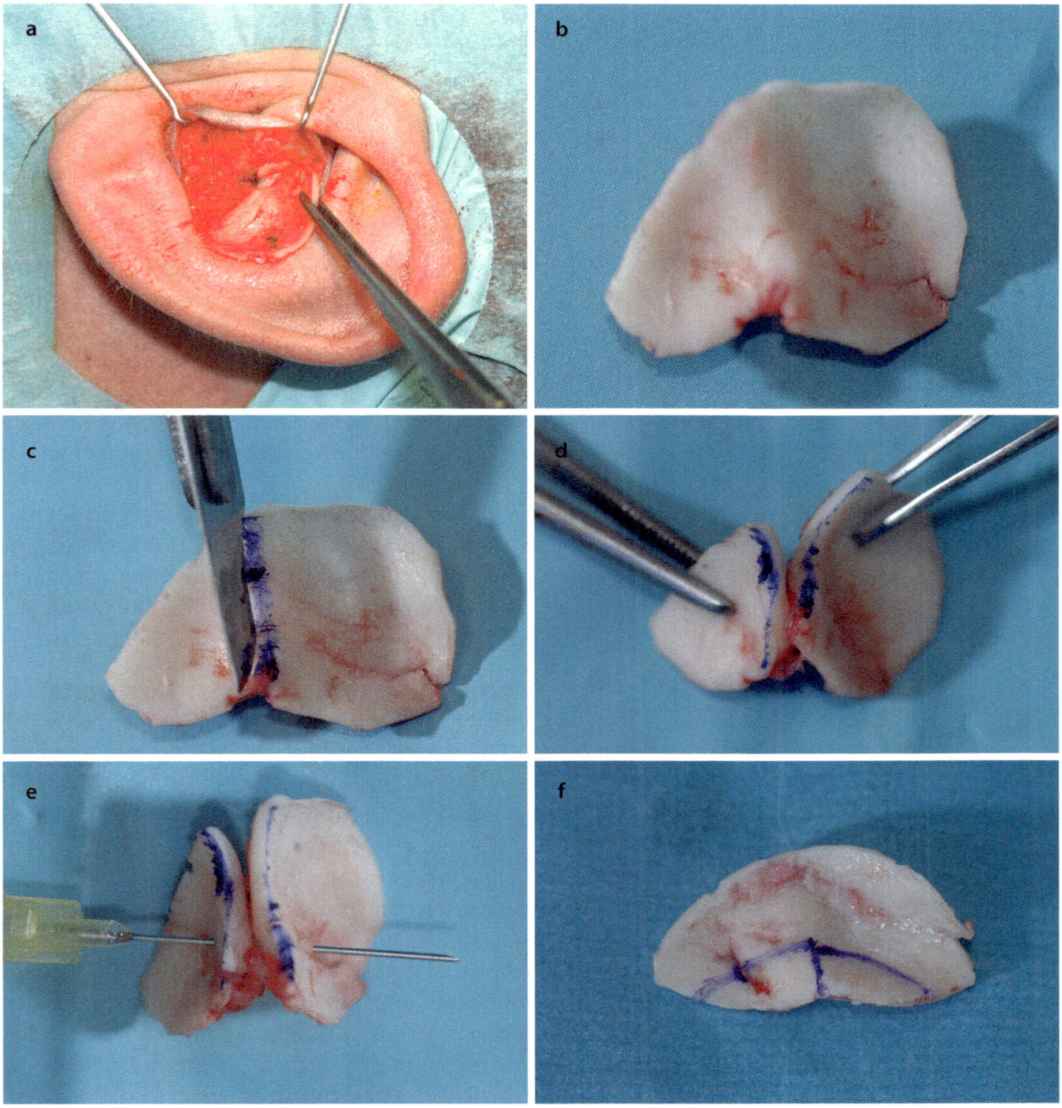

Fig. 9.3 **a**–**f** Shaping the conchal bowl cartilage for reconstructing the medial crus. **a** Harvesting conchal bowl cartilage. **b** Conchal cartilage showing two concavities and a convexity. **c** Incision on the convexity. **d** Split conchal cartilage. **e** How to use them as a "hay-stack" for medial crural grafting. **f** The dimensions for medial crural grafting

Key Points

- Try and take the cartilage in a single piece without shattering, so that it can be shaped based on the surgical requirements.
- Once harvested, take a bit of time to think and plan the design of the grafts as per the surgical needs.
- Do not waste any cartilage. Anything left behind can be used as a diced or crushed cartilage.
- To reconstruct a lateral alar region with either a lateral crural strut or batten on one side, it is wise to harvest from the opposite conchal bowl.
- The edges of the cartilage should be bevelled to prevent any sharp edges.
- If posterior approach is used be extremely careful NOT to damage the anti-helical fold, by marking it with methylene blue-soaked needle.

- In our experience, pressure dressing for 12 hours is more useful than using multiple stab wounds and stitching a piece of gauze which does not help and also cause some pigmented scarring at the stab sites.
- Be aware that there are reported incidences of keloid formation at the scar site. This risk should be discussed with the patient, particularly while doing the anterior approach [13].
- Fine tissue handling of cartilage without causing damage to the edges of the cartilage with skin hooks or toothed forceps is vital.

Conclusion

- In conclusion, conchal cartilage is a good source of pliable autologous material and if taken from both ears will suffice for most nasal reconstructions.

9.3 Harvesting Helical Rim Graft

9.3.1 Introduction

Helix of the ear is another good source of cartilage graft without changing or damaging the helical rim anatomy. The advantage of helical rim graft would be to get a soft, pliable cartilage graft which can be used either as a functional graft or as a folded double-layered structural graft.

Helical rim is a nice anatomical area for auricular cartilage harvest, when all the sources of grafts have been exhausted particularly in multiple revision surgeries. It can be very time-consuming and may need harvesting on both sides. The only disadvantage being the graft is quite thin and not a lot of material can be harvested. Nevertheless, it is a useful graft to keep up your sleeve when required [14].

As far as I am aware, it is not very well reported in the literature.

9.3.2 Indications

- Can be used as a spreader graft for functional reasons.
- Can be used as a folded piece of double-layered cartilage or two helical rim grafts can be sutured together and then used as structural grafts for caudal septal extensions.
- Can be used as a single piece to achieve a smooth dorsum to buffer the dorsum after hump removal, similar to the use of crushed septal cartilage (CATS) grafts.
- Can also be used to reconstruct the "SIL" and columella when used as two separate grafts on either side of the columella as a "hay stack".
- Can also be used as double layer, to act as a Batten graft or as a strut graft for strengthening the lateral crus, although a single layer will be too soft for this purpose.

9.3.3 Anatomical Considerations

The lateral aspect of the most projecting part of the pinna is the helical fold, and this fold forms the lateral most boundary of the helix. The area to harvest the helical graft is in this superior-lateral aspect of the helix, just medial to the folded helical margin and tucked away just under the helical fold. This area of helix is slightly concave and also pliable and smooth, the only disadvantage being it can be very thin. The harvesting area is limited to the area of "scapha" of pinna between the helical rim and the anti-helical fold. This area roughly looks like a triangle, but in practice a rectangular piece of cartilage (Fig. 9.4) can be safely harvested without causing any damage to the helical fold. The upper extent of the anti-helical fold divides into a superior and inferior fork forming the navicular fossa in between. This navicular fossa will form the medial boundary of the scapha of the pinna. The graft is harvested lateral to the superior rim of the anti-helical fold, staying lateral to the navicular fossa and staying medial to the helical rim margin, taking care not to damage either the helical rim or the anti-helical fold.

9.3.4 Surgical Technique: Harvesting the Graft (Posterior Approach) (Fig. 9.5a–i)

- The graft has to be removed through a posterior approach only, keeping the scar in the back. Unlike conchal bowl harvest, an anterior approach is not advisable, as the scar cannot be hidden.
- First mark the area of the cartilage excision in the "scaphoid" fossa of the pinna on the anterior aspect. Make sure this is not involving the helical or anti-helical fold of pinna, to avoid unnecessary damage to the cartilage.
- The margins of the graft are marked on the lateral superior aspect of the pinna based on the anatomical knowledge as mentioned above. This is done from the front of the pinna, so that the desired length and width of cartilage can be removed, without causing a cosmetic deformity of the pinna.
- The access to the superior most part of the scapha can be gained by lifting the hood of the helical fold by skin hooks. Since the exposure is from the back of the pinna, to identify the cartilage borders to be excised, the excision margin is marked out from the anterior aspect of the pinna, (to avoid damage to the anti-helical convexity), with a needle dipped in methylene blue as shown in Fig. 9.5a.
- Now inject and hydro-dissect the anterior skin of the marked area with a local anaesthetic of your choice. This step will help in dissecting the cartilage "off" the skin without damaging the overlying skin.
- After this, a longitudinal incision is made in the back of the pinna overlying the cartilage area to be excised, so that the scar is not visible from the front. A single curved incision is made in the posterior aspect of pinna in the middle of the markings, taking care not to come too close to the free border of pinna. This is to avoid any localised deformities of the contour margins of the pinna.
- The skin is dissected away from the underlying cartilage and methylene blue mark-

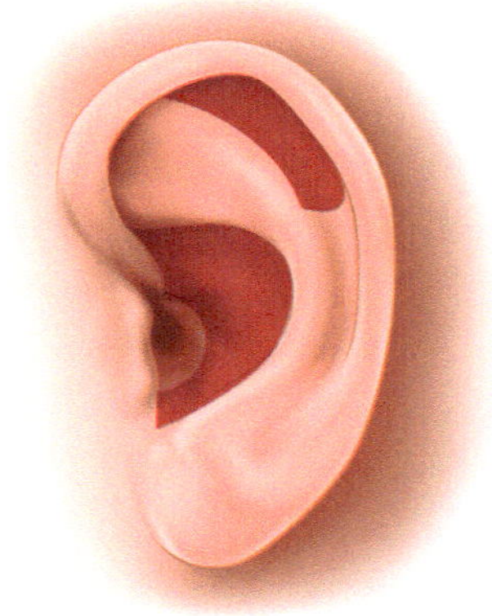

Fig. 9.4 Schematic representation of the left pinna showing the two shaded areas with the navicular fossa in between. The upper shaded area below the helical fold is the "scapha" of the pinna where helical rim cartilage is harvested. The lower shaded area is the conchal bowl of the pinna

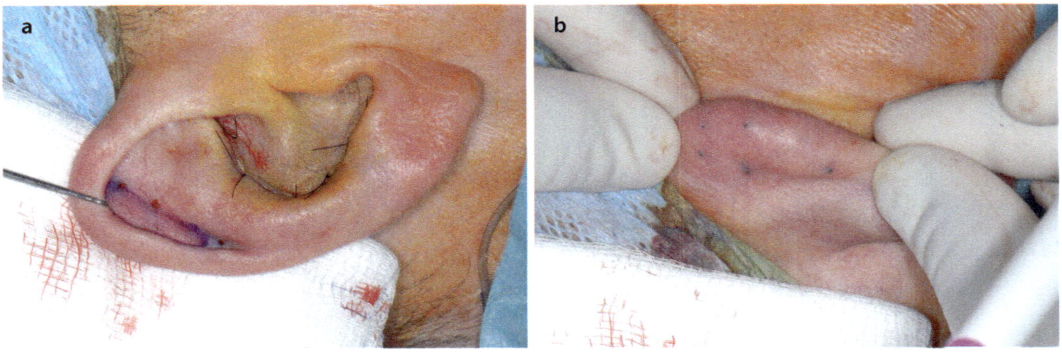

Fig. 9.5 a–i Sequential steps in harvesting helical rim cartilage from the right pinna through a "posterior" approach

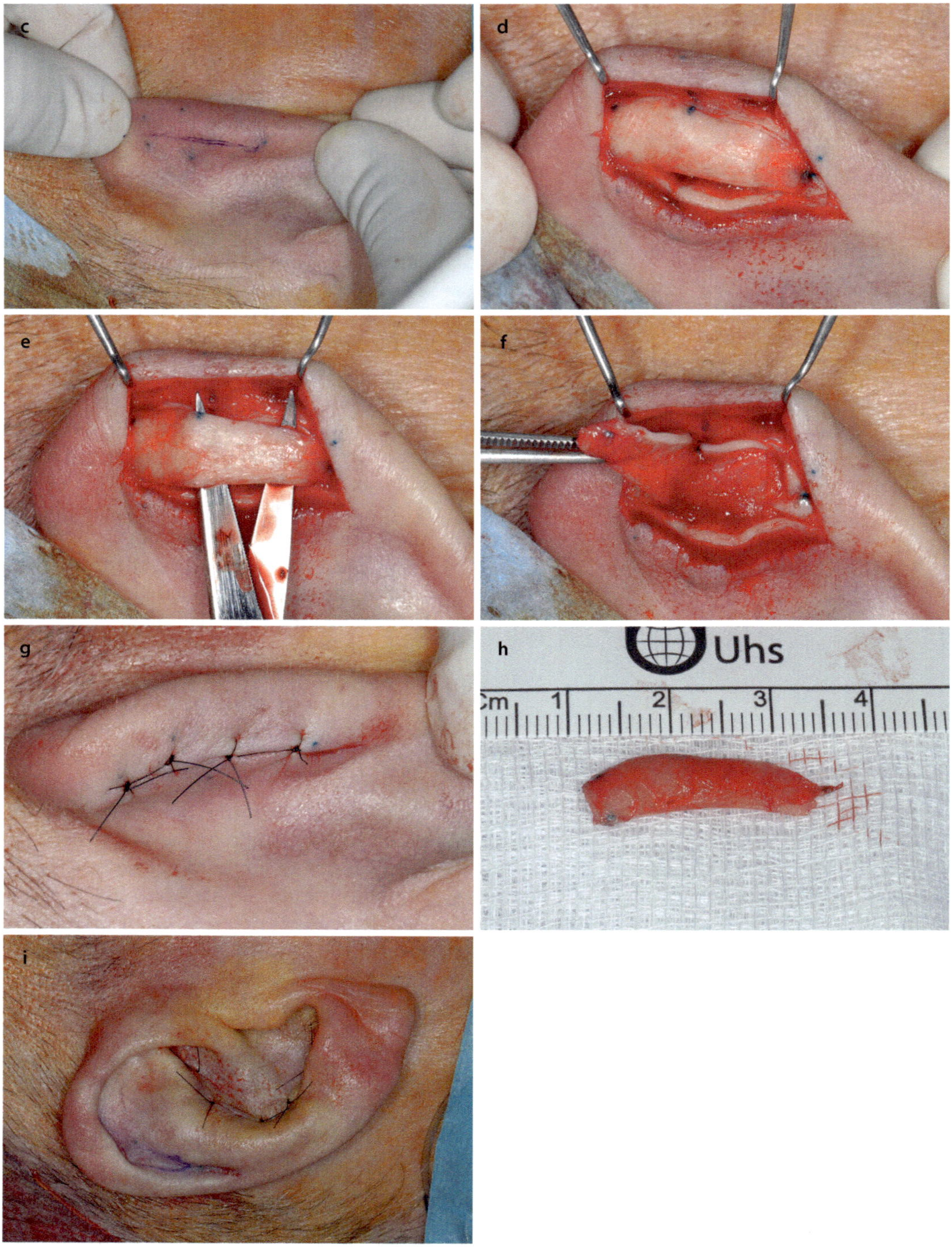

9

■ **Fig. 9.5** (continued)

ings at the margins of cartilage to be excised are exposed.
- The cartilage is then incised along the length of the graft running in parallel. Then with a curved scissors, the anterior skin is lifted (initial injection of the local anaesthetic to the anterior skin will help in lifting the skin), taking care not to injure the anterior skin. I have button holed once only in an international meeting live surgery! (If you button hole the anterior skin, nothing lost, as this may act as a drain).
- Once the anterior skin is elevated along the entire segment of the cartilage to be excised, then with a curved scissors the superior and inferior margins are released in a curvy fashion contouring to the shape of the helical rim as shown in ◘ Fig. 9.5e.
- Then the superior and inferior incision is made and the cartilage graft is freed and stored in saline.
- It is preferable to use absorbable sutures like 5-0 Biosyn for skin, as it can be very difficult to remove sutures in the post-operative period.
- The skin is closed gently taking care to take the bite just at the edge and not to bunch up the skin which again can cause a contour deformity of the pinna.
- Please note, only the skin is approximated and NOT the cut cartilage edges.
- Usually after removing the helical cartilage, there is more bruising and discolouration seen anteriorly over the helical rim than a conchal bowl cartilage harvest. Patient should be well counselled regarding this as it may take few weeks to settle.
- Apply pressure bandage for 12 hours in the post-operative period.
- In our unit we routinely give acyclovir 200 mg five times a day for 5 days in the post-operative period, as for some reason there is reactivation of herpes simplex virus in patients needing helical rim graft rather than with conchal bowl harvest. We have seen it in many patients to be a coincidence.

9.3.5 Shaping and Designing the Grafts

- The harvested graft size is usually around 25 mm × 8 mm (depending on the size of the pinna) and is rectangular in shape and the cartilage is slightly concave on one side and convex on the other with the thickness around 2–3 mm, which is more softer than the conchal or septal cartilage.
- Folding the cartilage lengthwise or width wise gives strength by using a double layer.
- It can be used as a folded piece by partially incising the cartilage.
- It can be folded in the middle *length wise* where the length of the cartilage is preserved with added strength, which then can be used for columella or septal extension grafts.
- It can also be folded in the middle *width wise* where you will be able to get a smaller length but a double stronger piece, which then can be used for spreader or strut grafts or batten grafts.
- Similarly, two helical rims from both ears can be added together to get both length and strength.

Key Points

- Not an easy technique to master. Can be very footery.
- Use skin hooks and take care not to damage the skin edges.
- Make sure the excision lines are clearly marked in the cartilage so that they are visible from the back.
- Try and take the cartilage in a single piece, so that it can be shaped based on the requirements.
- Try to hydro-dissect the overlying skin, which will help in elevating the skin without damage.
- Take extreme care NOT to damage the helical or anti-helical fold margins.
- For some reason, there is a risk of reactivation of herpes simplex virus with helical rim graft harvest. Hence, we give

acyclovir in these patients for 5 days in the post-operative period.
- Patient should be counselled that the site where the graft has been harvested will be bruised and discoloured for few weeks, visible from the front.

Conclusion
- In conclusion, helical rim cartilage is a good source of pliable autologous material and if taken from both ears can be used for a variety of reconstructive options as mentioned above.
- They are an easy and alternative source of nasal grafts, particularly in multiple revision surgeries where it is more likely the conchal cartilages are already harvested and used rather than the helical rim.

9.4 Harvesting Fascia Lata Graft

9.4.1 Introduction

Fascia lata graft is a tough layer of soft pliable membranous graft material, which can be versatile in its use particularly in revision procedures to cover small blemishes in the bony cartilaginous framework, which cannot be satisfactorily corrected. It is also very helpful in revision surgeries where the overlying skin is very thin and discoloured and helps in the vascularity of the overlying skin. Temporalis fascia [15, 16] and temporo-parietal fascia can also be used [17]. Based on our personal experience, fascia lata is a better option than temporalis fascia as it is tougher and available in plenty to harvest. The only down side being a scar in the thigh. Fascia lata is the membranous deep fascia of the thigh which is thicker and tougher than the temporalis fascia and is located in the thigh and gluteal region encircling the thigh muscles. This fascia is there in abundance and is a useful source of graft material in secondary and also in some cases of primary rhinoplasty. Beware, that tensor fascia lata is a deeper muscle and should not be confused with the superficial fascia lata. Although these are not used for structural reconstructions, they are good for covering minor irregularities of the dorsum, small volume augmentations and also as a means of adding thickness to the flap in patients with thin skin envelope. We have been using more and more of the fascia lata grafts in revision procedures particularly with skin changes to smoothen the nasal dorsum and we are finding more indications to use this graft, as we come across more complex nasal deformities needing revision surgery.

9.4.2 Indications

- Ideally indicated in revision rhinoplasty procedures as an adjunct to cartilage grafts to camouflage small dorsal irregularities [18, 19].
- Ideally in revision rhinoplasty patients with very thin overlying skin with hyperaemic skin changes to cushion the skin and improve the vascularity (Fig. 9.6a–c).
- Thin skin with irregular dorsum with tiny cartilage blemishes (Fig. 9.6d).
- As a sole procedure in correcting the cosmetic deformity of mid- dorsal deprojection (dorsal augmentation) in patients with active vasculitis with granulomatosis where major reconstructive procedures are contra-indicated and may be more likely to fail as well. In these group of patients, the use of fascia lata graft through a simple dorsal tunnelling is easier, quicker with better outcomes even if they have active disease where reconstructive surgery is contra-indicated. This procedure all be it, not a reconstructive one, can still be very uplifting mentally for a patient with extensive dorsal collapse.
- For cosmetic nasal dorsal camouflage, in patients with very large septal perforation causing dorsal de-projection.
- For nasion/radix augmentation, small pieces of rolled up fascia lata grafts can be used for selectively augmenting the nasion. In this situation either done alone or in conjunction with a rhinoplasty, the use of fascia lata offers an added advantage of giving a smoother and softer nasion, where glasses can rest smoothly.

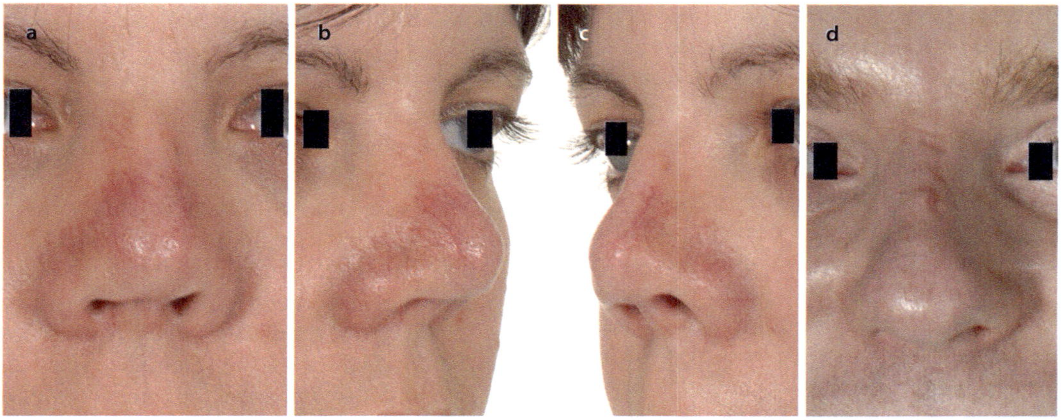

Fig. 9.6 **a–c** Erythematous skin over the dorsum after revision surgery. **d** Thin irregular skin over the dorsum

- Fascia lata can also be sued to create a pocket for diced cartilages for augmentation of the dorsum, the so-called Turkish delight [20, 21].
- Can also be used in between layers of cartilage grafts if multiple layers of cartilage grafts are needed to augment the dorsum to prevent cartilage grafts sliding on each other.

9.4.3 Contra-indications

- Patient's wishes to avoid a scar in the thigh.
- Patient on anticoagulants, as there is a high risk of deep space haematoma.
- Neuralgia of the thigh with sensory issues.

9.4.4 Designing the Graft

- As a single-layered graft for the nasal dorsal and side walls camouflage to cover the blemishes after dorsal bony hump reduction to prevent irregular bony edges felt through the overlying skin. The advantage of this graft over crushed septal cartilage is that this graft is smooth and can be draped over the entire dorsum and side wall of the nose to smoothen defects over a larger area, whereas the crushed cartilage graft may not be enough to cover a larger area.
- Parallel-layered sheeting (just like steri-strips for the outside), particularly for the dorsal cushioning.
- As multiple small pieces, particularly for the nasion augmentation in low radix. It is used as small pieces ((5 mm × 5 mm) of multi-layered fascia lata graft, particularly for augmenting the nasion in a low radix as an isolated procedure. If it is multiple-layered folded graft for the nasion, it will be nice to dry the graft over a metal cup with hot water underneath. A dried graft can be folded easily into layers and more user friendly and not slippery due to the underlying fat globules.
- Can be used as a rolled multi-layered fascia lata graft for augmenting the nasion in a low radix.
- Can also be used as a rolled, tubed cylinder with crushed cartilages inside and augment a de-projected nasal dorsum, the so-called Turkish delight. The advantage of this being the crushed cartilage can confirm smoothly to the contours of the dorsum inside this fascia envelop making the graft soft and pliable and give a more cosmetically acceptable dorsum.
- Can be used as a "moist" or a "dry" graft. We prefer to use multiple small pieces of moist graft for the nasion and use dried fascia lata graft layers for the dorsal reconstruction.
- In patients with active polyangitis with granulomatosis causing dorsal de-projection due to loss of cartilage, complex reconstruction with cartilage is not advisable. Fascia lata graft can be used to

address the nasal dorsal de-projection in these patients with active disease. These group of patients usually have septal perforation superiorly, and they do not have intact septal cartilage above the perforation for a mid-dorsal reconstruction with spreader. Moreover, these patients often end up with a dorsal graft which is mobile and does not integrate with the dorsal tissues. So a good alternative in these patients is to use multi-layered fascia lata graft instead, inserted through a small stab incision at the anterior septal angle, by deflecting the conjoined medial crus away from the midline. This is a fantastic option, in patients with active disease requesting surgery for short-term minimalistic outcomes. The long-term stability of this graft is also quite acceptable in patients with active polyangiitis. In this situation it is usually wise to cut the graft into small pieces of 2 cm by 1 cm and roll them with the muscular side facing outside to prevent fat side slipping. The advantages being that the multiple small pieces of fascia lata graft are less likely to slide out when pressure is applied to the dorsal skin, and many pieces can be used separately and manipulated separately along the dorsal line to achieve the desired cosmetic effect. Even if one or two pieces slide out through the incision lines, they can be easily removed, without affecting the outcome of the procedure.

9.4.5 Surgical Technique (Fig. 9.7a–i)

- The amount of fascia lata required for use in rhinoplasty is usually a rectangular piece around 4 cm by 2 cm.
- The fascia lata graft is taken from the thigh on the lateral aspect along a line extending from the greater trochanter to the lateral aspect of the knee. The fascia lata is harvested about 2 cm in front of this line at the upper third of the thigh. The incision is about 2–3 cm long and made around 8–10 cm below the greater trochanter of the femur. It can also be done through multiple small stab incisions if a bigger piece is needed. By staying around 8–10 cm below the trochanter, injury to the superficial branches of the lateral cutaneous nerve of the thigh is avoided. This is a purely sensory nerve which can cause mononeuropathy and neuralgia if damaged. Avoid making the incision very high close to the iliac crest due to cosmetic reasons.
- Imagine the thigh as a cylindrical structure divided into four quadrants, the graft should be harvested in the antero-lateral quadrant of the thigh. This is because of ease of working against bulging convexity of the thigh muscles.
- Once the skin incision is made, there is usually a thick layer of fat before you reach the fascia. The fat should be dissected and a long self-retaining retractor can be used to keep the fat away to the sides.

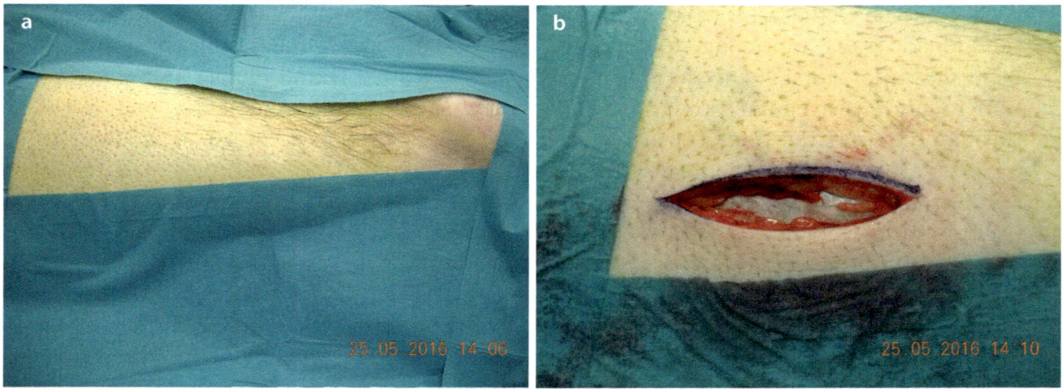

Fig. 9.7 **a–i** Sequential steps in harvesting fascia lata graft from the right thigh

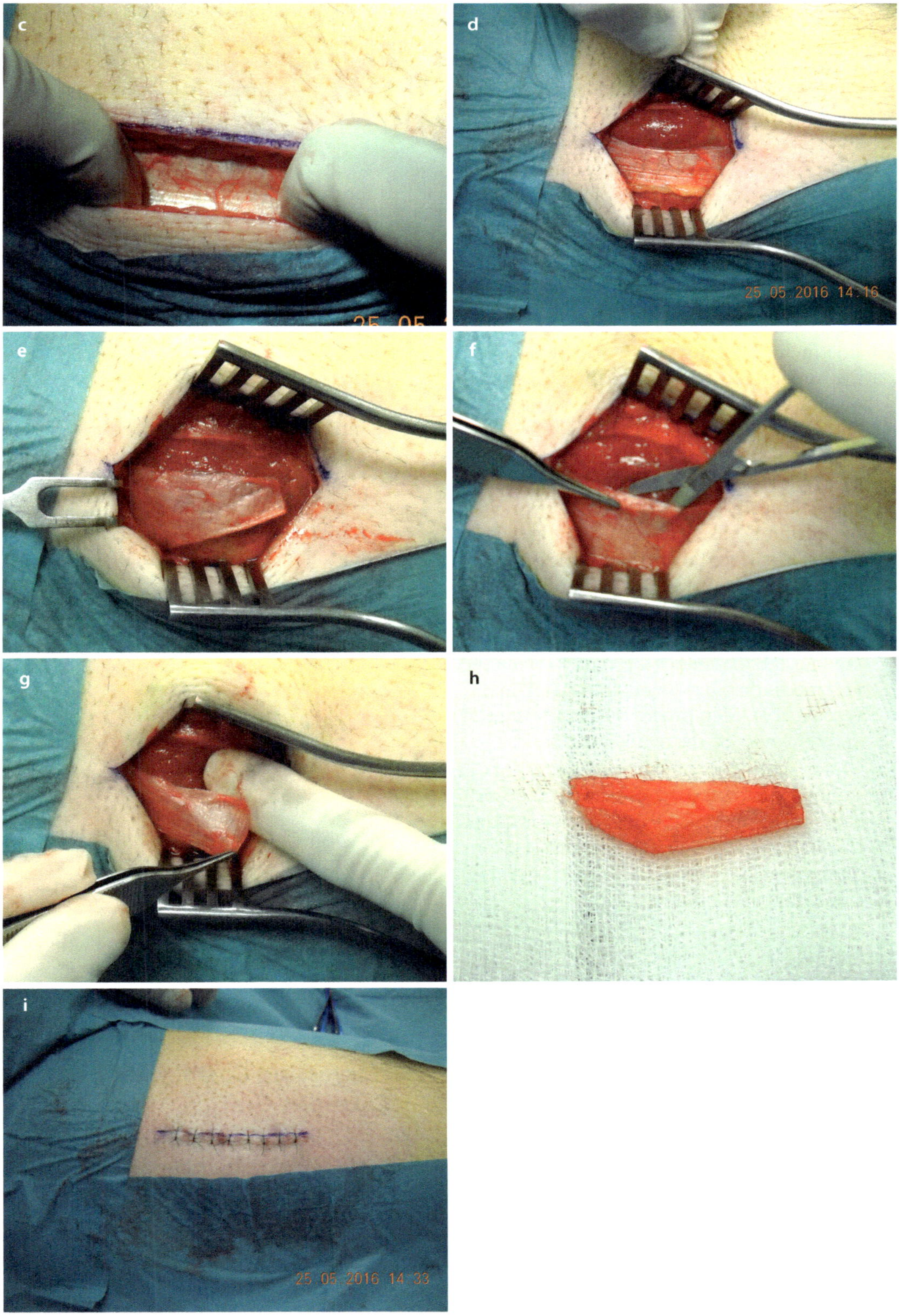

Fig. 9.7 (continued)

- Once the required amount of fascia lata is exposed, usually a rectangular piece with length wise running along the vertical direction of the thigh, make two incisions along the greater length of the rectangle about 4 cm long. Then a curved dissecting scissors is used to lift the fascia from the underlying muscles. Finally make two incisions on either side and remove the fascia. The bleeding is controlled and the thigh incision closed in layers with or without a corrugated drain.
- The fascia lata has two sides, the deeper side facing the muscle is non-slippery and the superficial side facing the subcutaneous fat is slippery.
- Once the fascia is off the thigh, it is stretched out on a metal cup and allowed to dry for ease of use. There is no difference clinically whether used dry or wet, but certainly easier to use if it is dry.
- The deep surface facing the muscle is usually laid on the nasal skeleton facing the osseo-cartilaginous framework and the superficial layer of the fascia lata overlying the subcutaneous fat goes under the skin. Leaving the fat side under the dorsal skin helps in the vascularity and improves the discolouration and thickness of the overlying skin.
- Make sure too much overlying fat is thinned meticulously, otherwise the graft can be slippery, particularly sprouting through the edges of the various incisions lines when pressure is applied to the dorsum while using the nasal splints.

Key Points

- Harvesting fascia lata graft is fairly simple. Beware there is lot of fat before you reach the fascia. Large self-retaining retractors are helpful in the procedure.
- Make sure the thigh incision is in the right place to avoid injury to the lateral cutaneous nerve.
- Once the graft is applied, be careful to suture all the muco-cutaneous incisions closely; otherwise, a gentle pressure over the dorsum will squeeze the graft through even a small opening.
- Make sure the excess underlying fat is carefully removed as much as possible, otherwise the graft can slip out particularly, when pressure is applied to the dorsum in an open approach.
- If securing the graft as a single layer, it is advisable to lay down the graft over the dorsum by making sure the graft is well spread out under the skin and not rolled at the edges. If used as a single sheet make some perforations in the graft which allows drainage of tissue fluid.
- If it is multiple-layered folded graft for the nasion, it will be nice to dry the graft over a metal cup with hot water underneath. A dried graft can be folded easily into layers and more user friendly and not slippery due to the fat globules.
- Make sure adequate haemostasis in the thigh, before closure. Avoid unnecessary damage to underlying muscles while dissecting the fascia off the muscle. A pressure dressing applied overnight helps.

Conclusion

Fascia lata graft is a tough layer of soft pliable membranous graft material, which can be versatile in its use particularly in revision procedures to cover small blemishes in the bony cartilaginous framework, which cannot be satisfactorily corrected. It is also very helpful in revision surgeries where the overlying skin is very thin and discoloured and helps in the vascularity of the overlying skin.

9.5 Harvesting Costal (Rib) Cartilage Graft

9.5.1 Introduction

Costal cartilage graft from the rib cage is an abundant and good source of graft material for reconstructing major deformities of the nose requiring lots of cartilage. For a nasal surgeon, knowing the surface anatomy of the rib cage can be confusing in the beginning, but it is easier to harvest with no major issues. Be aware that this is a tough material and cause warping and hence constantly changing. We prefer harvesting sixth rib cartilage. Although there is plenty of cartilage available, and considered as a first choice for severe saddle nose [22, 23], this is not the author's preferred choice for reconstruction until otherwise there is no other option. We have seen more post-operative issues with costal cartilage grafting than ear cartilage grafts. The costal cartilage is firmer and good for septal reconstructions, but when used for dorsal augmentation can cause sharp edges, unacceptable stiffness, ("frozen nose") [24] high visibility, not integrating with underlying soft tissues and resulting in mobility of the graft under the dorsal skin, which can be very annoying after a good augmentation. Patients do not like the mobility of the graft particularly when they wear glasses. It is sometimes wiser to avoid these side effects even if the augmentation is sub-optimal with other methods of grafting. There is a donor site morbidity and risk of damage to the underlying lung and also external scar over the chest. Some patients develop long-term neuralgia of the intercostal nerves. As mentioned, it is definitely a good source of cartilage and can be done quicker than taking multiple conchal and helical rim cartilages to get the same amount of cartilage. The thickness of the external skin should also be taken into account while using rib cartilage to avoid any unnecessary sharp edges showing through. Each patient should be assessed after thorough discussion of the pros and cons of different graft materials [25]. We prefer to use both helical and both conchal cartilages (◘ Fig. 9.8) as a first choice in reconstructing a collapsed dorsum rather than rib cartilage for the above reasons. In our unit, we use rib graft only in less than 5% of the patients, virtually limiting the procedure only to septal reconstructions and not for the dorsum. This is based on our personal experience, and this will vary with the experience of different surgeons and different population groups.

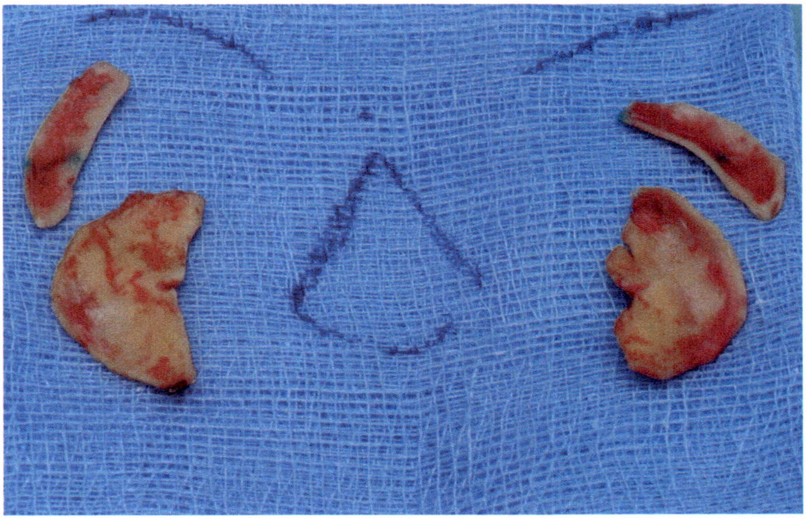

◘ **Fig. 9.8** Showing the extent of cartilage volume that can be harvetsed from conchal and helical parts of the pinna for dorsal nasal augmentation

9.5.2 Indications

- Dorsal augmentation in patients with severe dorsal collapse.
- Good for septal reconstructions.
- Can be used as a spreader graft for functional reasons.
- Can be used as a structural graft for caudal septal extensions and dorsal septal extension.
- Can be used for lateral crural struts and batten.
- In revision surgeries when all the other sources of cartilage harvest are exhausted.

9.5.3 Surface Anatomy

It is preferable to use the anterior costal cartilage of the sixth rib. A mental picture of the surface anatomy of the rib cartilage is essential. Most nasal surgeons starting to do this operation feel uncomfortable due to lack of knowledge on surface anatomy of the rib cage. Once the surgeon understands the surface anatomy of the chest wall, then the procedure becomes easier. Identify two vertical lines, one is the *lateral sternal line*, which is a vertical line at the lateral border of the sternum (not the mid-sternal line).The other one is the *mid-clavicular line*, a vertical line dropped from the mid-clavicular point. (Please note that the vertical line dropped through the nipple is slightly lateral to the mid-clavicular line). *So the lateral extent of the incision should stop medial to the nipple.* Also note a horizontal line drawn on the chest through the two nipples is at the lower border of the fifth rib. *So the incision should be one rib below the nipple line* (Fig. 9.9). Once these two vertical lines are marked, feel the lower most rib cage border between the two lines. This is usually the seventh rib. Go one rib above, which is the sixth rib. The incision is then centred at this point. The incision is usually around 3–3.5 cm depending on the

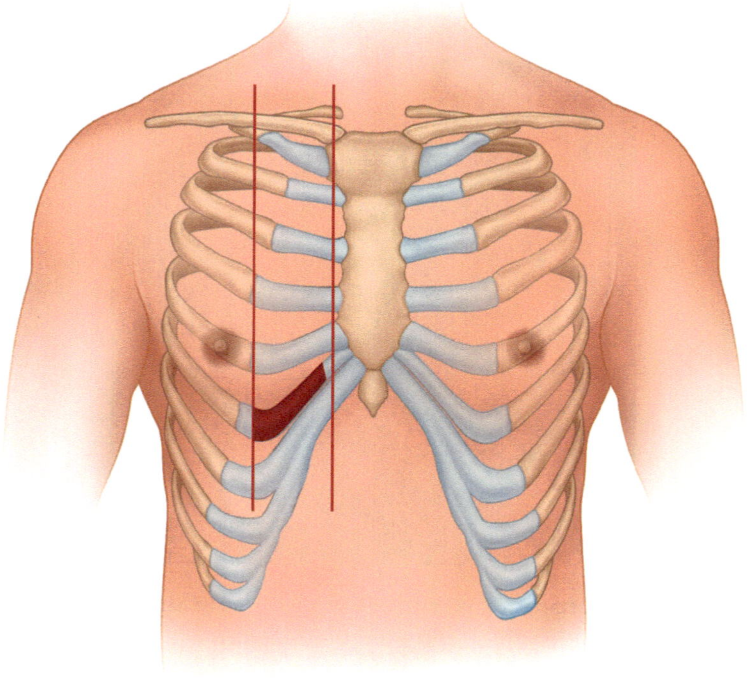

Fig. 9.9 Schematic representation of the surface anatomy of the chest wall for rib graft harvest with the red-shaded area on the right side representing the graft

experience of the surgeon. Remember not to come too close to the sternum. Roughly avoid coming close to the sternal edge staying 2 cm away, from the mid-sternal line as the cartilage is wider and also there is a caudal attachment of the sixth rib to the cephalic border of the seventh rib, which will make the dissection difficult if you are close to the sternum. Similarly going too far laterally towards the mid-clavicular line will take you into the bony rib. Also coming too close to the sternum, the pectoralis muscles will come in the way. Similarly going too far laterally towards the mid-clavicular line will take you into the bony rib.

9.5.4 Surgical Technique

- The surface landmarks as mentioned above are marked on the patient's chest with the *patient in the pre-anaesthetic room sitting up*. A curvy horizontal line is drawn at the lower border of the sixth rib between the lateral sternal line and the mid-clavicular line, about 3 cm long. The side of the harvest will be decided by the patient's wishes, preferably right side. Once a decision is made to harvest the rib cartilage, it is advisable to do this first before starting the nose.
- The surgery is usually done under general anaesthetic.
- The skin incision is made and the underlying fascia and transversalis muscles are gently incised over the palpable cartilage of the sixth rib with a Colorado needle diathermy.
- No attempt should be made to cut the intercostal muscles between the ribs.
- Then the perichondrium over the rib cartilage is incised along the line of skin incision after a self-retaining retractor is placed. Anterior sub-perichondrial dissection is done very gently taking care not to breach the perichondrium. Then the perichondrium is incised both laterally and medially depending on the length of the graft needed. The anterior sub-perichondrial dissection is continued posteriorly with a rib stripper or a curved elevator taking care not to breach the posterior perichondrium and injure the parietal pleura.
- Then the cartilage is incised at the edges depending on the length needed and lifted out gently with an Allis forceps, protecting the underlying soft tissues and lung with a malleable retractor.
- Once the cartilage is removed, the soft tissues are closed in layers after haemostasis. Before closing, it will be wise to use some water in the wound to make sure there is no air escape on positive ventilation.
- If so, it is not a major issue, put a drain in and do a purse string suture and ask the anaesthetist to inflate lung maximum and then pull the drain out as you tighten the purse string and have a post-operative chest X-ray to rule out pneumothorax.
- Inject long acting local anesthetic of your choice in the wound for pain control and close with sub-cuticular 5-0 ethilon.

9.5.5 Shaping and Designing the Grafts

Shaping the graft is done depending on the requirements. It will be advisable to score the cartilage and split them vertically and allow it to settle for 30 minutes and meanwhile proceed with the rest of the nasal surgery to allow for warping issues. Soak in broad-spectrum antibiotic before using.

Key Points

- Knowing the surface anatomy is the key to avoid apprehension.
- As mentioned above, we tend to use costal cartilage only when no other source of cartilage is available.
- It is quite good for septal reconstructions to give adequate projection and also for septal extension grafts.
- Be aware it can cause lot of post-operative issues with poor integration, excess mobility, slipping and not sitting in the right place when used for dorsal reconstructions. It is one of the author's causes of revision surgeries.

- There are some inherent problems with rib cartilage due to convexity of the anatomy of the cartilage and also because of the thickness. They can change shape called warping. This can be reduced by making multiple vertical cuts in the cartilage and allow it to rest for a minimum of 30 minutes before using in the nose.
- Try and take the cartilage in a single piece, so that it can be shaped based on the requirements. Do not damage the intercostal muscles as they can cause neuralgia. Careful approximation of skin edges is important as the scar is visible in the chest.
- Take care to prevent post-operative pneumothorax.
- They can cause tip rigidity when used for tip reconstructions.

Conclusion

- Costal cartilage is a good source of abundant autologous material and if used judiciously will suffice for most septal and some dorsal reconstructions.
- They are an easy and alternative source of nasal grafts, particularly in multiple revision surgeries where it is more likely the conchal cartilages are already harvested.

9.6 Cartilage Crushing and Handling

9.6.1 Introduction

Crushed cartilage is a versatile tool in camouflage grafting in rhinoplasty. We will discuss how to crush and use leftover cartilage pieces to maximise the outcomes of rhinoplasty surgery. The types of cartilage we use for reconstruction of nasal tip are predominantly from the nasal septum, conchal or helical rim ear cartilages and rarely rib cartilages. Only the septal cartilage and rib cartilage need to be crushed or diced if necessary, but not the helical rim or conchal cartilage. Aural cartilages, both conchal and helical, are a type of "elastic" cartilage whose matrix contains elastic fibres and elastic lamellae, in addition to the normal components of hyaline cartilage matrix. They are more flexible and softer. Costal cartilages and septal cartilages are more firm and they are called "hyaline" cartilages, characterised by a homogenous amorphous matrix containing predominately Type 2 collagen and ground substance. Hyaline cartilages may be used as a solid, diced or crushed pieces, whereas elastic ear cartilages are soft and does not need to be crushed.

9.6.2 Indications

- Septal cartilage is a fairly strong hyaline cartilage and a fair amount of septal cartilage can be harvested leaving behind an "L" strut, without de-stabilising the septal support. It can be used as a flat straight piece for structural support or can be used to camouflage using either diced septal cartilage or crushed septal cartilage.
- It is strongly advisable to routinely use crushed septal cartilage for dorsal camoflouage, in all primary osseo-cartilaginous hump reductions to prevent any future irregularities showing through the skin – the so-called CATS graft (*C*artilaginous *A*utogenous *T*hin *S*eptal graft) [26, 27].
- In patients with thin scared skin and discoloured skin to buffer and improve the vascularity of the skin.
- To cover the incision lines when cutting the lateral crus, in procedures like lateral crural overlap or lateral crural steal.
- To cover suture knots over the cartilages, when the end of sutures come to lie directly under the overlying skin.
- To cover the supra-dorsal region particularly after a shield graft.
- Instead of crushing, the cartilage can be diced with a dicer and wrapped in surgical, the so-called Turkish delight and can be used for dorsal augmentation [28].

9.6.3 Surgical Techniques of Cartilage Crushing and Handling (◘ Fig. 9.10a–g)

- If the septal or rib cartilage need to be crushed, then a metal cartilage crusher is used. This is made of heavy metal with a strong base and a heavy metal flap lid which can be flipped over the base as shown in ◘ Fig. 9.10b.
- If the cartilage needs to be diced, it can be done easily on a block with a sharp knife or a dicer blade.
- The cartilage is kept inside the crusher and few drops of saline is added to the cartilage and the lid placed over the cartilage. Keep a padded wet swab (◘ Fig. 9.10a) on top of the metal lid and hit hard with a mallet. It is surprising how much strength is needed to crush the septal cartilage.
- Once the cartilage is crushed like a meshwork, it is gently lifted from the crusher with a Freer's elevator as shown in ◘ Fig. 9.10g. There is no need to secure this thin layer of cartilage as they are quite immobile due to the meshwork nature.

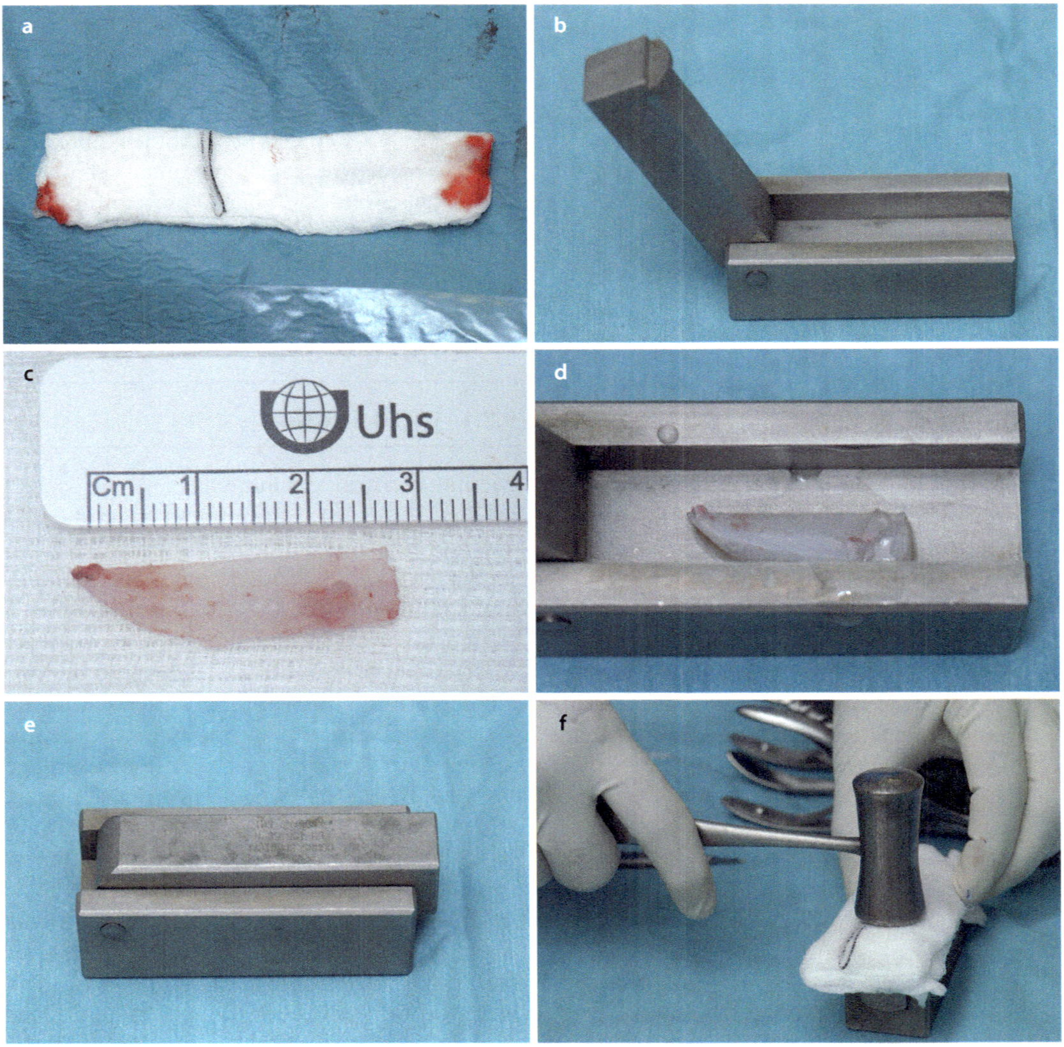

◘ **Fig. 9.10** **a–g** Sequential steps in the technique of cartilage crushing and handling

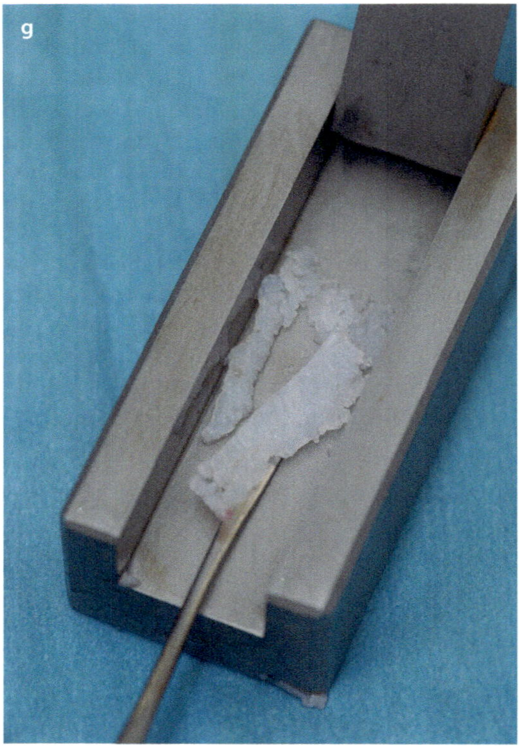

Fig. 9.10 (continued)

- The mesh of crushed cartilage is about 2 mm thickness and is trimmed to make an oval-shaped graft and held with a long non-toothed forceps and is fed under the external flap of skin and the skin draped back. Then run the wet gloved finger over the dorsal profile and mould the graft around the dorsum.
- To cover the supra-dorsal depression, they can be used in layers to cover the defect.
- To cover the lateral crus, a small patch of a single layer of crushed cartilage is more than enough to prevent any free cut ends of cartilage showing through.

Key Points Fig. 9.10g

- Only septal and costal cartilage need to be crushed. Conchal or helical cartilage need not be crushed.
- Always use wet swabs above and below the crusher to dampen the noise. Warn the theatre and anaesthetic staff about the noise.
- Be aware that a certain amount of force is needed to crush the cartilage. Keep checking the degree of softness needed before you stop.
- Also add drops of water to the cartilage before crushing. This keeps the cartilage hydrated.
- It is always advisable to use crushed cartilage grafts for the dorsum after any dorsal reduction even in primary noses to avoid post-operative dorsal irregularities.

Conclusion

- Try and use thin layer of CATS graft for all primary dorsal reduction work to prevent post-operative dorsal irregularities.
- This concept of using crushed cartilage to buffer and smoothen dorsal irregularities even in primary rhinoplasty is a clever one to prevent future revisions.

9.7 Medial Crural Columellar Strut Graft (MCCSG)

9.7.1 Introduction

Medial crural columellar strut graft (Fig. 9.11a, b), as the name suggests, it is a structural graft aimed to support the two media crura and hence strengthen the columella and improve the tip support. It is a structural graft where a piece of cartilage inserted in the columella is secured to the two medial crura with running sutures forming a structural support as opposed to a "columellar strut" which is just a piece of cartilage inserted in the columella through a pocket and not secured to the medial crura. Be aware of different nomenclatures used by different surgeons when they mean different things. A straight piece of the posterior septal cartilage leaving an "L"-strut is an ideal graft material for the columellar strut. To call it a medial crural columellar strut graft [29], the piece of cartilage should be anchored to the

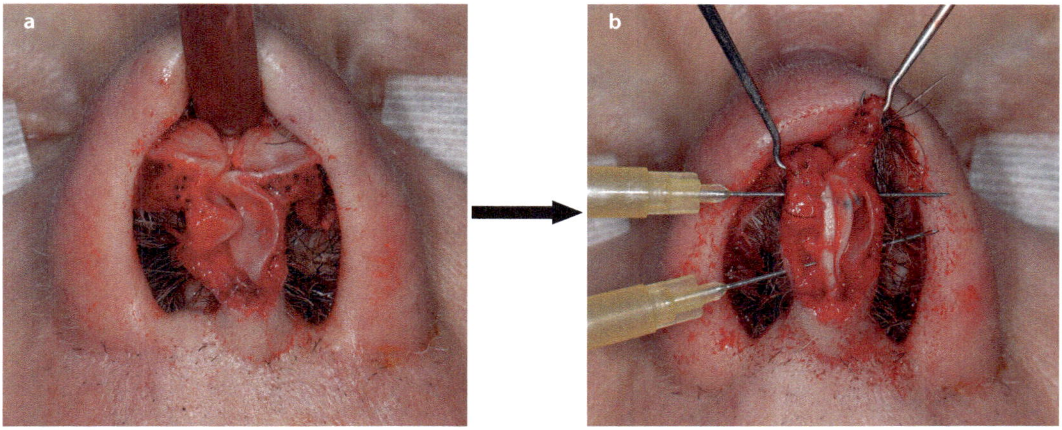

Fig. 9.11 a, b Medial crural columellar strut graft being used to straighten the damaged medial crura and increase the tip support and projection

medial crus, acting as a stent to strengthen and support the medial crus. This is usually performed as part of the complex nasal caudal septal reconstruction. But this cartilage graft is often used as a separate "unsecured free standing" piece of cartilage in the columella and called as "columellar struts". This is more unstable than when secured to the medial crura. It is important to understand the nomenclature based on what exactly the procedure is intended to achieve. Other alternatives to support the caudal septum being a tongue and groove advancement or a septal extension graft depending on the diagnostic algorithm.

9.7.2 Indications

- This graft helps to support the tip complex.
- It helps to increase the tip projection in a de-projected tip [30].
- Lengthens the nose from the nasion to the tip by increasing the tip projection.
- To support a week and fractured medial crus, either unilateral or bilateral.
- To support a week and absent caudal septum.
- This graft helps to widen a very thin columella.
- To correct caudal columellar retraction and vertical shortening of columella.
- To correct a deformed medial crus either on one side or both sides.
- It helps in tip ptosis and may rotate the tip up as well, if done in isolation.

9.7.3 Contra-indications

In patients needing columellar strut grafts, there is often a retracted columella with vertical shortening and thickening with narrow external valve inlet and functional obstruction and a de-projected nasal tip. There is always a conflict between achieving good functional results against achieving good cosmesis. Be aware that these grafts increase the thickness of the columella and thereby further narrow the external valve inlet. This can make any functional issues worse, particularly when there is a pre-existing external nasal valve weakness due to lateral alar in-drawing. Sometimes these effects can be offset with the extra projection of the tip achieved by the graft which can open the valve region. This thought process should be taken into account during the reconstructive options. A degree of caution is necessary in patients with external lateral nasal valve weakness needing this graft, with shortened and already thickened columella.

9.7.4 Surgical Technique (Fig. 9.12a–d)

- The ideal dimensions of the columellar strut in a Caucasian nose is around 12 mm height by 6 mm width and by 2 mm in thickness.
- The sources of material for this type of graft are usually a straight piece of posterior or ventral septal cartilage, rib cartilage or two pieces of helical rim cartilage sutured together.
- Adequate exposure of the medial crus is achieved, preferably through an open approach.
- The first step is to secure the posterior superior border of medial crus together with a medial crural fixation suture. This not only brings the two crura together, but also prevents posterior migration of the columellar strut.
- The columellar strut is then secured between the two medial crus staying just below the dome with either 2–3 simple sutures (5-0 vicryl or PDS sutures) or a couple of vertical mattress sutures. Avoid a long single vertical mattress suture to prevent cutting through and vertical crinkling of the caudal septal mucosa [14, 31–33].
- Make sure the sutures are placed well away from the free caudal border of the medial crura, so that caudal splaying of the medial crus is preserved and undue narrowing of the edge of the columella is avoided.
- Once the caudal strut is in place, make sure the anterior superior border is made slightly convex and blunt, by excising a small semilunar piece of the cartilage so that there is no sharp edge at the tip. This also helps in creating an aesthetic double-break to the tip.

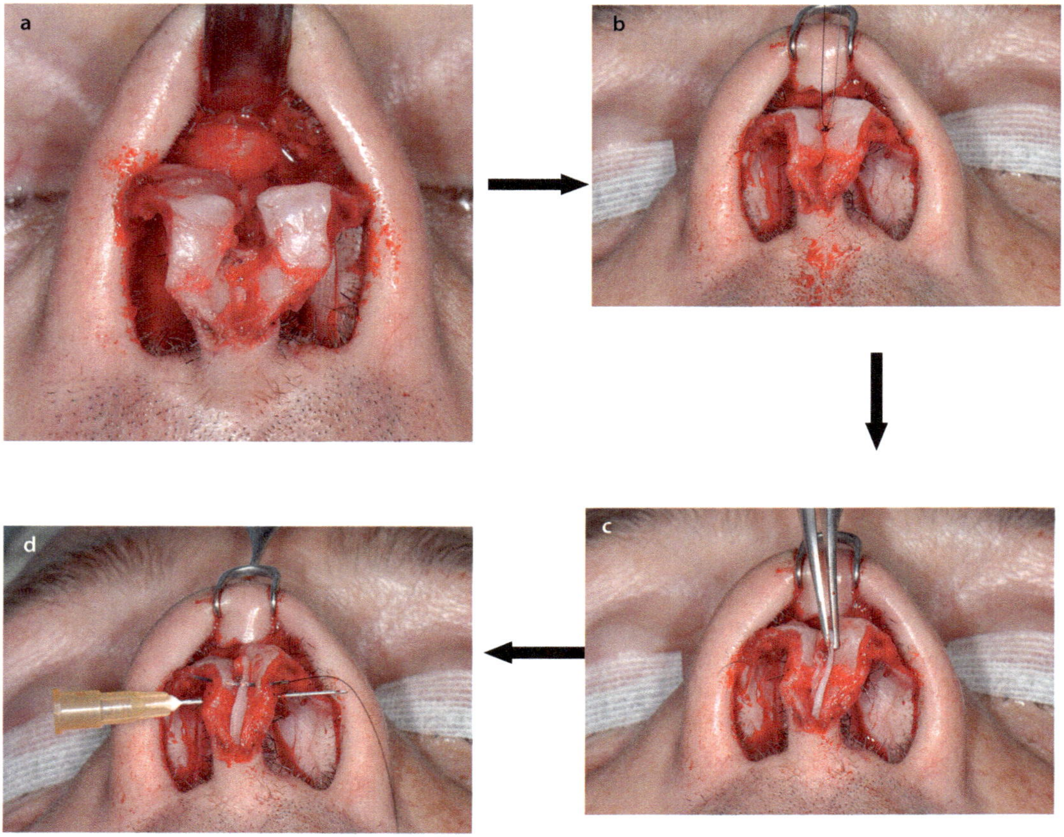

Fig. 9.12 **a–d** Sequential steps in the technique of medial crural columellar strut graft (MCCSG). ("Reproduced with kind permission from Refs: [31, 33]")

- Make sure the height of the columellar strut cartilage does not project above the junction of the medial crus with the intermediate crus.
- The antero-inferior part of the cartilage may or may not extend or sutured to the anterior nasal spine depending on the expected outcomes.
- May need a shield graft antero-superiorly at the anterior septal angle to correct any infra-tip lobule blunting.
- As mentioned above in selected patients, particularly elderly with de-projected and under rotated tip causing nasal obstruction, a quicker option would be to create a columellar pocket and insert a piece of septal cartilage, (columellar strut) without the need to suture it to the medial crura, which will help to increase the projection and improve the airway.
- The direction of the columellar graft can be changed from vertical to horizontal angle to correct caudal septal deviations and stabilise them in the midline, the so-called controlled columellar strut described by Tebbetts.

9.7.5 Surgical Sequence

If it is done as part of nasal reconstruction, the following sequence is preferable with cephalic trim of the lateral crus, followed by dorsal reduction if needed. Then middle vault reconstruction should be done (e.g. spreader grafts) if needed. Then only the medial crural fixation suture should be done, followed by the columellar strut.

Key Points

- Be aware medial crural columellar strut grafts can cause widening of the columella, hence patient should be counselled of this before surgery.
- Be aware not to suture the free anterior border of the medial crus in front of the strut, as this will cause not only blunting and unacceptable "pencil thin" columella anteriorly, but also thickened columella posteriorly, narrowing the external valve region and also causing functional obstruction. Always structure and function should be balanced.
- Make sure there is no sharp antero-superior edge to the columellar strut and if necessary use a shield graft as well antero-superiorly to create a nice smooth infra-tip lobule complex.

Conclusion

- Before deciding to use this graft, you need to think for what purpose you are using it rather than just relying on the terminology which for different surgeons means different things!
- Open approach is preferable, if done with more complex procedures and allows you to secure the graft to the rest of the septum if necessary, as a dorsal or caudal extension grafts.
- Can also be done as an isolated procedure in selected patients for various reasons, including patient's preference, anaesthetic time, etc.

9.8 Caudal Septal Extension Graft (CSEG)

9.8.1 Introduction

Caudal septal extension graft (CSEG) is a structural graft first described by Byrd [34, 35], aimed to support the caudal septum and also add to the length of the caudal septum thereby increasing the length of the nose and also increasing the tip projection and to address a retracted columella.

As the name suggests, it is an extension to the existing caudal septal cartilage, securing the additional piece of graft to the existing caudal septal cartilage to extend and correct the length of the existing septum. This can be used to correct both the vertical height and the dorsal length of the existing nasal septal cartilage by adding a piece of cartilage to the caudal septum as an extension. To call this a caudal extension graft, the extended piece needs to be secured to the remains of the caudal septum to create a single septal cartilage unit. The cartilage may or may not be anchored to the anterior nasal spine depending on the requirements. The length of the cartilage can also be varied extending superiorly up to the nasal tip to correct the nasal tip projection and also to support the nasal tip structurally. But by doing this, it can add to rigidity of the nasal tip. These are ideally indicated in a short, less projected caudal septum with columellar shortening causing a grossly retracted nasal tip, with a secondary over rotation of the tip [36].

9.8.2 Indications

- To primarily reconstruct if the caudal septal cartilage is lacking in excess of 5–6 mm from the columellar margin.
- To support and extend the length of the caudal septum.
- To increase the tip projection.
- To correct caudal columellar retraction.
- To increase the length of the nose.
- To widen a very thin columella.
- To correct nasal tip deformities associated with cleft lip.

9.8.3 Contra-indications

Be cautious in using this technique in patients with external lateral nasal valve weakness due to lateral crural concavity. Any additional thickening of the columella caused by the septal extension graft can cause functional restriction of airflow at the external valve area and will worsen the functional valve obstruction caused by a pre-existing external nasal valve weakness, particularly in the presence of lateral alar in-drawing.

9.8.4 Surgical Technique (▫ Fig. 9.13a–g)

- Septal extension grafts are ideally suited for the retracted columella. Ideally, 2–4 mm of columellar show is acceptable for cosmetic purposes. If the columellar show is "true" (i.e., no alar retraction) and less than 1 mm due to lack of caudal septal cartilage, septal extension grafts are advisable.
- Usually done through an open approach as part of complex reconstruction of a deprojected short and over rotated nose.
- If done as a sole procedure, the caudal end of the septum can be exposed through a trans-columellar incision.
- An ideal graft site would be the posterior part of the septal cartilage leaving behind an "L" strut. But some of these patients may not have enough cartilage in the septum to start with. In these patients, costal cartilage is harvested. The graft to be used should be straight and not deviated.
- The ideal dimensions of the graft will be around 12 mm vertical height and 2 mm thickness. The antero-posterior width of the cartilage graft varies as much as it is necessary taking into consideration the degree of overlap needed for stabilisation.
- The graft is secured to the posterior edge of the existing septum with figure of 8 pivot sutures [37] to prevent vertical movements and to withstand torsion forces.
- There should be about 3–4 mm overlap between the graft and the caudal end of the septum. This will ensure that the graft is placed securely. Another way of anchoring the graft will be to use a bilateral spreader grafts and extend them down with a space in between like a dove tail [38, 39] and secure the anterior superior edge of the graft into the slot. There are pros and cons of each technique based on the clinical findings.
- Ideally the graft should not be visible post surgery. The graft is placed in such a way that it does not protrude caudal to the medial crus.
- If dorsal extension grafts or extended spreader grafts are also needed, it is better to do them first and then do the caudal septal extension after. It is safer to anchor the anterior superior end of the septal extension graft superiorly to the space created between the spreaders like a "dove-tail" inter-locking joint. This adds to the stability of the tip.
- For purposes of additional stability, the graft can be sutured to the medial crura [40], making sure that the edge of the graft does not protrude beyond the caudal edge of the medial crura [14, 31, 32].

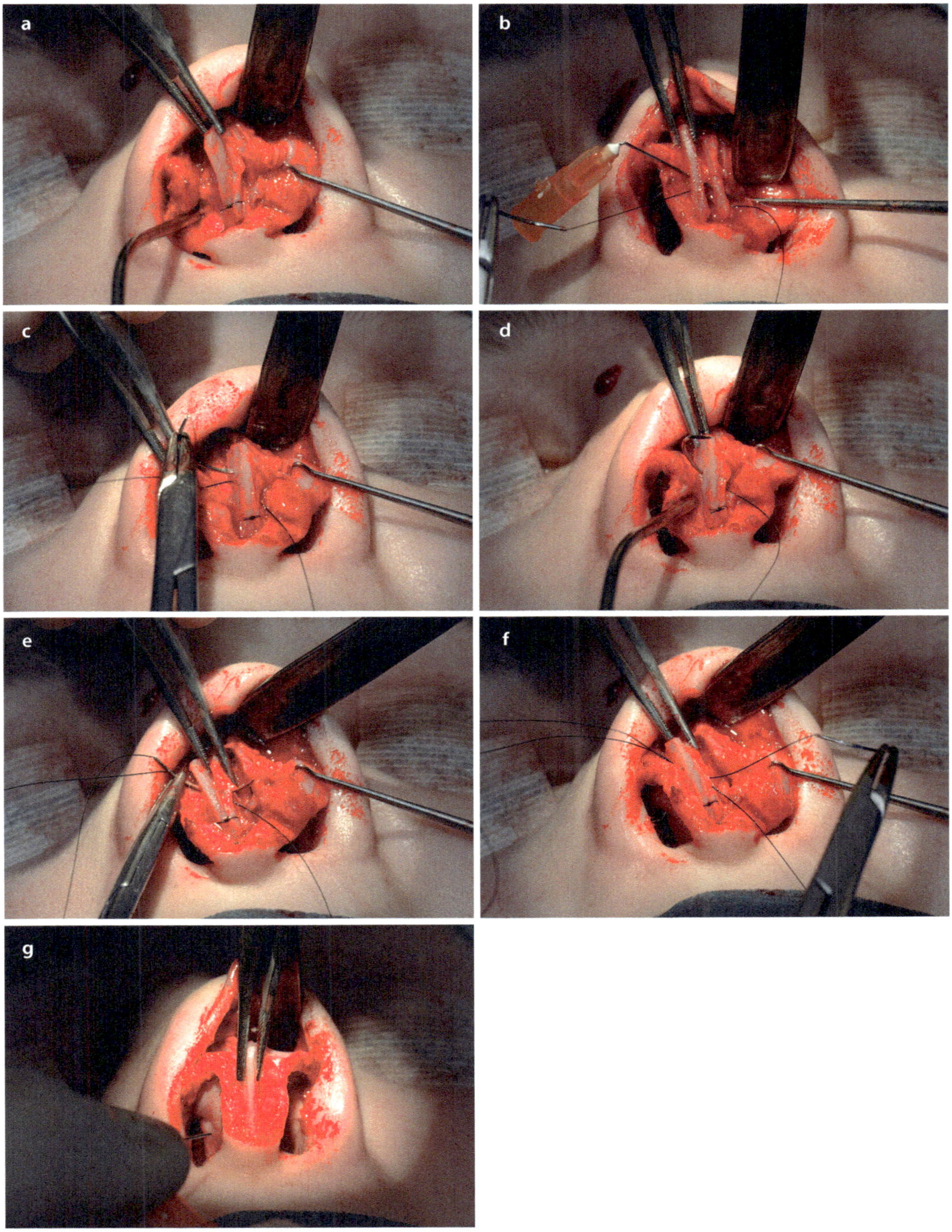

Fig. 9.13 **a–g** Sequential steps in the surgical technique of caudal septal extension graft being secured to the existing caudal septum and also being anchored to the anterior nasal spine

- Care should be taken to make sure that the septal graft does not extend above the level of the dome of the lower lateral cartilage.
- One disadvantage with this technique is that the patient will have a relatively stiff nasal tip with very limited tip recoil. The patient should be adequately counselled before the surgery. It can also cause thickening of the anterior septum causing a degree of functional obstruction in the external valve region.
- Sometimes it is worth doing a shield graft as well to "soften" the infra-tip lobule of the nasal tip.
- Be also aware that if the caudal extension graft is not in the midline and if the medial crura is sutured to the graft, it can turn the tip to one side causing tip asymmetry.

9.8.5 Surgical Sequence

This procedure is usually done in a short petit nose with caudal and dorsal de-projection with a slightly over rotated tip resulting from lack of caudal and dorsal septum. It is usually better done through an open approach for easy access. Existing septum should be straightened first and the necessary cartilage graft should be harvested either from posterior septum or rib cartilage. Then dorsal extension done first if needed followed by caudal extension. Then if needed dorsal grafting is done finally.

Key Points

- Any deformities or deviations of the caudal septum should be corrected and the caudal septum should be absolutely in the midline, before any form of septal extension can be considered. Otherwise, there is a risk of the tip being pulled to the side of the caudal septal deformity. Be aware of secondary tip deformities which can be a problem if the existing caudal septum is not straight.
- Patient should be adequately counselled that the tip recoil will be lost and the tip will be stiffer and some patients do not like this.
- It is often required to insert a shield graft to smoothen the new anterior septal angle after performing a septal extension to avoid an excessively pointed nasal tip.
- At the end of the procedure, it is advisable to use small plumping grafts to buffer the columella.
- Be aware if the columella is already thickened and shortened, adding a piece of cartilage can cause further thickening and narrowing of the external nasal vestibular region causing functional obstruction at the external nasal valve region.

Conclusion

- Straightening the caudal septum and strengthening the caudal septum are the two most important prerequisites for achieving positive long-term outcomes in nasal tip reconstruction.
- Caudal septum extension graft by definition aims to act as an extension of the rest of the nasal septal cartilage, hence need to be anchored to the rest of the septum.
- This needs to be distinguished from free columellar graft which acts as a support to the soft tissue columella only, hence subject to distraction forces.
- Adequate pre-planning and harvesting of a straight piece of cartilage is vital. This can be from rib cartilage if a large piece is required.
- In conclusion, a septal extension graft will tend to increase the definition of the tip, and will help in some degree of rotation of the tip downwards and will also improve the projection of the nasal tip.

9.9 Bilateral Spreader Graft (BSG)

9.9.1 Introduction

Bilateral spreader graft (BSG) was originally described by Jack Sheen [41] to "spread" and open the space between the high mid-dorsal septum and the upper lateral junction aiming to improve the internal nasal valve "function". It also acts as a "structural" graft to support the mid dorsum and lateral dorsal "K" area. Be aware of terminologies like "mini spreaders" and "auto spreaders". In our unit we tend to use spreader grafts more and more for structural reasons than functional improvement. In our experience, this procedure gives consistent results to improve the nasal airway in the selected group of patients. They are cartilage grafts roughly around 12 × 4 × 2 mm in dimension used to augment the space between the medial border of the upper lateral cartilage and the high dorsal septal cartilage at the internal nasal valve region. This is performed on both sides to improve the functional nasal capacity in the internal nasal valve region [42, 41]. Although this is a fairly established and accepted procedure to open the internal valve, recently there are studies questioning this hypothesis. Clinically we have found that this procedure does make a big difference to the nasal function. Though this procedure is meant to improve the internal nasal valve function, it also offers structural stability to the mid dorsum in patients with collapsed dorsum. In patients with unilateral internal valve problems, it is still advisable to insert the graft on both sides to avoid any distortion and prevent asymmetry in the mid dorsum. The material mostly used for spreader grafts are autologous septal cartilage. "Auto spreaders" are used when the dorsal section of the upper lateral cartilage is preserved during hump reduction and turned into the internal nasal valve region keeping the mucosa intact to increase the space in the internal valve region.

9.9.2 Indications

- The main indications for the use of spreader grafts in the nose is to *improve the nasal function* in patients with functional internal valve narrowing, thereby causing the classical "hour-glass" narrowing (◘ Fig. 9.15) of the mid-dorsal aesthetic lines.
- To offer purely *structural* mid-dorsal support in the reconstruction of the collapsed dorsum of the nose in patients with extensive fronto-nasal trauma causing severe mid-dorsal collapse of the nose, de-projection and over rotation of the tip. Most of these patients who require this form of surgery have some degree of structural damage to upper lateral cartilages and the dorsal septum. It seems illogical to use augmentation material directly on to the dorsum without reconstituting the dorsal support. We now routinely use bilateral spreader grafts in patients with severe nasal collapse of the dorsum (even in those without nasal valve dysfunction) to give *structural stability* to the mid dorsum and offer a stable platform before dorsal cartilage augmentation. This concept has evolved based on our observation of patients who had dorsal reconstruction with and without spreader grafts done for nasal valve defects. We found that patients who had spreader grafts had much better long-term stability of the dorsal reconstruction.
- To correct a very high dorsal septal deviation. Here the graft acts as a scaffold to support the septum.
- To correct a severely twisted mid dorsum due to gross septal deviation.
- Used to stabilise the "K" area collapse in the mid dorsum as seen on the right side in ◘ Fig. 9.14 [43].
- To support the internal valve region, following reduction of a large very thin nasal dorsal hump in an ethnic or familial nose. This is done prophylactically to prevent post-operative internal nasal valve collapse after reduction rhinoplasty (◘ Figs. 9.16 and 9.17).
- If rhinoplasty is contemplated in a petit nose with a combination of short nasal bones, wide and long upper lateral cartilage, again it is advisable to use bilateral spreader grafts prophylactically to prevent any future internal nasal valve issues.

9.9.3 Contra-indications

- Literally none in the right group of patients, hence patient selection is important.

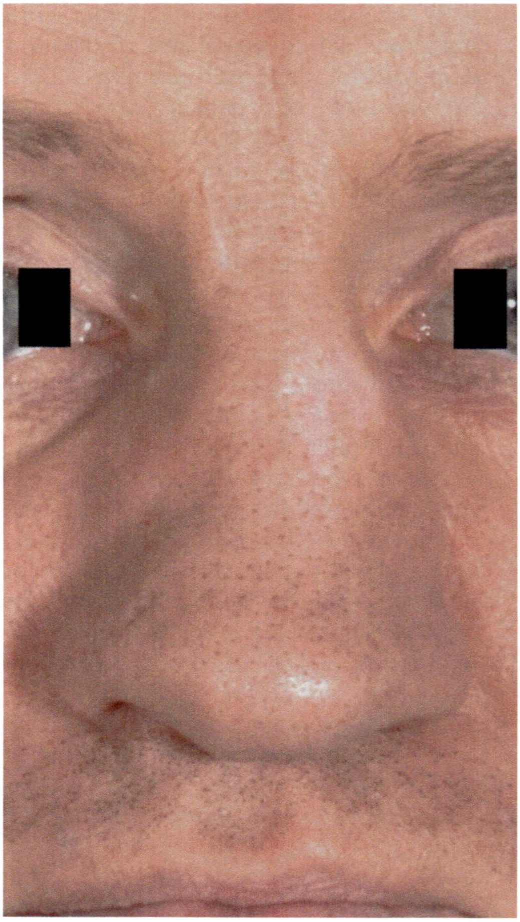

Fig. 9.14 Frontal view showing a twisted mid dorsum with "K" area collapse on the right side

- If done purely for functional reasons, patients should be warned of increase in the width of the nasal mid dorsum.
- As with all rhinoplasty procedures, one must weigh the consequences of balancing the structure with function.
- If the patient does not wish a wider mid dorsum.

9.9.4 Surgical Technique

- Accurate pre-operative assessment is the key. An ideal patient would be someone with mid-dorsal de-projection with an hour-glass narrowing of the mid dorsum with very narrow angle between the upper lateral cartilage and the dorsal septum.

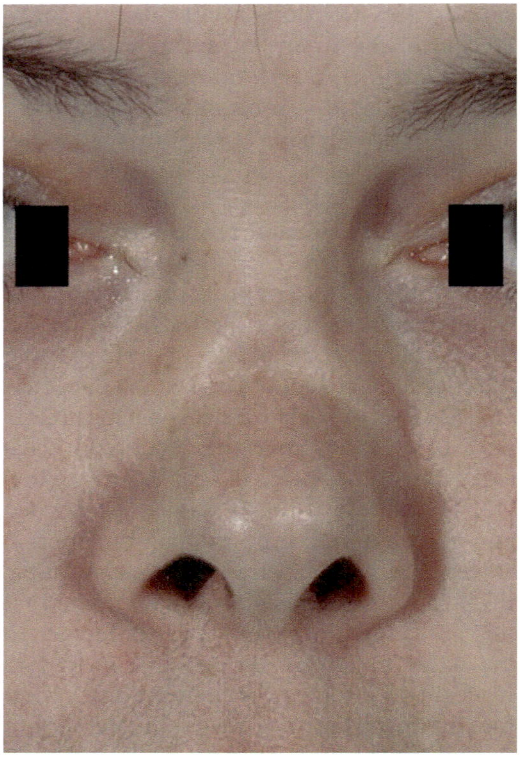

Fig. 9.15 Frontal view showing bilateral collapsed mid dorsum with "hour-glass" narrowing of the internal nasal valve region. ("Reproduced with kind permission from Ref: [32]")

- Endoscopic examination of the internal nasal valve region for high dorsal deviations of septum is important for assessing the valve function.
- In the author's view, Cottle's test which improves the nasal airway on pulling the cheek skin out is a non-specific test, which is positive in most people even without nasal valve obstruction. Lifting the caudal border of the upper lateral cartilage with a probe (probe test or modified Cottle's test) and measuring the subjective improvement in breathing on a visual analogue scale is of more practical value in the decision-making in diagnosing internal valve narrowing.
- Look at the width of the nose in the mid-dorsal level by analysing the dorsal eye brow to tip line. Usually patients with internal nasal valve obstruction on both sides have an external narrowing of the width of the mid dorsum and in extreme cases an

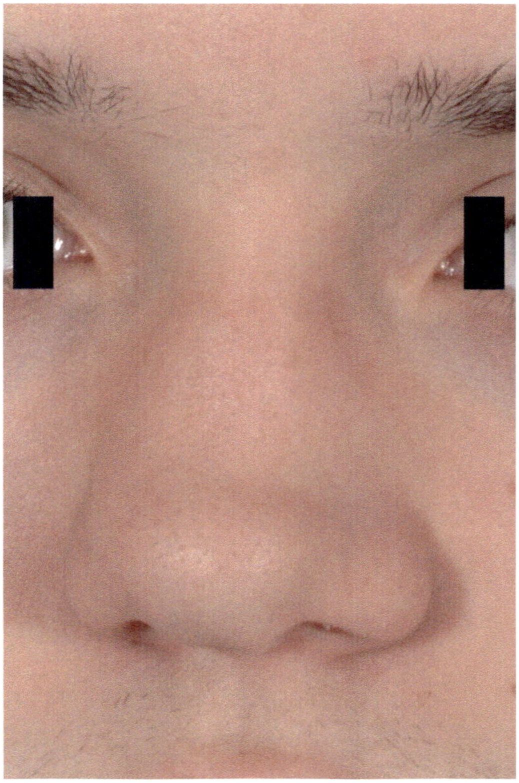

Fig. 9.16 Frontal view showing bilateral asymmetrical collapse of the internal valve following frontal trauma

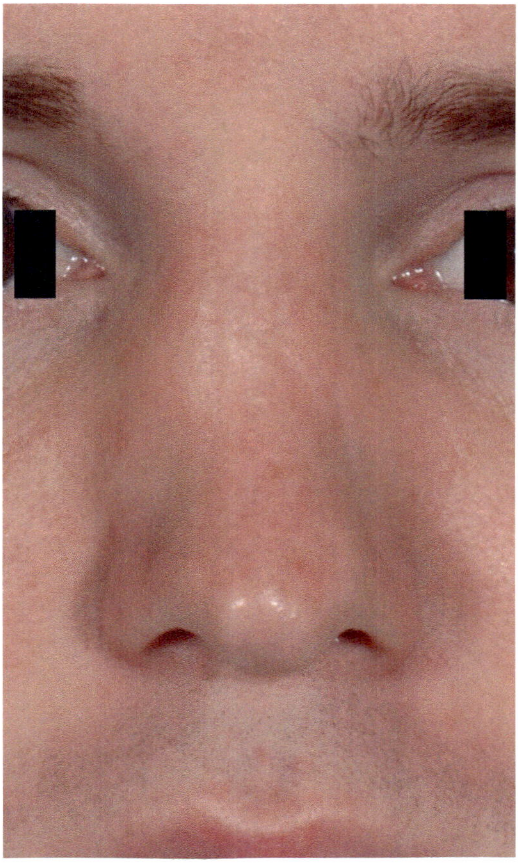

Fig. 9.17 Frontal view showing twisted nose and bilateral internal valve collapse following over resection of the dorsal hump

"hour-glass" narrowing of the dorsal aesthetic lines from the eyebrow to the tip.

- In unilateral cases, there is usually a depression of the lateral "K" area at the junction between the upper lateral cartilage and nasal bone. This is common in patients with a twisted nose where the nasal bony complex points in one direction and the lower two-thirds of the cartilage including the tip is pointing in the opposite direction. The side of the concavity is usually the side where the internal valve is narrow.
- Ideally septal cartilage from the posterior and ventral septum is harvested in a dimension of 12 mm length, by 4 mm width and 2 mm thickness (Fig. 9.18e).
- Can be done either through an open or closed approach, although open approach helps in precise placement and securing of the graft.
- If the bulk of the lateral crus need to be reduced, do the cephalic trim first before doing the spreaders, as it creates an optimum space to work on the dorsum (Fig. 9.18b).
- The mucosal flaps over the septal cartilage is raised on both sides, and the junction between the upper lateral cartilage and the dorsal septum is exposed.
- The upper lateral is separated from the dorsal septum medial to the "T" bar of the dorsal septum as close to the septal cartilage (Fig. 9.18c). This is done in the sub-muco-perichondrial layer of the septal cartilage so that the mucosa over the upper lateral cartilage and septal junction is preserved. If for some reasons septal flaps are not raised, then the mucosal junction between upper lateral and the septum is spared by accurately incising the junction extra-mucosally from the sky view.

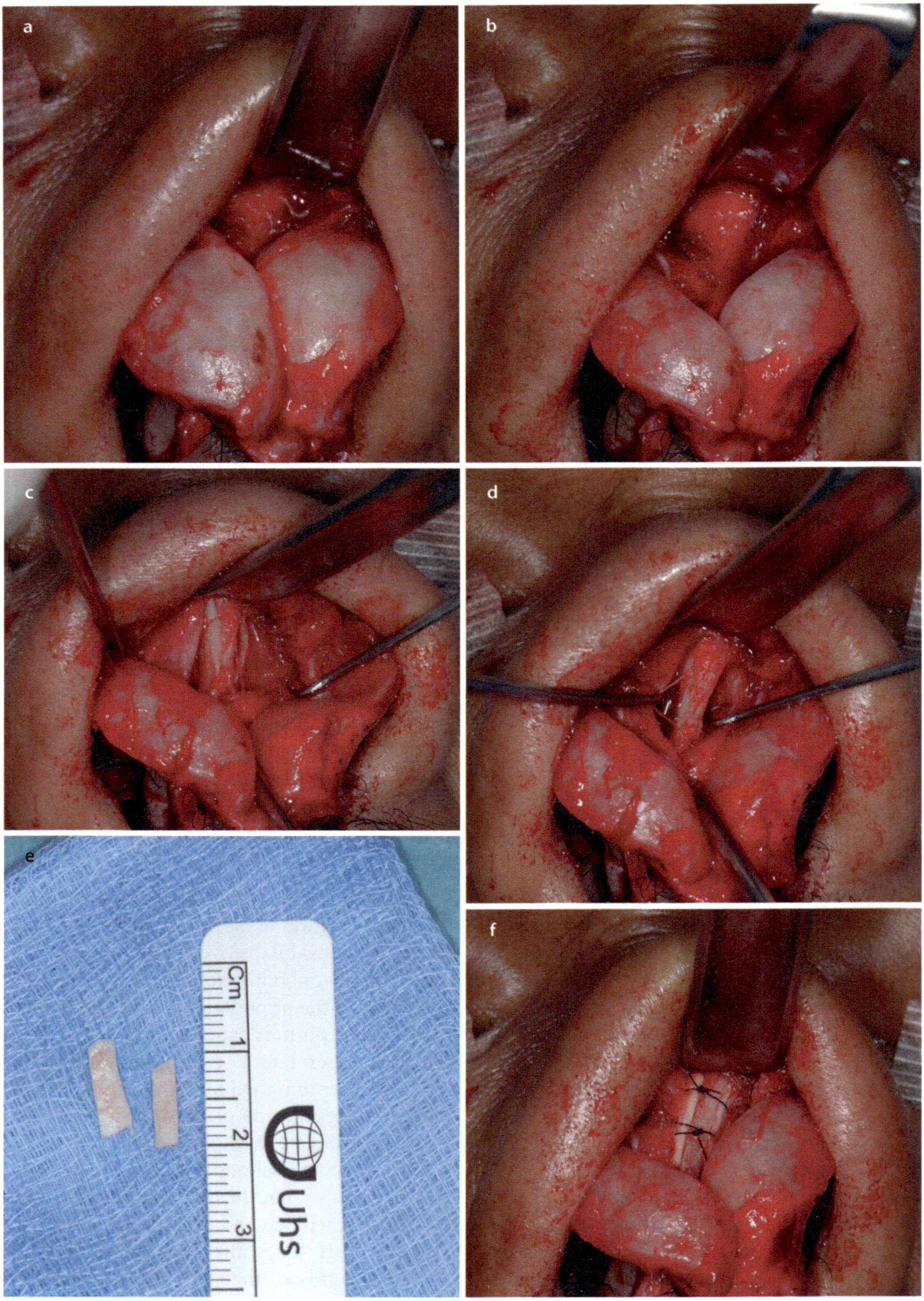

Fig. 9.18 **a–f** Sequential steps in the insertion of bilateral spreader grafts between the mid-dorsal septum and the upper lateral cartilage

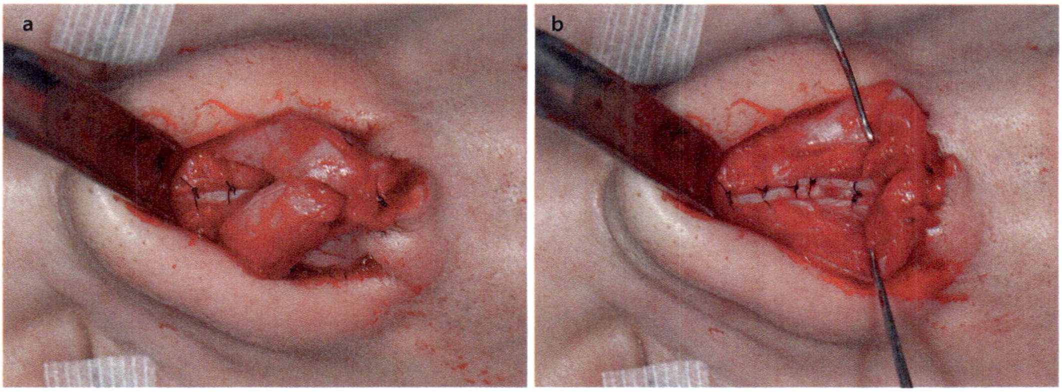

Fig. 9.19 a, b Spreader grafts in place in another patient

- The spreader grafts are inserted one at a time and secured in place with 5-0 ethilon suture either as a single suture or as two simple sutures on either side.
- Sometimes the length of the spreader grafts may need to be extended depending on the requirements as seen in another patient in Fig. 9.19b.

9.9.5 Surgical Sequence

Spreader grafts are to be done only after dorsal hump reduction if needed. If cephalic trim is indicated, it will be wise to de-bulk the lateral crus at this stage as it gives easier access to the mid dorsum. This should be followed by caudal septal and tip work if needed.

Key Points

- Generally preferable to be done through an open approach, but can also be done through an internal sub-mucosal approach. It can be a fiddly procedure for the beginner. Particular issue being the graft is either too big or taking two unequal pieces.
- Once inserted in the space between the upper lateral cartilage and the dorsal septum, the cartilage tends to jump out before you use the suture. The way to address this issue will be to "cut into" the lower border of the upper lateral cartilage in a lateral direction for a millimetre or two, so that the top end of the space is slightly rectangular and helps to accommodate the width of the graft more securely and does not push the graft out of the space. This gives enough stability for the graft before using the sutures. The graft can also be secured with hypodermic needles before suturing.
- It will be wise to use spreader grafts as a "basement" graft in patients requiring augmentation of mid dorsum. This gives added stability to the dorsal camouflage grafts if used later to augment mid-dorsal collapse.
- In patients with unilateral internal valve problems, it is still advisable to insert the graft on both sides to avoid any distortion and prevent asymmetry in the mid-dorsal aesthetic lines.

Conclusion

- Thus, spreader grafts are cartilage grafts roughly 12 × 4 × 2 mm in dimension, usually done on both sides to widen (spread) the space between the upper lateral cartilage and the high dorsal septal cartilage to improve the function of the internal nasal valve region.
- Although it improves the subjective nasal function, we use this technique more and more for structural stability of the mid dorsum rather than functional improvement.
- This is a time-tested procedure in our practice, and we think that this technique is here to stay.

9.10 Extended Bilateral Spreader Grafts

9.10.1 Introduction

Extended bilateral spreader grafts are used to offer mid-dorsal and lower dorsal support in the reconstruction of the collapsed nasal dorsum in patients with extensive fronto-nasal trauma causing severe mid-dorsal collapse of the nose, de-projection and over rotation of the nasal tip and a short nose. As the name suggests they are an extension of the spreader grafts, which usually are restricted to the mid dorsum between the septum and the upper lateral cartilage. By supporting the mid dorsum and extending the support down the lower dorsal septum of the nose, they not only help in improving the function of the internal nasal valve region but also structurally provide support to the lower dorsal septum of the nose and the tip in the external valve area.

9.10.2 Indications

- To increase the anatomical cross section of the internal nasal valve region by opening the internal nasal valve and improving the nasal valve function.
- To support the dorsal septum in the mid and lower dorsum till the anterior septal angle thus helping in the structural support of a de-projected dorsum of the nose.
- To straighten a high caudal dorsal deviation of the nasal septum.
- To correct a severely twisted S-shaped nasal dorsum.
- After reduction rhinoplasty, in patients with very thin dorsal profile lines and a large dorsal hump up to the anterior septal angle and to prevent any post-operative functional valve area issues at a later date.
- For reconstruction of structural integrity of the mid and low dorsum of the nose prior to dorsal grafting, since most of these patients who require this form of surgery have some degree of structural damage to dorsal cartilages and dorsal septum as well.
- Extended spreader grafts also offer an effective anchoring point antero-superiorly in securing the nasal tip cartilages in an over projected and de-rotated position thereby helping to increase the tip projection and bring the tip down.
- It can be also be used to increase the length of a short nose in the profile line.
- Bilateral extended spreader grafts can also be used as a viable alternative to septal extension grafts [44].

9.10.3 Contra-indications

- Should be used cautiously when compared to spreader grafts.
- Patient selection is important, but beware this can cause rigidity to the nasal dorsum and tip.
- Beware extending the graft on both sides down to the tip can cause thickening of the nasal septum anteriorly and restricting the flow in the external valve region.

9.10.4 Sources of Cartilage Graft

- Posterior septal cartilage.
- Costal cartilage.
- Double-layered sandwiched helical rim cartilage.

9.10.5 Surgical Technique (◘ Fig. 9.20a–g)

- Ideally septal cartilage from the posterior and ventral septum is harvested in a dimension of roughly 25 mm length, by 4 mm width and 2 mm thickness, depending on the requirements. The other alternative being costal cartilage graft.
- Advisable to do through open approach, when compared to spreader grafts as these are longer and difficult to secure through an internal approach.
- The septal flaps over the septal cartilage is raised on both sides, and the junction between the upper lateral cartilage and the dorsal septum is exposed.

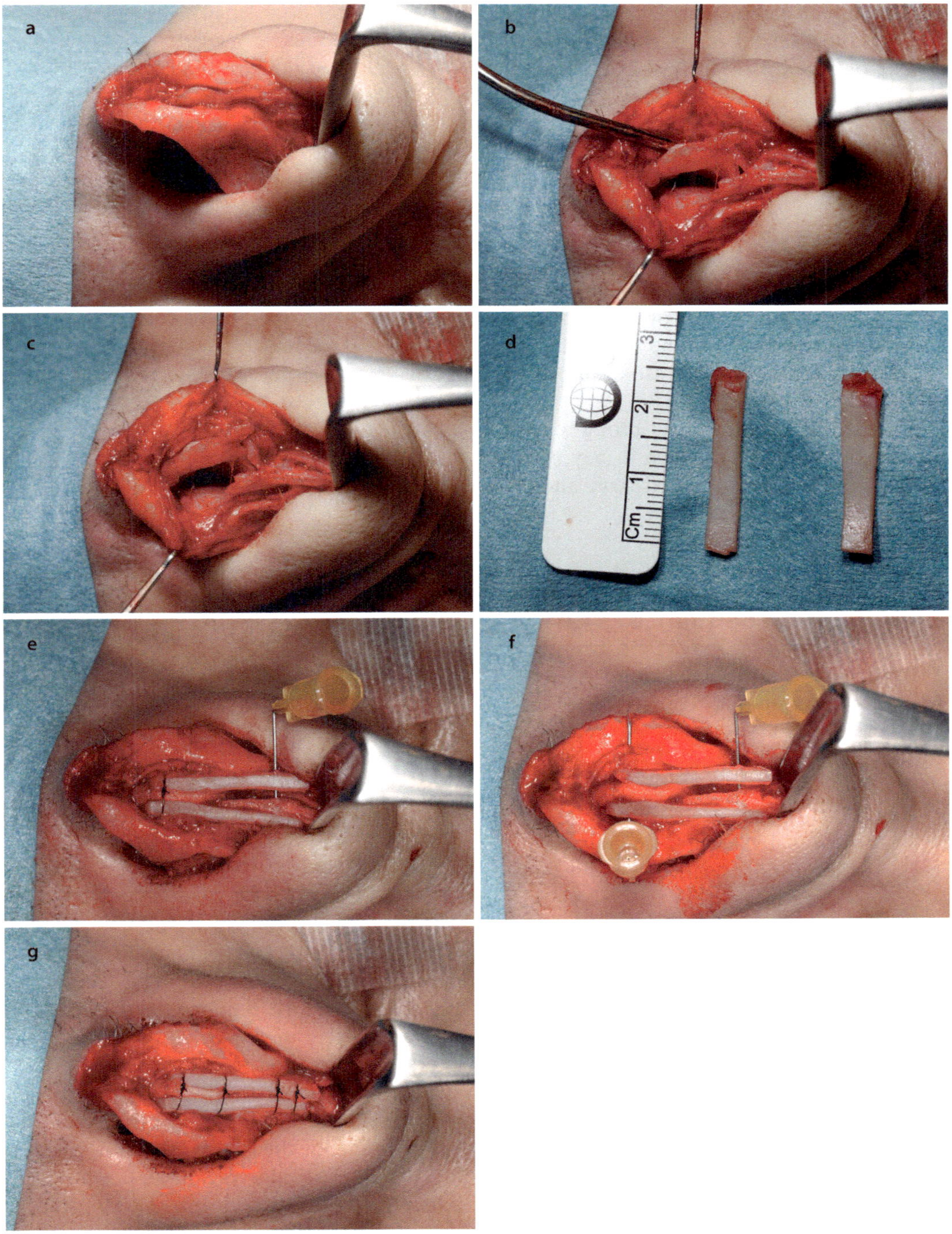

Fig. 9.20 **a–g** Sequential steps in the insertion of extended bilateral spreader grafts extending from the mid-dorsal level to the anterior septal angle of the nasal septum

- The upper lateral cartilage is separated from the dorsal septum medial to the "T" bar of the dorsal septum as close to the septal cartilage.
- The spreader grafts are inserted one at a time and secured in place with a suture of your choice. We use 5-0 ethilon suture either as a single suture going through both grafts or as two simple sutures on either side.
- The anterior extension of the spreader graft beyond the lower border of the upper lateral cartilage should be bevelled to prevent thickening of the graft at the external nasal valve region.
- Often if the extension is brought to the anterior septal angle, then it may need to be supported by a caudal strut and or a caudal extension graft.

9.10.6 Surgical Sequence

This procedure should be done only after any dorsal hump reduction is performed. Tip work should be done after the spreader grafts.

Key Points

- Beware that extending the graft down to the anterior septal angle and the tip will cause stiffening of the tip and can cause thickening of the external nasal valve region and can cause functional nasal valve obstruction as well.
- This when done along with caudal septal extension graft is an ideal replacement for an "L" strut, the advantage of this being you can change the angle between the dorsal and caudal pieces of cartilage, which cannot be done in the "L" strut once fashioned.
- The thickness should be kept not more than 2 mm; otherwise, there can be too much widening of the dorsal profile lines.
- Always take care to bevel the anterior extension of the spreader graft beyond the lower border of the upper lateral cartilage, if not it will end up in a thickening of the external nasal valve region antero-superiorly, interfering with nasal function and structural annoyance to the patient.
- In patients with unilateral internal valve problems, it is still advisable to insert the graft on both sides to avoid any distortion and prevent asymmetry in the mid-dorsal aesthetic lines and prevent any tip asymmetry developing at a later date.
- Be aware they cause rigidity to the nasal tip, which should be discussed in the pre-operative counselling stage and documented.

Conclusion

- Extended spreader grafts are basically an extension of spreader grafts extending the graft and support down from the middle vault to the anterior septal angle and the tip.
- Generally preferable to be done through an open approach, which will also help in the tip work.

9.11 Lateral Crural Strut Grafts (LCSG)

9.11.1 Introduction

The lateral crural strut grafts (LCSG), (◘ Fig. 9.21a–c), were first described by Gunter and Friedman [45]. They are versatile grafts used to reinforce and strengthen the lateral alar region collapse due to weak lateral crus. As the name suggests, it offers structural support to a weak lateral crura acting like a strut and thus helps to prevent the "in-drawing" of the lateral crus thus supporting the external alar region. As opposed to batten graft, lateral crural strut graft is placed between the existing weak or damaged lateral crus and the underlying alar mucosa. In the author's experience, this is the best technique available to correct the lateral alar weakness successfully. Ideally this graft is placed between the remnants of the lateral crus and the underlying alar mucosa and the procedure

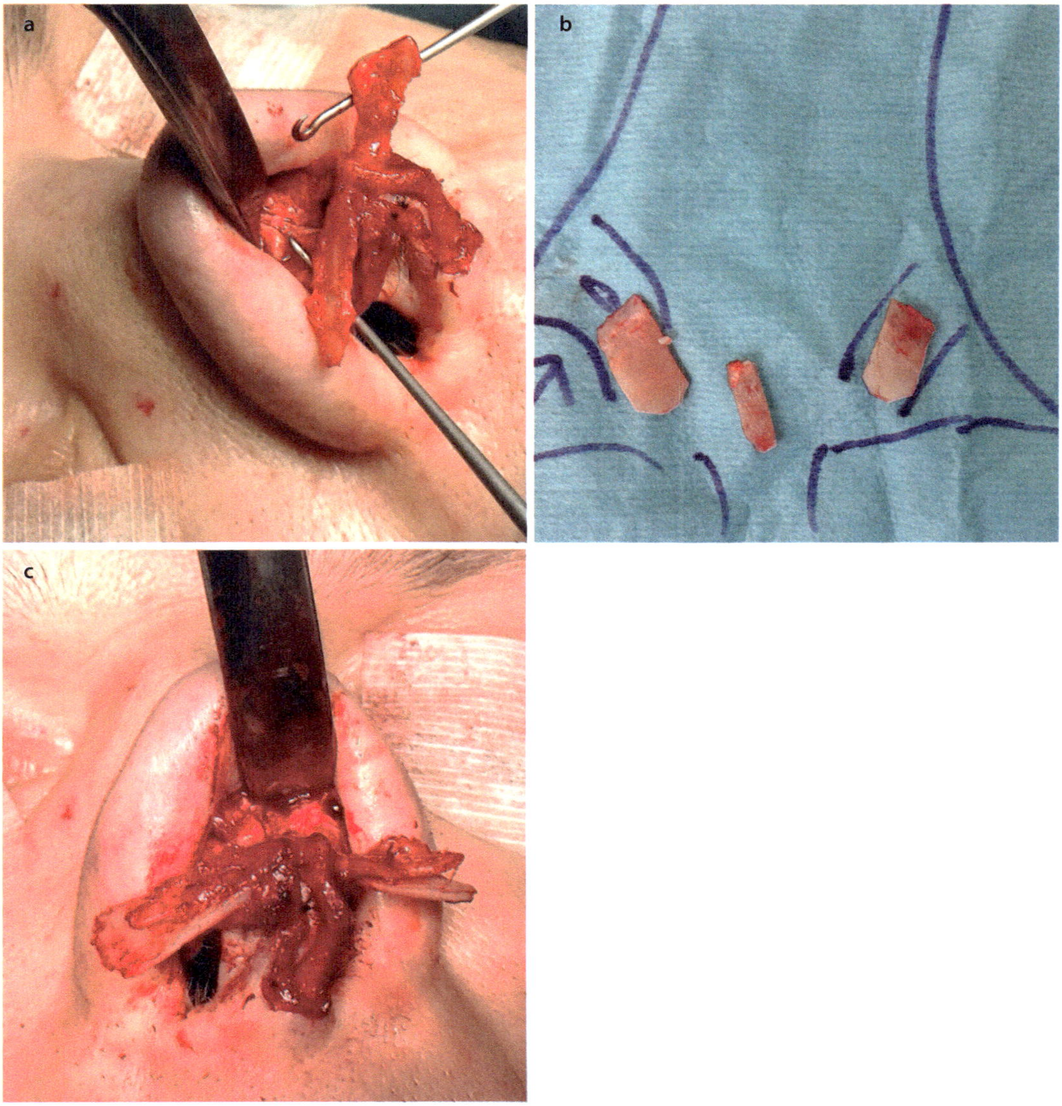

Fig. 9.21 **a–c** Lateral crural strut grafts. **a** The weak and damaged lateral crus on both sides. **b** Schematic representation of lateral crural strut grafts and columellar strut. **c** Lateral crural strut grafts being secured under the existing weak lateral crus on both sides

involves releasing the alar mucosa from the lateral crus and creating a space under the lateral crus for enclosing the graft. It can be done through a tunnel created from the alar margin or the lateral crus be completely lifted away from the alar mucosa and re-secured back again (Fig. 9.21c). This "sutured graft complex" can be used not only to support the lateral crura but also to change the direction of the lateral crura in an "arc" from medial to lateral and also to physically push and rotate the nasal tip down in an over rotated tip. This is different from alar batten graft which is placed over the lateral crus underlying the skin envelope and cannot be used as a structural graft to de-rotate the tip or alter the position of the lateral crus. By supporting and strengthening the lateral crura, the strut grafts also corrects the collapse of external nasal valve and alar pinching in the lateral alar region. Hence, this surgery not only helps in structural reconstruction of lateral crus but also supports the function in the external nasal valve region.

9.11.2 Indications

- Deficient and weak lateral crura, unilateral or bilateral (Fig. 9.21a). These patients present with alar weakness and alar "in-drawing" on inspiration. It is extremely difficult in these patients to differentiate lateral crural weakness from other causes of alar collapse. The issue could be in the lateral crus or in the scroll region above or in the alar margin below the lateral crus or simply due to lateral crural cephalic migration. LCSG works only in patients with alar weakness due to defects in lateral crus.
- The diagnostic clues pointing to lateral crural weakness (as the cause of alar collapse) are the severity of the alar collapse, the more severe the collapse the more possibility it is due to lateral crural weakness. Look for localised concavity in the alar region or localised defects in the lateral alar region which are usually due to defects in the lateral crus. Also an important diagnostic clue for lateral crural weakness as the cause of alar weakness is tip deviation to the same side (Fig. 9.23a, b) [46, 43]. This is because of relatively stronger opposite lateral crus pushing the tip to the affected side. This can happen only if the lateral crus is weak.
- Over rotation (upward) of the nasal tip (Fig. 9.23a), where lateral crural strut grafts can be used to strengthen the lateral crus, de-rotate and push the tip down as a strut.
- Very thin lateral crus which is either convex out with or concave out with.
- Over-resected lateral crus (Fig. 9.24b) in revision surgeries or lateral crural weakness due to previous vertical dome division (Fig. 9.22).
- The underlying mucosa of the vestibule should not be scarred and be easily dissectible.
- It can be used to correct the functional issues associated with a bulbous parenthesis tip due to a cephalic malposition of the lateral crus, where the strut can be used to change the position of the remnants of the lateral crura.
- It is a good technique to correct alar margin collapse and can be effectively used to bring the alar margin down and out.
- It can be used unilaterally or bilaterally depending on the deformity of the lateral crus.

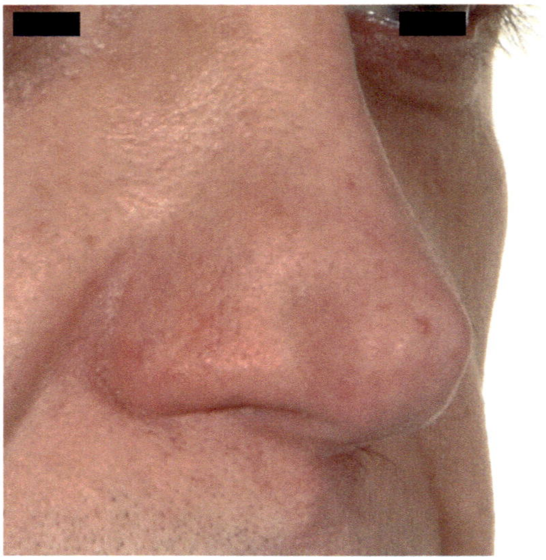

Fig. 9.22 A Lateral view showing interrupted right lateral crus

9.11.3 Contra-indications

- Multiple revision surgeries with scarring of the vestibular mucosa.
- Associated webbing or vestibular stenosis.
- If the dorsal aesthetic line is already quite wide at the alar-tip region.
- There is a potential risk of causing a lateral alar bulge, which should be discussed with the patient at the counselling stage.

9.11.4 Surgical Technique (Fig. 9.25a–h)

- *Be aware that patients present clinically with lateral alar weakness and functional obstruction of the ala on inspiration and not lateral crural weakness. It is up to the*

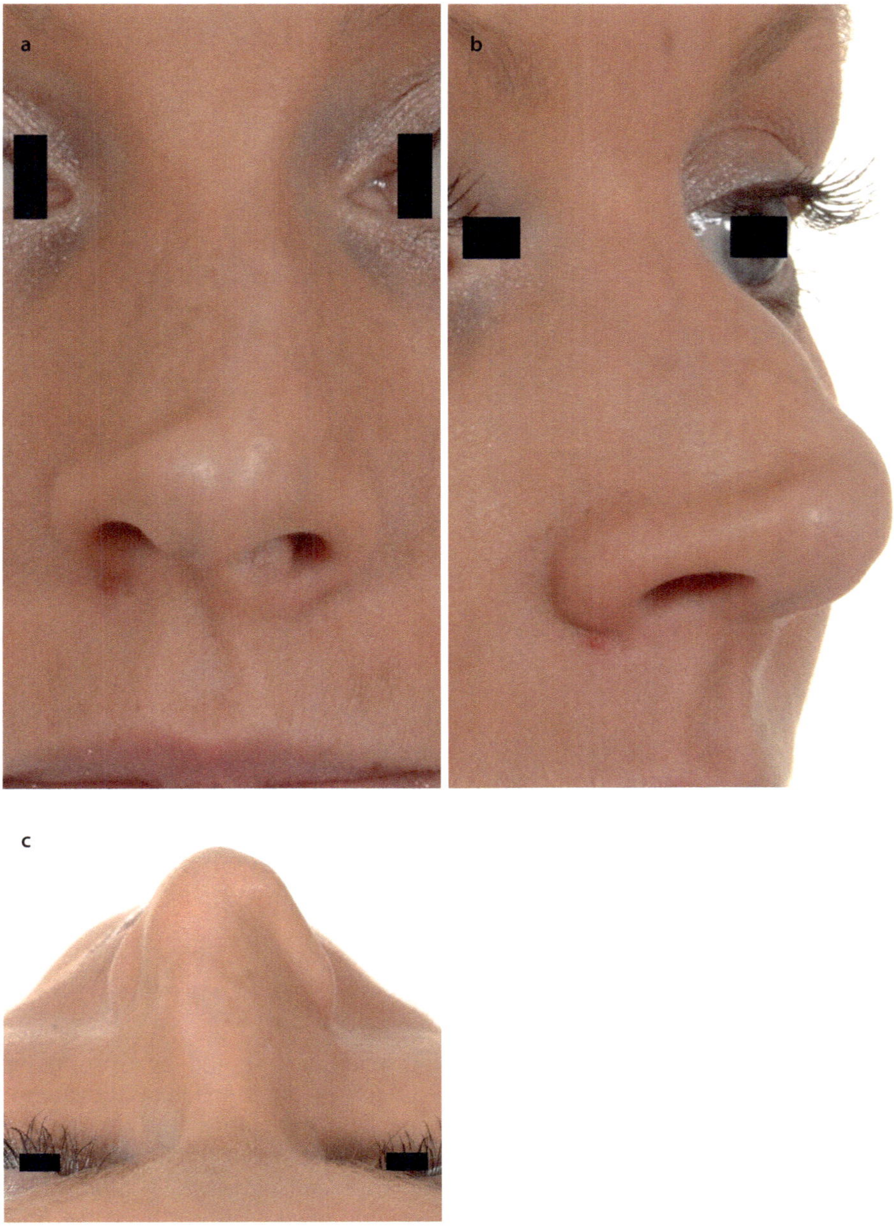

Fig. 9.23 **a–c** Right lateral crural weakness causing right alar collapse with tip tilt towards the same weaker side. Please note that this tip deviation is not because of the caudal septum ("Reproduced with kind permission from Ref: [46]")

surgeon to diagnose lateral crural weakness as a cause of lateral alar weakness [46–49]. Lateral alar pinching or weakness is commonly due to weak lateral crus, but could also be due to weakness in the scroll region above the lateral crus or below the lateral crus near the alar margin or a combination of all these. In the author's experience, the

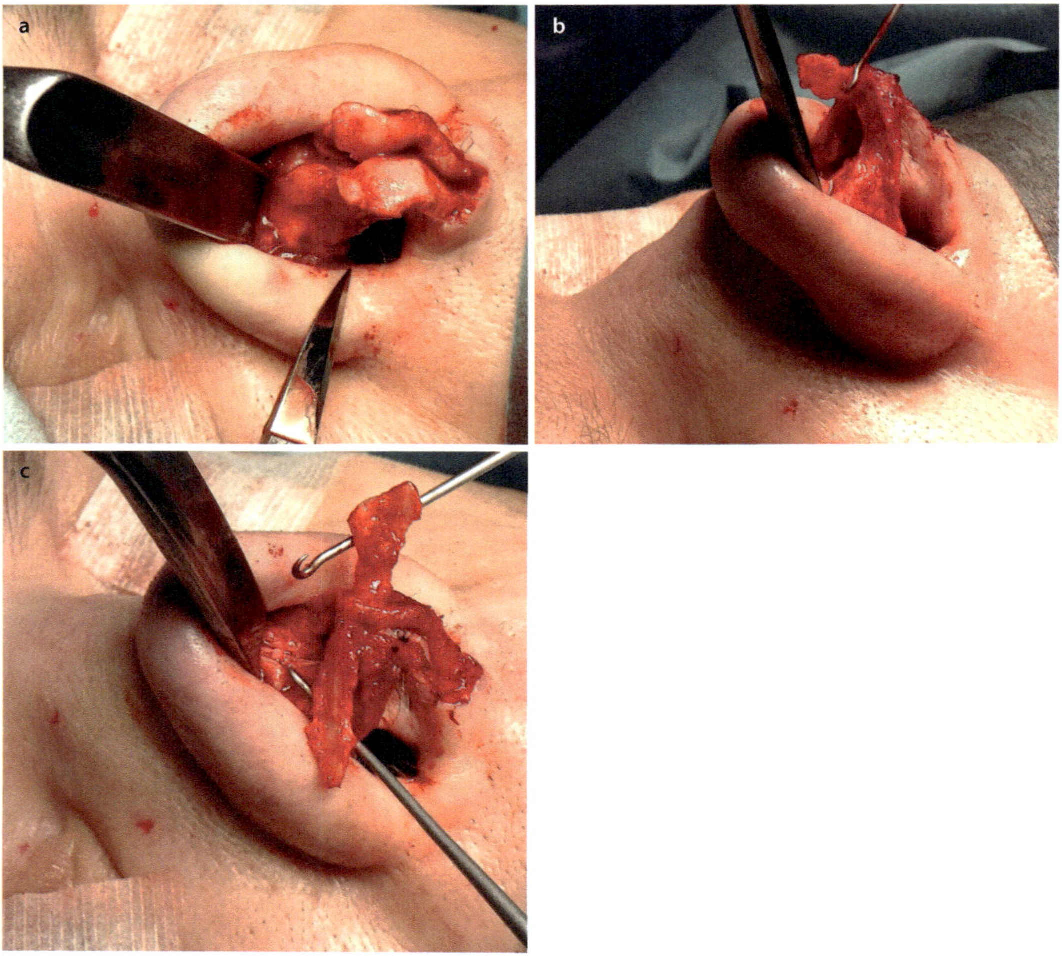

Fig. 9.24 a–c Open view showing bilateral damaged lateral crus dissected off from the underlying mucosa

LCSG works only in alar collapse due to weak or damaged lateral crus and not in scroll weakness or alar margin weakness.

- This procedure is one of the preferred options for lateral crural weakness as opposed to batten grafts.
- This is best done through an open approach. Open approach also helps to confirm whether the issue is in the lateral crus and if so what type of defect.
- The ideal width of a strut graft should be around 6–8 mm and not much more than that. The length of the graft depends on how much lateral crural length is left behind. This can vary from 8 to 12 mm. The caudal border and the medial extent of the strut should be ideally bevelled. A strut graft should be firm enough to strengthen the remains of the lateral crus and help push down the tip, hence preferably taken from septal cartilage or thin down costal cartilage. A slightly convex conchal bowl cartilage from the opposite side can be suited as well, but may not be firm enough, but can provide a good cosmesis.
- The presence of intermediate crus is important for tip definition after lateral crural strut grafts.
- Once the findings of lateral crural weakness or defect is confirmed through an open approach, hydro-dissection is done by injecting local anaesthetic in the alar mucosa underneath, thus helping to create

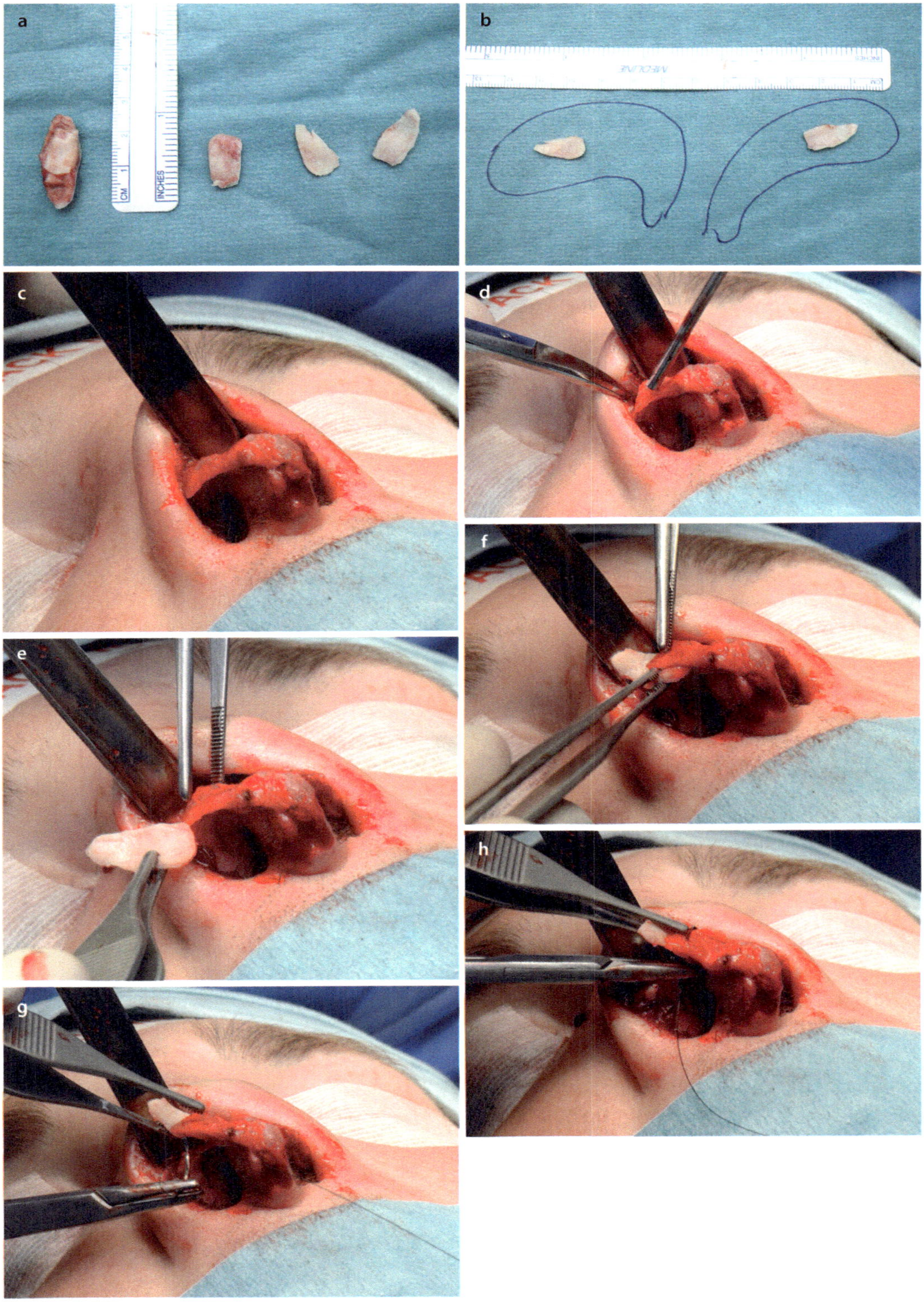

Fig. 9.25 **a–h** Sequential steps in the use of lateral crural strut grafts harvested from the nasal septum

a space between the under surface of the lateral crural cartilage and the mucosa of the alar region.
- Then the entire lateral crura is dissected off the underlying mucosa by careful dissection with iris scissors without damaging the underlying mucosa.
- The plane below the lateral crus can be approached from all four directions either superiorly, inferiorly, laterally at the scroll or medially close to the dome.
- The direction of approach depends on the defect in the lateral crus and also the indications for doing the lateral crural strut graft. There are pros and cons of approaching through all four directions.
- If there are defects in the lateral crus like a fracture line, then it will be wise to go through the defect in the cartilage and use this approach to "go under" the cartilage.
- Be aware not to approach the lateral crus from the inferior border as you run the risk of superior retraction of the alar margin with increased columellar show, which cannot be satisfactorily brought down by any revision procedure.
- Usually there is a fracture line just lateral to dome in more than 80% of our patients with trauma, and we prefer to go through the fracture line and then establish continuity after placing the graft underneath the lateral crus.
- The whole lateral crus can be dissected off if only small remnants are present. The strut cartilage is secured to the remains of the lateral crus cartilage with 5-0 vicryl through-and-through sutures.
- If the lateral crural strut graft is also used to bring down or push the tip forward and down or used to alter the position of the lateral crus due to cephalic migration, then it is wise to keep the inferior margin of the lateral crus attached to the alar mucosa, so that it can be used as a lever to push the alar margin or the tip down as a strut force and change the angle of vector.
- The width of the strut graft will be usually bigger than the damaged crus if the indication is right and in this situation when the strut grafts are secured to the remains of the lateral crus, the edges of the overlying lateral crus should be bevelled and not be seen on the outside once the skin is draped.
- On completion, it will be advisable to use crushed cartilage onto the suture site.
- Be aware that it can give "rigidity" to the nasal tip. The strut grafts are used with straight pieces of septal cartilage or costal cartilage graft. Hence, it adds thickness and heaviness to the lateral crus, thus running the risk of widening of the nasal alar region, and rigidity to the tip.
- LCSG can also add weight to both the lateral crura and can push the tip down (◘ Fig. 9.21c), particularly if the medial crus is weak and not adequately supported. To avoid this issue, this procedure is usually combined with columellar strut as well. It can also cause thickening of the lateral alar region causing external nasal valve narrowing with subjective nasal obstruction and functional external nasal valve obstruction. Patients can also complain of "feeling a lump" inside the lateral alar region.

9.11.5 Surgical Sequence

Open approach is preferable. Septal work and graft harvesting should be done first, followed by bony dorsal work. This should be followed by internal valve surgery (spreader grafts) if needed. Finally medial crural work and caudal septal strengthening should be done followed by tip work and finally lateral crural strut grafts before closing the skin flap.

Key Points
- Strut grafts are ideally indicated in weak or fractured and discontinuous lateral crura. The grafts should be thin and not too thick, which can cause rigidity to the nasal tip.
- Septal cartilage would be the ideal choice, and the graft should preferably not wider than 8 mm in width. The length can be up to 12–14 mm.
- There is also a potential risk of causing a lateral alar bulge, although less likely compared to an alar batten graft. This should be discussed with the patient at the counselling stage.

- It is important to secure a caudal strut or put medial crural flare control sutures to improve the conjoined medial crural strength before using a strut graft, otherwise there is a risk of loss of tip projection and under rotation due to the weight of the lateral crural strut.
- Do not dissect the inferior border of the lateral crus from the alar margin mucosa until otherwise needed, as it can cause retraction of the alar margin.
- If the lateral crural strut graft is also used to bring down or push the tip forward and down or used to alter the position of the lateral crus due to cephalic migration, then it is wiser to keep the inferior margin of the lateral crus to the alar mucosa intact so that you can use it to lever and push the alar margin or the tip down as a strut force and also change the angle of vector.
- The whole lateral crus should be dissected off if only small remnants are present and the strut cartilage is secured to the remains of the lateral crus cartilage with 5-0 vicryl through-and-through sutures.
- The strut graft can be individually attached to the remnants of the damaged lateral crus and then sutured to the alar mucosa at the desired level or can be done through a single through-and-through suture going through the remnants of the lateral crus, the strut and the alar mucosa in one go.

Conclusion

- Strut grafts are structural grafts to reconstruct a weak ala due to a weak lateral crus so that it can give stability to the lateral alar wall and also withstand the inspiratory forces and help in restoring the external nasal valve function.
- Ideally it should be thin enough to support the lateral crus but at the same time strong enough not to cause rigidity to the nasal tip.
- Usually needed in revision procedures where there has been over-resected lateral crus.

9.12 Alar Batten Graft

9.12.1 Introduction

The word batten (Bat-Ten) means a long flat strip of metal or wood used to hold something in place. Batten grafts were described to support and stabilise a week lateral ala causing functional nasal obstruction at the external nasal valve. Alar batten graft, as the name suggests, is supposed to offer structural support to a weak lateral ala acting like a flat strip of metal or wood. The cartilage is usually harvested from the opposite conchal bowl to suite the anatomical orientation. *As opposed to lateral crural strut grafts, the batten grafts sit between the overlying skin envelope and the lateral crus. It cannot be placed entirely on a weak and damaged lateral crus as it can be counterproductive*. It can be placed at exactly where the alar pinching and weakness is, usually at the lateral alar region where there is no cartilage. *It does not work if the lateral crus itself is weak and damaged*. In our hands the indications for batten grafts are very limited, as it adds to the problem than solving the external nasal valve issues. The long-term outcome is consistently poor if done in the wrong patient. The surgical principle is flawed in a way if the lateral crus is weak, like building a first floor when the ground floor is already weak. Sometimes the outcome is much worse, by not only making the nasal obstruction worse by adding the cartilage which in turn pushes the alar region inside, but also ends up giving the patient unwanted cosmetic bulge in the ala.

9.12.2 Indications

- Lateral alar weakness, causing alar pinching, either unilateral (◘ Fig. 9.26a), or bilateral made worse on inspiration (◘ Fig. 9.26b). Some studies show excellent results [50, 51], but in our experience batten grafts works in patients with alar collapse due to weakness above or below the lateral crus and not involving the lateral crus.

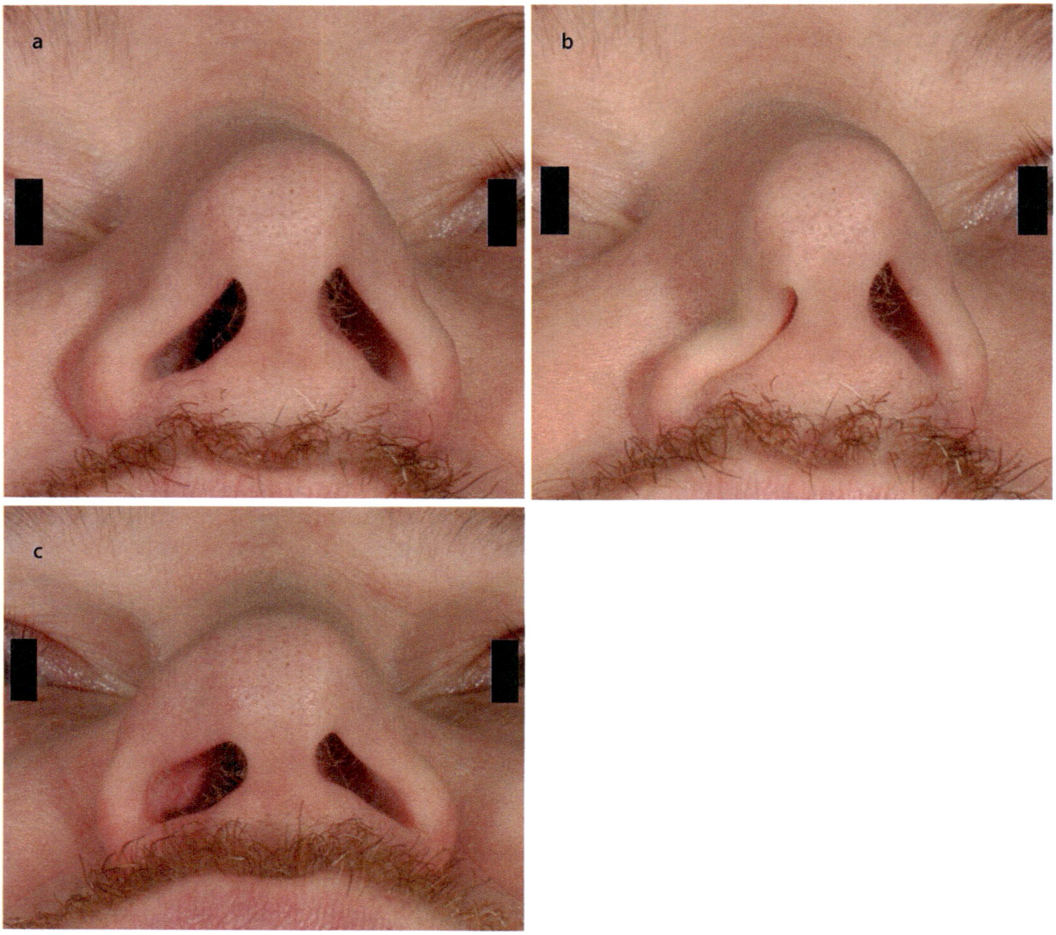

Fig. 9.26 **a** Weak right ala on quiet breathing. **b** Collapsed right ala on inspiration. **c** Wide ala on the right side after batten graft placement

- An intact, but cephalically migrated lateral crus.
- The width of the lateral crus should be at least 4–5 mm.
- There should be no discontinuity in the structure of the lateral crus.
- Usually performed in association with alar rim graft.

9.12.3 Contra-indications

- Batten grafts do not work if lateral crural weakness is due to a concavity or discontinuity in the lateral crus, particularly if there is a vertical fracture line just lateral to the dome on the affected side.
- If there is only a thin strip of lateral crus left or if the width of the lateral crus is less than 4–5 mm, or completely missing, as seen in revision surgeries following over resection.

9.12.4 Sources of Graft Material

- Conchal cartilage graft from the opposite conchal bowl would be the ideal choice (Fig. 9.27a–c).
- Sometimes thin septal cartilage can be used.

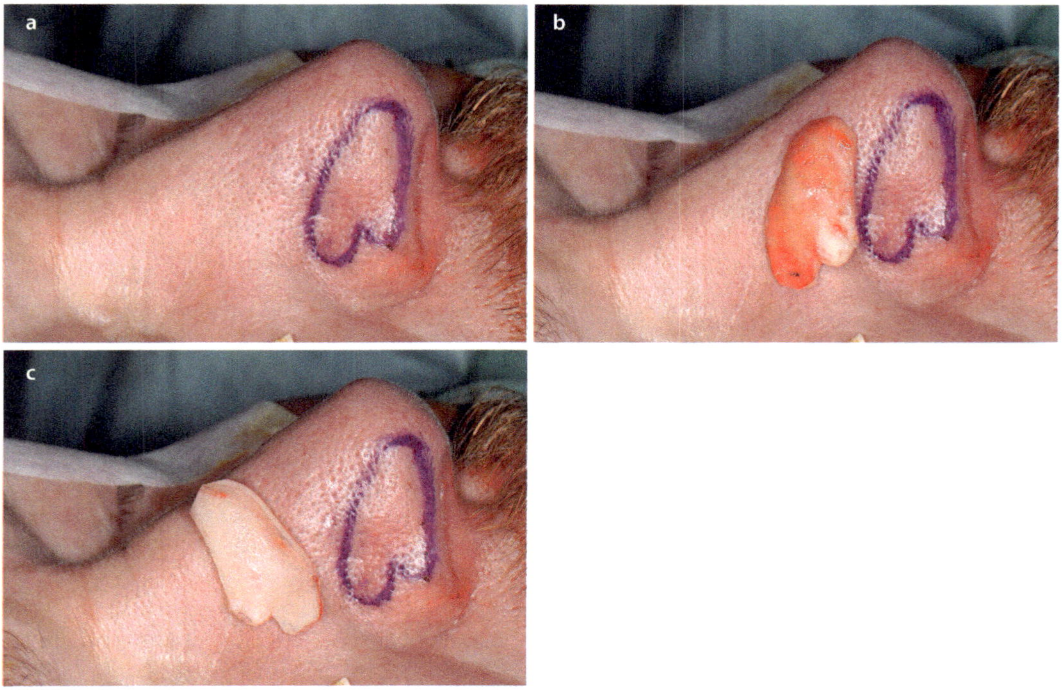

Fig. 9.27 a–c The shape and position of the alar batten graft on the right side

- Helical rim cartilage folded lengthwise can also be used as a batten graft.
- Polyethylenes or PDS sheets can be used. We personally don't use them to avoid any unwanted post-operative issues, particularly if it gets infected.

9.12.5 Surgical Technique (Fig. 9.28a–j)

- The batten grafts can be done through a closed approach creating a pocket at the point of maximum weakness in the lateral ala and inserting the graft. The problem with this technique is that the anatomical site of the problem cannot be ascertained and if the patient has alar weakness due to a damaged lateral crus, the issue of nasal obstruction can be made worse.
- This diagnostic dilemma can be avoided if done through an open approach where the diagnosis can be confirmed and the right surgery can be planned. We prefer to do this procedure through an open approach, as sometimes multiple grafts may have to be used and sutured in place.
- Ideally the area of maximum concavity in the alar region is marked out before, with the patient in quiet breathing and also forced inspiration. This way the surgeon can mark out the exact area where the graft should sit in.
- The skin flap is elevated through an open approach or done through a closed approach to expose the entire lateral alar region. Overlying soft tissues are dissected away to expose the cartilage.
- The diagnosis is confirmed when done through an open approach and the correct choice of surgical technique can be made. Make sure the lateral crus is weak BUT intact. Be aware that a damaged or partly missing lateral crus will NOT be helped by batten graft. In this situation, a better choice would be a structural lateral crural strut graft.
- Ideal graft material will be from the septal cartilage, which is firmer and straighter than the conchal cartilage.

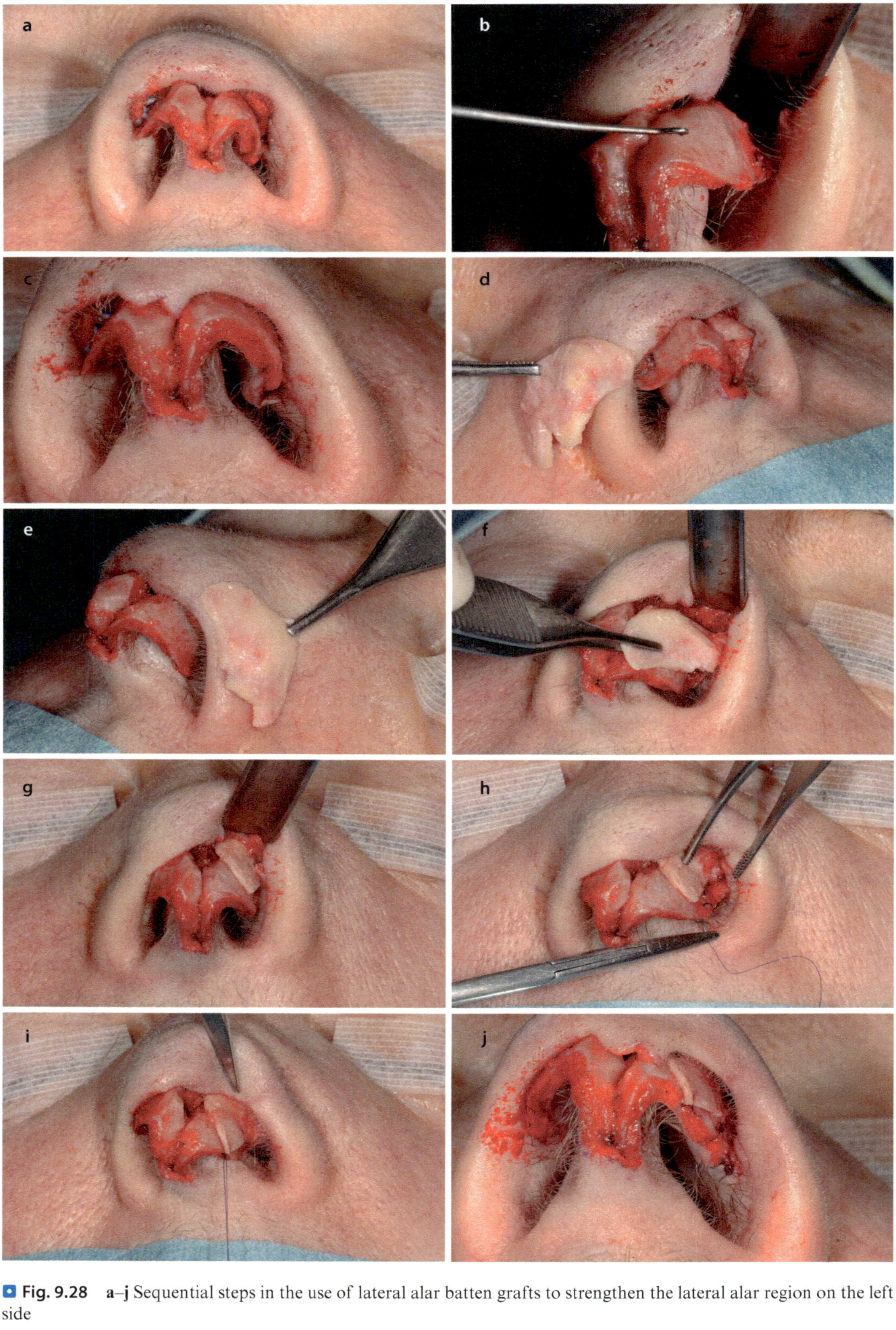

Fig. 9.28 **a–j** Sequential steps in the use of lateral alar batten grafts to strengthen the lateral alar region on the left side

- If conchal bowl cartilage is harvested, it is preferable to harvest from the opposite side and fashioned as shown in ◘ Fig. 9.28e. It is advisable to have the lateral side fashioned as a double bulge, one shorter and one longer, the longer section used as far laterally as possible over riding the pyriform aperture.
- Before inserting the batten graft laterally, a small stab incision is made in the mucosa of the pyriform aperture and the superior lateral bulge is inserted through the mucosal stab along the plane of the lateral crus. The shorter lateral bulge is placed inferiorly and the longer lateral bulge is placed superiorly over the bone in the pyriform aperture and the junctional area is hitched against the bony pyriform aperture.
- The medial half of the cartilage is then placed over the lower half of the lateral crus overriding as much as two-thirds of the length and sutured to the lateral crus with vertical mattress sutures going through-and-through the mucosa with 5-0 vicryl suture.
- If done through closed approach, the pocket is custom fit as laterally as possible and there is no necessity to secure the graft with a suture.

Key Points

- Problems can arise with alar batten graft in the form of an asymmetric bulging in the lateral alar region, and alar ballooning particularly if the overlying skin is thin. Patient should be warned of the cosmetic bulge in the lateral alar region. Even if the breathing is better, patients do not like this asymmetry. This can last up to 6 months. Otherwise you may end up in an unhappy patient who can breathe but end up in a cosmetic deformity, which they did not have before!
- Sometimes the weight of the batten graft adds to the lateral crus weight and pushes it down inside. This happens if the the graft is too medially placed or too superiorly placed, or placed over a weak or fractured lateral crus, causing more obstruction and may end up in an unhappy patient who cannot breath and also have a cosmetic bulge in the lateral nose. Be aware of achieving a balance between structure and function.
- A superiorly placed batten graft can cause the alar margin to drop down beyond the inferior border of the batten graft and thus forming a hood at the lateral alar margin causing in-drawing on inspiration. Sometimes, this is seen even if the batten graft is in the right position. Hence, it is advisable to do this procedure along with alar marginal rim graft to prevent patients coming back again with alar hooding at a later date.
- Be aware that the soft triangle can get distorted and wider with batten graft exerting an upward pull.
- It is also advisable to do this procedure on both sides even if the indication is only on one side, as asymmetries both in structure and function can result at a later date following surgery on one side.

Conclusion

- Correcting lateral crural abnormalities can be complex and can lead to diagnostic challenges.
- A clear surgical algorithm based on the discussion above will help in choosing the correct surgical technique.
- If the lateral crura is intact, but if the weakness is either above or below the lateral crus, then the best choice would be a batten graft.
- If the lateral crura is wide, weak and concave, but structurally intact, the best choice would be a lateral crural turn in or out flap.
- If the the lateral crus is missing, fractured or if the width is less than 6 mm then consider lateral crural strut grafts.

9.13 Alar Marginal Rim Grafts

9.13.1 Introduction

Alar marginal rim grafts [29], as the name suggests, are indicated where there is an alar marginal weakness and in-drawing of the inferior alar margin causing functional obstruction in the external valve region associated with inspiratory in-drawing and nasal alar collapse [52]. This may be either due to primary damage to the caudal border of the lateral crus, or could be due to soft tissue alar retraction or due to cephalic migration of the lateral crura. As the name suggests, it offers structural support to a weak alar margin rim. They are thin long pieces of cartilage around 12 mm in length and not more than 4 mm wide placed at the alar margin through a stab incision laterally at the alar vestibule region and inserted in a subcutaneous tunnel. The alar marginal graft can be fashioned as a separate piece or as a part of the alar batten graft. Quite often alar margin weakness is associated with upward retraction of the alar margin causing an excess columellar show. Be aware that the alar marginal rim grafts will only prevent inward movement of the alar margin rim on inspiration, but will not correct the upward retraction of the alar margin. To bring down the alar margin, we need to use a lateral crural strut graft.

9.13.2 Indications

- Alar marginal collapse or weakness as seen in ◘ Fig. 9.29a, usually unilateral, may be bilateral, usually secondary to trauma either surgical or non-surgical.
- Alar hooding of skin and soft tissues unilateral or bilateral, due to superior retraction of underlying cartilaginous framework.
- Cephalic migration of the lateral crus due either to scarring or due to change in the orientation of intermediate crus leaving a larger area in the lateral alar region left uncovered by cartilage.
- To correct soft triangle scarring or retraction or excess triangulation of soft triangle due to upward migration of the intermediate segment of the lower lateral cartilage.
- Sometimes the use of a strong batten graft at a higher level can cause soft tissue hooding of the alar margin with loss of support and inspiratory in-drawing.

9.13.3 Contra-indications

Alar retraction and weakness due to loss of overlying skin and also underlying mucosa with resulting lack of soft tissue cover, as seen after localised full-thickness traumatic defects, surgical excision and burns/scalds.

9.13.4 Sources of Graft Materials

- Conchal bowl cartilage from the opposite ear.
- Helical rim graft from the same or opposite ear.
- Sometimes a composite graft from the root of the helix may be needed if there is an associated loss of overlying skin.

9.13.5 Diagnostic Algorithm

- For considering alar marginal grafts, there should be a collapse of the alar margin (◘ Fig. 9.29a). Look at the alar margin on inspiration and expiration and compare with other side. If so, the extent of the length of the collapse should be noted. Is it extending up to and beyond the soft triangle? Any weakness of the lateral crura and the junctional areas between the upper lateral cartilage and the lower lateral cartilage should be noted as well.
- Palpate the soft triangle region and measure the distance from the skin margin from the apex of the nostril in the basal view to the lower concave margin of the intermediate segment of the lower lateral cartilage.
- As seen in ◘ Fig. 9.29a, there is a retraction and collapse of the right alar margin on inspiration when compared to the left ala. There is a collapse at the soft triangle region either due to weak intermediate crura and disconnection or just simply an upward migration of the lower margin of the intermediate segment of the lower lateral cartilage away from the skin margin causing excess triangulation of the already existing soft triangle.

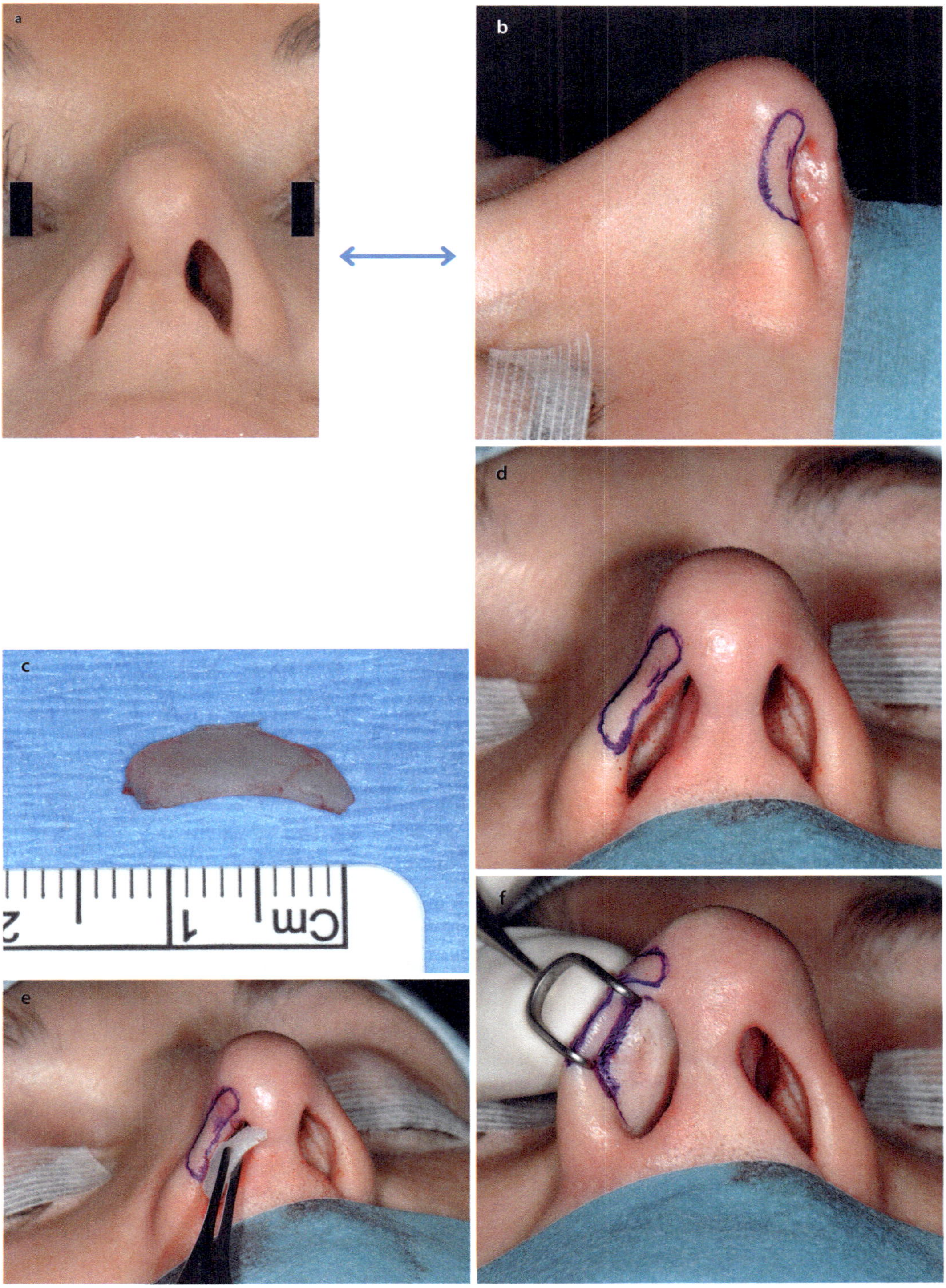

Fig. 9.29 **a–j** Sequential steps in the use of lateral alar marginal rim grafts to strengthen the lateral alar margin on the right side. ("Reproduced with kind permission from Ref: [43]")

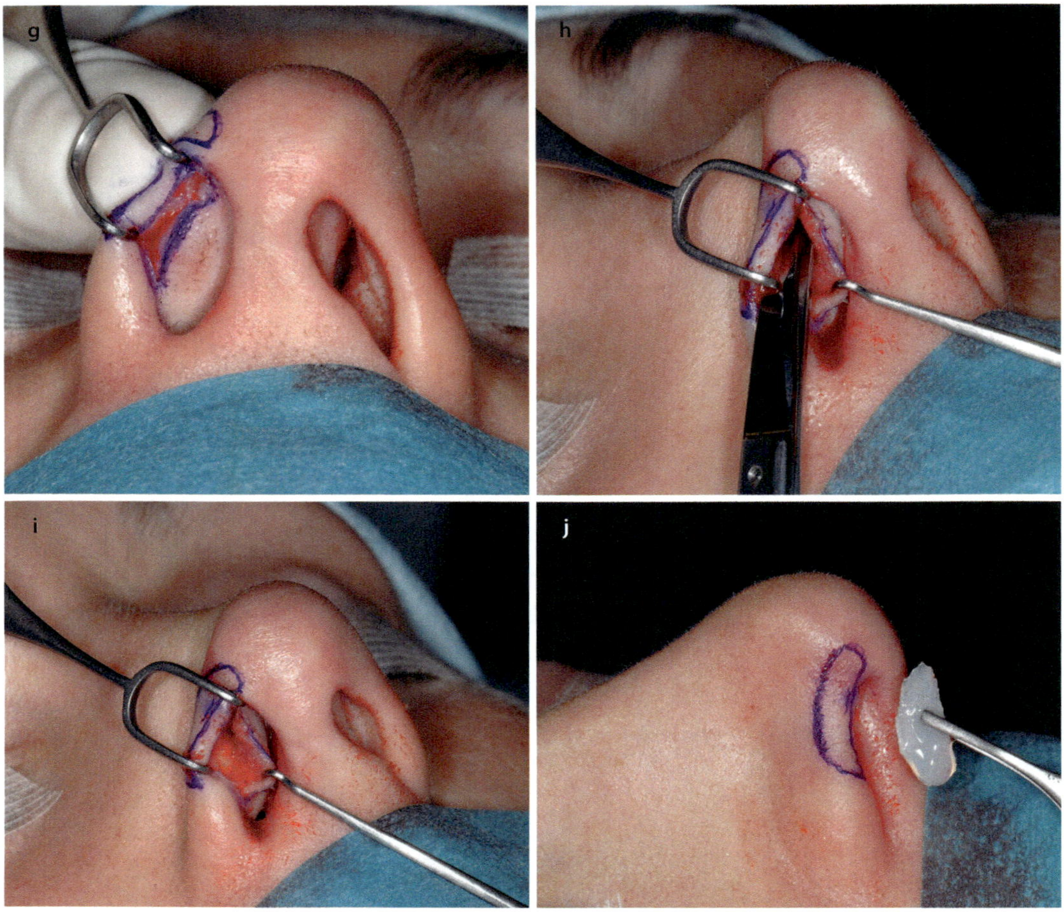

▣ Fig. 9.29 (continued)

9.13.6 Surgical Technique (▣ Fig. 9.29a–j)

- Before planning the surgical procedure, a decision is made whether this is required in isolation or as part of an alar batten graft.
- If it is done in isolation as in ▣ Fig. 9.29a, the approach is either through a small stab incision in the lateral alar region and using a subcutaneous tunnel up to the soft triangle or through a horizontal alar marginal incision following the cutaneous alar margin and not along the lower margin of the lateral crural cartilage.
- A smaller incision is made when compared to the length of the graft. The soft tissues are elevated in a plane below the cutaneous fat of the ala. The tunnel should be of the equal length and width of the graft, although the outer incision should be less than the length of the graft. Once the space is dissected, the graft is shaped and inserted first towards the nasal tip and rest of the graft is pushed into the posterior pocket and then the marginal incision closed with absorbable 5-0 vicryl.
- The graft is usually harvested from the conchal bowl of the contralateral ear and shaped to the required size.
- If the procedure is performed as part of nasal tip reconstruction through an open approach, then the graft should be placed precisely at the alar margin and secured by interrupted 5-0 ethilon sutures as there is

a risk of superior migration of the graft when done through open approach. This problem is not there when a specific pocket is created allowing the size of the graft to fit into the pocket.

9.13.7 Complications

Bruising, swelling and thickening of the alar margin which in turn can cause nasal obstruction.

Long-term scar contraction as well.

Key Points

- Remember alar rim grafts can ONLY be used to push the lateral alar margin outwards and NOT downwards! Upward migration of the alar skin margin due to scarring or secondary to loss of tissue cannot be compensated by the alar rim grafts.
- If patients require alar batten graft or lateral crural strut graft, it is always advisable to do an alar rim graft as well, as reinforcing the lateral crus can have a negative effect on the alar margin, even if the margin is not weak initially.
- If it is done as a sole procedure, it is advisable to create a smaller pocket and use a bigger graft, so that there is no need to secure the graft, but if it is done as part of a more complex reconstruction through open approach, it is advisable to stitch the graft in place.
- Remember alar margin is an area, where normally there is no cartilage, but a cartilage framework is needed to reinforce the area, when it is weak.
- If it is done as the only procedure, make the incision in the lateral alar region as close to the margin and do an avascular dissection, avoiding bleeding as any blood clots later can cause fibrosis and loss of cartilage strength.
- Make sure the medial end of the graft does not override the domes as this will introduce a cosmetic bulge at the tip and also a step. But at the same time, the medial end should not fall short of lateral border of the intermediate crus.
- Shaping of the graft is important with adequate width and roughly a dome shape. The medial border should be tapered smoothly so that it does not override the intermediate crus and the dome.

Conclusion

- Alar marginal rim grafts are structural grafts to reconstruct a collapsed alar margin. It aims to give stability to the lateral alar rim to withstand the inspiratory forces and helps in restoring the external nasal valve function.
- In conclusion the alar rim grafts are used in reconstructing a collapsed alar margin, where the graft is used to bring the alar margin "OUT" and not "Down".
- Ideal cartilage material would be from the conchal bowl, which will conform to the shape of the alar margin. Long strip of cartilage with narrow width (12 mm by 4 mm) will be ideal.
- It should be thin enough to support the alar margin but at the same time strong enough not to cause rigidity of the nasal tip.

9.14 Lateral Crural Reciprocating Graft

9.14.1 Introduction

Lateral crural reciprocating graft is a clever technique used to correct a "concave" lateral crus with normal width and normal strength. It can also be done in a concave strong lateral crus with a discontinuity or fracture of the lateral crura close to the dome. Please note the rest of the lateral crus should be structurally intact. In post-traumatic lateral crural concavity, the commonest site we have found the fracture line is just next to the dome with the rest of the lateral crus being pulled in due to negative inspiratory forces. *Thus the key considerations for correcting a lateral crural concavity are the width and structural integrity of the lateral crus.* In this technique, the lateral crus is turned on its side so that the outer concave surface is "turned in" as the lateral crus is rotated on its long axis. This technique not only helps to correct the lateral crural concavity, but also helps in improving the nasal function at the external valve region.

9.14.2 Indications

- It is a versatile technique to be considered if there is a lateral crural concavity due to a single fracture (◘ Fig. 9.30a), just lateral to the dome, but with otherwise structurally intact lateral crus with normal width.
- Concave lateral crus with concavity limited to the middle of the lateral crus (◘ Fig. 9.30a).
- Width of the lateral crus should be limited to 10–12 mm and not too wide.
- Adequately preserved lateral crural cartilage with no multiple fractures or defects.
- Lateral alar "in" drawing with valve obstruction due to concave lateral crus. The most likely scenario in a traumatic nose with concave lateral crus is as shown in ◘ Fig. 9.30a, when there is a longstanding fracture line just lateral to the dome and constant negative forces of inspiration causes the concavity, making the functional obstruction worse.
- Usually this deformity is also associated with a twist in the nasal dome with a tip deviation to the affected same side due to the unopposed action of the opposite normal lateral crus. The affected side may also show a localised asymmetric over projection of the dome and under rotation when compared to the opposite normal side.
- There could also be a dorsal curvature of the lower third to the opposite side near the tip due to associated problems with the caudal dorsal septum.

9.14.3 Contra-indications

- Multiple fractures of lateral crus, associated with a very narrow and week medial crus.
- Very wide lateral crus with a width of more than 12 mm.
- If the concavity of the lateral crus is not central but well localised either to the medial or lateral aspect of the lateral crus.

9.14.4 Surgical Algorithm

The alternative procedure to consider in these patients is a lateral crural strut graft. The clinical findings which make you decide to do a lateral crural reciprocating graft is the *width* and the *absence of any fractures* or scarring of the lateral crus. If the concavity of the lateral crus is associated with a normal width of between 10 and 12 mm and adequate strength, then the LCRG is indicated. Instead if the width is in excess of 12 mm and the concavity is because of the excess width rather than any weakness or discontinuity of the lateral crus then a cephalic turn in flap (as described by Dr. Fazil Apayddin from Izmur) would be ideal [53]. Please refer to the ▶ Chap. 18 on surgical algorithms in dealing with lateral crural deformities.

9.14.5 Surgical Technique (◘ Fig. 9.31a–l)

- Open approach is ideal for access, as it helps to confirm the findings and also helps in executing the technique.
- This can be done by two ways, the concave segment of the lateral crus can be dissected off the underlying mucosa and flipped over pivoting at the scroll region or the concave segment can be completely excised and turned inside out as a separate piece (◘ Fig. 9.31f) and sutured back end to end.
- The lateral crus is incised at the junction between the intermediate crus and the lateral crus. If there is a fracture line just lateral to the intermediate crus, go through the fracture line.
- Care is taken not to go through the alar mucosa. Dissection is facilitated by hydrodissection.
- The cartilage is dissected off the underlying mucosa till the lateral aspect near the scroll.

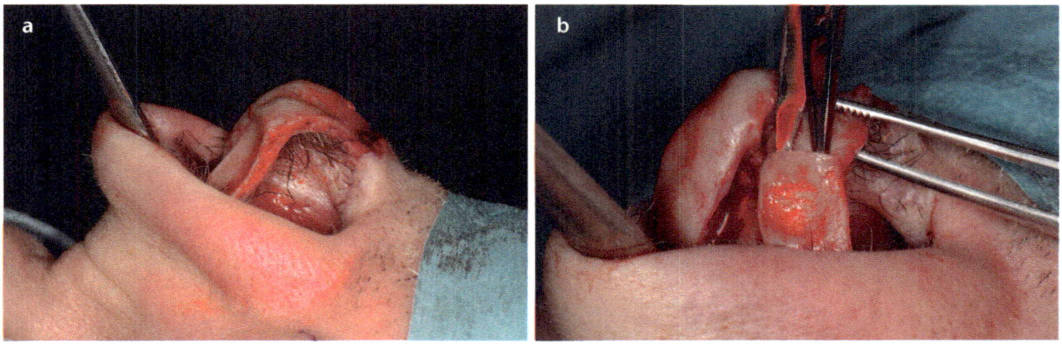

Fig. 9.30 **a**, **b** Concave lateral crus due to a fracture line just lateral to the dome on the right side

- Once lateral extent of the lateral crus is reached, the dissection is tapered to a small point medial to the "scroll", so that the lateral crus is still attached and not completely free.
- Once the lateral crus beyond the incision line is completely lifted from the underlying skin, then the lateral crus is vertically turned around 180 degrees around its longitudinal axis avoiding any torsion and stitched back to the Intermediate crus with two or three simple 5-0 ethilon sutures.

9.14.6 Surgical Sequence

Lateral crural work should always be preceded by columellar reconstruction and medial crural work.

If the same patient needs a tip narrowing procedure like an inter-domal or trans-domal suture, then be aware that this may cause stress on the lateral crural suture lines.

Key Points

- Surgical planning is the key, depending on the clinical findings. It is always better to have an algorithm in your mind to correct different deformities of the lateral crus before the surgical intervention.
- Care must be taken to dissect the lateral crus, without damaging the alar mucosa.
- Attention to the suture line is important, keeping it as a simple suture than a mattress suture.
- Always use non-absorbable suture when suturing two edges of cartilage together close to the mucosal edge of the ala.
- If the lateral crus is wider, you may need to use two separate simple sutures, rather than a single suture in the middle.
- Since the suture line is quite medial close to the nasal tip, cut the knots very close and cover them with crushed cartilage.
- Patient should be counselled that the concavity in the alar region might become convex.
- Take care to preserve the scroll region, avoiding any damage to the scroll fat with too much dissection or diathermy.

Conclusion

Thus lateral crural reciprocating graft is used if the lateral crus is of normal width, but still strong and concave without multiple fractures or weakness and scarring. Other options like lateral crural strut graft and lateral crural turn in flap should also be considered depending on the clinical findings.

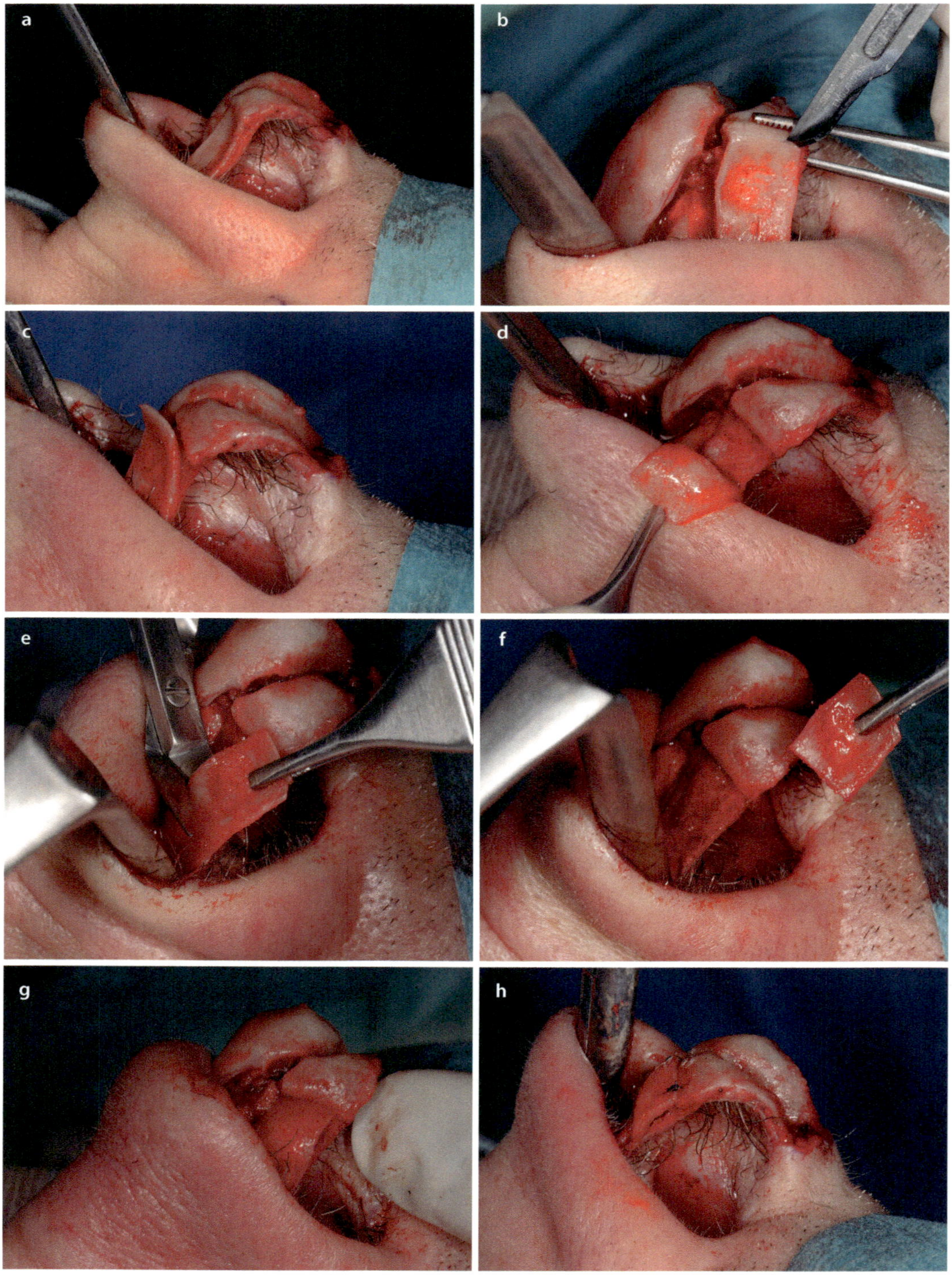

Fig. 9.31 **a–l** Surgical sequence showing the steps of lateral crural reciprocating graft to correct a concave lateral crus

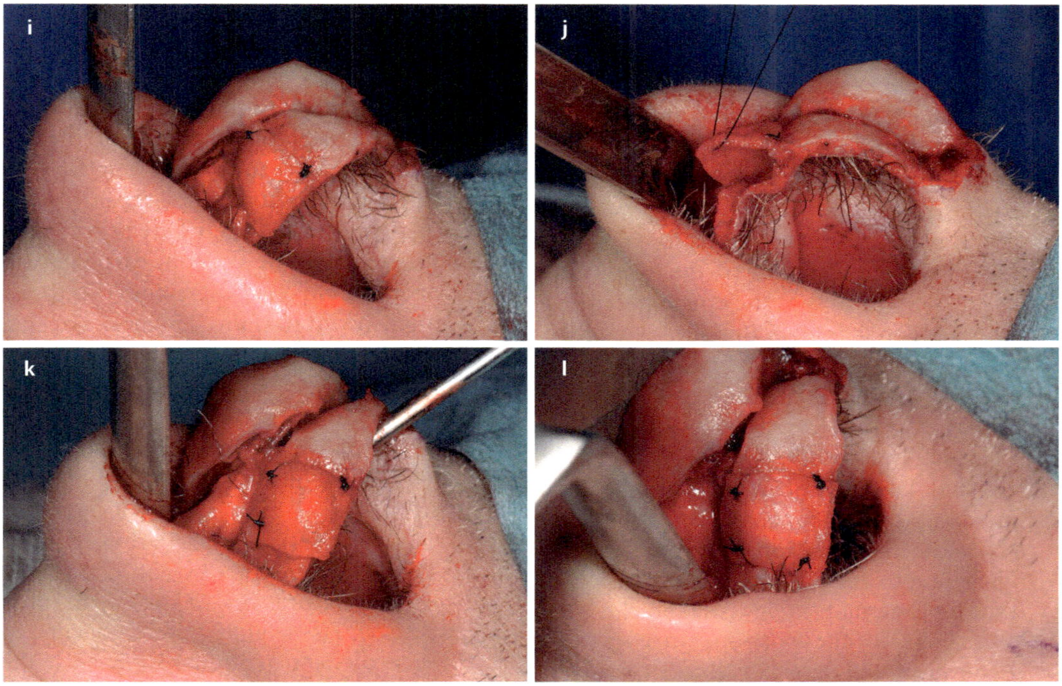

Fig. 9.31 (continued)

9.15 Dorsal Double-Layered Boat Graft

9.15.1 Introduction

This graft is the one most commonly used for augmenting a mid-dorsal collapse of the nasal dorsum. This graft is a work horse for nasal dorsal reconstruction of a de-projected and collapsed dorsum. Be aware this is not a structural graft, but a camouflage graft. Ideally we use a two-layered conchal bowl cartilage for most of the dorsal reconstructions. Sometimes rib cartilage can be used, but it can be rigid and non-pliable and does not integrate with the soft tissues of the dorsum and become mobile, particularly in patients wearing glasses would be a problem.

9.15.2 Indications

- Dorsal augmentation for a de-projected mid-nasal dorsum due to nasal trauma or previous surgery involving the dorsal cartilaginous septum with loss of dorsal septal support.
- To rebuild the nasal dorsal profile in an over-resected nasal dorsum after a rhinoplasty.
- Mid-dorsal collapse secondary to septal haematoma and infection.
- Mid-dorsal collapse secondary to septal perforation either traumatic or post surgery.
- Mid-dorsal collapse due to loss of septal support due to a granulomatous process.

9.15.3 Contra-indications

- There are no contra-indications, although when indicated in mid-dorsal collapse, it is advisable to put this over a solid structural base of bilateral spreader grafts.
- Also need to be careful of post-operative infections in patients with septal perforations. In our experience, there is an increased risk of post-operative infection of the graft in patients with septal perforation.

9.15.4 Surgical Technique (Fig. 9.32a–j)

- Cartilage is harvested from the conchal bowl of the pinna (Fig. 9.32a). This is a deep concave area of the pinna just lateral to the cartilaginous part of the external auditory canal. (See chapter on conchal bowl harvest). The root of the helix (crus of the helix) starts at the concha abutting into the conchal bowl dividing them into a slightly larger concave "cavum" concha inferiorly and a smaller concave "cymba" concha superiorly.
- It is usually advisable to remove the whole conchal bowl cartilage as a single unit including cavum concha and cymba concha, as partial resection can cause the overlying skin to stick around the cut edges of the cartilage making it visible in the conchal bowl in the post-operative period. If however, only a small sliver of conchal cartilage is needed, care must be taken to bevel the remaining edges. The cartilage can be harvested via *anterior approach or posterior approach.*
- Generally multiple layers of conchal cartilage is needed for adequate dorsal augmentation (Fig. 9.32c). If costal cartilage graft is used, the cartilage is used as a single layer and shaped to the right size and allowed to warp for 30 minutes before use and soaked in an antibiotic solution prior to use.
- If conchal cartilage is used, a decision is made to harvest on one or both sides, depending on the degree of dorsal augmentation required.
- Usually with one conchal bowl cartilage with an average thickness of around 2–3 mm, we can build either a two-layered or three-layered graft building up to a vertical height of up to 5 mm (Fig. 9.32f).
- Similarly by staggering the layers one below the other, the length of the graft can be anywhere between 3 and 4 cm.
- The layers are designed or mapped out in the conchal bowl cartilage depending on the requirements, as shown in Fig. 9.32c. Generally we use the longer cavum concha forming the uppermost layer and the shorter second layer formed by the cymba concha and the intermediate segment used as an inferior third layer, if necessary. Generally two layers are enough for most reconstructions. The length of the adult Caucasian nose to be reconstructed is usually around 4 cm, whereas the maximum length of the conchal cartilage will be only around 3 cm maximum. So to get a length of more than 3.5 cm of conchal cartilage you may have to stagger lengthwise the two layers of cartilage so that the length of the graft is extended.
- Be aware that the superior layer should match the length of the defect to be reconstructed.
- If multiple layers of grafts are used, they are held together either by non-absorbable 5-0 ethilon sutures [54, 55] or any licensed tissue glue. Tissue glue is preferable due to the ease of their use and also because the sutures can cut through cartilage and can make the framework weaker. On the other hand, sutures may be helpful to anchor the graft in the right place.
- If tissue glue is used always check the local guidelines before using and be careful to wash off any extra glue in saline, and it will be wise to soak the cartilage in a broad-spectrum antibiotic of your choice before using.
- If done through open approach, the graft can be secured in place with 5-0′ PDS or vicryl sutures. If done through internal approach, a selective pocket is made so that the graft sits nicely in the pocket.

9.15.5 Surgical Sequence

To achieve long-term predictable outcomes, it is advisable to stabilise the mid dorsum by bilateral spreader grafts, before using the dorsal grafts. As dorsal de-projection is associated with a short nasal bones, a lateral straight high to low osteotomies are advisable to narrow the wide base and get some dorsal bony height/projection before using dorsal conchal graft for augmentation. Usually

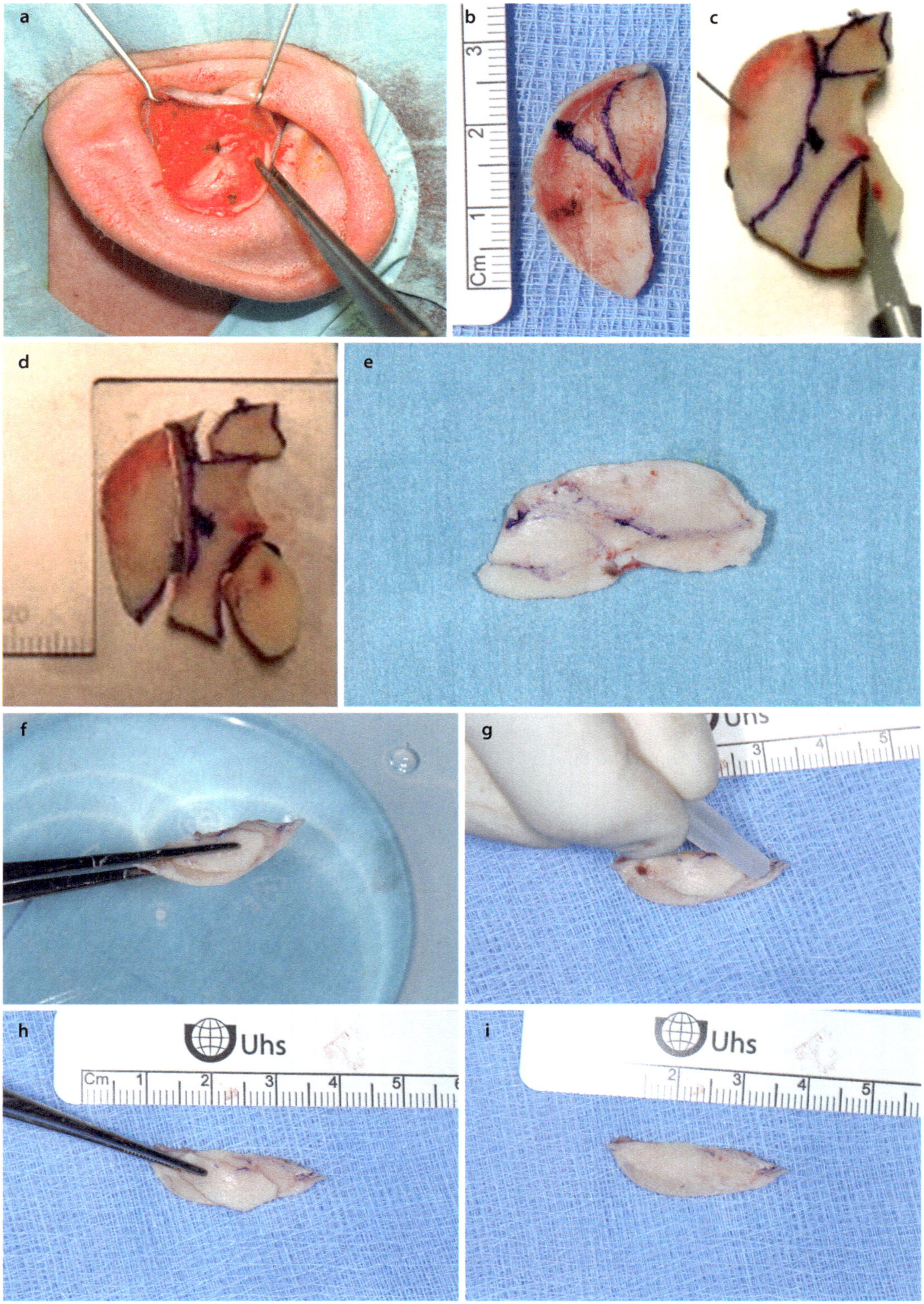

Fig. 9.32 **a–j** Surgical sequence showing the steps of dorsal double-layered "boat-graft" fashioned from the conchal bowl cartilage of the pinna

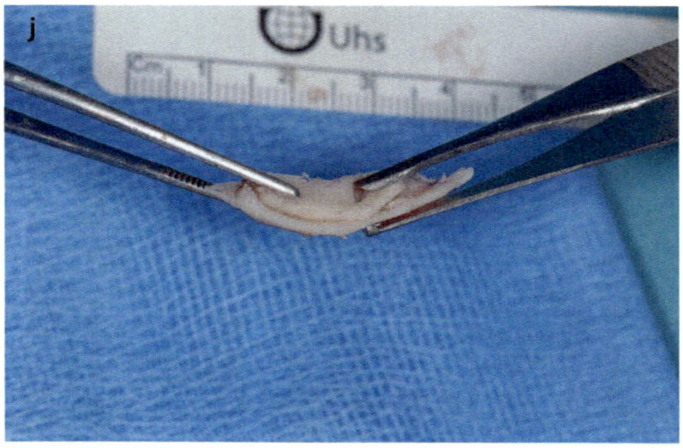

Fig. 9.32 (continued)

a straight high to low lateral osteotomy is preferred than a curved osteotomy, so that extra projection of the frontal process of the maxilla and the nasal bones can be achieved even though there is a risk of medialisation of inferior turbinates. Tip work should be done prior to augmentation to establish the projection height of the tip before augmenting the mid-dorsal height.

9

Key Points

- Preferably done through an open approach, so that any ancillary procedures like spreader grafts can be easily done as well, at the same time. The approach also makes it easy to secure the graft in the right place.
- Care must be taken to bevel the edges of the cartilage so that there is a smooth transition in the sides of the graft.
- Per-operative antibiotics are indicated in the presence of septal perforation.
- It is preferable to do a stabilising spreader grafts before dorsal camouflage.
- Be aware that rib cartilage may be quicker to harvest on one side than bilateral conchal bowl harvest, but rib cartilage may be difficult to shape and is firm and not be satisfactory in patients with thin contracted skin and do not integrate very well with the dorsal framework.

Conclusion

The dorsal conchal graft is a versatile option to augment the mid dorsum. It is easy to harvest and easy to execute with consistently positive outcomes.

9.16 Cartilaginous Autogenous Thin Septal Graft (CATS Graft)

9.16.1 Introduction

Cartilaginous autogenous thin septal (CATS) graft was first described by McKinney, from Northwestern University School of Medicine, Chicago [56]. This graft is taken from the septal cartilage and it is thin and narrow; it is used to smoothen any dorsal irregularities, after a septo-rhinoplasty, be it primary or secondary procedure. This is not a structural graft, but a camouflage graft used to camouflage and prevent any residual dorsal irregularities during the healing process after dorsal reduction. It can be used with or without crushing as required. It is more of a prophylactic value to avoid any dorsal irregularities in the postoperative period, which is one of the commonest reasons for a revision rhinoplasty. Literally we use this in all primary rhinoplasties where dorsal reduction is done to prevent any unwanted dorsal irregularities requiring revision surgery at a later date.

9.16.2 Indications

- To cover any dorsal irregularities after hump reduction and re-shaping the nasal bony dorsum.
- To avoid any unwanted depressions or dents appearing in the mid-dorsal region during the healing process few months after surgery.
- To establish a smooth continuous dorsal profile line between the nasal bony dorsum and the cartilaginous dorsum.

- Advisable to do this in patients with thin overlying skin with or without overlying pigmentation to camouflage and strengthen the dorsal soft tissues. This is a very useful way of buffering a very thin and discoloured dorsal skin after multiple previous surgeries.
- We recommend the use of this graft routinely in all revision rhinoplasties and also even in primary rhinoplasty to prevent any future issues.

9.16.3 Contra-indications

- Might not be possible to harvest septal cartilage in all patients, particularly in revision surgeries where there is not enough septal cartilage or the septal muco-perichondrial planes cannot be raised without causing further damage to the septum.
- In patients with large septal perforations.
- In patients with multiple revision surgeries where the dorsal flaps cannot be raised.
- Even in these above-mentioned situations, the concept is still valid using any other cartilage and use them as a thin crushed cartilage graft on the dorsum.
- If there is any of the above-mentioned contra-indications, we prefer to use a small patch of fascia lata or temporalis fascia particularly in revision rhinoplasties with thin overlying and discoloured skin.

9.16.4 Surgical Technique (◘ Fig. 9.33a–i)

- Most patients requiring this graft would need septal work to be done as well. Hence these patients will have the septal muco-perichondrial flaps raised on both sides. Usually the ventral 4–5 mm of the septal cartilage which is dislocated from the maxillary crest is used. A typical piece removed from the ventral septum is boat shaped rather than rectangular shape so that the anterior nasal spine region support is maintained.
- Before the segment is used, the piece of cartilage should be of uniform thickness. The triangular base should be shaved off and kept in a cartilage crusher and crushed gently, up to a point where it is still firm and not become not too soft. An ideal cartilage would be a 4 mm strip of ventral septum removed after a septoplasty.
- Ideally a cartilage crusher is used as above. It is made of heavy metal and surprisingly considerable force is used to crush the cartilage.
- It can be used as a thin crushed cartilage or can be crushed and used as a fine mesh graft.
- Septal cartilage is best suited for the purpose as it holds a degree of stability even after crushing. If not available any other cartilage can be used. If helical or conchal

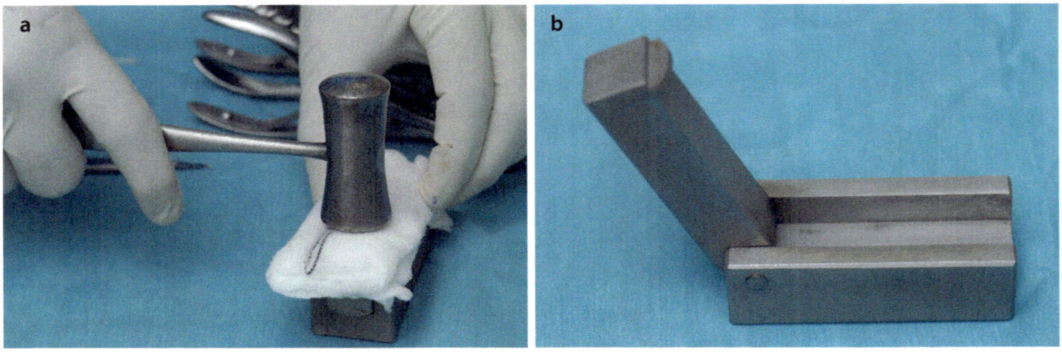

◘ **Fig. 9.33** a–i Surgical sequence showing the steps of cartilaginous autogenous thin septal graft (CATS) crushing, handling and used as a dorsal camouflage graft before closing the skin flap

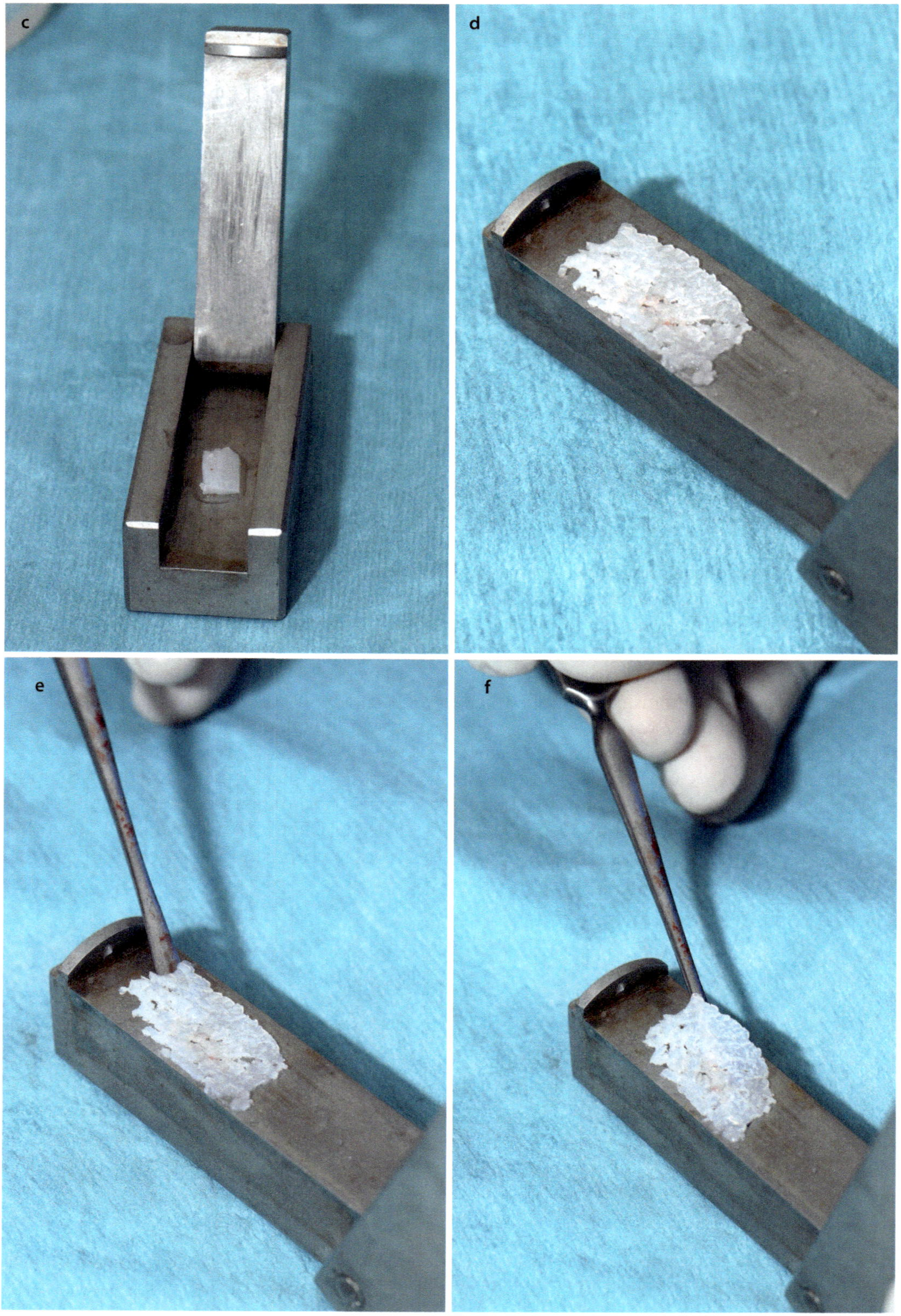

Fig. 9.33 (continued)

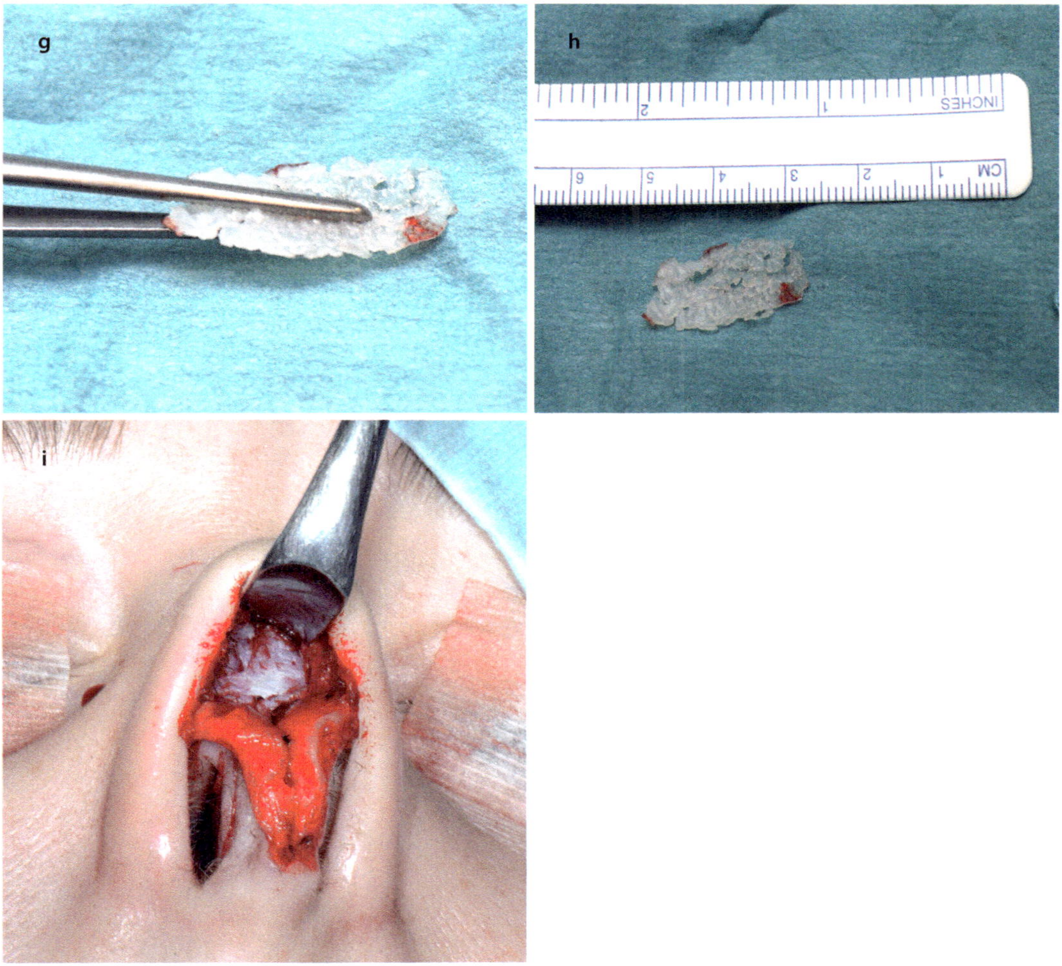

Fig. 9.33 (continued)

cartilage is used, there is no need to crush them. If crusher is not available, you can crush the cartilage with a heavy curved artery forceps and break the resilience all along the length of the cartilage.

- Alternatives are layered fascia lata, particularly used if there is a thin, scarred and pigmented dorsal skin in multiple revision rhinoplasty patients.

9.16.5 Surgical Sequence

This should be used as a LAST step before closing the flap and gently moulded into the dorsum with a wet swab. It is NOT advisable to do anything further in the nose after this is done.

Key Points

- Try and use a thin layer of CATS graft at the end of all primary reduction dorsal work to prevent post-operative dorsal irregularities. This concept makes it a wonderful added tool to avoid future revisions.
- Cartilage crushers are used for crushing the septal cartilage. High force will be needed to achieve the desired effect. When crushing the septal or rib cartilage grafts, use wet swabs both above and below the crusher to buffer the noise. Always warn the theatre staff about the impending noise. You will be surprised how much noise this can create.

- Use Freer's elevator to lift the crushed cartilage rather than forceps and then use long non-toothed forceps to insert the graft over the dorsum.
- A viable alternative, if no septal cartilage is available, is to use the excised cephalic portion of the lateral crus without the need for crushing.

Conclusion
This is a very clever concept which takes extra few minutes at the end of the procedure to avoid future revision procedures and heartache to the surgeon.

9.17 Columellar Plumping Graft (CPG)

9

9.17.1 Introduction

Columellar plumping grafts, as its name suggests, helps in plumping the columella which is retracted and scarred. Columellar plumping grafts are used to camouflage any minor retraction of the columella at the columellolabial angle region (◘ Fig. 9.34), thereby plumping the columella out. It is also used to correct small irregularities showing through the columella after a caudal strut or caudal septal extension procedure as a buffer. *Although it adds to the volume of columella, it is not an alternative for a "volume loss" of the columella.* These are additional techniques to camouflage and are NOT structural support grafts for the tip; can also be used to correct small areas of puckered skin in the columella. This is not an alternative to caudal septal reconstruction or a columellar strut, but acts as an adjunct to smoothen the columella.

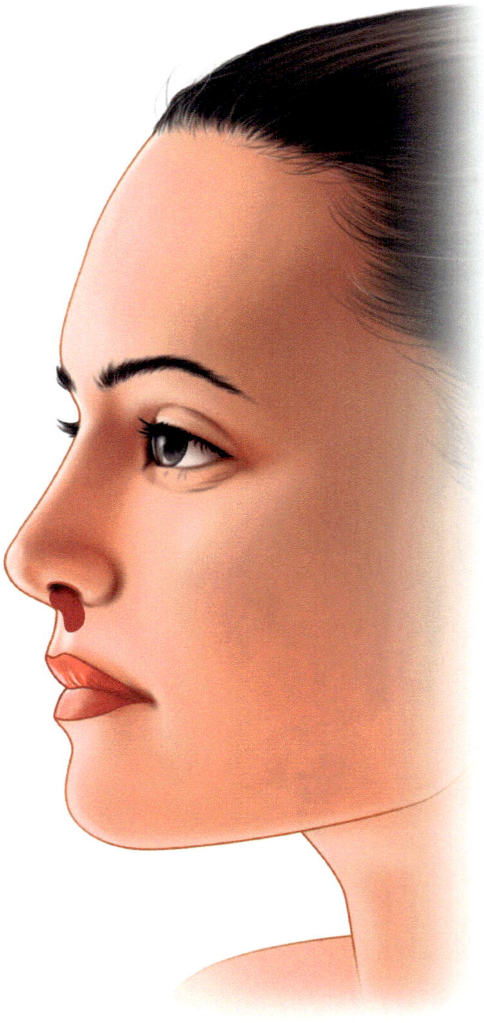

◘ **Fig. 9.34** Schematic representation of the ideal site for the placement of a columellar plumping graft

9.17.2 Indications

- The most common indication is usually a traumatic patient who had multiple previous trauma or surgery, with a retracted columella.
- Patients with a vertical cleft along the length of the columella (◘ Fig. 9.35a), associated with a degree of retraction and volume loss of columella.
- Usually done along with a caudal septal reconstruction with an extension graft.
- Also helps in smoothening small puckered scars in columellar skin.

9.17.3 Contra-indications

- No specific contra-indications in the right patient.
- Non-availability of cartilage pieces.

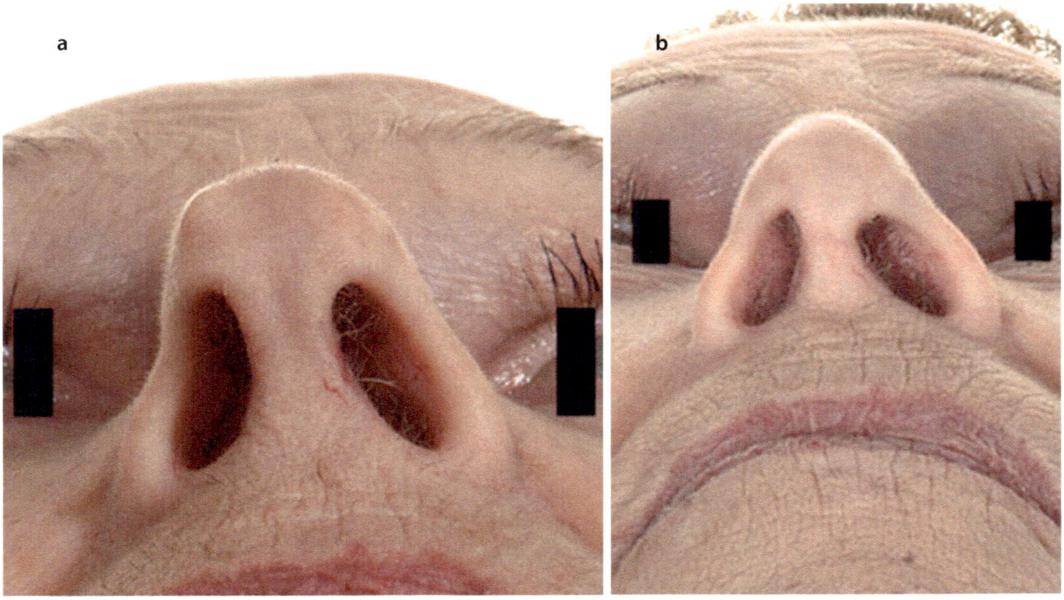

Fig. 9.35 a, b Basal view showing volume loss in the columella and is an ideal indication for the placement of a columellar plumping graft as an adjunct to any form of caudal reconstruction

9.17.4 Surgical Technique

- Usually done as an adjunct to a caudal septal reconstructive procedure, like a caudal septal extension graft or a columellar strut graft to correct volume loss.
- More recently this plumping of columella is done as an isolated procedure, using fillers, although the volume augmentation with fillers will be temporary and may be sought with other potential complications and does not address the primary structural issue.
- If there is a volume loss of columella along with loss of structural support needing extensive septal reconstruction procedure, then, it is better to do this through an open approach as part of the caudal septal reconstruction.
- As an isolated procedure, it can be done through a vertical marginal columellar incision.
- The type of grafts used is usually a crushed or diced septal cartilage, but a lateral crural cartilage cephalic strip which was excised during a cephalic trim can be very well suited to plump the columella.
- Plumping graft need not be secured in place with sutures and usually kept in place in small closed pockets between the medial crus or between the medial crural footplate and the overlying columellar skin of the naso-labial angle.
- It will be easier to insert the graft after the alar marginal incisions are closed, when done through an open approach.
- Used in multiple pieces to plump areas where it is needed (Fig. 9.35).

9.17.5 Surgical Sequence

It is advisable to do the medial crural reconstruction if necessary and strengthen the medial crus and bring them together to create a conjoined medial crus before using the plumping graft.

Key Points

- Literally none.
- Even a little over correction does not matter.
- Do not use large pieces of firmer uncrushed cartilages.

- When done along with septal extension grafts, it helps to avoid sharp edges of cartilage showing through.
- These are quick adjunctive procedures to be aware of during a rhinoplasty surgery which will make bigger impact to your results.

Conclusion

This is a simple and effective technique to smoothen the columella in the basal view and to avoid any unwanted sharp edges of the cartilage and also to correct small puckered scars. Although it does help to add volume, it is not a structural graft for caudal septal reconstructions and tip support.

9.18 Cartilage Augmentation and Projection (CAP) Grafts

9.18.1 Introduction

"Cap" grafts are "cartilage augmentation and projection" grafts used to camouflage any depression and loss of dorsal profile height in the supra-tip region. This is particularly indicated after an increase in tip projection, which can result in a depression in the supra-tip region. As the name suggests is shaped like a "cap" or a hat and is positioned in the supra-tip lobule (◘ Fig. 9.36) as an on-lay graft [57] just cephalad to the maximum projecting points of the tip, *essentially occupying the supra-tip lobule of the tip* thus helping to fill any minor depressions or concavity and help in the smooth transition of the dorsal profile line from the nasion to the tip defining points. These are used to camouflage small defects following a rhinoplasty and are NOT structural support grafts. It is advisable to gently crush the cartilage and make it soft before placing the graft. These grafts are more commonly used in Asian rhinoplasty requiring augmentation particularly for revision procedures [58, 59, 60, 61, 62].

9.18.2 Indications

- To camouflage the concavity in the supra-tip lobule region. This usually happens in any surgical procedure like a septal extension graft, done to increase tip projection. Happens typically when a bulbous tip is narrowed, causing increased projection when compared to the rest of the dorsal profile line. The surgeon should be aware that narrowing a bulbous tip will increase the tip projection as well, and this will cause a concavity of the dorsal profile line in the supra-tip lobule segment. In this situation, it is important to plump the cephalic side of the tip cartilages with a cap graft as there is a dead space in the supra-tip lobule created due to increase in the projection at the tip.
- Cap graft may also indicated when a shield graft is used for increasing tip projection.
- Lack of cartilage or defective cartilage well localised only to the anterior septal angle of the septum.
- Cap graft also helps to establish a smooth dorsal profile line transition from the nasion to the tip-defining points. The graft helps to allow the transition from the mid-dorsal profile line to the supra-tip lobule profile line.
- Graft material should be either crushed or diced rather than a single piece of thick cartilage graft as the supra-tip space is a dynamic space where the tip can rotate into. Hence, this space should not be rigid and non-pliable (◘ Fig. 9.36).

9.18.3 Contra-indications

Avoid overfilling the supra-tip lobule space. Hence not indicated if there is a tension nose with excess anterior septal angle or after an extended dorsal spreader grafts or after septal extension grafts.

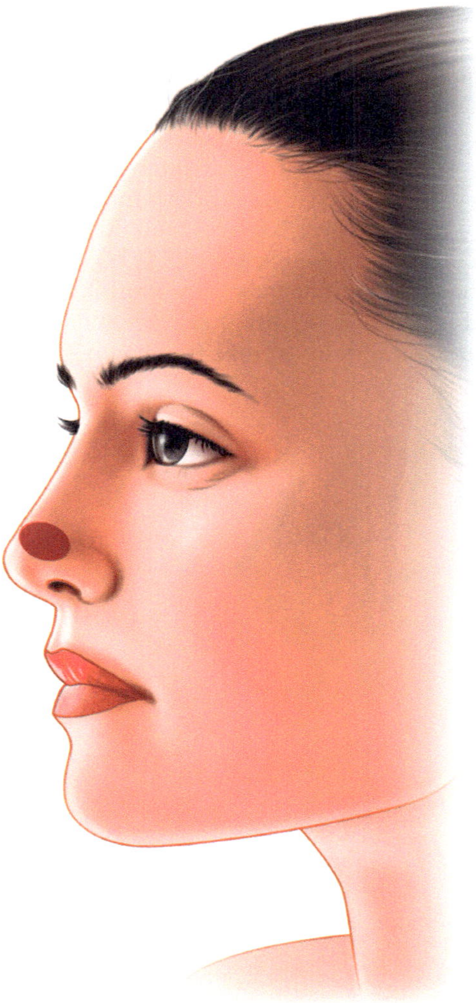

■ **Fig. 9.36** Schematic representation of the ideal site for the placement of a "cartilage augmentation and projection" (CAP) graft

9.18.4 Sources of Graft Materials

It is usually taken from crushed septal cartilage or the auricular cartilage of the conchal bowl or the helical rim. Crushed septal cartilage is the best for cap graft. Sometimes we can use leftover fascia lata as well. I would not advice fascia lata to be harvested specifically for a cap graft, in view of the time and morbidity involved. Literally any piece of leftover cartilage, be it soft and pliable can be used as a cap graft.

9.18.5 Surgical Technique

- Crushed cartilage is used in small pieces to fill the gap in the supra-tip lobule caused by the tip elevation by gently packing the space in the midline, behind the posterior superior border of the tip complex.
- Usually either crushed septal cartilage or ideally a soft pliable cephalic trimmed lateral crural cartilage is used. The ideal patient requiring a cap graft also would have had a bulk reduction of the tip cartilages; hence, plenty of cephalic portion of the lateral crus would be available to be used as a cap graft.
- Make sure the underlying mucosa is not breached during the rhinoplasty process.
- If nasal tip narrowing needed to be done, do that first so that the tip projection point is finalised before using the cap graft.
- Similarly, if using a shield graft and a cap graft, it is advisable to use the shield graft first and decide on the projection of the tip and then fill the supra-tip lobule section with the cap graft.
- There is no need to secure the graft as the only free crushed pieces of small cartilages are used. The graft is just left in place and the flap replaced (■ Fig. 9.37).

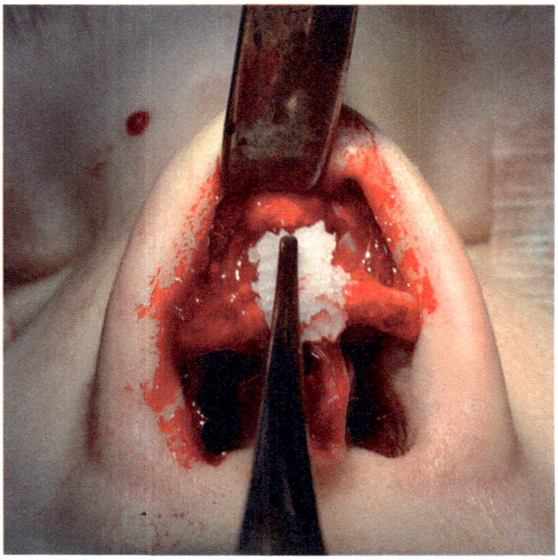

■ **Fig. 9.37** Open approach view showing the final placement of a "cartilage augmentation and projection" (CAP) graft before replacing the skin flap

9.18.6 Surgical Sequence

If done through an open approach, place it on the supra-tip region after the alar marginal incision had been sutured on both sides, so that the space is tight and there is no room for movement of the graft.

Key Points

- These are quick adjunctive procedures to be aware of during a rhinoplasty surgery which will make bigger impact to your results.
- It is a nice procedure to keep up your sleeve to re-establish the dorsal profile line after tip projection. Both septal crushed cartilage and resected cephalic portion of lateral crus can be used, but any available cartilage can be used.
- Used in multiple pieces to plump the supra-tip lobule segment.
- The graft should be ideally soft and pliable rather than firm. Hence, crushed cartilages are used instead of diced cartilages. Avoid using large pieces of cartilages as you run the risk of sliding and sharp edges.
- Avoid over correction so that the dorsal profile line is not altered by an elevation rather than a depression in the transition zone between the dorsal profile line and the tip.

Conclusion

These camouflage grafts can make a big difference to the dorsal profile lines and used as ancillary procedures after a septorhinoplasty. An aesthetic sense of when to use it cannot be explained but need to be experienced like a sculptor!

9.19 Shield Graft

9.19.1 Introduction

"Shield graft" was described by Jack Sheen in 1984 [1]. These are on-lay grafts. Although called a shield, they need not have to look like a shield. This graft is used to support the columella and increase projection of the nasal tip. This graft is placed in the infra-tip lobule segment and can be extended into the columella. The general shape of the graft roughly looks like a "shield", having a superior wider portion and a slightly tapered inferior portion. The graft is placed covering the *infra-tip lobule segment* when there is infra-tip blunting at the tip columellar junction (Fig. 9.38), as seen in the lateral profile view. This graft is ideally used to increase the tip projection and create an aesthetic "double-break" of the tip [63, 1].

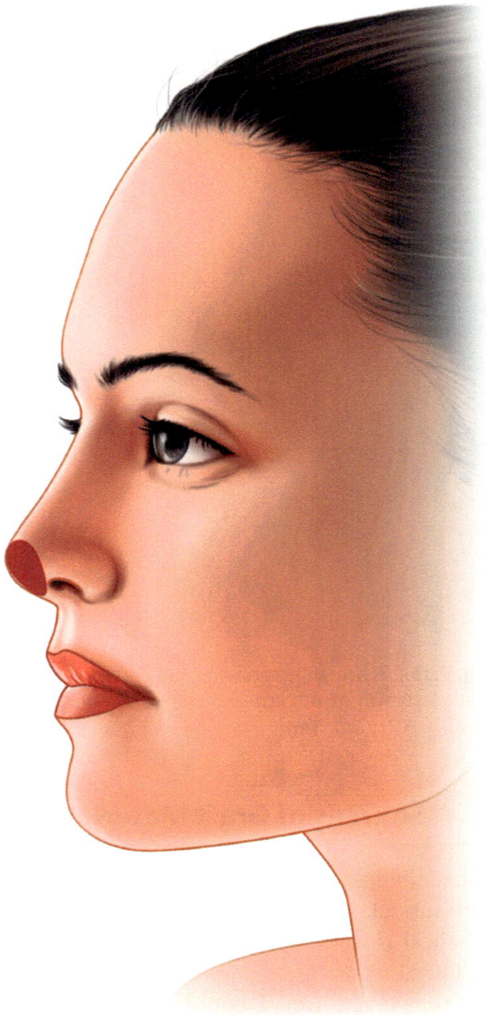

Fig. 9.38 Schematic representation of the ideal site for the placement of a "shield graft"

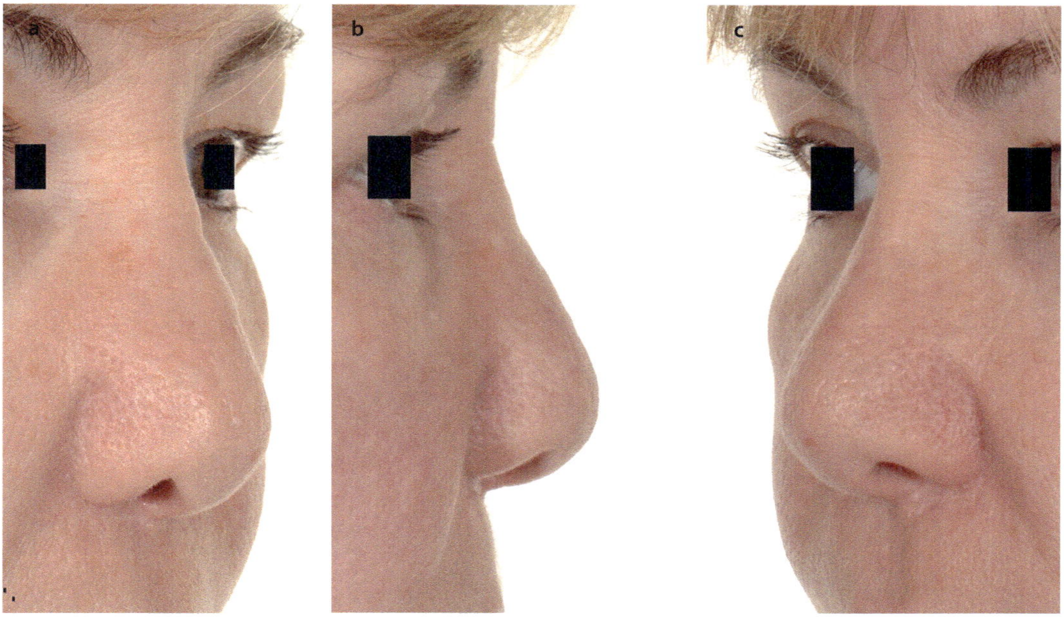

Fig. 9.39 **a–c** "Infra-tip" blunting which is an ideal indication for a shield graft. **a** Right three-fourth view. **b** Lateral view. **c** Left three-fourth view

9.19.2 Indications

- Major infra-tip blunting as seen on the lateral view with loss of projection (Fig. 9.39b), loss of definition on frontal view and short length of the nose.
- Thus shield grafts are used to address infra-tip lobule blunting and increase the projection of the tip in the profile view, thereby increasing the length of the nose.
- Augment the infra-tip lobule, thereby increasing the tip projection as well.
- Ideally indicated in an under projected tip with a much thickened skin.
- Also used to augment columella, in patients with retracted columella, when used as a long extension into the columella segment.
- Improves the definition of the tip by balancing the supra-tip and infra-tip lobule segments and helps to create an aesthetically pleasing "double-break" of the tip complex.
- Corrects an over rotated infra-tip lobule segment, particularly when there is an over resection of the anterior septal angle in a revision rhinoplasty patient.
- As mentioned above, this graft need not look like a shield.

9.19.3 Contra-indications

- Patients with very thin and discoloured pigmented skin, with atrophic changes due to multiple surgical procedures.
- Contracted overlying skin. Know your limitations. The overlying skin has to stretch, if not pulling the skin down over the graft can cause a polly beak.

9.19.4 Surgical Technique (Fig. 9.40a–j)

- Usually done through an open approach as an ancillary procedure. In isolation can be done through an internal approach, as described by Jack Sheen who used sutures to anchor the graft in the right place by passing them through the overlying skin. Sheen used this graft to augment the infra-tip lobule of the tip to correct infra-tip blunting and loss of loss of aesthetic double-break.

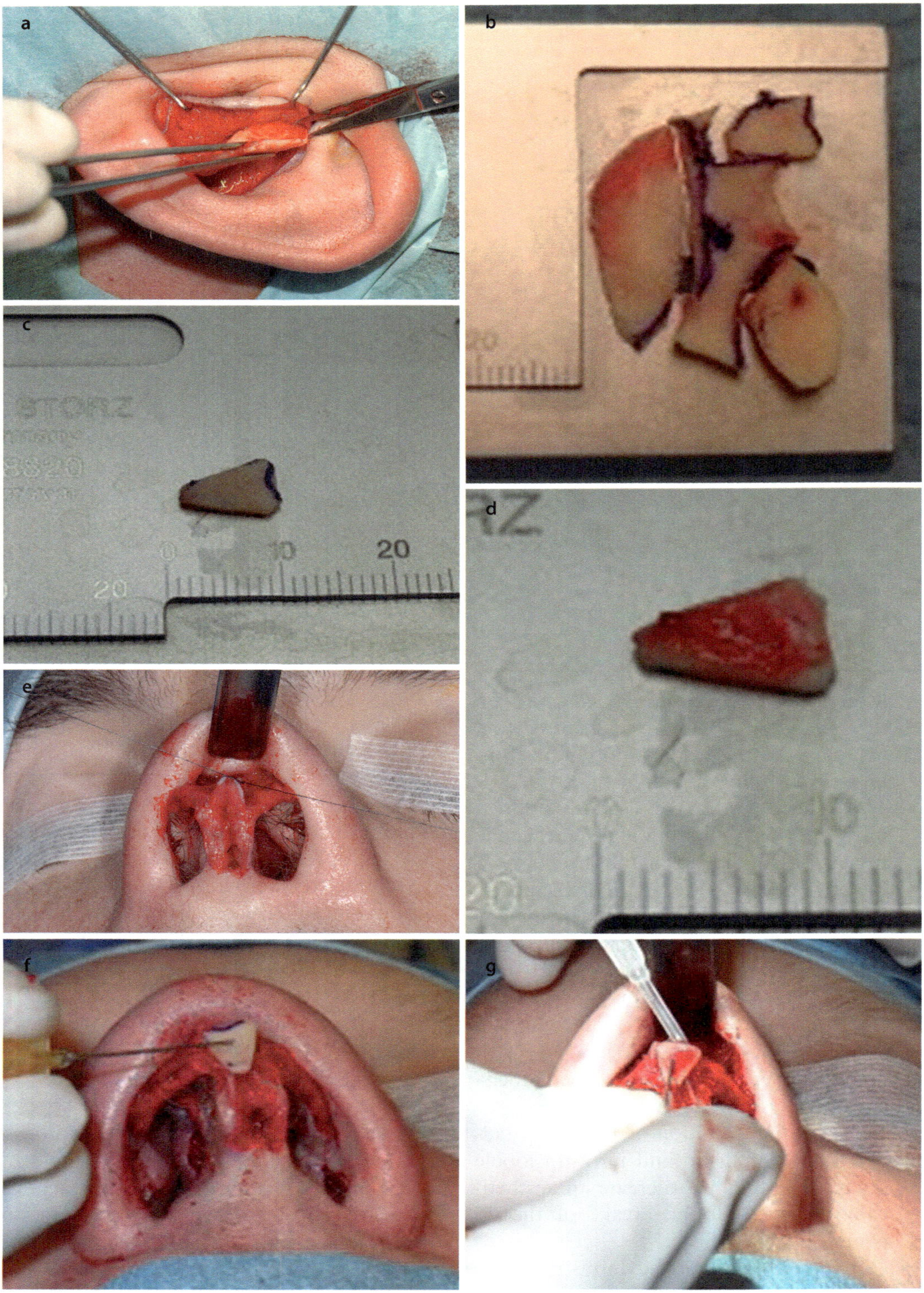

Fig. 9.40 a–j Surgical sequence showing the steps of shield graft harvest from conchal cartilage, fashioning and placement in the infra-tip lobule segment with sutures

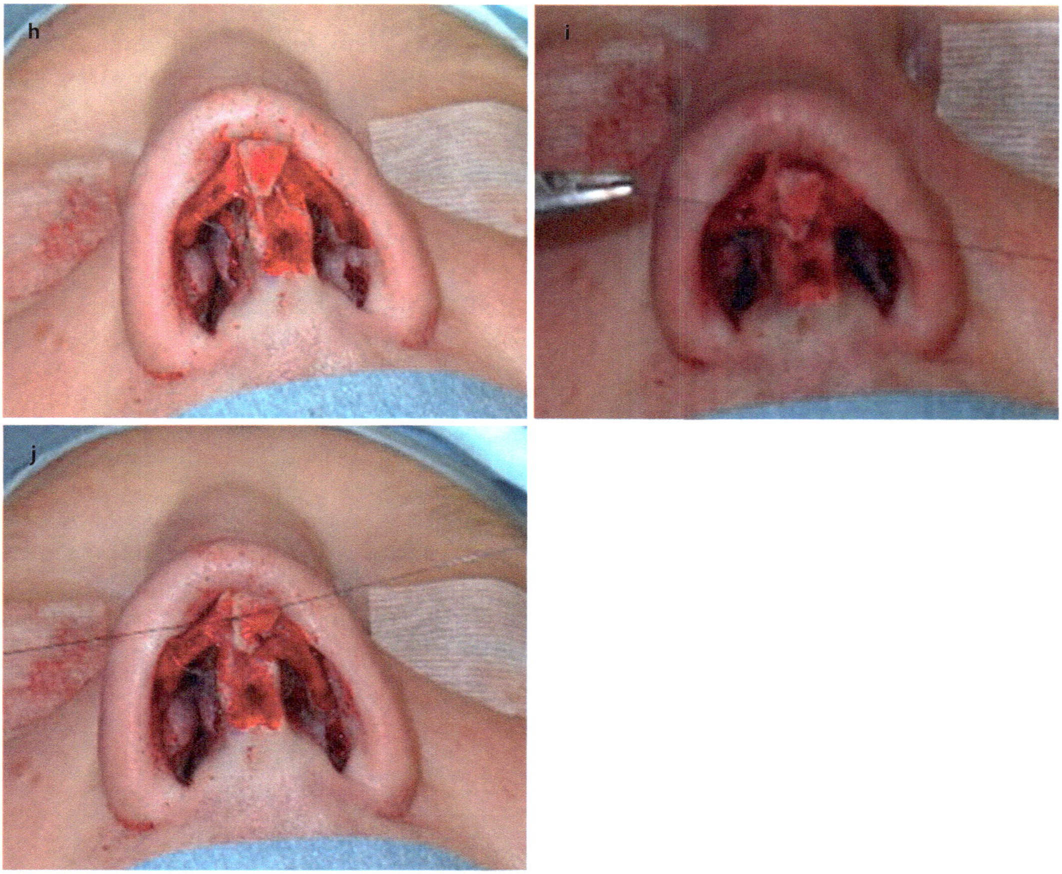

Fig. 9.40 (continued)

- Conchal bowl cartilage is the ideal cartilage for a shield graft. If septal cartilage is used, make sure the edges are bevelled and made pliable by thinning and gently crushing them with artery forceps.
- Although shaped like a shield, it need not be a shield. It can extend from the infratip lobule to the entire columellar segment inferiorly.
- The dimensions are usually around 4–5 mm width superiorly, 2 mm thickness, but length can vary and hence inferior extension may vary depending on the requirements, but generally around 8 mm in vertical length.
- The author is not a big fan of shield graft as there are viable alternatives to increase the projection like columellar strut grafts and tip suturing techniques. The tip grafts can have issues with fixing in the right place, distorted position and sharp edges showing through an overlying thin skin.
- The graft should be shaped like a shield with a wider width at the cephalic end and a narrow side pointing towards the columella.
- Care must be taken to shape the cartilage to the right size and also make sure the edges are smoothened and bevelled to avoid any sharp edges.
- Once the dorsal and septal work is done and tip work completed, a decision is made whether to use the shield graft. Hold the shaped cartilage in the infra-tip lobule segment in the right position with an Adson's tissue forceps to achieve adequate projection as well. The best way to secure a shield graft before using the sutures is

to use a hypodermic needle, as shown in Fig. 9.40f. A drop of compatible tissue glue can be used to stabilise the graft as well. When using tissue glue, always check local guidelines. Sutures can then be used to stabilise the graft as well (Fig. 9.40j).
- Any unwanted sharp edges or over projection should be bevelled and shaved off and may have to use some crushed cartilage for camouflage.

9.19.5 Surgical Sequence

Usually performed after caudal and dorsal septal work and after strengthening the medial crura if necessary. This is basically done towards the end of the procedure.

Key Points
- Stabilising the grafts in the correct position is difficult before using sutures and can be very footery. Hence use small hypodermic needles and licensed tissue glues for stabilisation.
- When using sutures do not tighten too much on one side before anchoring the other side as there can be difficulty in distributing the tension on the sutures equally on both sides. The moment a suture is placed on one side of the graft, the tension in the knot can tilt the graft to that side introducing asymmetry.
- Avoid overfilling the infra-tip lobule space.
- Be careful in stabilising the graft in the right place.
- In patients with thin skin, sharp edges can show through. Hence, extreme care needed to bevel the edges.

Conclusion

This graft can be done either through open or closed approach and can be very tricky to use and may cause more issues then solving issues. We personally do not use this graft very often, as it is fraught with many technical issues, if not executed properly. If done for increasing the projection, there are more predictable alternatives than a shield graft.

9.20 Radix Graft

9.20.1 Introduction

Radix is the area of the root of the nose joining the facial skeleton. The term "nasion" is also used to denote this junctional area at the root of the nose. Although there is a distinction between nasion and radix anatomically, it is of no clinical value. Radix grafts are used for camouflage and not used as a structural graft. Radix grafts are on-lay grafts. As the name suggests, it is used to augment the radix at the root of the nose. It is not a support graft but a camouflage graft used to increase the projection of the nose in the profile line at the radix, thus increasing the length of the nose.

9.20.2 Indications

- Radix grafts are used to reconstruct the radix or nasion region of the nose. The take off point of the nose should be roughly at the inter-pupillary line or just above it. One of the indications for a radix graft *is a shallow radix with a de-projected nasal dorsum* at the nasion or radix level on a lateral profile view. In patients with shallow radix, the "take off" point of the nose is lower and the rest of the dorsum below may appear to have a pseudo hump. In this situation, it is important to correct the nasion and not to remove the pseudo-hump, which may result in a disastrous "washed out" appearance of the profile line of the nose in line with the forehead.
- Since these type of patients present as a revision procedure, we tend to use multiple layers of fascia lata for radix augmentation, in view of the graft being soft,

pliable and aesthetically more pleasing. Sometimes crushed cartilage can be firm and non-pliable at the nasion, particularly in patients wearing glasses.

9.20.3 Contra-indications

No major contra-indications in the right patient, although when using larger pieces of cartilage which are not crushed properly may show through if the overlying skin is thin.

9.20.4 Choice of Graft Material

Usually crushed or diced septal cartilage is used. Fascia lata can be used as multiple small layers or virtually any piece of cartilage even rib cartilage crushed or diced can be used.

9.20.5 Surgical Technique

- The procedure if performed alone can be done through internal approach after raising the dorsal flap. But if done as a part of a rhinoplasty can be done through open approach.
- The graft material depends on the availability and whether the procedure is being done in isolation or as a part of a total nasal reconstruction.
- Pieces of diced or crushed cartilage from the nasal septum or conchal bowl cartilage can be used for dorsal augmentation, packed inside a membranous sheath of either temporalis fascia or fascia lata.
- Using many layers of fascia lata gives a better cosmetic result than the crushed or diced cartilage, and this has the added advantage of being able to be moulded into irregular concavities of the radix, particularly when they are done as a sole procedure. The only disadvantage is the donor site scar.
- The skin over the radix should be lifted. If done through an internal approach, there is no need to do an inter-cartilaginous incision from the alar region. Instead it will be quick and easy to put a medial crural clamp and flip the conjoined medial crus to one side away from the midline to gain access to the anterior septal angle in the midline. A small stab is made at this point in the midline and the overlying skin is lifted without damaging the inter-cartilaginous region of the lateral nasal alar region.
- Do not dissect too much skin into the frontal region as the post-operative oedema and facial distortion is directly proportional to this. Keep the radix pocket to an ideal size when doing an internal approach.
- Then the radix bed is made rough by gentle rasping of the bony periosteum with a diamond rasp. This allows the graft to stick to the bone without any slippage.
- The graft is then placed on the radix bed inside the pocket and skin re-draped back. It is always better to over correct, as there will always be a volume loss, particularly when using fascia lata grafts.

9.20.6 Surgical Sequence

Usually done towards the end of the rhinoplasty procedure before closing the skin flap.

Key Points

- Always be aware of the take-off point of the nose (nasion). This should be at the inter-pupillary line. If it is well below, augmenting the nasion would be an ideal option.
- Multiple pieces of crushed cartilage from the septal remnants are perfectly fine for this graft.
- If fascia lata is used, it is advisable to use small multiple pieces of fascia lata about 10 mm by 5 mm and used as several layers and not as a single layer.
- Multiple smaller pieces of fascia lata works very well (particularly when the overlying skin is discoloured and scarred) both from patient's acceptance (softness and pliability) and the ease of use, the only issue being donor site morbidity.
- If using fascia lata, do not use a single large piece as it runs the risk of sliding out through suture lines when pressure

is applied to the dorsum. If there are multiple pieces, even if one small piece comes out, it does not affect the final outcome. Hence, the need for over correction if fascia lata is used.
- Once the grafts are in place, it is gently pressed down with Steri-strips without too much pressure.
- If done through closed approach, always create an "exact" pocket so that the graft sits in place without any displacement.

Conclusion

It is an easy and effective procedure which can have a profound positive effect on the dorsal profile line.

Key Points Box

- Nasal tip grafts are used both for structure and function.
- Grafting in nasal tip surgery is usually reserved for secondary rather than primary rhinoplasty.
- Be aware grafts can introduce variables in the surgical outcome.
- There are an array of graft materials available, but autologous materials are safer in the long run to achieve sustainable results.
- Be aware tip is a stable, but mobile structure and any grafting in the tip runs the risk of increasing the stiffness of the nasal tip and causing rigidity to the nasal tip region.

References

1. Sheen JH. Tip graft: a 20-year retrospective. Plast Reconstr Surg. 1993;91:48–63.
2. Balaji N. Top tips in nasal tip surgery, ENT-FPS UK Newsletter— Feb 2018 –Issue 6.
3. Murrell GL. Auricular cartilage grafts and nasal surgery. Laryngoscope. 2004;114:2092–102.
4. Daniel RK. Rhinoplasty and rib grafts: evolving a flexible operative technique. Plast Reconstr Surg. 1994;94:597–609.
5. Adamson PA. Grafts in rhinoplasty: autogenous grafts are superior to alloplastic. Arch Otolaryngol Head Neck Surg. 2000;126:561–2.
6. Toriumi DM. Autogenous grafts are worth the extra time. Arch Otolaryngol Head Neck Surg. 2000;126:562–4.
7. Romo T 3rd, Kwak ES, Sclafani AP. Revision rhinoplasty using porous high-density polyethylene implants to re-establish ethnic identity. Aesthet Plast Surg. 2006;30:679–84.
8. Boenisch M, Nolst Trenité GJ. Reconstructive septal surgery. Facial Plast Surg. 2006;22(4):249–54.
9. Lee M, Callahan S, Cochran CS. Auricular cartilage: harvest technique and versatility in rhinoplasty. Am J Otolaryngol. 2011;32:547–5523.
10. Boccieri A, Marano A. The Conchal cartilage graft in nasal reconstruction. J Plast Reconstr Aesthet Surg. 2007;60:188–94.
11. Kim JY, Yang HJ, Jeong JW. A new technique for conchal cartilage harvest. Arch Plast Surg. 2017;44(2):166–9.
12. Lee M, Callahan S, Cochran CS. Auricular cartilage: harvest technique and versatility in rhinoplasty. Am J Otolaryngol. 2011;32:547–52.
13. Lan MY, Park JP, Jang YJ. Donor site morbidities resulting from conchal cartilage harvesting in rhinoplasty. J Laryngol Ototol. 2007;131(6):529–33.
14. Balaji N. Non-suture techniques in nasal tip reconstruction. Romanian J Rhinol. 2014;4(13):37–44.
15. Baker TM, Courtiss EH. Temporalis fascia grafts in open secondary rhinoplasty. Plast Reconstr Surg. 1994;93:802.
16. Miller TA. Temporalis fascia grafts for facial and nasal contour augmentation. Plast Reconstr Surg. 1988;81:524.
17. Sheen JH. Temporoparietal free fascia grafts in rhinoplasty (discussion). Plast Reconstr Surg. 1984;74:475.
18. Karaaltin MV, Orhan KS, Demirel T. Fascia lata graft for nasal dorsal contouring in rhinoplasty. J Plast Reconstr Aesthet Surg. 2009;62(10):1255–60.
19. Karaaltin MV, Batioglu-Karaaltin A, Orhan KS, Demirel T, Guldiken Y. Autologous fascia lata graft for contour restoration and camouflage in tertiary rhinoplasty. J Craniofac Surg. 2012;23(3):719–23.
20. Erol OO. The Turkish delight: a pliable graft for rhinoplasty. Plast Reconstr Surg. 2000;105(6):2229–41.
21. Daniel RK, Calvert JW. Diced cartilage grafts in rhinoplasty surgery. Plast Reconstr Surg. 2004;113(7):2156–71.
22. Sheen JH. The ideal dorsal graft: a continuing quest. Plast Reconstr Surg. 1998;102:2490.
23. Gibson T, Davis WB. Distortion of autogenous rib grafts: its cause and prevention. Br J Plast Surg. 1957;10:247–74.
24. Tasman A-J. Rhinoplasty-indications and techniques. GMs Current Top Otorhinolaryngol Head Neck Surg. 2007;6:Doc09,Online publication.
25. Daniel RK. Rhinoplasty and rib grafts: evolving a flexible operative technique. Plast Reconstr Surg. 1994;94:597–609.
26. McKinney P. An aesthetic dorsum: the CATS graft. Clin Plast Surg. 1996;23(2):233–44.

27. McKinney P, Loomis MG, Wiedrich TA. Reconstruction of the nasal cap with a thin septal graft. Plast Reconstr Surg. 1993;92(2):346–51.
28. Erol OO. The Turkish delight: a pliable graft for rhinoplasty. Plast Reconstr Surg. 2000;105(6):2229–41.
29. Toriumi DM. New concepts in nasal tip contouring. Arch Facial Plast Surg. 2006;8(3):156–85. –for strut and columnar stabilising grafts.
30. Pastorek NJ, Bustillo A, Murphy MR, Becker DG. The extended columellar strut-tip graft. Arch Facial Plast Surg. 2005;7(3):176–18.
31. Sil A, Ravichandran S, Balaji N. Non- suture techniques in posttraumatic nasal tip reconstruction. ENT Audiol News. 2010;19(2):109–12.
32. Balaji N, Ravichandran S. Assessment of nasal valve obstruction: a new nasal "wall" subunit concept. ENT Audiol News. 2012;21(4):111–3.
33. Balaji N. Suture techniques in nasal tip reconstruction. Romanian J Rhinol. 2014;4(14):105–10.
34. Byrd HS, Andochick S, Copit S, et al. Septal extension grafts: a method of controlling tip projection shape. Plast Reconstr Surg. 1997;100:999–1010.
35. Ha RY, Byrd HS. Septal extension grafts revisited: 6-year experience in controlling nasal tip projection and sshape. Plast Reconstr Surg. 2003;112: 1929–35.
36. Toriumi DM. Caudal septal extension graft for correction of the retracted columella. Op Tech Otolaryngol Head Neck Surg. 1995;6:311–8.
37. Oh SH, Kang NH, Woo JS, et al. Stabilization of unilateral septal extension graft using pivot locking suture. J Korean Soc Aesthetic Plast Surg. 2008;14:156–60.
38. Tebbetts JB. Primary rhinoplasty: a new approach to the logic and the techniques. St. Louis: Mosby; 1998.
39. Tebbetts JB. Shaping and positioning the nasal tip without structural disruption: a new, systematic approach. Plast Reconstr Surg. 1994;94: 61–77.
40. Guyuron B, Varghai A. Lengthening the nose with a tongue-and-groove technique. Plast Reconstr Surg. 2003;111:1533–9.
41. Sheen J. Spreader graft: a method of reconstructing the middle nasal vault following rhinoplasty. Plast Reconstr Surg. 1984;73:230–9.
42. Vuyk HD. Cartilage spreader grafting for lateral augmentation for the middle third of the nose. Faces. 1993;3:159–70.
43. Balaji N, Ravichandran S. Assessment of nasal valve obstruction: a new Glasgow nasal "wall" subunit concept. ENT Audiol News. 2012;21(5):86–7.
44. Guyuron B, Varghai A. Lengthening the nose with a tongue-and-groove technique. Plast Reconstr Surg. 2003;111(4):1533–9.
45. Gunter JP, Friedman RM. Lateral crural strut graft: technique and clinical applications in rhinoplasty. Plast Reconstr Surg. 1997;99(4):943–52.
46. Okhovat S, Balaji N. An algorithm for the management of lateral crural pathology. J ENT Master Class. 2018;11(1):45–53.
47. Spielmann PM, White PS, Hussain SS. Surgical techniques for the treatment of nasal valve collapse: a systematic review. Laryngoscope. 2009;119(7):1281–90.
48. Vaezeafshar R, Moubayed SP, Most SP. Repair of lateral wall insufficiency. JAMA Facial Plast Surg. 2018;20(2):111–5.
49. Tsao GJ, Fijalkowski N, Most SP. Validation of a grading system for lateral nasal wall insufficiency. Allergy Rhinol (Providence). 2013;4(2):e66–8.
50. Becker DG, Becker SS. Treatment of nasal obstruction from nasal valve collapse with alar batten grafts. J Long-Term Eff Med Implants. 2003;13:259–69.
51. Toriumi DM, Josen J, Weinberger M, Tardy ME Jr. Use of alar batten grafts for correction of nasal valve collapse. Arch Otolaryngol Head Neck Surg. 1997;123:802–8.
52. Rohrich RJ, Raniere J Jr, Ha RY. The alar contour graft: correction and prevention of alar rim deformities in rhinoplasty. Plast Reconstr Surg. 2002;109(7):2495–505.
53. Apaydin F. Lateral crural turn-in flap in functional rhinoplasty. Arch Facial Plast Surg. 2012;14(2):93–6.
54. Lovice DB, Mingrone MD, Toriumi DM. Rhinoplasty and septoplasty. Grafts and implants in rhinoplasty and nasal reconstruction. Otolaryngol Clin N Am. 1999;32:113–41.
55. Becker DG, Becker SS, Saad AA. Auricular cartilage in revision rhinoplasty. Facial Plast Surg. 2003;19:41–52.
56. McKinney P, Loomis MG, Wiedrich TA. Reconstruction of the nasal cap with a thin septal graft. Plast Reconstr Surg. 1993;92(2):346–51.
57. Peck GC. The onlay graft for nasal tip projection. Plast Reconstr Surg. 1983;71:27–39.
58. Won TB, Jin HR. Revision rhinoplasty in Asians. Ann Plast Surg. 2010;65:379–84.
59. Toriumi DM, Swartout B. Asian rhinoplasty. Facial Plast Surg Clin North Am. 2007;15:293–307.
60. Jin HR, Won TB. Nasal hump removal in Asians. Acta Otolaryngol Suppl. 2007;558:95–101.
61. Jin HR, Won TB. Nasal tip augmentation in Asians using autogenous cartilage. Otolarygol Head Neck Surg. 2009;140:526–30.
62. Collawn SS, Fix RJ, Moore JR, Vasconez LO. Nasal cartilage grafts: more than a decade of experience. Plast Reconstr Surg. 1997;100:1547.
63. Gunter JP, Landecker A, Cochran CS. Frequently used grafts in rhinoplasty: nomenclature and analysis. Plast Reconstr Surg. 2006;118(1):14e–29e.

Non-suture and Non-grafting Techniques in Nasal Tip Rhinoplasty

Contents

N. Balaji, *Textbook of Nasal Tip Rhinoplasty*, https://doi.org/10.1007/978-3-030-48157-5_10

Learning Objectives
- To understand different non-grafting and non-suture techniques in nasal tip reconstruction.
- To understand the pros and cons of each technique.
- To understand the indications and surgical techniques of the techniques used, both for structural and functional rhinoplasty.

10.1 Introduction

Nasal tip plasty is one of the most demanding and complex operations in facial plastic surgery. The surgery demands not only creating ideal structural changes in the cartilaginous skeleton of the nasal tip, but also the overlying soft tissue should re-drape on the cartilaginous skeleton for the aesthetic outcome to be obvious. In the previous chapters, the various suture and grafting techniques have been described as a primary technique in tip surgery which would alter in isolation or in combination, the definition, rotation and projection of the nasal tip. In this chapter, we will describe the non-suture and non-grafting operative techniques of nasal tip plasty, as the primary tool for reconstruction. Although these techniques have been grouped together as "non-suture techniques" and "non-grafting techniques", they are not stand-alone techniques and invariably used in conjunction with suture and grafting techniques to achieve the desirable outcomes. Sutures do offer additional secondary support and are indispensable in most techniques.

10.2 Cephalic Trim of the Lateral Crus of the Lower Lateral Cartilage

10.2.1 Introduction

Cephalic trim of the lateral crura of lower lateral cartilages is the most commonly performed non-grafting and non-suture nasal tip procedure to reduce the bulk and re-define the nasal tip. Usually is done in conjunction with other suture techniques to narrow or define the nasal tip. The cephalic border of the lateral crus of the lower lateral cartilage is excised on both sides symmetrically preserving enough width of the lateral crus to sustain the external nasal valve function. There is a considerable variability in the width of the lateral crus between different patients and also between two sides in the same patient. This is more so in revision procedures. Hence, leaving behind symmetrical rim strips of lateral crus is of paramount importance.

> How much to excise is not important, but how much to leave behind is important. It is essential to leave a minimum of 8 mm of lateral crural cartilage to prevent external nasal valve collapse and alar pinching.

It is important to leave behind symmetric rim strips on both sides. Sometimes the cephalic border is too wide either on one or both sides causing wide symmetrical bulbous tip or causing asymmetric bulbous tip and pushing the dorsal septum and the tip to the opposite side. Care is taken to excise the "rolled in" cephalic border to achieve the desired outcomes. It is all the more important if a degree of rotation is expected from the procedure.

10.2.2 Indications

- To reduce the bulk of the nasal tip in patients with wide nasal tip (Fig. 10.1).
- To create a space between the two cephalic margins of the lateral crus, so that the nasal tip can be rotated into. It has a marginal effect on upward tip rotation. By excising the cephalic border of both lateral crus there is a space created in the midline into which the reconstructed unified tip complex can be rotated into and secured if necessary with sutures.
- As a pre-requisite before using sutures, to narrow the tip and increase the tip projection in a wide, de-projected nasal tip.
- To address an asymmetrical lateral crural rim strips, cephalic trim achieves a symmetrical rim strip on both sides, creating tip symmetry between the two sides.

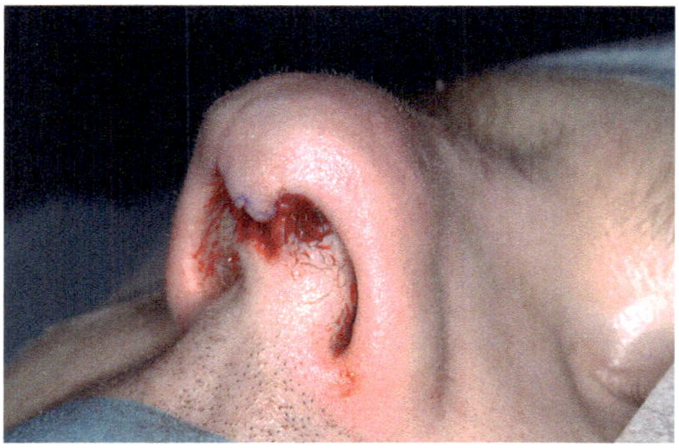

Fig. 10.1 A bulbous nasal tip

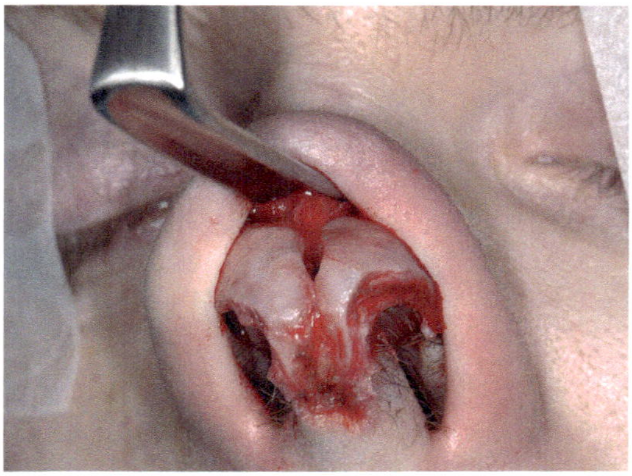

Fig. 10.2 An open approach view of the wide lateral crus

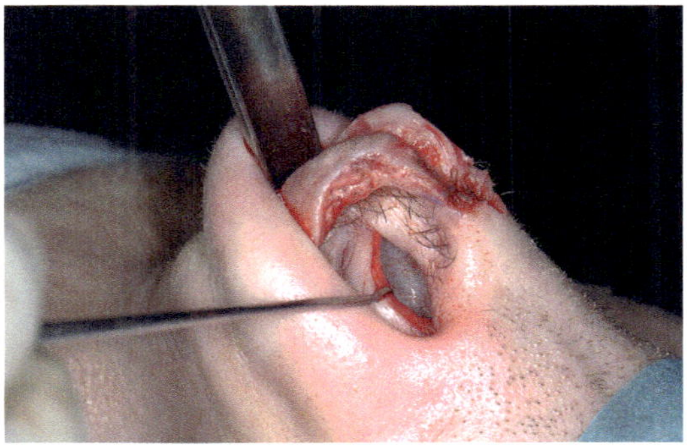

Fig. 10.3 Both "open" approach and hemi-trans fixation approach in the same patient

10.2.3 Contra-indications

- If the width of the lateral crus is narrow and less than 6 mm.
- If technically not feasible to do, due to scar tissue in multiple revision surgeries.
- Narrow and cephalically migrated lateral crus, as any excision of the width of the lateral crus in these situations can cause alar margin to retract up.
- If there is lateral alar weakness or pinching.

10.2.4 Surgical Technique

- The key is to expose adequately both lateral crura including the caudal and cephalic borders through an open approach (Figs. 10.2 and 10.3) or tip delivery techniques.
- The surface of the cartilage is exposed after removal of any overlying scar tissue.
- The excess width of lateral crus can cause either a symmetric or asymmetric bulbous tip. Sometimes, the cephalic border is not definable easily. This may be due to or associated with "rolling in" of the cephalic border due to excess width of the lateral crus. If so, this will cause tip widening not only due to the excess width, but also due to the rolled in segment pushing into the space between the septum and the two lateral crura. Cephalic trim helps to remove this "rolled cephalic edge" as well. Care must be taken to excise this "rolled in" cephalic border as well to achieve tip definition and symmetry. It is all the more important if a degree of rotation is expected from the procedure.
- Hold the inferior border of the lateral crus, with an Adson's tissue forceps at the desired level and with a gentle to and fro traction look for the rolled edge (if present) at the cephalic margin (Fig. 10.4a–d).
- The amount to be left behind (usually 8 mm) is measured and Adson's tissue forceps is used to hold the lateral crus gently at the measured level. Take care to leave 8 mm, but not less than a minimum of 6 mm.
- Then with a 15 blade knife, the cartilage is incised carefully at the desired level usually running parallel to the lower margin of the lateral crus but not going through the mucosa, starting the blade from lateral to medial, as there is a risk of damage to the elevated skin flap if not careful when coming from medial to lateral. Make sure the incision is not taken too far laterally.

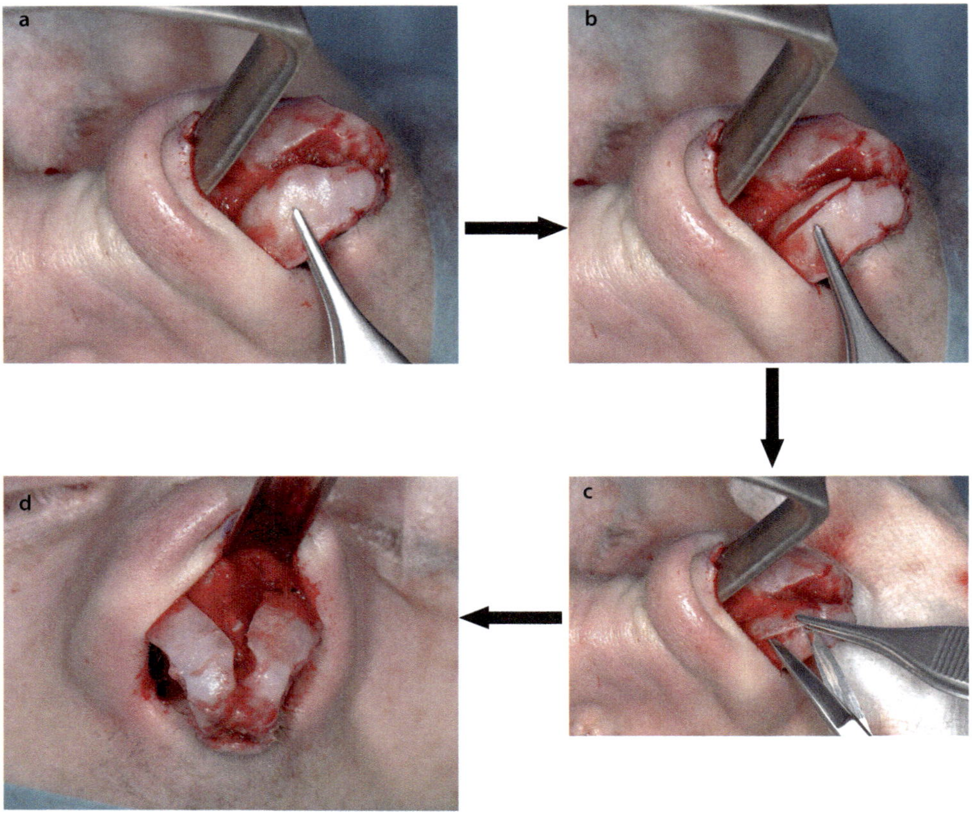

Fig. 10.4 **a–d** Open approach view of the nose showing the sequence of cephalic trimming of the lateral crus. (Reproduced with kind permission from Refs. [1–3])

- Then with a sharp curved scissors using a technique of "small snips and big spreads", the cephalic portion of the cartilage is separated from the underlying mucosa and excised [1–3].
- The cephalic excision line should be parallel to the caudal border of the lateral crus with a gentle convexity leading to the intermediate segment staying 2 mm lateral to the dome. The space created allows the tip to rotate into, thus increasing the rotation. Take care not to cut into the intermediate crus at the dome and stay few millimetres lateral.
- The lateral limit of excision depends on the indications and generally advisable not to go too far laterally staying around 4 mm medial to the scroll region, as any bleeding or cautery at that point can be counterproductive.
- When nearing the dome, it is advisable to gently curve the line of excision to prevent unwanted alteration in the tip dynamics. A sharp "beak" of cartilage left behind at the junction of the new superior margin of the lateral crus and the intermediate crus will prevent tip rotation into the space created.
- Care should be taken not to damage the mucosa of the alar vestibule. If the underlying mucosa is buttonholed or damaged, it is advisable not to panic and leave it without suturing the mucosa. Suturing the damaged mucosa will cause scarring and will end up in unwanted retraction of the alar margin.
- It is vital to remember that the tip rotation following cephalic trim does not happen on the table or in the immediate post-operative period, but can happen up to 6 months post surgery due to scar con-

traction in the space created which helps to pull the tip up marginally.

- Finally, it is important to make sure that you have left behind symmetrical rim strip width of lateral crus on both sides with a minimum width of 8 mm to prevent any functional issues at the external nasal valve region.
- This standard technique will suffice in majority of nasal tip surgery, but be aware that there are lot of variations in the doing the cephalic trim, which will help in certain situations. The reader is advised to refer individual monographs [4].

10.2.5 Surgical Sequence

- As mentioned above it is usually done first when planning tip plasty, before any sutures. Reducing the width of the lateral crus to an optimum level also helps in the handling of the alar cartilages with sutures and takes less tension on the sutures, to get the same desired effect. This is usually followed by medial crural fixation suture and then followed by domal sutures.
- If needed, doing this procedure first before a hump reduction makes it easier to visualise the nasal dorsum and also helps in the actual resection of the hump by reducing the need for retraction of the lateral crus thus creating more space to work on the dorsum. These sequences make the operation looks sleek and save time as well, thus avoiding unwanted wasted movements.
- The same principle is followed before any dorsal septal work as well. Prior cephalic trim, if needed, makes the dissection of the dorsal septum easier and the use of spreader grafts can also be done with ease due to more space available to work, following the cephalic trim.

Key Points

- Make sure to leave *symmetrical and parallel rim strips* on both sides. If the left behind rim strips of the lateral crus are asymmetrical and not parallel, then it will affect the outcome.
- Leave a minimum of 8 mm of the lateral crus to prevent alar collapse [5].
- Try not to damage the underlying alar mucosa. If damaged, do not suture the hole in the mucosa until otherwise it is too big.
- Do not leave a sharp edge between the new superior border of the lateral crus and the intermediate crus, but if you do the tip will still be wide with two lateral crus trying to push against each other, giving less favourable outcomes.
- When done through an open approach, it is important NOT to raise the skin flap over the lateral extremes of the lateral crus and over the sesamoid cartilages, particularly in a patient with a hanging columella. A "free floating" lateral crus in this situation can migrate to a cephalic position in the post-operative period as quickly as in few weeks due to the weight of the conjoined medial crus and this will result in a cosmetically unacceptable "nostril show". This is a "preventable" deformity which is very difficult to correct in a revision procedure.
- Beware of doing this procedure in a cephalically migrated lateral crus, although not an absolute contra-indication if associated with excess width. This may cause upward retraction of alar margin.
- Be careful not to excise the cephalic portion too far laterally near the scroll region and also avoid too much diathermy too far laterally to prevent scarring and alar collapse in the post-operative period.
- Do not throw away the excised portions, which can be used to soften both the dorsum and tip regions as additional grafts. I tend to use the left over pieces at the end to soften the dorsum and the tip profiles [6].

Conclusion

This is one of the most commonly used tip procedure in nasal tip rhinoplasty and is an effective technique to reduce the bulk of lateral crus in a wide bulbous nasal tip. This procedure is also done as a prerequisite before using tip sutures to narrow the tip.

10.3 Lateral Crural Incision and Overlap

10.3.1 Introduction

This is an "*incisional technique*", not to be confused with any excisional techniques involving the lateral crus. The two lateral crura form the two supero-lateral limbs of the nasal tip tripod. This technique is considered if there is a need to reduce the length of the lateral crus and shorten the lateral crus. Done on both sides, this reduction in the length of the lateral crus has an effect on the upward rotation of the nasal tip and the projection and also to a lesser extent have an effect on the nasal tip definition [7].

10.3.2 Indications

- This technique performed alone on both sides rotates the tip up and de-projects the nasal tip to a larger extent. It works well for an over projected tip with significant under rotation (Fig. 10.5a, b) and droopiness of the tip [8].
- Also indicated in large over projected noses where dorsal reduction should be combined with de-projection of the nasal tip as well. When done in conjunction with bilateral medial crural overlap, de-projects the nose without any element of rotation.
- To correct localised bulges or weakness in revision or traumatic tip deformities associated with tip asymmetry (Fig. 10.6a). For

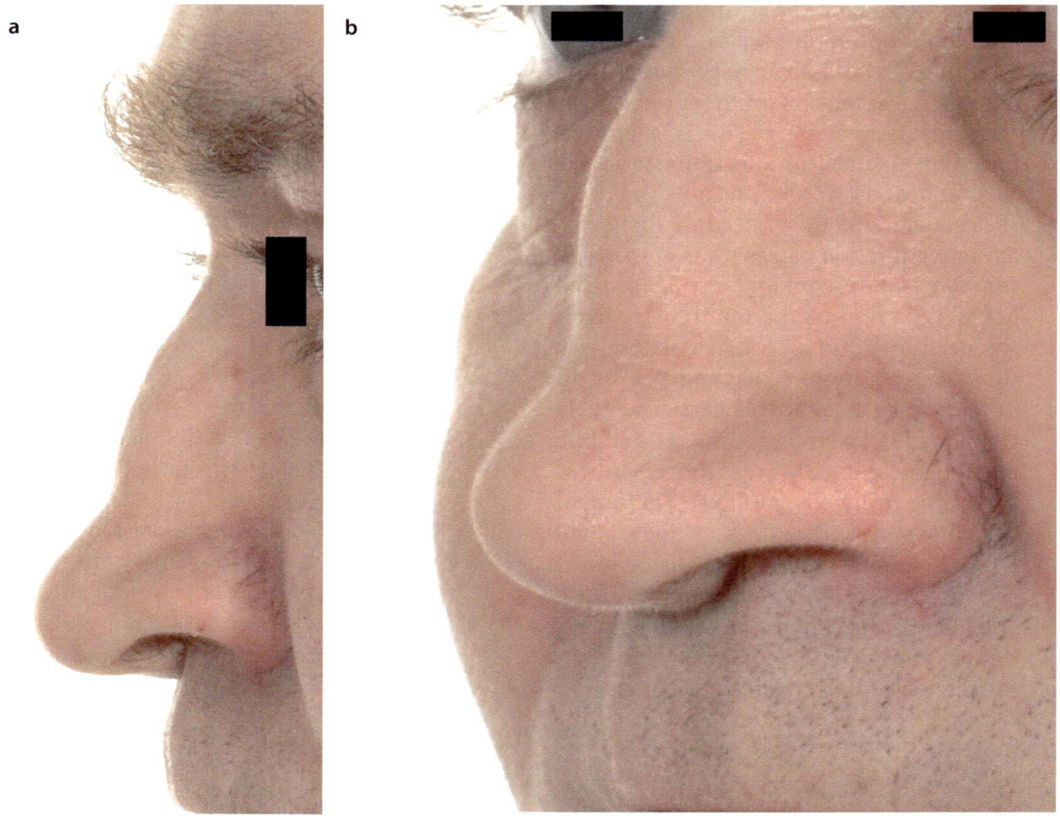

Fig. 10.5 **a**, **b** Droopy ptotic tip. **a** Lateral view. **b** Three-fourth view

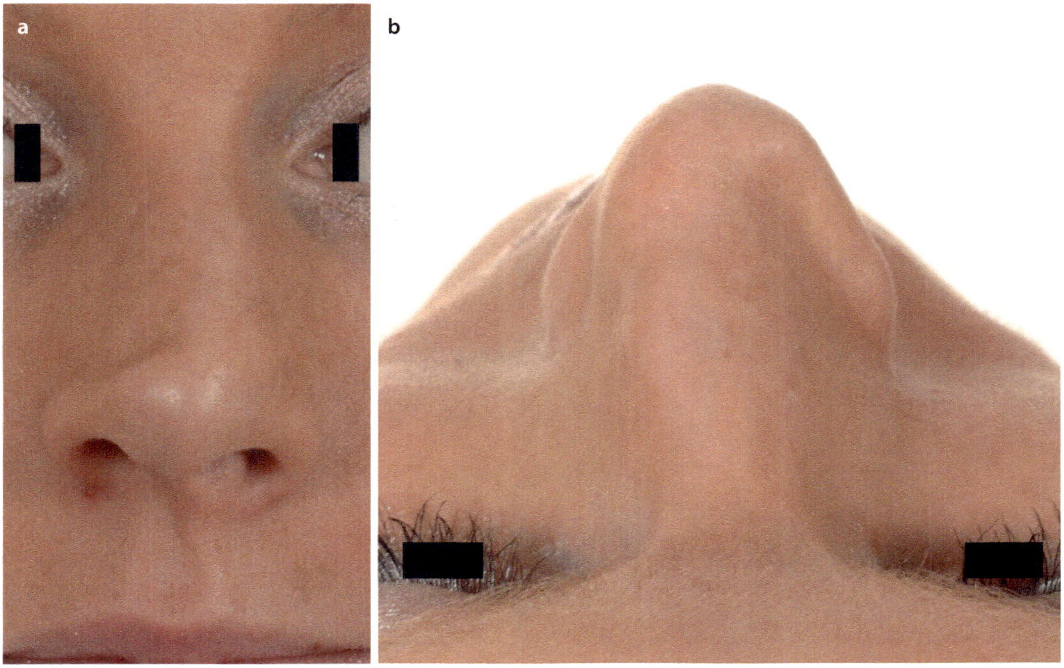

Fig. 10.6 **a**, **b** Concave right lateral crus with tip deviation to the same affected side. **a** Frontal view. **b** Sky view

example, if there is an asymmetrical nasal tip with foreshortening of the length of lateral crus due to a fracture lateral to dome on one side, the opposite side is usually longer. In this situation, it is done on the longer normal side (left side in Fig. 10.6b) to shorten the length of the lateral crus without altering the tip rotation or projection.

10.3.3 Contra-indications

- In young patients, there is a risk of abnormalities of cartilage edges showing through.
- Patients with very thin skin, again for the same reason mentioned above.
- If technically not possible to do, due to scarred alar skin preventing elevation of the skin.

10.3.4 Surgical Procedure

- Open approach offers adequate exposure, also offers the ability to address different deformities of the lateral crus on opening the flap.
- Once the decision is made to do the procedure, the incision site is marked on the lateral crura, well away from the dome.
- An incision is made on each side, taking care only to go through the lateral crural cartilage and not the underlying mucosa (Fig. 10.7a). One way of doing this is to change the angle of knife by using an Adson's forceps at the marked site and tilting the lateral crus outwards and using the knife against one of the tongs of the Adson's forceps, as shown in Fig. 10.9. This manoeuvre is safe and allows the surgeon to make a controlled incision of the lateral crus at an angle so that any direct injury to the mucosa underneath is prevented. Hydro-dissection with a local anaesthetic will also help in the dissection of the cartilage away from the underlying mucosa.
- The cartilage incision extends vertically from the cephalic to caudal margin of the lateral crus and results in a medial and a lateral segment as shown in Fig. 10.7a. Great care is taken not to cut the underlying mucosa. If this happens, it can be repaired but runs the risk of alar collapse

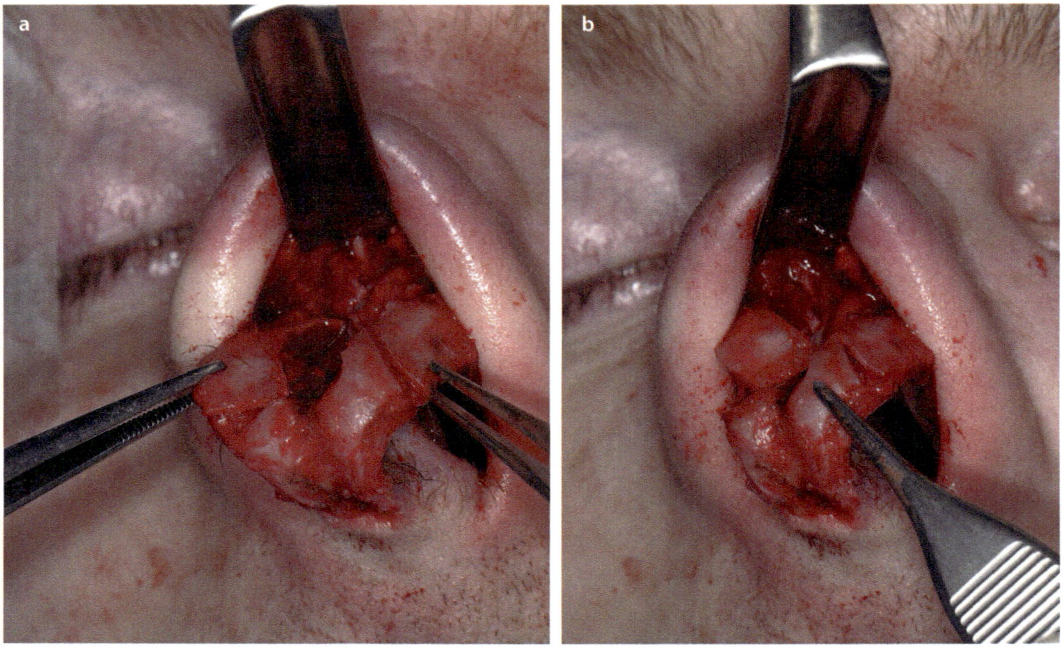

Fig. 10.7 **a**, **b** Lateral crural incision and overlapping the medial segment. (Reproduced with kind permission from Refs. [1–3])

and functional narrowing of external nasal valve region.

- Then the medial segment of the cut edges of the lateral crus is then lifted from the underlying alar mucosa (Fig. 10.7b) and advanced over the lateral aspect of the lateral crus [1–3, 9] and secured with a horizontal mattress suture using 5-0 vicryl to achieve the desired shortening of the lateral crus and upward rotation of the tip. In view of the shortening of the cartilage, there is always some mucosal folds underneath which will settle over time. Please note that the lateral segment of the incised lateral crus is left undisturbed. Otherwise, the desired tip de-projection and over rotation of the tip will not happen.
- Where to incise and how much to overlap goes with experience and to be tailored to the desired effect. As a general rule of thumb, the maximum advancement should be no more than 4 mm to avoid tip distortion.
- If going through the alar mucosa, it is advisable to use 5-0 absorbable vicryl vertical mattress sutures to overlap the two segments going through and through the alar mucosa. Be aware this can cause a slight bulge at the overlap site. The two cartilage segments can be sutured with non-absorbable 5-0 ethilon, if the underlying mucosa is completely freed.
- Finally it is always worthwhile putting some pieces of crushed cartilages over incised tip cartilages particularly in patients with thin skin.
- The lateral crus close to the scroll should never be breached.

10.3.5 Surgical Sequence

- Usually preceded by dorsal work.
- Consider cephalic trim of lateral crus to reduce the width of the lateral crus to an optimum size before proceeding for lateral crural overlap.
- Then do the overlap of lateral crus.
- Usually it is advisable to start working from the medial crus to lateral crus. But if lateral crural overlap or excision is planned to de-project the position of the new tip,

do the medial crural fixation suture and if necessary medial crural flare control suture first following which, do the lateral crural overlap.
- It is generally *not advisable* to do a trans-domal or inter-domal suture after lateral crural overlap as they will put tension on the lateral crural suture site. This need to be thought of in the planning stage.

Key Points
- The site of incision is very important. It should be a minimum of 6–7 mm lateral to the dome, although the exact placement is governed by the site and shape of the pathology in the lower lateral cartilage.
- Too lateral an incision, fails to achieve an adequate result in terms of de-projection and rotation, and too medial an incision results in a loss of tip definition.
- The incision line must be placed at the same place symmetrically on both sides and at 90 degrees to the caudal margin of the lateral crus and not at an angle.
- Beware, once the lateral crural cartilage is incised, the medial segment will tilt upwards due to the downward pull of the nasal tip. So when suturing back make sure they are sutured in the same orientation, if done only to reduce the length of the lateral crus.
- The edges can also be moved up or down overlapping up to 75%, but not less than that, if we are expecting a degree of rotation as well. If lesser amount of cartilage is overlapped, the sutured site becomes unstable.
- Skin thickness must be considered. In people with thin skin, the cartilage overlap may not produce a cosmetically favourable result and may cause a visible bulge.
- The other alternative to this procedure is excising a lateral crural segment and end-to-end anastomosis of the lateral crus.
- Do not dissect too far laterally close to the scroll region, otherwise this can cause damage to the scroll fat and accessory cartilages causing alar pinching.
- While suturing the cartilage fragments together, make sure the edges are approximated properly to prevent any rotation or pivotal movements.
- Try not to damage the underlying vestibular mucosa of the lateral crus.

Conclusion

The lateral crural overlap is an effective procedure to reduce the length of the lateral crus, thereby de-projecting and over rotating the nasal tip as well. These are powerful techniques not to be taken lightly, not a common procedure to be performed within the gamut of rhinoplasty surgery.

10.4 Lateral Crural Excision and Advancement

10.4.1 Introduction

This is an *"excisional" technique* not to be confused with any incisional techniques. This technique is a powerful way of reducing the length of the entire lower lateral cartilage from the scroll to the medial crural footplate, similar to the lateral crural overlap, but without the additional bulge in the lateral alar region. This technique achieves a reduction in the length of the lateral crus and hence the reduction in the length of the entire lower lateral cartilage, similar to the incision and overlap technique. This reduction in the length of the lateral crus has a profound effect on the position of the nasal tip, moving the tip up and also towards the face causing de-projection and over rotation. *This will happen only if the lateral scroll region of the lateral crus is left undisturbed. Beware this technique cannot be combined with tip narrowing sutures like trans-domal or inter-domal sutures, as they cause traction on the lateral crural suture line*. Thus it restricts the amount of tip narrowing (if the patient also needs one) that can be achieved with sutures, hence affecting the nasal tip definition as well. It is usually done on both sides to achieve a nasal tip balance in the midline. Very rarely done on one side if there is a unilateral bulge in the lateral crura and tip turn. In this situation, it is usually done on the stronger and longer side which is usually the side opposite to the tip deviation. This situation is due to long-standing localised fractures or weak segments in the lateral crus. The maximum limit of excision should be ONLY 4 mms, beyond which unnatural tip rotation and tip blunting will occur, which is not easily rectifiable. Generally, excision techniques are considered in circumstances only in males with thicker skin and slightly older population group where the skin has the ability to camouflage small irregularities at the suture site. In recent years, we have been doing this procedure for younger patients with thinner skin and over projected lower two-thirds of the nose, without any major issues [8].

10.4.2 Indications

- This is indicated in an overly projected large ethnic noses with large tip cartilages with significant under rotation. This technique performed alone helps to rotate the tip upwards lifting it up to a larger extent along with a degree of de-projection, taking the nose back to the face [10].
- When done in conjunction with bilateral medial crural overlap, de-projects the nose without any element of rotation.
- Usually done on both sides, but sometimes may have to be done alone on the so-called "normal" side in a clinical scenario of an asymmetrical nasal tip turn to one side due to weak lateral crus and unopposed action of the normal other side (◘ Fig. 10.8a). In

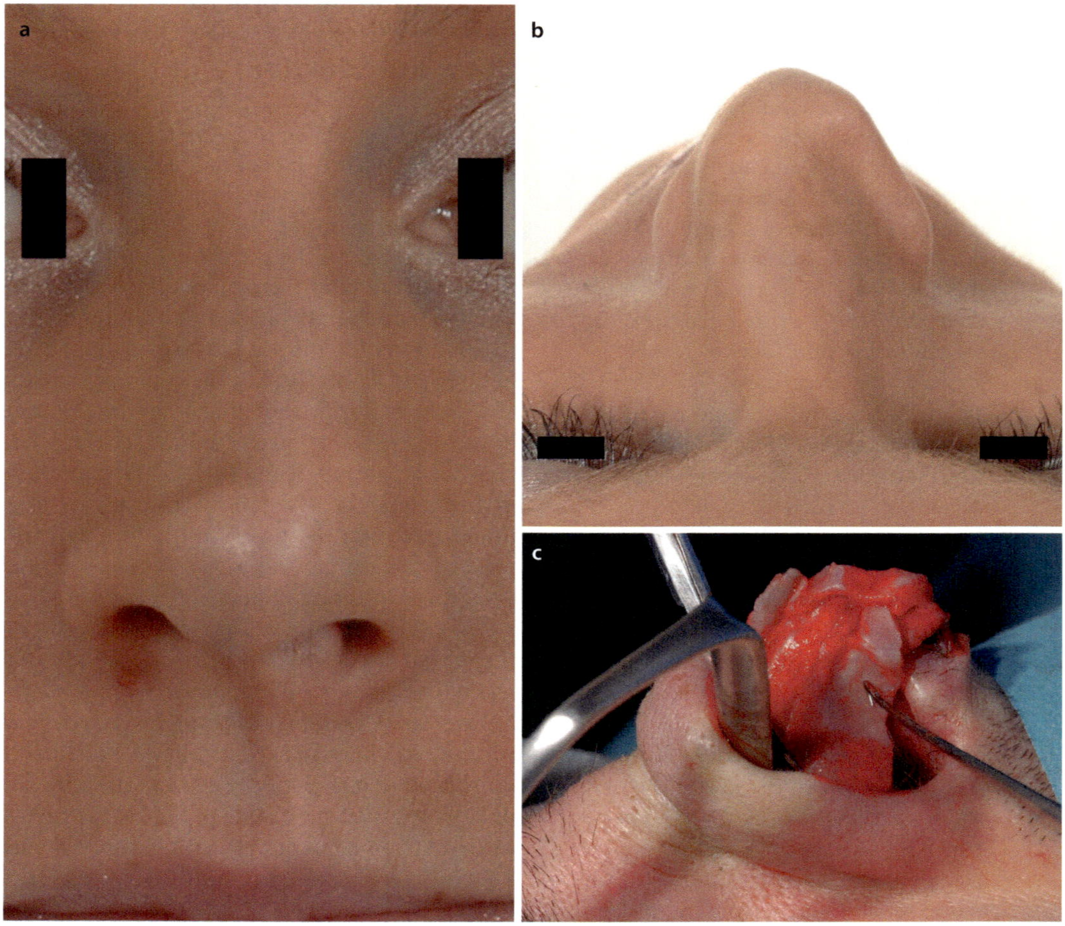

◘ **Fig. 10.8** **a–c** Concave right lateral crus with tip deviation to the same affected side. **a** Frontal view. **b** Sky view. **c** Open view of a concave lateral crus with a fracture on the right side this situation, there is usually a foreshortening of the length of lateral crus on the affected side due to a fracture lateral to dome on one side, and the opposite normal side is usually longer and stronger and convexing up pushing the weaker tip across the midline to the weaker side. In this situation apart from strengthening the abnormal lateral crus with a strut graft, it is advisable to do a minimum lateral crural excision on the opposite normal side to counterbalance the nasal tip position (see chapter on case studies).

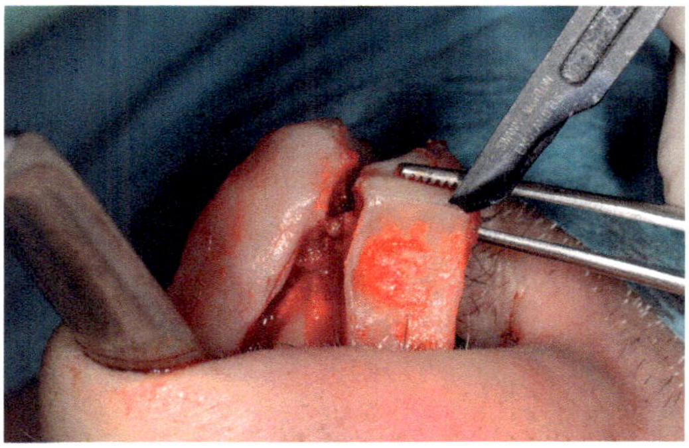

Fig. 10.9 Open approach view showing the angle of the knife towards the Adson's forceps tilting the lateral crus outwards and using the knife against one of the tongs of the Adson's forceps to avoid mucosal injury

10.4.3 Contra-indications

- Younger patients with thinner skin.
- Technical difficulty in raising the alar skin from the underlying thin scarred alar cartilages.
- Missing segments of lateral crus.
- If domal sutures are definitely indicated to narrow the tip, then it will be advisable to avoid this technique and think of an alternative technique.

10.4.4 Surgical Steps

- Open approach offers adequate exposure and also the ability to address different deformities of the lateral crus.
- The lateral crus is exposed on both sides. Once a decision is made to shorten the lateral crus by excising a segmental width of the lateral crus, the segment which need to be excised is marked out on the lateral crus well away from the dome and also not too close to the scroll region. Ideally centered around the middle of the lateral crus. As mentioned above, the maximum width which needs to be excised should be not more than 4 mm each side. The medial edge of the excision site should be at least 5–6 mm away from the intermediate crus.
- The segment of lateral crus to be excised is held by the prongs of the Adson's forceps and slightly tilted laterally and the medial part of the incision is made first. Great care is taken not to cut the underlying mucosa. If this happens, it can result in alar collapse and pinching which although can be repaired, but at the cost of lateral alar weakness, scarring and functional narrowing of external nasal valve region. One way of avoiding direct damage to the underlying mucosa of the lateral crus is to change the angle of the knife towards the Adson's forceps, tilting the lateral crus outwards and using the knife against one of the tongs of the Adson's forceps, as shown in the Fig. 10.9. Incising the cartilage directly carries the risk of going through the cartilage and the underlying mucosa together. This is a useful manoeuvre which is safe and allows the surgeon to make a controlled incision of the lateral crus, so that any direct injury to the mucosa underneath is prevented.
- The cartilage incision extends from the cephalic to caudal margin of the lateral crus and results in a proximal and a distal lateral crural cartilage segment. Please note as soon as an incision is made in the lateral crus, the two cut edges becomes asymmetric in its position (as clearly seen on the right side in Fig. 10.10b) due to the orientation of the lateral crus. This should be taken care of in approximating the two edges.
- The marked segment of the lateral crus which need to be excised is dissected free of the underlying mucosa, and a maximum of 4 mm is excised with an angled scissors, making sure the segment is strictly rect-

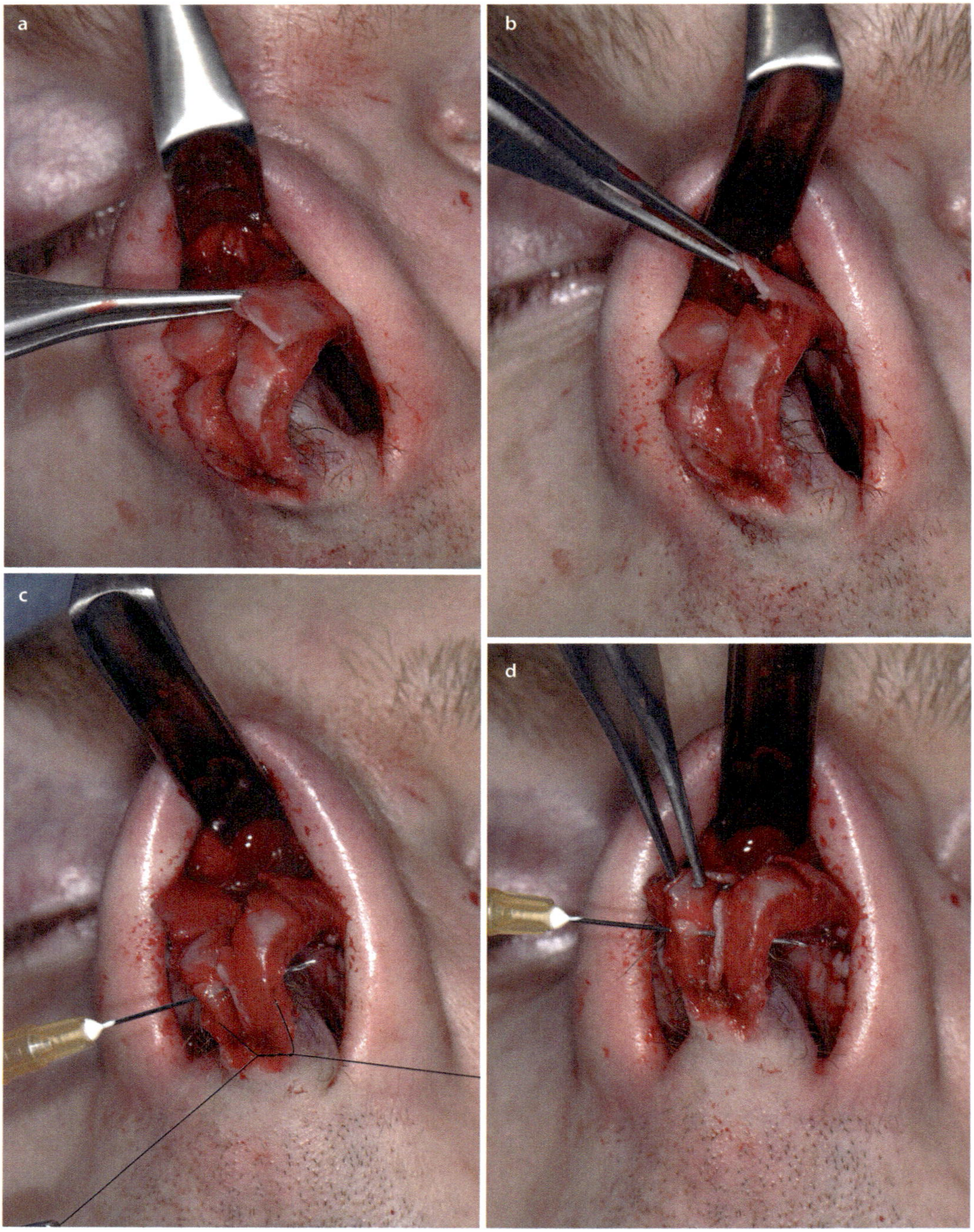

Fig. 10.10 **a–d** Open approach view showing the surgical sequence of lateral crural excision and advancement technique along with a columellar strut. (Reproduced with kind permission from Refs. [1–3])

angular with both the medial and lateral incision lines strictly parallel to each other. The excess mucosal folds underneath will settle over time.

- How much lateral crus to excise and which bit of lateral crus to excise depends on the experience of the surgeon and of course the deformity and should be tailored to the desired effect. As a general rule of thumb, the maximum excision should be no more than 4 mm to avoid over rotation of the tip.
- After excising the segment of the lateral crus on both sides, the continuity of the lateral crus is re-established with two simple 5-0 ethilon or PDS sutures to bring together the two segments. One suture is placed at the cephalic border of the lateral crus, and another at the caudal border of the lateral crus and sutured end to end without any vertical sliding. Make sure the suture is snipped very close to the knot as this suture is superficial under the skin [1–3, 9].
- Since the lateral scroll region is a fixed point and the medial tip region is mobile, this will de-project the tip back and over rotate the tip if done in isolation. Hence, it is important that the lateral aspect of the lateral crus should be left undisturbed.
- Finally it is always advisable to put some pieces of crushed cartilages over incised tip cartilages particularly in people with thin skin.
- Once this procedure is done, then it is advisable to consider either a medial crural suture or a columellar strut (■ Fig. 10.10d) to secure the height of the medial crus in a lower de-projected site.
- Once this procedure is performed, NO attempt should be made to narrow the tip with inter-domal or trans-domal suture, as these sutures will put strain on the lateral crural suture line, which in turn can snap the suture line, resulting in an alar collapse.

10.4.5 Surgical Sequence

- Always consider cephalic trim to reduce the width of the lateral crus to an optimum size before proceeding for lateral crural excision.
- Then do the excision and suturing of the lateral crus.

Key Points

- Beware this is an excision technique. Hence, it is a destructive technique with the disruption of the continuity of the lateral crus. It should be used ONLY in extreme circumstances by experienced surgeons. Lot of thought process should go into this depending upon the deformities you are planning to correct.
- The site of excision of the lateral crus is very important. Too lateral excision will result in damage to the scroll region and may cause damage to the scroll fat and accessory cartilages causing alar pinching. Too medially placed excision results in distortion of the nasal tip.
- The amount of excision should NOT be more than 4 mm; otherwise, there is a risk of over rotation of the tip and anterior nostril show.
- The excised segment should be parallel. Two segments should be approximated nicely without overlap.
- The suture should be a simple suture, just enough to approximate the cartilages edges and NOT too tight to cause overlap. The knots should be camouflaged with crushed cartilage, to avoid shown through the skin.
- Patient's age, sex and skin thickness must be considered. In people with thin skin, the cartilage suture junction may not produce a cosmetically favourable result and may cause a visible bulge.
- Beware, as soon as the cartilage is cut, the cut edges will rotate and will not be parallel to each other due to the direction and the resulting pivotal movement. So do not panic. After excising the segment, take care while suturing the cartilage fragments together making sure the edges are approximated properly to prevent any rotation or pivotal movements of the two segments in the lateral crus.
- Once this procedure is done, DO NOT attempt to narrow the tip with an inter-domal or trans-domal sutures, which

will put strain on the lateral crural suture site with resulting irregular cartilage show or resultant weakness, or discontinuity in the lateral crus.
- Finally be careful in avoiding damage to the vestibular mucosa underlying the lateral crus by handling the tissues gently and using the blade at an angle.

Conclusion

Be aware that this technique involving the lateral crus is a destructive technique which should not be taken lightly without prior consideration of all the pros and cons involved in correcting a particular tip deformity.

10.5 Lateral Crural Steal: Vertical Dome Division (VDD)

10.5.1 Introduction

Collectively, vertical dome division (VDD) refers to one of many methods of vertically dividing the lower lateral (alar) cartilage at or just lateral to the dome and approximating the medial segments against each other and sutured together to increase tip height and tip definition. The classic "Goldman tip", popularised by Goldman in 1957 as a method of refining the tip, is an *incisional technique* (not to be confused with any excisional techniques), which involved complete division (incision) of the alar cartilage 2 to 3 mms lateral to the dome along with the underlying mucosa and the medial cut ends turned towards each other in the midline to achieve tip projection without the use of columellar struts. This was an interrupted strip technique involving the cartilage and mucosa which interrupts the integrity of the lateral crus. This fell into disrepute due to being a destructive technique and resulting in tip irregularities, bossae formation and also functional lateral alar collapse. However since the tripod concept, the principle of VDD has seen a resurgence, (thanks to Simmons) with the exception being to preserve the underlying vestibular skin. *There are various modifications of vertical dome division, which are all incisional techniques involving ONLY the lateral crural cartilage and NOT the underlying alar mucosa*, as opposed to the original Goldman tip technique, which involved incising both cartilage and mucosa. Hence, it is less destructive than the original Goldman tip procedure [11]. If the incision is made just lateral to the intermediate crus of the dome, it becomes a form of *lateral crural steel*, as part of the lateral crura which is medial to the incision is incorporated into the newly established projected tip, thus extending the length of the medial crus doing effectively the job of a medial crus strut graft [12, 13].

10.5.2 Indications

VDD is a versatile technique which has undergone several modifications since its first description by Goldman. Ideal indication being a moderate to severe under projected wide nasal tip (◘ Fig. 10.11) with suboptimal definition and rotation. Simon's modification involves making the incision lateral to the dome and turning the medial segments towards each other to increase tip projection (lateral crural steal). One other modification (Lipsett) involves making the incision medial to the dome in the medial crus. This would result in decreasing tip projection [14]. These techniques of VDD and its modifications are not to be tried by inexperienced surgeons as they do not produce consistent results in the author's view [15].

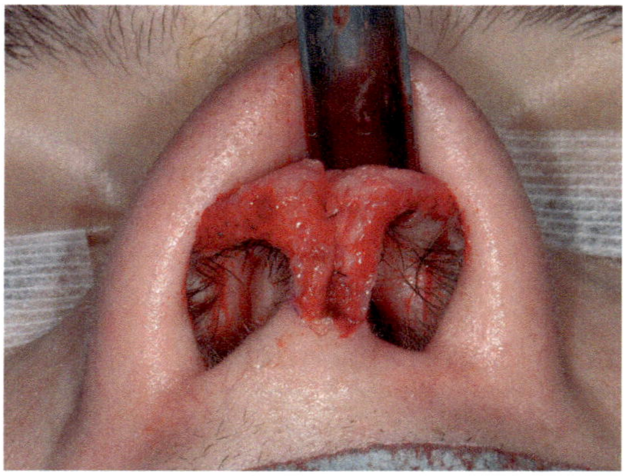

◘ **Fig. 10.11** Open approach view showing a broad under projected tip

10.5.3 Contra-indications

- In younger age.
- Thin overlying skin.
- Scarred contracted skin.
- Revision procedures.
- Weak lateral alar cartilages with functional weakness of the alar margin.

10.5.4 Surgical Steps of Lateral Crural Steel (▣ Fig. 10.12a–g)

- Best achieved through an open approach.
- Most commonly performed is the Simon's modification where, essentially the medial crural height is increased by stealing from the lateral crus (hence called lateral crural steal).
- To achieve this, the vestibular skin is undermined from the under surface of the lower lateral cartilage, for at least 5–7 mm to allow for mobilisation of the cartilage.
- Then the direction of medial crus should be changed from the coronal to sagittal plane if necessary using medial crural flare control sutures.
- The lateral crus is then divided closer to the intermediate crus, depending upon how much projection to achieve, sparing the underlying mucosa and advanced on to the medial crus (*without dividing the integrity of alar mucosa*) [1, 2].
- This procedure is then repeated on the contralateral side, and a new dome is created at a higher level than the existing dome using a horizontal mattress suture.
- It is advisable to use a lateral crural strut to bridge the gap in the lateral crus and also to use a shield graft in front of the new tip to camouflage any sharp edges. May also need a CAP graft in the supra-tip region.
- Place some crushed septal cartilage or resected cephalic portion of the lateral crus over the lateral alar mucosa, from where the lateral crus was lifted. This will avoid some "shouldering" effect of the eye-brow tip line at the level of the lateral alar region.

10.5.5 Surgical Sequence

Do the septal work first, followed by a cephalic trim if lateral crus is wide and bulky. Then do the dorsal work and then secure the medial crus together with a medial crural fixation suture if necessary and then the lateral crural steal is performed as a final procedure before closing the flap.

Key Points

- Firstly before considering this procedure, think of available alternatives which can achieve the same result without disrupting the continuity of the lateral crus. Other procedures, which can increase projection, include trans-domal sutures and inter-domal sutures and grafting techniques like a columellar strut and caudal septal extension grafts.
- Remember this procedure is an incisional disruptive technique and there is a potential to cause lateral alar collapse, and hence should be used with extreme caution by beginner surgeons.
- If a decision is made to do the procedure, it will be advisable to modify the technique by preserving the underlying mucosa and NOT to do the originally described Goldman technique.
- Cutting the mucosa and cartilage results in loss of the lateral crural arch, causing devastating alar pinching and shouldering of the lateral crus. Functionally this will result in alar collapse which will be very difficult to manage surgically.
- Always camouflage the sharp cartilage edges and the sutures with some crushed septal cartilage and also camouflage the small depression created over the lateral alar mucosa, which is devoid of the lateral crural cartilage either with crushed septal cartilage or ideally the resected cephalic portion of the lateral crus.

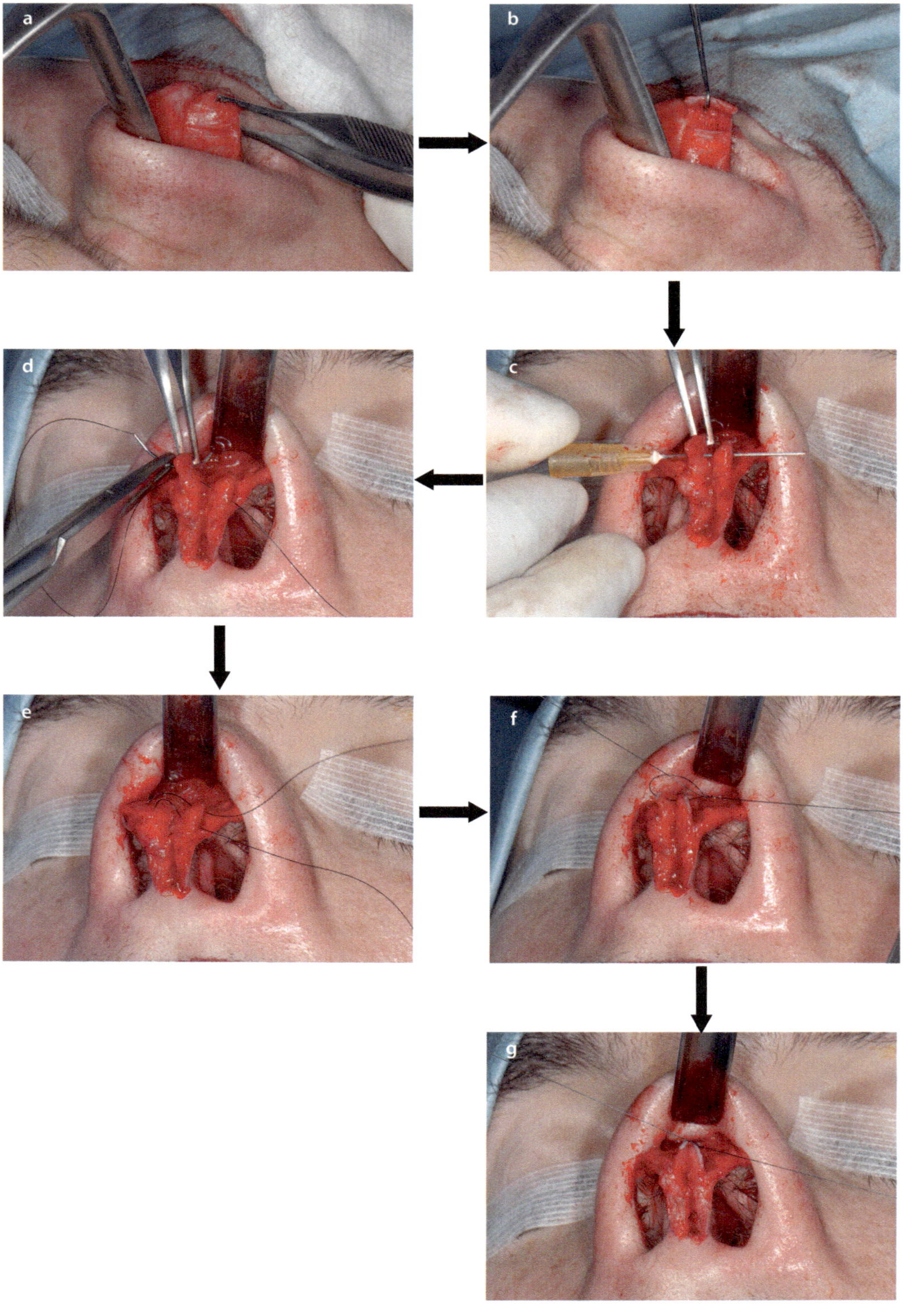

Fig. 10.12 **a–g** Open approach view showing the surgical steps of lateral crural steal. (Reproduced with kind permission from Refs. [1, 2])

Conclusion

This technique has been modified and frequently confused with the original description of Goldman tip technique. Some modifications of vertical dome division is still favoured by some surgeons as a very effective technique to achieve adequate tip projection and /or to de-project the tip as well. This technique is not advisable for beginner surgeons.

10.6 Intermediate Crural Excision and Re-Approximation

10.6.1 Introduction

Intermediate crural segment excision involves excision of a segment of the intermediate crus without damaging the underlying mucosa. The continuity of the lateral and medial crus is re-established with 5-0 ethilon sutures or PDS. This is a powerful technique to reset the nasal tip position straight back (de-projection) without altering the rotation. This can be done in patients with intrinsically long antero-posterior length of the lower lateral cartilage mostly genetic and mostly ethnic noses like north Indian/Punjabi/Pakistani/Arab noses. The other alternative to reduce tip projection (to take the tip towards the face) without altering the rotation of the tip would be to do a concurrent lateral crural overlap and a medial crural overlap (done at the same time). There are pros and cons of both the techniques. As opposed to this combined procedure, we call this intermediate segment excision as a "Direct Dome Technique". As per the "tripod" concept, this technique brings down the base of the tripod (dome of the nasal tip) without individually altering the length of the two lateral crura and the conjoined medial crura separately. It can also be used to correct some localised knobbly deformities of the nasal tip domes. Be aware of doing this procedure in young patients with thin skin envelope.

10.6.2 Indications

- Large over projected nasal tip along with over projected nasal dorsum (◘ Figs. 10.13 and 10.14). In these patients Intermediate crural resection and re-approximation done along with dorsal reduction helps in decreasing the size of the nose and restoring symmetry.
- Isolated over projected tips (◘ Fig. 10.15a–c), along with over rotation with the patients complaining of a "Pinocchio" type of nose. This situation may be due from birth or due to excess dorsal resection following a rhinoplasty, without concomitant tip de-projection.

Bilateral large bossae formation over the nasal tip, usually genetic or post-traumatic (◘ Fig. 10.16).

Large noses with thicker skin and older patient.

10.6.3 Contra-indications

- Young patient.
- Very thin skin.
- Multiple revision procedures.

10.6.4 Surgical Steps (◘ Fig. 10.17a–i)

- Adequate exposure is important through an open approach.
- If needed, a cephalic trim of lateral crus is done prior to intermediate crural resection to reduce the bulk of the lateral crus.
- Intermediate crura (segment) is marked out (maximum 3–4 mm width) to be excised and excised without damaging the underlying mucosa.
- Underlying mucosa should be dissected free not only over the area of cartilage to be excised, but also on either side of it for 2 mm so that there is a sub-mucosal space to put 5-0 ethilon non-absorbable sutures between the lateral crus and medial crus.

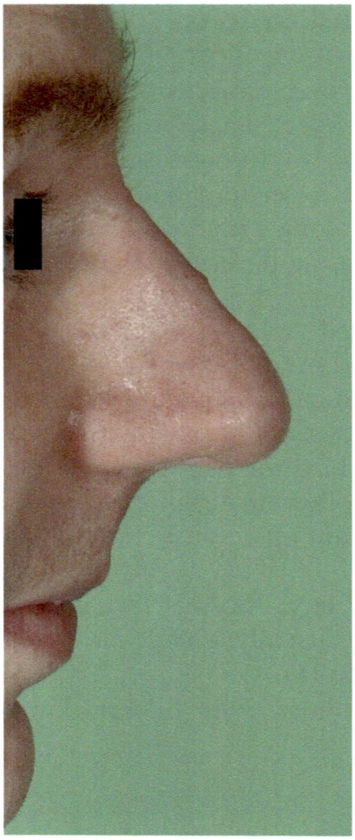

Fig. 10.13 Lateral view showing isolated over projection of the nasal tip

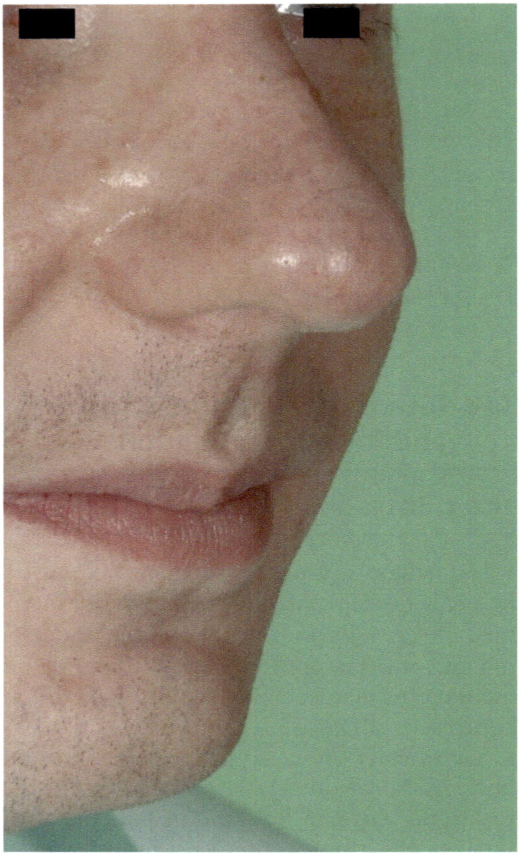

Fig. 10.14 Three-fourth view showing isolated over projection of the nasal tip

10

- Now stabilise the medial crus on both sides by passing a small hypodermic needle through them.
- Then excise the intermediate crus as shown in the Fig. 10.17h
- The continuity between the medial crus and the lateral crus is then re-established by two simple sutures, one cephalic and one caudal. Avoid horizontal mattress sutures as they cause the edges to lift up.
- Crushed septal cartilage or the soft cartilage excised from the cephalic portion of the lateral crus is used to cover the knots over the dome.

10.6.5 Surgical Sequence

Dorsal reduction should be done first, if indicated, followed by cephalic trim of lateral crus. Then the medial crura should be stabilised with hypodermic needle. Then the intermediate crus is resected and the continuity of the lateral crus established with sutures. Once this is done, do not do inter-domal or trans-domal sutures, as they will cause tension on the suture lines.

Key Points

- Beware this is an excisional technique, but preserving the vestibular mucosa. Hence, it is a destructive technique with the disruption of the continuity of the lateral crus. It should be used ONLY in extreme circumstances after assessing the pros and cons.
- Patient's age, sex and skin thickness must be considered. In people with thin skin, the cartilage suturing may not produce a cosmetically favourable result and may cause a visible irregularities.

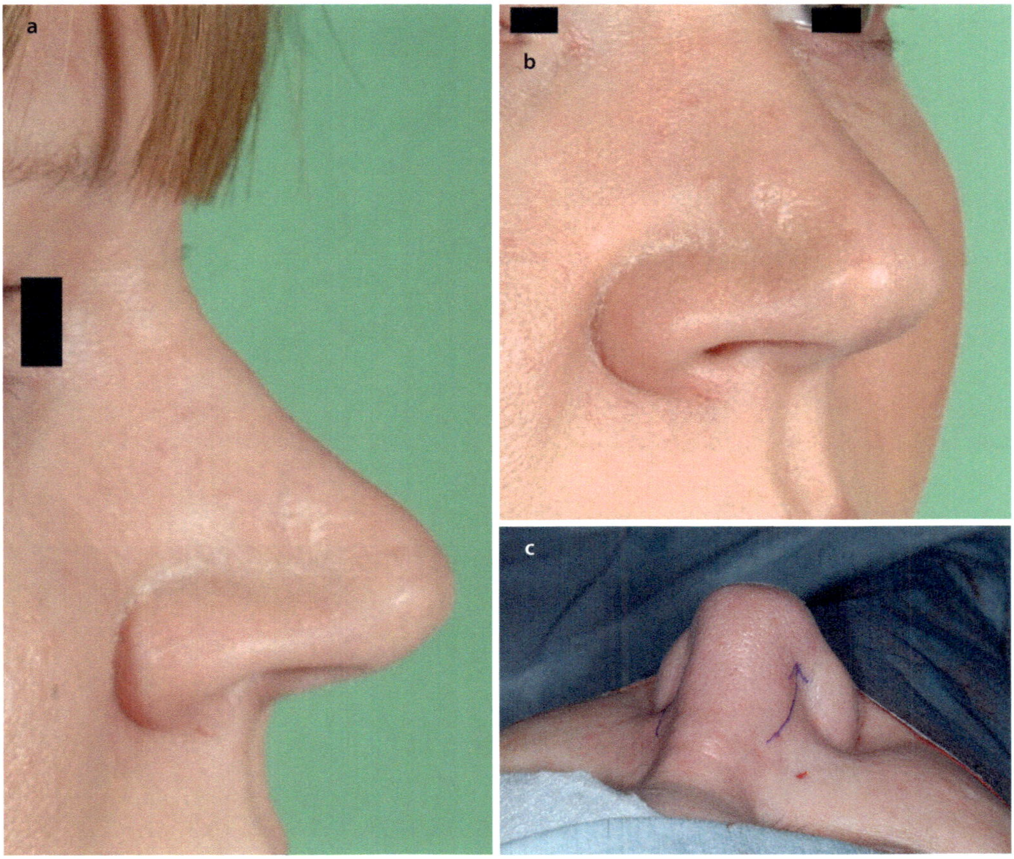

Fig. 10.15 **a–c** Isolated over projection of the nasal tip after dorsal reduction. **a** Lateral view. **b** Three-fourth view. **c** Sky view

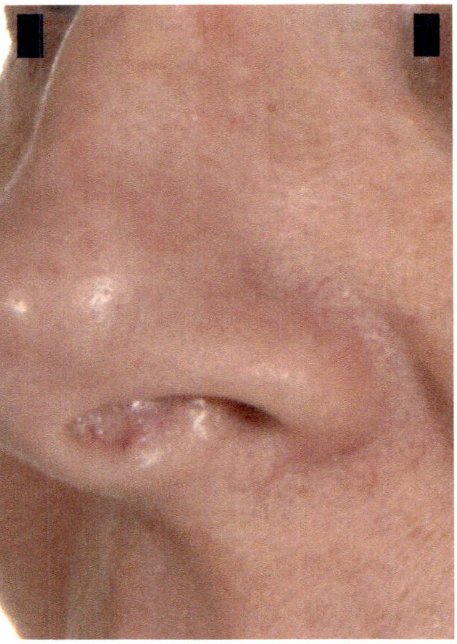

Fig. 10.16 Three-fourth view showing isolated over projection of the nasal tip with bilateral bossae formation

- The site of excision of the intermediate crus is very important. Too lateral excision will not achieve the desired effect of de-projection. Too medially placed excision will result in distortion of the nasal tip and infra tip blunting.
- The amount of excision should NOT be more than 4 mm maximum (usually around 2 mm); otherwise, there is a risk of under projection and widening of the tip.
- The excised segment should be parallel. Two segments should be approximated nicely without overlap with simple sutures.
- The suture should be just right to approximate the cartilages edges and NOT too tight to cause overlap. The knots should be camouflaged with crushed cartilage, to avoid shown through the skin.

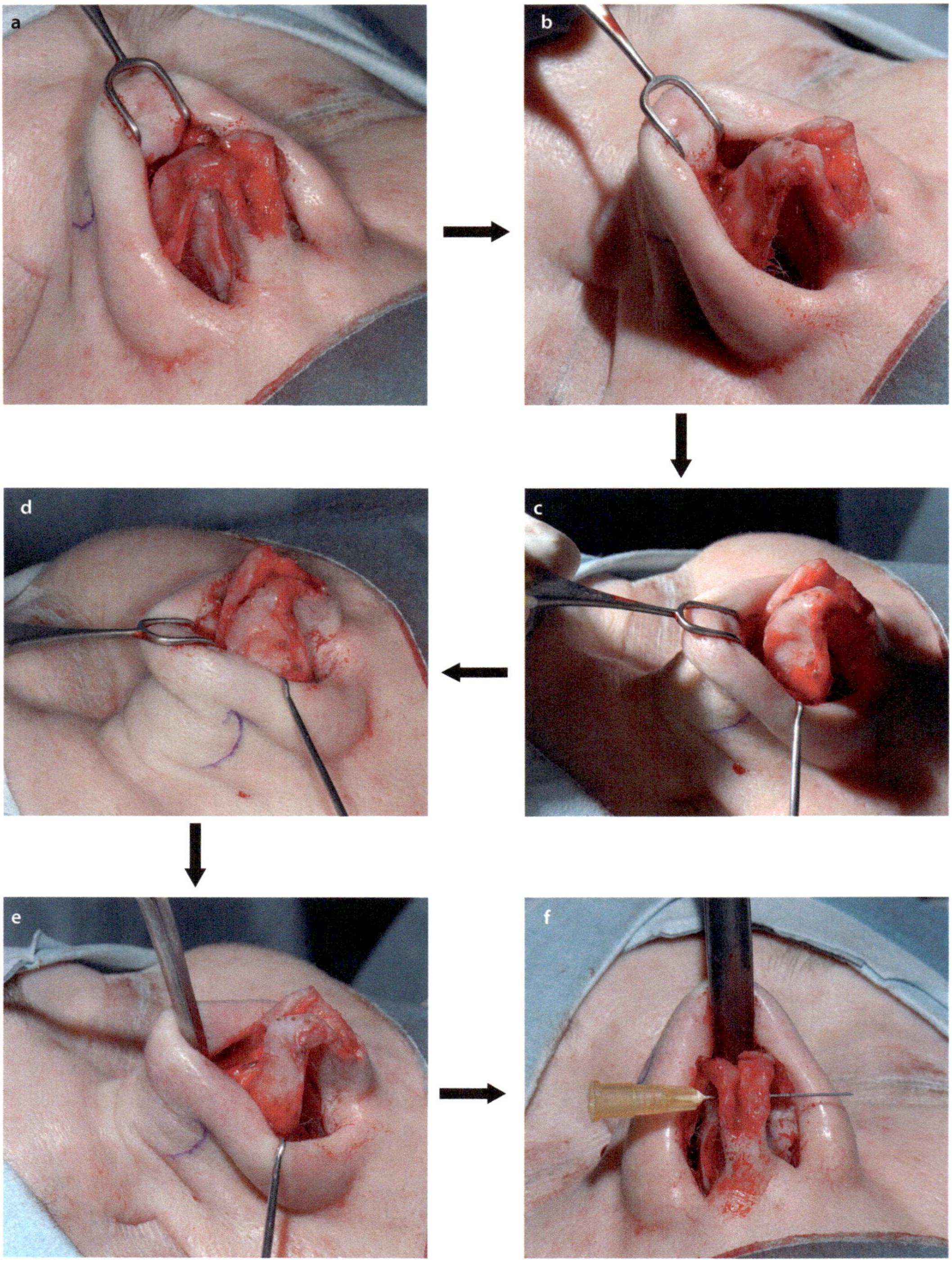

Fig. 10.17 **a–i** Open approach view showing the surgical sequence of intermediate crural excision and advancement to de-project the tip to the face

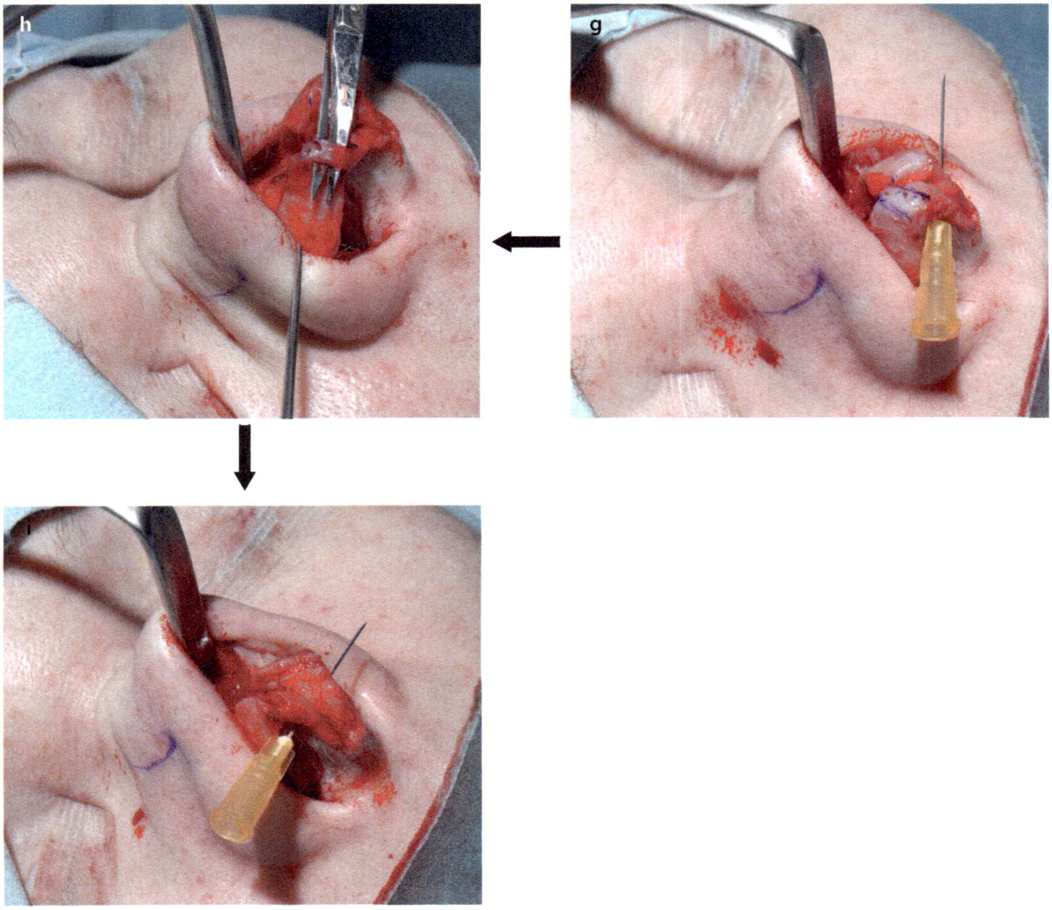

Fig. 10.17 (continued)

- Beware, as soon as the cartilage is cut, the cut edges will rotate and will not be parallel to each other due to the direction and the resulting pivotal movement. So do not panic. After excising the segment, take care while suturing the cartilage fragments together making sure the edges are approximated properly to prevent any rotation or pivotal movements of the two segments in the lateral crus.
- Once this procedure is done, DO NOT attempt to narrow the tip with an inter-domal or trans-domal sutures, which will put strain on the lateral crural suture site with resulting irregular cartilage show or resultant weakness or discontinuity in the lateral crus.
- Finally be careful in avoiding damage to the vestibular mucosa, underlying the lateral crus by handling the tissues gently and using the blade at an angle.

Conclusion

This is a very effective technique in de-projecting a large tip back to the face with quicker operating time. Beware it is still a destructive technique, disrupting the continuity of the lateral crus. We used to do this only in slightly older patients with thicker skin so that any underlying cartilage irregularity is not shown through. But in selected patients we have been using this technique more and more for effective de-projection of the tip, in younger age group as well, with predicable long-term results.

10.7 Cephalic Lateral Crural Turn "In" or "Out" Flap

10.7.1 Introduction

LC turn "in" or "out" flaps are used to reconstruct a very "**WIDE**" and concave but *structurally intact* lateral crus causing external nasal valve pinching, alar collapse and functional nasal valve obstruction. *The key considerations being the "width" and the "structural integrity" of the lateral crus.* External nasal tip deformities secondary to weak and concave lateral crura is one of the difficult scenarios to correct in nasal tip rhinoplasty surgery. Although there are various options like batten graft, lateral crural strut graft, lateral crural turn in flap, lateral crural reciprocating grafts, the decision to use which technique in which patient takes years of experience and training. We suggest reading the ► Chap. 18 on algorithms to address lateral crural deformities. In reconstructing lateral crural weakness with an extra piece of an autologous cartilage, there is always a fine balance between restoring function and restoring structure. It can restore the external valve function, but can cause unwanted lateral alar bulge. It can correct the concavity of the lateral crus but can cause "in-drawing" on inspiration due to the extra weight of the added cartilage. If there are localised areas of concavity in the lateral crus without any functional issues, small pieces of crushed cartilage can be used as separate lateral crural camouflage graft.

A normal but wide, lateral crus can become concave over a period of time, due to constant inward pull in a patient with a long-standing nasal obstruction due to a septal deviation or a thickened columella [16].

This concavity of the lateral crus can in turn cause external lateral nasal wall collapse on inspiration and cause further nasal obstruction. Sometimes it is difficult to know the cause and effect of these deformities, until otherwise you have been watching these patients over the years. This deformity can present with a cosmetic structural issue as well. The deformity may be either unilateral or bilateral. Mostly they are associated with an over projected nasal tip cartilages, where the length of the lower lateral cartilage is also longer than normal. The wider and longer lateral crus is subjected to more negative inspiratory forces than normal, resulting in a weaker concave lateral crus, which is not able to withstand the inspiratory forces. Any preexisting nasal obstruction due to other causes, like a caudal septal deviation or medial crural footplate prolapse into the vestibule of the nose, can also make the lateral crural weakness worse, narrowing the external nasal valve region further.

This concept of "cephalic lateral crural turn in flap" and folding the cephalic portion of the lateral crus either internally or externally over the remaining concave caudal portion of the lateral crus was first described by Fazil Apaydin from Izmir, Turkey [17]. The technique involved folding the cephalic portion of the wide lateral crus and turning it "in" after lifting the alar mucosa on the medial side. The cephalic portion of the lateral crus can also be folded out and stitched to the inferior segment of the lateral crus depending on the width of the lateral crura, leaving a flatter lateral segment near the scroll which acts as a spring out platform and helps to pull the inferior concave segment of the lateral crus out, thereby improving the airway. Thus this technique helps in achieving a better cosmetic outcome by addressing the concavity and also improving the function by keeping the external nasal valve open. There are pros and cons of folding the cephalic lateral crus "in" or "out" depending on the indications.

10.7.2 Advantages of Lateral Crural Flaps

- It is a "like for like" reconstruction of a concave lateral crus using the cephalic part of the lateral crus.
- There is no extra thickness of the lateral ala, as the concave area is corrected.
- There is no donor site morbidity.
- There is no sliding or slipping, associated with batten grafts or strut grafts.
- Quicker and less time consuming.

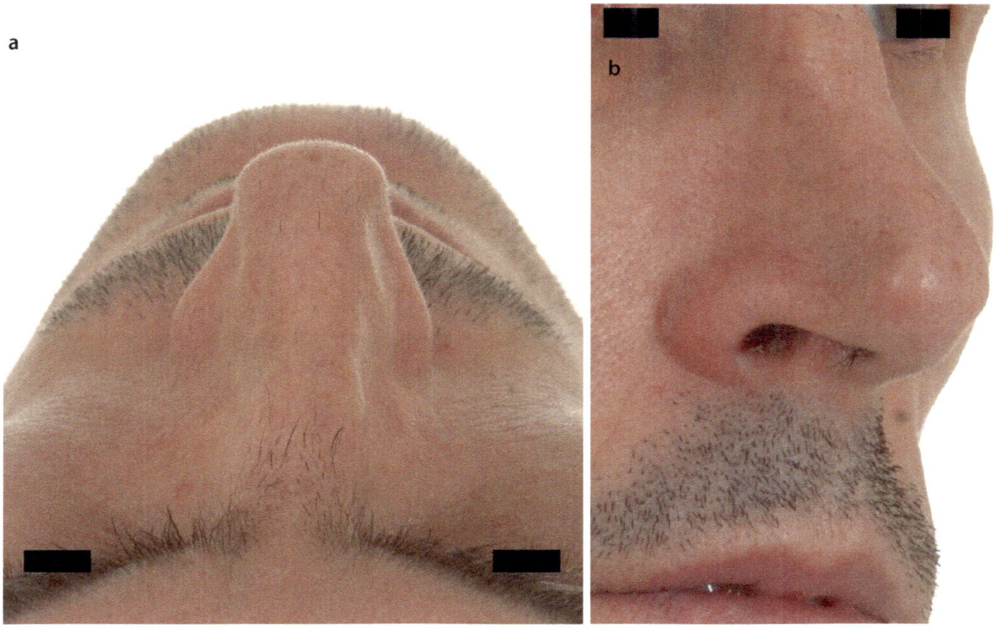

Fig. 10.18 **a, b** Sky view and three-fourth view showing bilateral external nasal valve collapse due to wide and concave lateral crus causing "in drawing" of lateral crus on inspiration resulting in alar pinching and functional obstruction

- As a variant of this "turn in" flaps, we prefer the "turn out" flap more often, due to the ease of surgery and less dissection involved in lifting the alar mucosa. When a turn "out" LC flap is done, it is advisable to leave intact a small area laterally (3–4 mm) of the cephalic border of the lateral crus. The rest of the cephalic border is turned out and secured. The lateral intact segment of lateral crura, then acts as a "spring" to pull the rest of the lateral crus out, thus also helping to increase the external nasal valve cross section and improve the nasal valve function. By folding the cephalic border laterally over the concavity, it also helps in correcting the alar concavity without any additional grafting.

10.7.3 Indications

- External nasal valve collapse due to intact but wide (vertical width of lateral crus more than 12 mm), thin and concave (Fig. 10.18a, b), lateral crus causing in drawing of lateral crus on inspiration resulting in alar pinching and external concave deformity.
- This technique works well in both unilateral or bilateral lateral alar concavity, usually associated with an over projected tip.
- Adequate strength of the lateral crus, as evidenced by an over projected tip.
- There should be no structural damage or discontinuity of the lateral crus. In this situation, other options like lateral crural strut grafts need to be considered.
- Preserved intrinsic strength and structure of conjoined medial crus.

10.7.4 Contra-indications

- Fracture discontinuity of the lateral crus at the dome.
- Weak conjoined medial crus.
- A combination of both the above deformities.

10.7.5 Surgical Technique of Lateral Crural Turn Out Flap (Fig. 10.19a–l)

- This technique is indicated in patients with collapse of the lateral alar region causing concavity and nasal obstruction.
- The options available would be to reconstruct this type of deformity with a batten graft, a lateral crural "turn out or in" flaps or a lateral crural reciprocating graft or a lateral crural strut graft. The indications for each are different.
- The selection of which technique to implement depends on the structure of the lateral crus, width, length and absence of any breaks in the cartilage as mentioned in the indications above [9, 18].

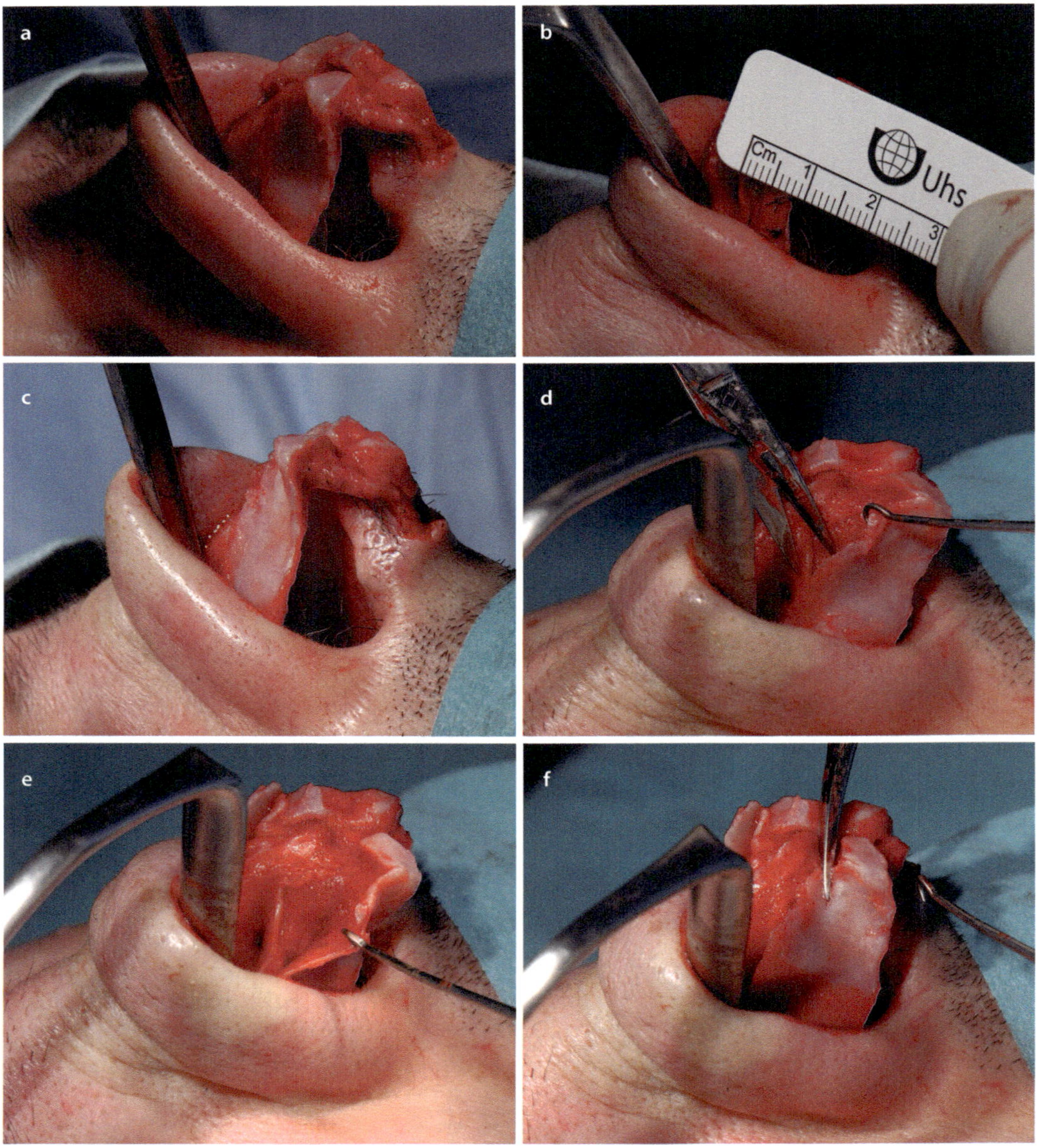

Fig. 10.19 a–l Open approach view showing the surgical sequence of lateral crural "turn-out" flap to address a concave and wide lateral crus causing functional obstruction

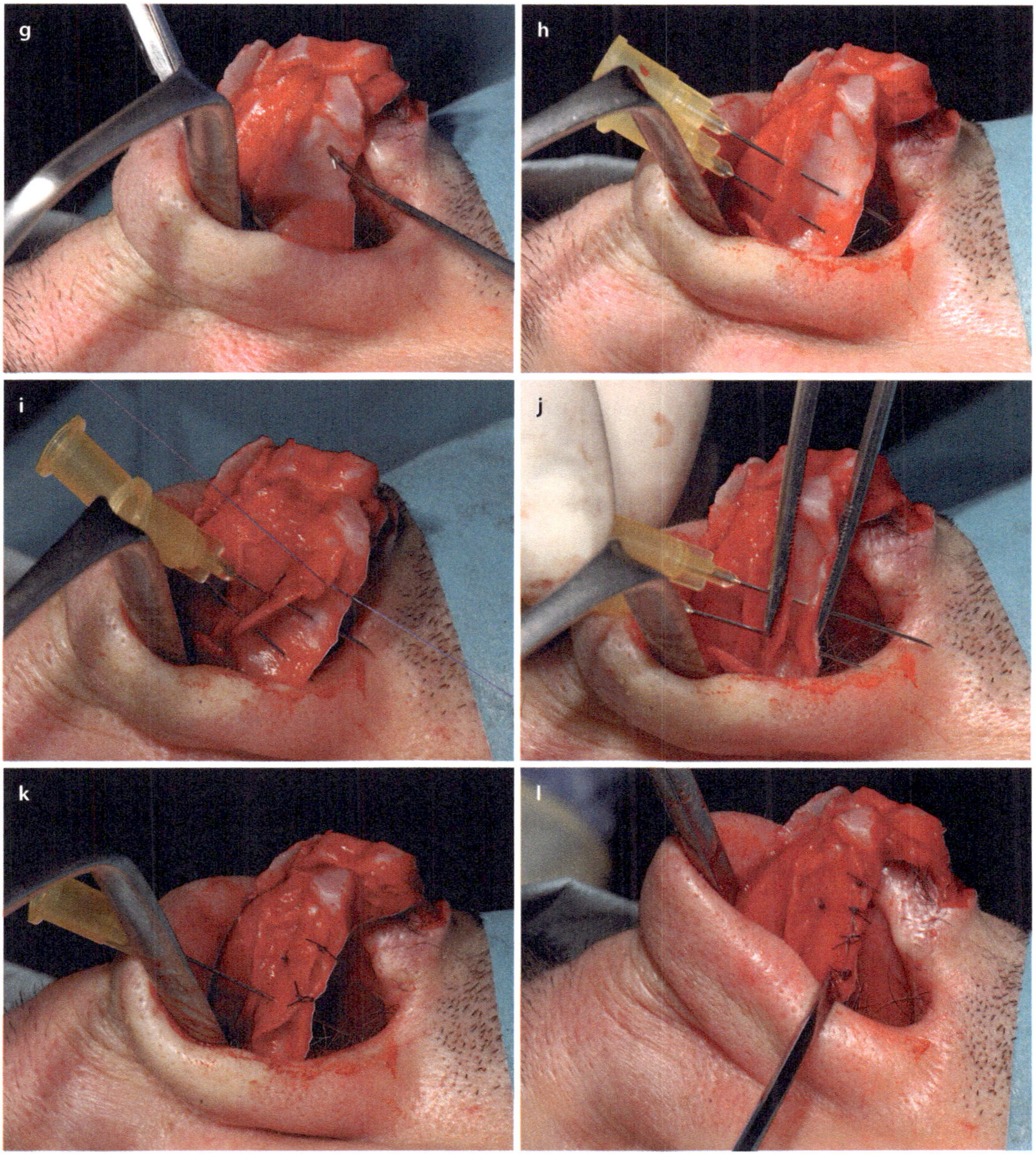

Fig. 10.19 (continued)

- The procedure is performed through an open approach with adequate exposure of the bony and cartilaginous framework of the nose. Open approach gives access and allows us to confirm the indication so that the right technique is done for the right deformity.
- The whole of the lateral crus from caudal to cephalic portion except the very lateral part of the lateral crus is skeletonised and overlying soft tissues are dissected off if necessary. The findings are confirmed. The lateral crus width should be wider, preferably well over 10 mm with concavity, but without any fractures, scarring or discontinuity. The conjoined medial crus should be intact. The intrinsic strength of the lateral crus should be preserved.

- The lateral crus is measured at the midpoint. A minimum distance of 8 mm is measured and the cephalic portion is dissected of the underlying mucosa with a curved sharp scissors, using a technique of small snips and big spreads.
- Then the medial side of the cephalic portion is snipped at an angle allowing it to fold on itself, except the most lateral portion of the lateral crus which is kept intact and flat.
- The cephalic portion is then folded "out or in", onto the caudal concave portion and secured with 5-0 absorbable through and through vicryl sutures. Non-absorbable sutures are not used in this area as the suture either goes through the mucosa or at least very close to the alar margin.
- The undisturbed lateral portion acts as a "spring out flap" to pull the rest of the lateral crus out, thus improving the nasal airway as well as correcting the structural concavity. Thus this procedure not only helps in the cosmetic camouflage of the lateral alar concavity, but also helps in improving the external nasal valve function.

10.7.6 Surgical Sequence

Lateral crural work should always be preceded by columellar reconstruction and medial crural work.

If the same patient needs a tip narrowing procedure like an inter-domal or transdomal suture, then this may cause stress on the lateral crural suture lines. This should be thought of in the initial planning stages of the surgery.

Key Points

- Surgical planning is the key depending on the clinical findings. It is always better to have a clinical algorithm to correct different deformities of the lateral crus before the surgical intervention.
- Care must be taken to dissect the cephalic border of the lateral crus away from the underlying mucosa, without damaging the alar mucosa.
- Care must be taken to maintain 8 mm of lateral crural cartilage to preserve the valve function.
- Care must be taken NOT to fold an excess of the cephalic portion as otherwise there will be alar margin retraction and columellar show.
- Remember to use absorbable sutures for the cartilage if the suture is close to the underlying mucosa.

Conclusion

Extreme caution is necessary in making a decision to use these "turn out or turn in" flaps of the lateral crus. The right indication should be a concave, wide but intact lateral crus width of nearly 12 mm and over. Excess folding of the cephalic border of the lateral crus can pull the caudal border up and can cause alar margin retraction.

10.8 Lateral Crural Rein Flap

10.8.1 Introduction

Lateral crural rein flap as the name suggests is a flap of cephalic portion of the two lateral crus brought together and pulled up like "reins" of the horse to lift the nasal tip and rotate it up. This can then be secured to the septal cartilage in the desired position. Be aware, since the rest of the lateral crus is intact, it can get distorted because of the upward pull of the flap. We have used this technique in only a handful of patients in over 1700 Caucasian noses. After this concept was put forward by Gruber [19–23], lot of other authors have published with different modifications.

10.8.2 Indications

- Droopy nasal tip with external valve weakness.
- Also helps in caudal migration of the lateral crus if it is malpositioned.
- By pulling the tip up, the remaining lateral crus may migrate down laterally, thus strengthening the lateral alar region.

10.8.3 Contra-indications

- Narrow cephalic portions of lateral crus.
- Scarred and discontinuous lateral crura.

10.8.4 Surgical Technique

- A cephalic flap of lateral crus is designed basically to lift a drooping tip by lifting the cephalic portion of the lateral crus like "reins of the horse". This procedure helps in lifting the ptotic tip with cephalic mal positioning of lateral crus.
- Open approach is the only way to do the procedure.
- The cephalic portion of the lateral crus is exposed completely and incised lateral to medial stopping 2–3 mm lateral to the dome.
- The incised cephalic portion is then dissected free of the underlying mucosa working lateral to medial, but keeping it in continuity with the intermediate and medial crus.
- The orientation of the two cephalic portions are then turned in a sagittal plane and "pulled up" like the reins of a horse.
- They are then moved up on either side of the septum pulling and thereby rotating the nasal tip upwards.
- The septal flaps should have been raised before and the cephalic portions stitched to the dorsal septal cartilage at the desired level.
- If necessary when there is an associated internal valve narrowing, the upper lateral can be separated from the dorsal septum three-fourths of the way and the cephalic portion of the lateral crura slid in between and stitched in place, thereby acting as a spreader graft providing an increased internal valve area as well.

10.8.5 Surgical Sequence

The septoplasty should be done first and septal flaps should be raised on both sides and dorsal work completed, and, if necessary, the upper lateral cartilage should be separated before doing this procedure.

Key Points

- Make sure the underlying mucosa is not damaged.
- Make sure the cephalic portion does not get totally separated from the rest of the lateral crus. The cartilage need to be incised and kept in continuity with the intermediate and medial crus.

Conclusion

As mentioned before, these are not considered as mainstream tip techniques which can achieve consistent results.

10.9 Medial Crural Overlap and Shortening

10.9.1 Introduction

The two medial crura forms the central conjoined limb of the nasal tip tripod and is one of the major tip support mechanisms. By incising and overlapping the two medial crura, we can reduce the length of the central limb of the tripod. This, in turn will not only de-project the tip but also under rotate the tip. If done with a lateral crural shortening procedure, this will de-project the tip without affecting the rotation.

This is an easier technique to do and mere incision of the medial crura is enough to de-project the tip due to the weight of the tip itself helping to overlap the cut segments.

10.9.2 Indications

- This manoeuvre helps in decreasing the height of the medial crus and thereby decreasing the projection of the tip on the face. It is a quite a powerful technique to de-project the tip.
- Indicated in large over projected noses (Fig. 10.20a, b) due to intrinsically large tip cartilages as seen more commonly in ethnic noses (north Indian, Arab, and Pakistani origin).

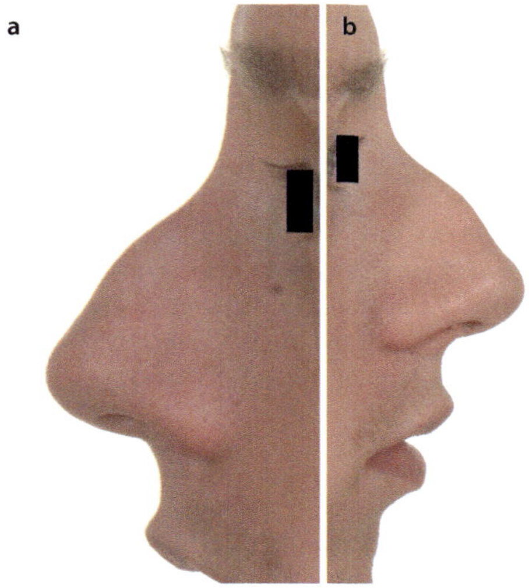

Fig. 10.20 **a**, **b** Large over projected nasal tip

- Should be done equally on both sides to achieve the desired effect, otherwise there will be unwanted tip deviation.
- Be aware that, if done alone it helps not only to de-project, but also under rotate the tip, particularly if the lateral crura is long.
- If done along with a lateral crural shortening procedures as well, only then it will help to de-project the nasal tip without altering the rotation.

10.9.3 Contra-indications

- In secondary revision rhinoplasty with scarring in the columella.
- Under rotated nasal tip with lack of tip support.
- If septal extension or columellar struts are considered as prime procedures.

10.9.4 Surgical Steps

- Adequate exposure is necessary of both the medial crura through an open approach.
- Decision is made if the medial crus needs to be advanced either with the overlying columellar skin or without the columellar skin.
- If there is an associated overhanging columella along with the over projected tip, then it is wise to move the medial crus with the overlying columellar skin.
- But in patients with no columellar show or over hanging columella, the skin over the medial crus should be lifted away from the cartilage and the cut edges jack knifed and advanced inferiorly towards the nasal spine. Sometimes just incising the medial crus horizontally is all that is needed to overlap the medial crus.
- The amount of medial crural overlap should be not more than 3 mm and should be sutured with non-absorbable fine sutures (e.g. 5-0′ ethilon). If the medial crus is advanced as a composite tissue along with columellar skin, then a fine absorbable suture are used.

10.9.5 Surgical Sequence

If planning to reduce the lateral crus as well, perform the medial crural overlap first and then the lateral crus length can be reduced accordingly.

Key Points

- This is a quite an easy technique and most of the time just incising the medial crus horizontally is all that is needed to de-project the tip.
- If the medial crural overlap is planned make sure the columellar incision is lower down in the columella almost towards the anterior nasal spine. When doing an open approach, avoid a superiorly placed columellar incision as this will prevent getting access to the entire vertical length of the medial crus.
- Reducing the height and overlapping the medial crus will increase the width of the columella, which may not be cosmetically acceptable and also will reduce the airflow in the external nasal valve region. Be aware that it can cause an unnatural bulge at the columello-labial junction, particularly in a patient with an over-hanging columella.

Conclusion

In conclusion, although this is an easier manoeuvre to decrease the tip projection, this needs to be used with caution along with lateral crural shortening procedure to avoid unwanted tip under rotation.

10.10 Medial Crural "Tongue in Groove" Advancement

10.10.1 Introduction

This technique helps to lift the hanging columella secondary to medial crural prolapse and advance them towards the caudal septum and secured to the caudal septum, thus strengthening the medial crural complex and also increasing the tip support. This technique thus helps to reduce overhanging columella and an excess "caudal show" in an under rotated and over projected tip. It recedes both the medial crura in a cephalic direction and anchors it to the caudal septum. This technique is not a commonly performed or needed in my practice. This concept of advancement was initially described by Guyuron [24], as a means of increasing the length of the nose.

10.10.2 Indications

- In patients with increased prominence of the caudal edge of the soft tissue columella with an increased columellar show and a bulky columella, tongue-in-groove technique can deliver a well-supported and a narrow columella. Kridel et al. have shown the importance of this technique in the management of the bulky columella with excess columellar flare [25].
- Long and slack medial crus which has lost the support of the anchoring medial crural ligaments either congenital or traumatic, with "hanging columella" (Fig. 10.21a).
- The caudal septum should be intact and in midline and the posterior border of the medial crus ideally should be 2–3 mm from the caudal border of the septal cartilage.

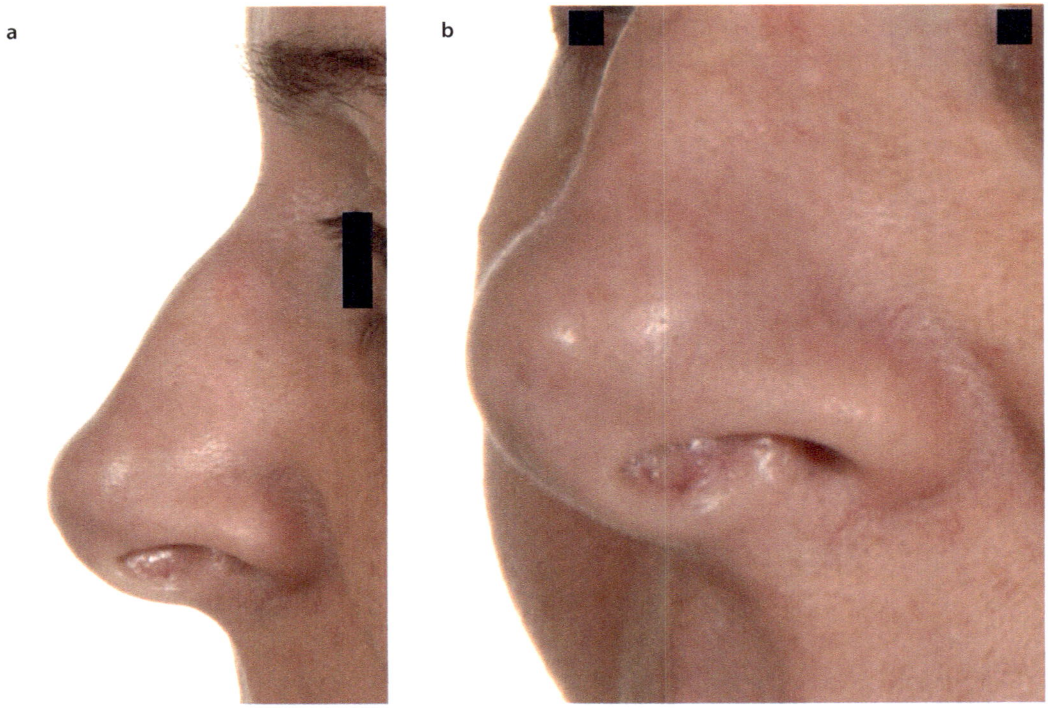

Fig. 10.21 **a, b** Long and slack medial crus which has lost the support of the anchoring medial crural ligaments either congenital or traumatic, with "hanging columella"

10.10.3 Contra-indications

- If the columella show is due to excess show of the medial crus due to fracture/discontinuity do not consider this procedure.
- Excess shortening of the caudal septum requiring a septal extension graft.
- If the caudal septum is not strictly in midline even after reconstruction.

10.10.4 Surgical Technique

- The first step is to straighten the caudal septum.
- Then the medial crura is exposed and mobilised from the overlying skin.
- The direction of the medial crus is changed from coronal plane to sagittal plane if necessary. The freed medial crura are advanced in a cephalic direction on either side of the caudal septum and sutured to the caudal border of septum to create a "tongue in groove complex" using through and through extra-mucosal sutures with 5-0 ethilon or through and through mucosal sutures with 5-0 vicryl (Fig. 10.22b).
- Do not trim the caudal septal cartilage before doing this procedure.
- Also too much advancement will cause alar retraction and columellar retraction and the tip lobule can rotate down.

10.10.5 Surgical Sequence

Straighten the caudal septum first before proceeding. Then cephalic trim of the lateral crus is performed if needed. Then judge the position of the tip and the strength and integrity of the lateral and medial crus. If lateral crural shortening is also planned, then do this at this stage and then do the medial crural advancement.

Key Points

- It is advisable not to recede the medial crus more than 2–3 mm maximum without distorting the columella.
- If tongue-in-groove de-projection is planned (which is also a technique to de-project the tip), *do not perform a caudal shave of the septum which is also a de-projecting technique,* as this will increase the distance you have to move the medial crus, resulting in columellar distortion.
- If the medial crural advancement is planned in a patient with over hanging columella, assessment of the "position"

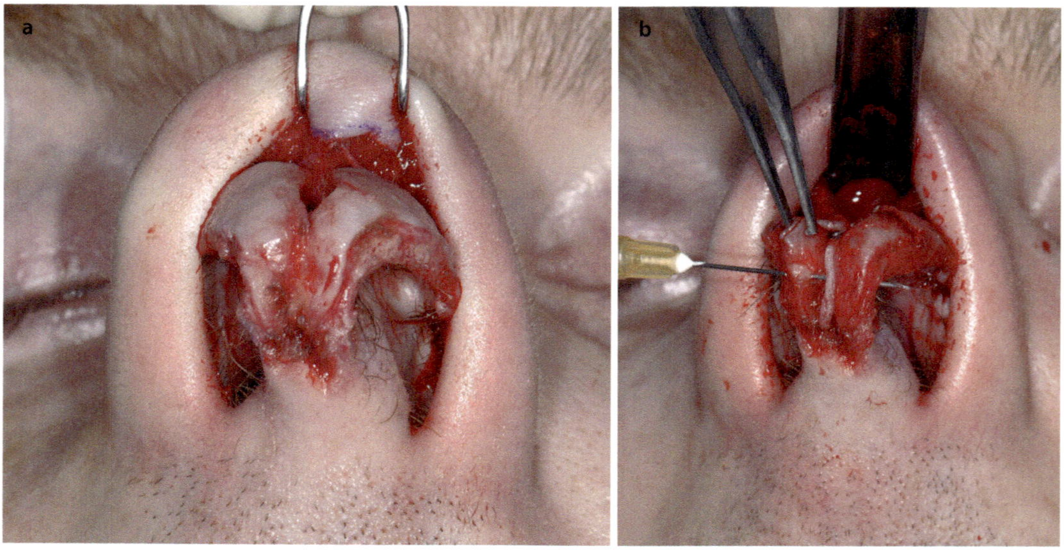

Fig. 10.22 **a**, **b** Open approach. **a** Overhanging medial crus. **b** With "tongue and groove advancement". (Reproduced with kind permission from Refs. [1, 2])

of the nasal tip is vital, before planning this procedure. If done when the tip is already in a slight under rotation, this procedure will make the under rotation worse. On the other hand if the tip position is slightly over rotated to begin with, then this procedure will also help to rotate the tip down.
- Beware if the caudal septum is still deviated to one side stitching the medial crus to it, it will turn the tip to that side.

Conclusion

This is indicated in an overhanging columella due to prolapse of medial crus. A decent caudal septal support is necessary and the caudal septum should be absolutely straight before advancing the medial crus as a "tongue in groove" advancement.

10.11 Nasal Sil Reconstruction with a Split Conchal Cartilage

10.11.1 Introduction

This is a new never been reported technique, which we have used in selected patients to increase the nasal tip projection with anatomical "like for like" reconstruction of the medial crus and the nasal sil region, with a split conchal bowl cartilage. We have done this in a small series of patients with an extremely de-projected nasal tip, shortening of columella and loss of nasal sil definition due to nasal trauma. Achieving an adequate nasal tip projection is an important parameter in an aesthetically balanced tip. This is a direct technique to increase the length of the conjoined medial crus (one limb of the tripod) thereby increasing the tip projection.

There are various alternative "indirect" techniques available to increase the tip projection, including strengthening the medial crus with a strut or septal extension graft. But the key difference is that, this "direct" technique not only reconstructs the medial crus, but also the nasal SIL region of the nasal base using split concave conchal bowl cartilage graft secured to the medial crus. This technique not only increases the columellar length and provides tip support, but also establishes a pleasing smooth, concave nasal SIL region with preservation of the anatomical thirds of the nasal base.

We selectively used this technique in a small series of post-traumatic patients and in patients needing revision surgery. In these patients we avoided the use of more extensive costal cartilage graft which are rigid and non-pliable and do not conform to the shape of the natural sil. We were able to achieve a concave sil region in these patients by using the natural concavity of the conchal bowl cartilage. As the incidence of post-traumatic nasal deformities are on the increase due to trauma, it is better to have multiple options of reconstruction in any abnormality and we recommend this technique as "one of the options" in reconstructing the nasal sil and establishing the columella height and the nasal base symmetry.

10.11.2 Indications

- Short columella due to loss of natural sil region of the lower thirds of the nasal base due to nasal trauma (◘ Fig. 10.23a).
- Extremely short columella due to lack of medial crus height (◘ Fig. 10.23b).
- To increase the tip projection and redefine the triangle of the nasal base establishing the lower third of the nasal base.
- This technique provides an alternative for other indirect ways of increasing the projection like septal extension grafts or columellar struts made from rib graft. This technique provides a "direct like for like" concave reconstruction of the sil region, at the same time increasing the projection as well. However the patient should be counselled that there will be an increase in width of the nasal columella due to the addition of extra pieces of cartilage.

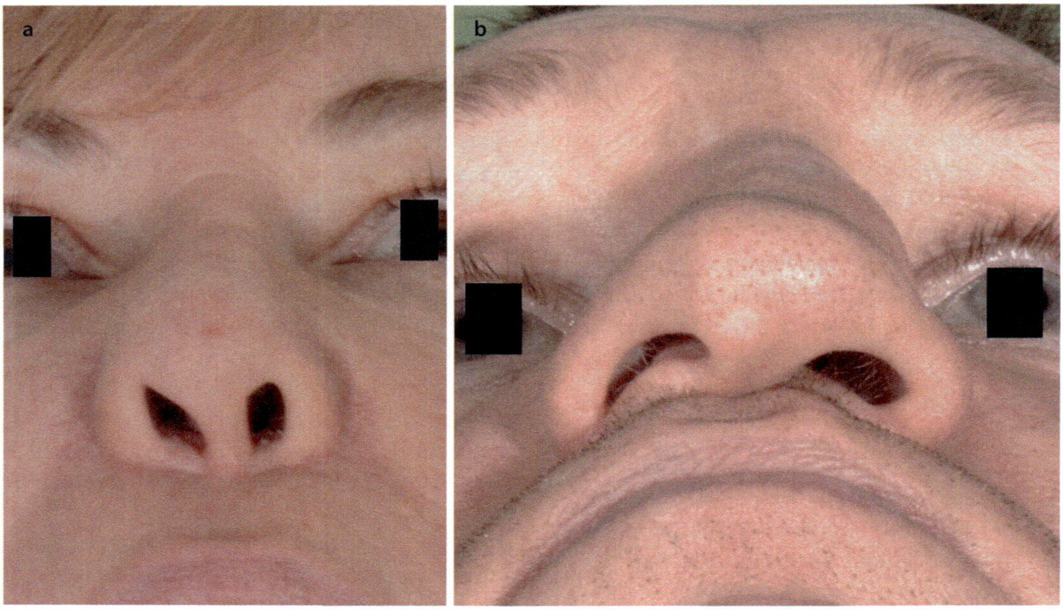

◘ **Fig. 10.23** **a** Distorted columella with loss of sil and distorted nostrils. **b** Extremely short columella due to lack of medial crus height

10.11.3 Contra-indications

- If the skin of the columella is scarred and deformed.
- If the columella is thickened with scar tissue.
- If the lateral alar margin is thicker and the external nasal valve aperture is already narrow.

10.11.4 Surgical Technique (◘ Fig. 10.24a–g)

- Adequate exposure is achieved through an open approach, flaps raised and the findings confirmed.
- The root of the helix creates a convex elevation anteriorly in the conchal bowl, separating the conchal bowl cartilage into a smaller concave superior cavum concha and larger concave inferior cymba concha.
- Next the entire conchal bowl cartilage is harvested either from right or left pinna. Once harvested from the pinna, the Conchal bowl cartilage is split horizontally at the convexity caused by the origin of the root of the helix into two separate concave units, one smaller superior concave “cavum” and a second larger inferior “Cymba” concha. The cartilage is then shaved to the required width (◘ Fig. 10.24b).
- After skeletonising the medial crural plate and freeing the skin over it, a space is created between the columellar skin laterally and the medial crura and soft tissue in the sil medially (◘ Fig. 10.24f).
- The split conchal segments are then reduced in width (thickness) and height to the desired measurements usually 3–4 mm width and up to 8 mm height.
- The two fragments of conchal cartilage, which can hold its concave shape, can then be sutured into the space created on both sides and sutured superiorly to the remains of the medial crural footplate and to each other, leaving the other end to spring naturally away from each other, looking like a haystack (◘ Fig. 10.24g).
- The cartilage can be thinned as necessary for reconstructing the sil region as a replacement for the medial crura.

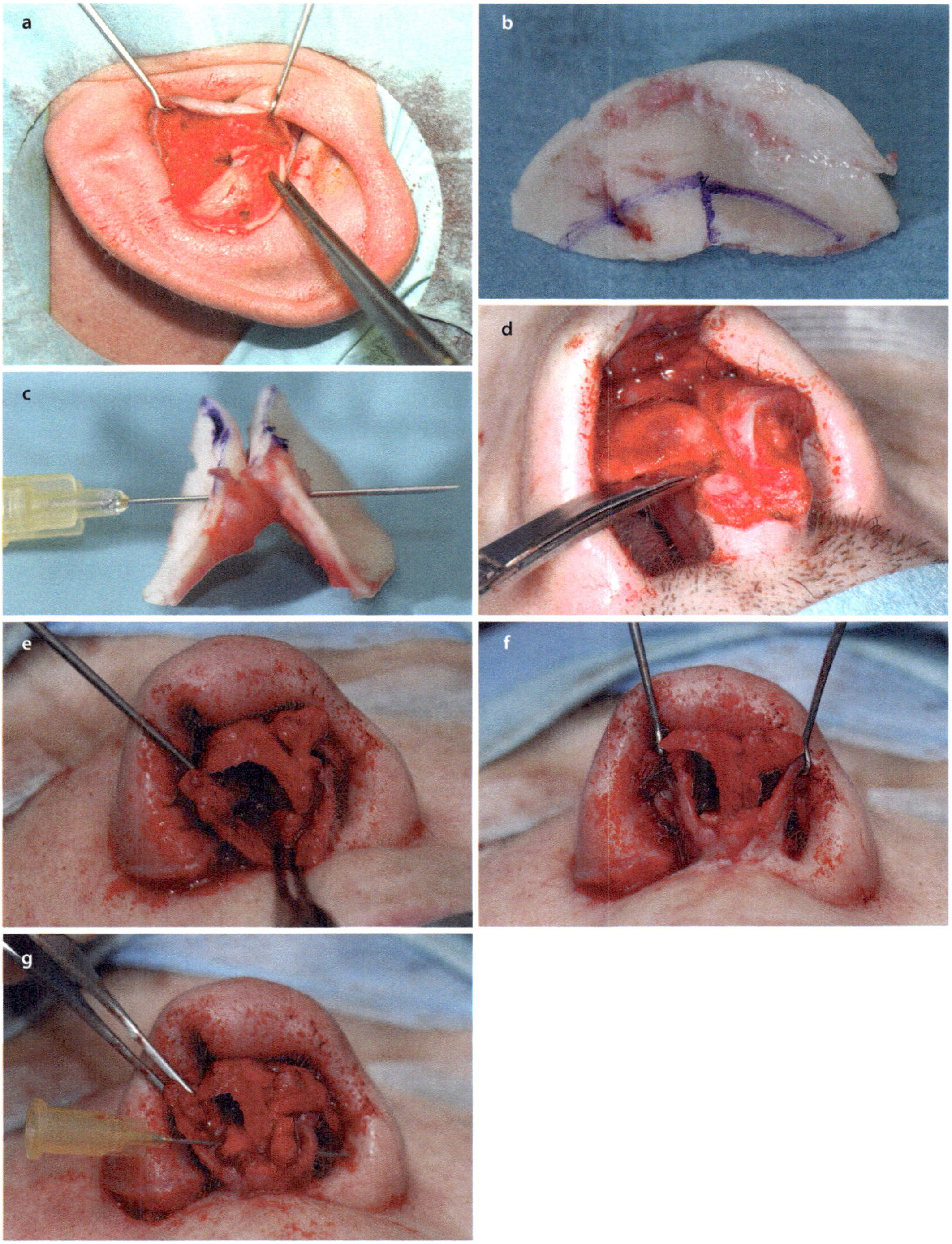

Fig. 10.24 **a–c** The use of split conchal graft and reshaping for nasal sil reconstruction. **d–g** The surgical sequence of using the split conchal cartilage for nasal sil reconstruction

- If necessary, the splayed wider segment in the sil region can be anchored on either side of the anterior nasal spine, thus recreating and reconstructing the sil region and also supporting the columella and increasing the length of the columella.

10.11.5 Surgical Sequence

Before deciding this technique consider alternatives like septal extension grafts, columellar struts, medial crural fixation and flare control sutures to gain columellar height and tip support and projection.

> **Key Points**
> Although this technique creates a smooth natural concave sil, the patient should be counselled that there will be an increase in width of the nasal columella due to the addition of extra pieces of cartilage. The added width of the cartilage in the columellar region may cause narrowing in the external nasal valve region with functional airway issues.

> **Conclusion**
> These are rare techniques which will help you in selected patients and not to be used as a routine, as there are viable alternatives as mentioned above.

10.12 Parenthesis Tip

10.12.1 Introduction

Parenthesis tip is a term given to a particular appearance of the tip when viewed from the frontal view, resembling the symbol of parenthesis like a double bracket {} as seen in the frontal view in the ◘ Fig. 10.25c. The origin is from Greek literature. This is usually due to a cephalic malposition or cephalic migration of the lateral crus. Normally the direction of the lateral crus points towards the lateral canthus of the eye (◘ Fig. 10.25a). On the other hand, if it points more medially towards the medial canthus, it is referred to as cephalic malpositioning of the lateral crus and is first described by Jack Sheen [26]. Due to a cephalic tilt in the lateral crus, it can cause an unnatural bulge higher up at the lateral aspect of the tip, almost causing a vertical bracket-shaped appearance to the tip, hence the term parenthesis. There is usually a "thumb-impression" of the lateral border of the lateral crus in the three-fourth view and more obvious if the skin is thin (◘ Fig. 10.25d). The mere presence of the cephalic migration does not mean that the tip is not aesthetically pleasing and need surgery. In fact they are common in certain ethnic populations in the Middle East and also in certain states in northern western India, like Maharashtra (anecdotal evidence). Cephalic malposition of the lower lateral cartilage (CMLLC) can result in not pleasing vertically placed lateral alar creases, wide boxy nasal tip, under rotated tip and external lateral alar weakness due to the cephalic migration of lateral crus from the usual position. Mohebbi describes three types of parenthesis tip, with bulbosity, with alar retraction and with alar collapse [27].

10.12.2 Indications for Parenthesis Tip Surgery

- Cephalic, vertical and medial migration of the caudal border of lateral crus as seen on the left side in ◘ Fig. 10.25d.
- Usually caused by trauma or revision surgery.
- Structural deformity of the nasal tip with a boxy de-projected, under rotated tip.
- Associated with functional alar weakness in the lateral alar region.
- Parenthesis tip is usually associated with under projection (◘ Fig. 10.25b). But rotation can vary usually under rotated, particularly if there is a traumatic damage to the tip.
- The length of the nose is related to the degree of under rotation.
- Parenthesis tip can be familial, particularly in patients from certain north western states of the Indian Sub-continent.

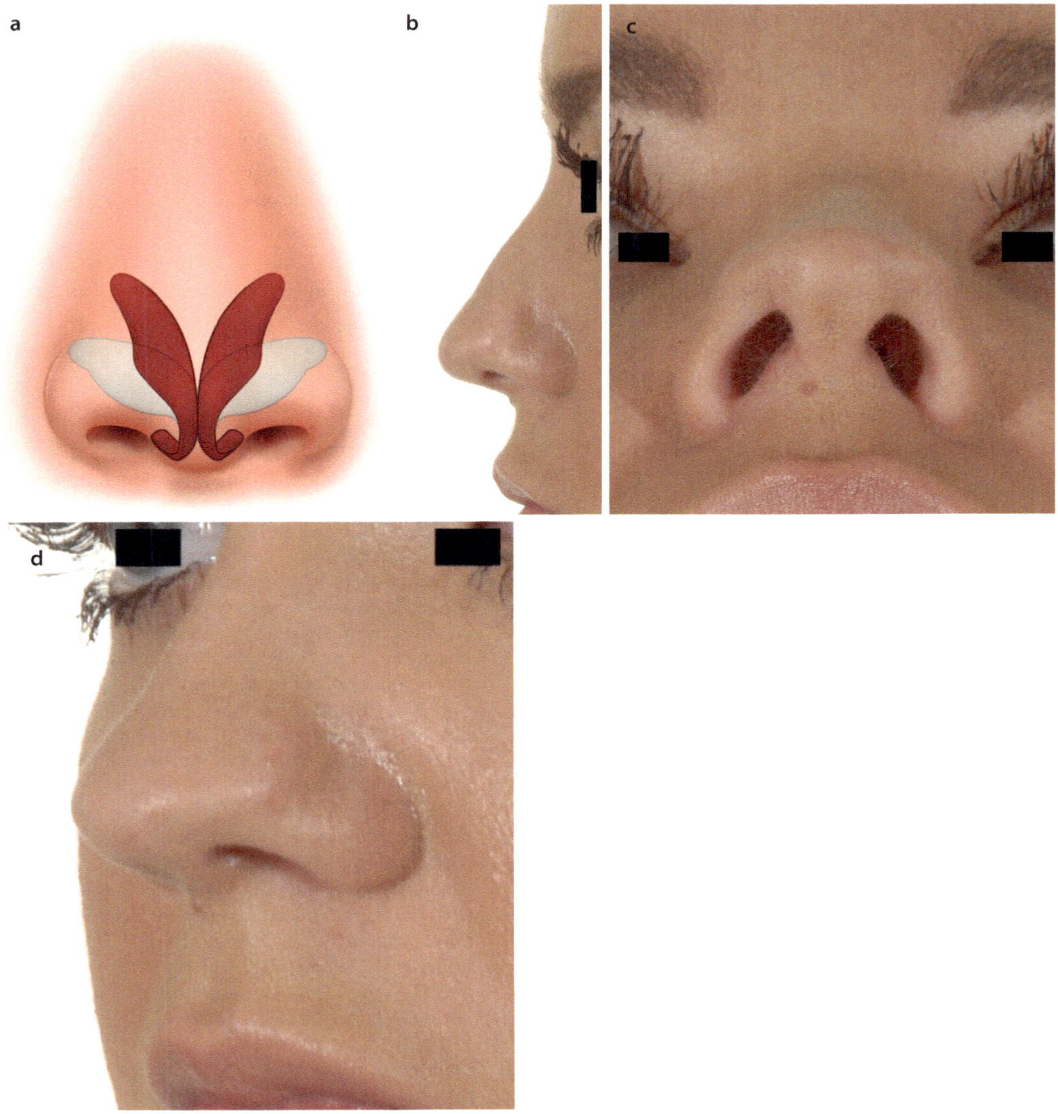

Fig. 10.25 **a** Schematic representation of nasal tip lower lateral cartilage showing the shaded area of the lateral crus pointing medially towards the medial canthus of the eye in a "parenthesis tip", instead of pointing laterally towards the lateral canthus of the eye. **b–d** Parenthesis tip. **b** Lateral view. **c** Frontal/basal view. **d** Lateral three-fourth view

10.12.3 Surgical Technique

- In the right patient with cephalic migration of the lateral crus associated with structural and functional deformity, it is best to do an open approach, as it is helpful to diagnose the problem and confirm the diagnosis as well.
- The lateral crus strength, length and width are assessed.
- No cephalic trim is performed.
- The lateral crus is elevated from the underlying mucosa completely till the tip and lifted out and down towards the alar margin.
- If the strength of the lateral crus is adequate with adequate width, then the elevated lateral crus is re-secured at a lower level by passing a 5-0 vicryl through and through sutures including the alar mucosa.

- If the strength of the lateral crus is poor, then the relocation is done along with a lateral crural strut graft (Gunter graft) harvested from the septal cartilage [28]. There are issues with adding a strut graft as there can be an additional bulge laterally [29].
- There are techniques described by Turkish surgeons without the need for strut grafts [27].
- Sometimes a low butterfly-like spreader graft might be needed near the tip to keep the lateral crus not to move back to the midline again. But all these add to the rigidity of the tip with extra graft material being needed.

10.12.4 Surgical Sequence

Usually done after dorsal and septal work and lateral crural work done last.

Key Points

Parenthesis tip can be familial.

- Accurate diagnosis is important.
- Only functional alar weakness with cephalic migration need to be addressed by surgery. Structural issues alone may not need correction.

Conclusion

Cephalic malposition should be thought of when patients present with alar weakness, although quite rare. It is usually secondary to revision surgery following over resection with scar tissue pulling the lateral crus up and medially. The diagnosis can easily be overlooked.

Key Points Box

- Apart from sutures and grafts, there are non-suture and non-grafting techniques available to achieve alterations in the tip definition, projection and rotation.
- Trimming the cephalic portion of the lateral crus is the commonest non-suture and non-grafting technique performed in nasal tip surgery.
- Although I have grouped them together as "non-suture techniques" and "non-grafting techniques", they are not stand-alone techniques and invariably used in conjunction with suture and grafting techniques to achieve the desirable outcomes.
- Sutures do offer additional secondary support and are indispensable in most techniques.

References

1. Sil A, Ravichandran S, Balaji N. Non- suture techniques in posttraumatic nasal tip reconstruction. ENT Audiol News. 2010;19(2):109–12.
2. Balaji N. Non-suture techniques in nasal tip reconstruction. Rom J Rhinol. 2014;4(13):37–44.
3. White PS, Ross PD. Open structure rhinoplasty. 2nd ed. Tuttlingen, Germany: Endo Press GmbH; 2012.
4. Nagarkar P, Stark RY, Pezeshk RA, Amirlak B, Rohrich RJ. Role of the cephalic trim in modern rhinoplasty. Plast Reconstr Surg. 2016;137(1):89–96.
5. Gruber RP, Weintraub J, Pomerantz J. Suture techniques for the nasal tip. Aesthet Surg J. 2008;28(1):92–100.
6. Rohrich RJ, Deuber MA. Nasal tip refinement in primary rhinoplasty: the cephalic trim cap graft. Aesthet Surg J. 2002;22(1):39–45.
7. Kridel RWH, Konior RJ. Controlled nasal tip rotation via the lateral crural overlay technique. Arch Otolaryngol Head Neck Surg. 1991;117:411–5.
8. Foda HM, Kridel RW. Lateral crural steal and lateral crural overlay: an objective evaluation. Arch Otolaryngol Head Neck Surg. 1999;125(12):1365–70.
9. Okhovat S, Balaji N. An algorithm for the management of lateral crural pathology. J ENT Master Class. 2018;11(1):45–53.
10. Foda HM. Management of the droopy tip: a comparison of three alar cartilage-modifying techniques. Plast Reconstr Surg. 2003;112(5):1408–17.
11. Kridel RW, Konior RJ, Shumrick KA, Wright WK. Advances in nasal tip surgery. The lateral crural steal. Arch Otolaryngol Head Neck Surg. 1989;115(10):1206–12.
12. Goldman IB. Surgical tips on the nasal tip. Eye Ear Nose Throat Mon. 1954;33:583–91.
13. Goldman IB. The importance of the mesial crura in nasal-tip reconstruction. Arch Otolaryngol. 1957;65:143–7.
14. Simons RL. Vertical dome division in rhinoplasty. Otolaryngol Clin North Am. 1987;20:785–96.
15. Chang CWD, Simons RL. Hockey-stick vertical dome division technique for overprojected and broad nasal tips. Arch Facial Plast Surg. 2008;10(2):88–92.

16. Ghidini A, Dallari S, Marchioni D. Surgery of the nasal columella in external valve collapse. Ann Otol Rhinol Laryngol. 2002;111(8):701–3.
17. Apaydin F. Lateral crural turn-in flap in functional rhinoplasty. Arch Facial Plast Surg. 2012;14(2):93–6.
18. Balaji N, Ravichandran S. Assessment of nasal valve obstruction : a new Glasgow nasal "wall" subunit concept. ENT Audiol News. 2012;21(5):86–7.
19. Gruber RP. Primary open rhinoplasty. In: Gruber RP, Peck GC, editors. Rhinoplasty: state of the art. St Louis: Mosby Year Book; 1993. p. 61–88.
20. Kuran I, Öreroğlu AR, Efendioğlu K. The lateral crural rein flap: a novel technique for management of tip rotation in primary rhinoplasty. Aesthet Surg J. 2014;347:1008–17.
21. Ozucer B, Ozturan O. Comments on "the lateral crural rein flap: a novel technique for management of tip rotation in primary rhinoplasty". Aesthet Surg J. 2015;355:NP125.
22. Bertossi D, Walter C, Nocini PF. The pull-up spreader high (PUSH) technique for nasal tip support. Aesthet Surg J. 2014;348:1153–61.
23. Bohluli B, Varedi P, Nazari S, Bagheri SC. Lateral crural suspension flap: a novel technique to modify and stabilize the nasolabial angle. J Oral Maxillofac Surg. 2013;719:1572–6.
24. Guyuron B, Varghai A. Lengthening the nose with a tongue-and-groove technique. Plast Reconstr Surg. 2003;111:1533–9.
25. Kridel RWH, Scott BA, Foda HMT. The tongue-in-groove technique in septorhinoplasty:a ten year experience. Arch Facial Plast Surg. 1999;1: 246–56.
26. Sheen JH. Aesthetic rhinoplasty. St Louis: CV Mosby; 1978. p. 264–5.
27. Mohebbi A, Azizi A, Tabatabaiee S. Repositioned lateral crural flap technique for cephalic malposition in rhinoplasty. Plast Surg (Oakv). 2015;23(3):183–8.
28. Toriumi DM, Asher SA. Lateral crural repositioning for treatment of cephalic malposition. Facial Plast Surg Clin North Am. 2015;23(1):55–71.
29. Ilhan AE, Saribas B, Caypinar B. Aesthetic and functional results of lateral crural repositioning. JAMA Facial Plast Surg. 2015;17(4):286–92.

Management of Nasal Septum: A "Step-Ladder" Approach

Contents

N. Balaji, *Textbook of Nasal Tip Rhinoplasty*, https://doi.org/10.1007/978-3-030-48157-5_11

Learning Objectives

- To learn the surgical principles in correcting a septal deformity.
- To learn the various ways of optimising the results of septoplasty.
- To learn grafting techniques to strengthen dorsal and caudal septum.
- To learn the stepladder approach of various surgical techniques available to straighten and reconstruct the septal cartilage.

11.1 Introduction

Correcting the nasal septal deformity is the key for a successful nasal tip rhinoplasty. It is akin to fixing the central pole before pitching a tent. Septum is made up of anterior cartilaginous portion and a posterior bony portion, made of ethmoid and vomer. Posterior superior ethmoid bone is thinner and straighter than the vomer and hence most used for bone grafts. The size, shape and position of the caudal septum determine the rotation and projection of the nasal tip. Secondary tip deformities are usually due to caudal septal issues and the sequence is to address the septum first before doing the tip work. The mid and posterior dorsal septum determines the dorsal profile line support and lack of this also can cause a mid-dorsal de-projection with upward rotation of the tip. Apart from the commonly performed septoplasty surgery, there are various other techniques available to straighten and support a damaged septum. We will start with the basics of septoplasty and go through various other techniques available to reconstruct the nasal septum and arrive at a "step-ladder" approach to the septal reconstruction.

11.2 Septoplasty

Septoplasty is the most common valve surgery performed to improve the nasal airway, by straightening the cartilaginous and bony septum. Deviations of the caudal septal cartilage are more difficult to correct than bony septal deviations [1, 2]. It is important to understand that septoplasty is also a key procedure to establish the structural integrity and position of the nasal tip. Septal surgery owes its beginnings to sub-mucous resection (SMR) described by Killian and Freer. SMR surgery is more radical involving elevating the muco-perichondrial layers on both sides, and excising the bent cartilage and closing the flap, leaving behind enough cartilage dorsally and caudally to support the nose. Septoplasty surgery, compared to SMR, is a conservative technique which involves straightening the septum with maximum preservation of the septal cartilage, with minimal excision.

Septal surgery is done either through an internal approach or an external approach.

An internal approach involves a hemitransfixation incision made at the caudal end of the septum (Freer's incision), usually on the side of maximum deviation as there is a scope to trim the redundant mucosa. If there is a gross caudal deviation, it is better to do the incision on the side of the dislocation for the same reason. The muco-perichondrial flaps are elevated on one or both sides of the septal cartilage. Raising the septal flaps on both sides does not affect the viability of the septal flaps nor does it increase the risk of septal haematoma. Once the septal flaps are raised and protected with nasal speculums, the ventral boat-shaped 3–4 mm wedge of septal cartilage sitting on the maxillary crest is removed after dislocating from the maxillary crest. This removed piece can be used for dorsal augmentation to smoothen the dorsal irregularities after a hump reduction. The caudal posterior septal angle is released from the nasal spine but not excised, preserving the height of the caudal septum. This can be re-secured back in the midline if needed. The next step would be to do a posterior chondrotomy to release the bony cartilaginous junction, which will further help in the mobilisation of the septum to the midline, the so called "swinging-door" technique described by Metzenbaum [3]. Becker described a "doorstop" technique where the ventral segment of the septal cartilage is dislocated and flipped to the side of the nasal spine opposite to the deviation and secured to the

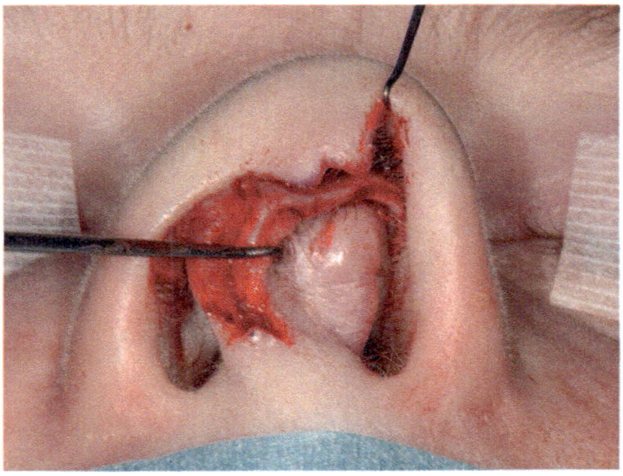

Fig. 11.1 Moderate caudal septal deviation to the left side

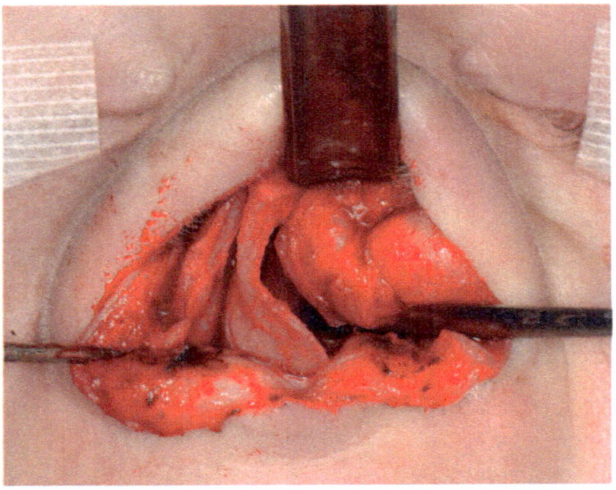

Fig. 11.2 Open approach showing "L"-shaped deviation of the cartilaginous nasal septum

spine, thus preserving cartilage [4]. Although many techniques have been described for correcting septal deformities, septoplasty is still a complex surgery (Figs. 11.1, 11.2, and 11.3) to get it right as it needs to be tailored to each patient individually depending on the anatomical findings. Individual septal cartilage fractures may need to be excised locally and stabilised. Once the caudal septum is centralised, it is best to suture the caudal septum to the anterior nasal spine region in the midline.

The following are some of the ancillary procedures which help to straighten the caudal septum and improve the outcomes in septal surgery.

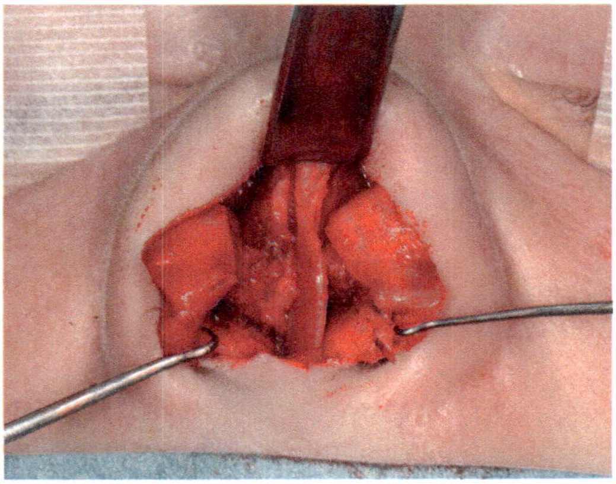

Fig. 11.3 Open approach showing septal repositioning in the midline

11.3 Suturing to Anterior Nasal Spine

To give stability to the caudal septum, it is advisable to secure the caudal septum to the anterior nasal spine with 5'o ethilon sutures or PDS. Once the caudal septum is medialised and in the correct position, then a decision is made to suture it to the anterior nasal spine, if there is a possibility of re displacement of the caudal septum. Suturing to the anterior nasal spine depends on the anatomy of the spine, which need not be a sharp projection, but have a wider base. The suture can go through the nasal spine horizontally if it is thin and sharp, and may need to make a hole in the bone with a small fissure burr. But if the spine is flat and wide, it is best to go vertically through the periosteum covering the spine (Fig. 11.4a–c).

If the suture has to go through the septal mucosa as well, then it is preferable to use PDS or vicryl (Fig. 11.5a–c).

11.4 Suturing to Mucosal Flaps for Stability

Sometimes the caudal septum can be secured to the septal mucosa temporarily just for support till the rest of the septal work is completed (Fig. 11.6a–c).

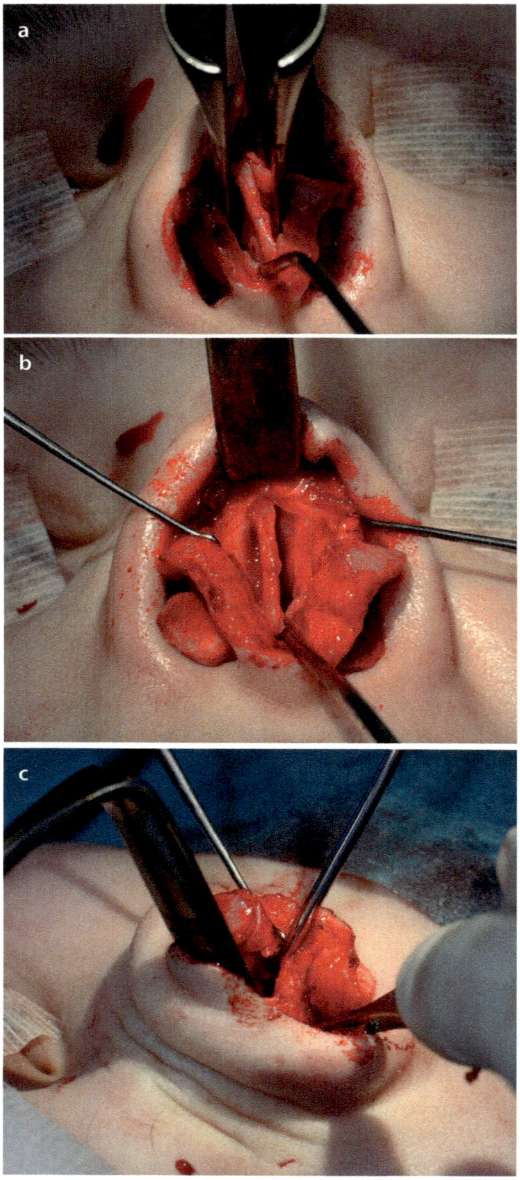

Fig. 11.4 a–c Suturing of the caudal septal cartilage to the anterior nasal spine

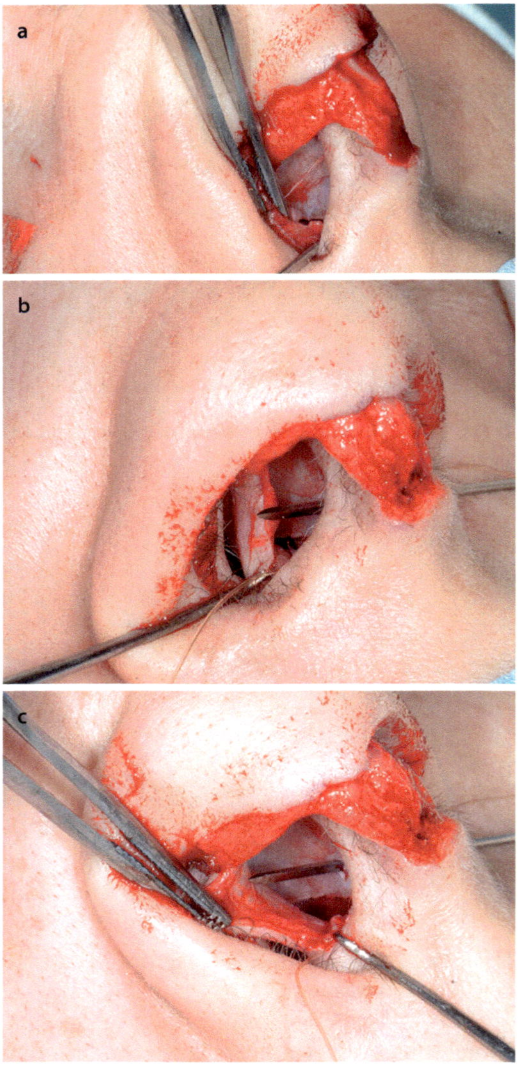

Fig. 11.5 a–c Anterior nasal spine suture going through the septal mucosa for additional stability

11.5 Caudal Septal Shave with or Without Soft Tissue Columelloplasty

Caudal septal shave and columelloplasty is done through hemi-transfixation incision as part of the septal surgery to correct the septal deviation. Sometimes septoplasty alone may not be able to straighten the caudal septum. This could be because of excess length and width of the septal cartilage, either traumatic or genetic trying to push the septum out of the columellar pocket as seen in severe long-standing caudal dislocations. In these situations, a good septoplasty may have to be combined with a caudal septal shave to reduce the anterior-posterior length of the septal cartilage. By reducing the length of the septum, it helps to "fit in" the columellar pocket better. This is also an effective technique to achieve a degree of de-projection of the nasal tip and shorten the length of the nose. Clinically it is usually

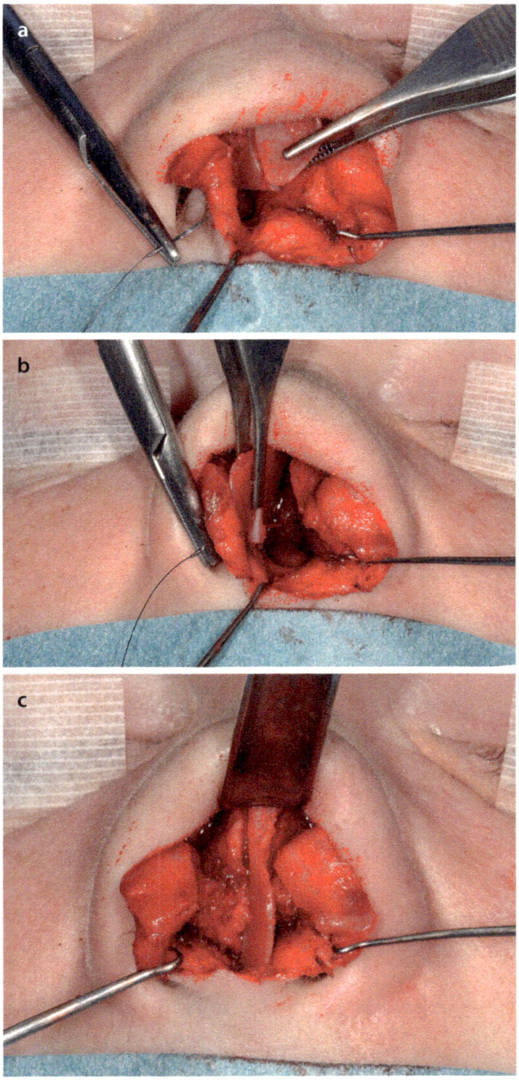

◘ **Fig. 11.6** a–c The straightened anterior septal cartilage stitched to the septal mucosa for stability

indicated in an over projected "tension nose" pulling on the upper lip and blunting the naso-labial angle. The aetiology of an over projected tension nose with blunting of the naso-labial angle is due to excess caudal septal cartilage at the spine region in about 85% of our patients. A smaller percentage is due to excess anterior bony nasal spine. This technique of caudal septal shave (◘ Fig. 11.7a–d) is an easier way of achieving small de-projection of the nasal tip in most patients with an excess caudal septum without affecting rotation.

The technique of parallel caudal septal shave is also indicated in large ethnic noses with over projection of the dorsum and the tip complex due to excess dorsal and caudal septum. This is usually done in conjunction with dorsal hump reduction in a reduction rhinoplasty in large noses with increased dorsal length. In revision noses with infra tip blunting with increased projection of the tip due to lack of septal cartilage near the anterior septal angle, a caudal shave of the septum with a triangle based inferiorly may be indicated to counter balance the tip. Of course this caudal shave of septal cartilage should not be considered in an already short nose with over rotated tips or if tongue and groove advancement of medial crus is planned to control an over hanging columella. Care should be taken not to excise caudal septal cartilage, beyond a maximum of 4 mm. Generally a "rule of thumb" in nasal tip and rhinoplasty work is an upper limit of 4 mm excision, particularly applicable to caudal septum and lateral crural excisions.

11.6 There Are Three Types of Caudal Septal Shave Possible

1. A parallel shave (◘ Fig. 11.8) of between 2 and 4 mm extending from the anterior septal angle to the posterior septal angle de-projects the tip without introducing any variability in rotation.
2. A triangular caudal shave with the base at the posterior septal angle/anterior nasal spine region can de-project the tip and at the same time can marginally under rotate the tip (◘ Fig. 11.8b).
3. A triangular caudal shave with the base at the anterior septal angle de-projects the tip and over rotates the tip (◘ Fig.11.8c).

Thus, if a parallel caudal septal cartilage segment is excised, de-projection is achieved without rotation of the tip. If a caudal septal triangle is excised based ventrally, the tip can rotate downwards along with de-projection. If the caudal septal triangle is excised with

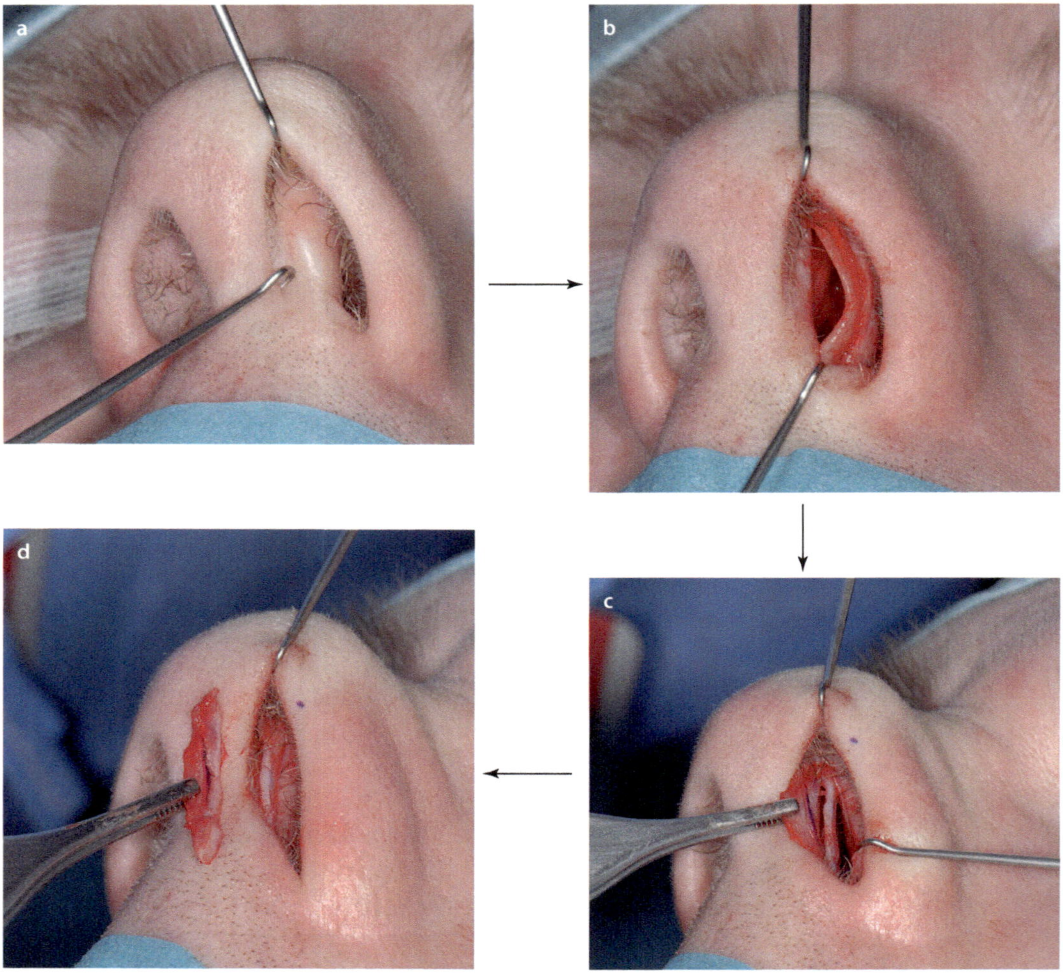

Fig. 11.7 **a–d** Caudal septal shave in a dislocated and over projected caudal septum. (Reproduced with permission from Refs. [5, 6])

the base of the triangle at the dorsal anterior septal angle, the tip will rotate upwards along with de-projection.

11.7 Soft Tissue Columelloplasty

This technique may be indicated to optimise the results of a good septoplasty, as an ancillary procedure. It is indicated in a long-standing columellar dislocation in an over projected nasal tip, stretching the septal mucosa and causing an excess on the side of the dislocation. Although this excess mucosa can settle down in most patients, in severe dislocations, if this excess mucosa is not trimmed, it can cause thickened columella narrowing the external nasal valve region. The excess septal mucosa is trimmed just enough and not to distort the columellar skin. The trimming of the septal mucosa on the dislocated side is usually done through the already made hemi-transfixation incision. It is trimmed as a smooth "D" shape, involving only the septal mucosa. Please make sure that the skin of the columella is not trimmed, as this will result in scarring and cause secondary tip deviation and tip distortion. Soft tissue mucosal trim-

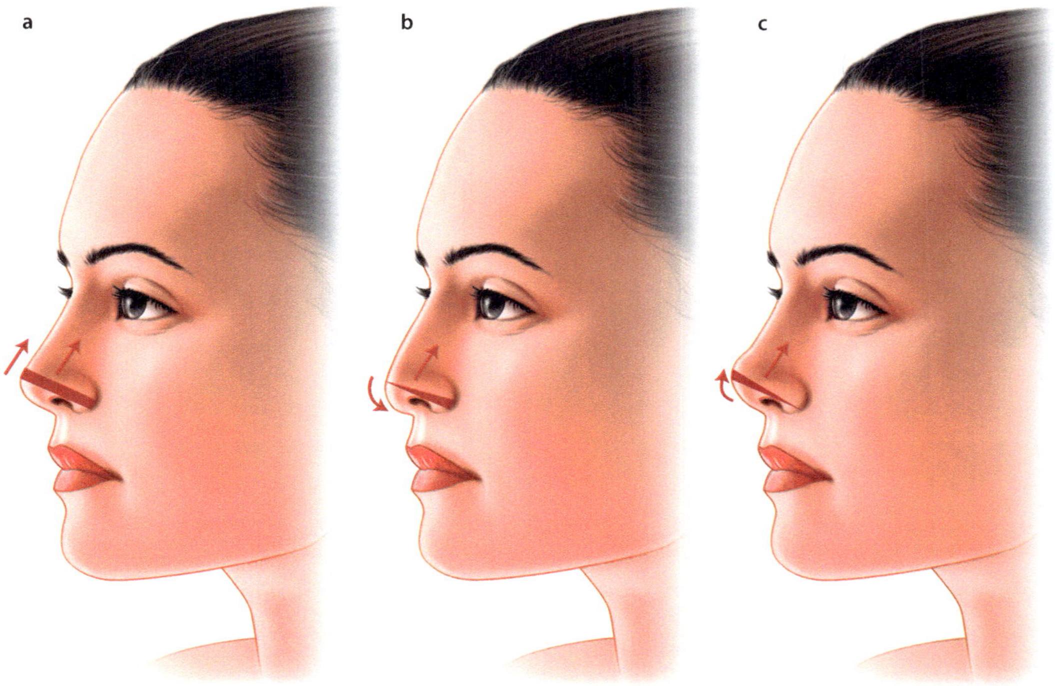

Fig. 11.8 **a–c** The effects of caudal septal shave. **a** A parallel shave causing de-projection. **b** A triangular caudal shave causing de-projection and under rotation. **c** A triangular caudal shave causing de-projection and over rotation of the tip

ming (Fig. 11.9a–d) should be done with extreme caution, again similar to cartilage excision doing it in small incremental steps. If a big piece of septal mucosa is excised, it will not be possible to close the hemi-transfixation incision without any distortion.

The key point while considering reduction of the caudal septal cartilage is "not to shave the caudal septum till the end of the operation", as you may sometimes have to consider a "tongue-in-groove" posterior advancement of the medial crura towards the caudal septum to de-project the nose. If the caudal septum is shaved early on in the procedure, it becomes difficult to move the medial crus towards the caudal septum without distorting the columella. If soft tissue columelloplasty is planned to take care not to excise the excess mucosa in one step, but instead a gradual stepwise excision is better, otherwise there will be tension on the suture line which may distort the tip.

11.8 Caudal Septal Struts

Caudal septal strut grafts [5, 6] can be harvested from the septal cartilage (Fig. 11.10a–c) leaving an "L" strut or shaped from costal cartilage and can be used to support and strengthen caudal septum and anchored with sutures either to the medial crus or to the existing posterior caudal septum. It can also be left free standing in a closed columellar pocket. Be aware, if it is secured to the medial crus it makes the tip rigid and looses the elastic recoil of the nasal tip.

11.9 Caudal Extension Grafts

Septal extension grafts, as the name suggests, is an extension to the existing caudal septal cartilage, securing the additional piece of graft to the existing caudal septal cartilage to extend and correct the length of the existing septum

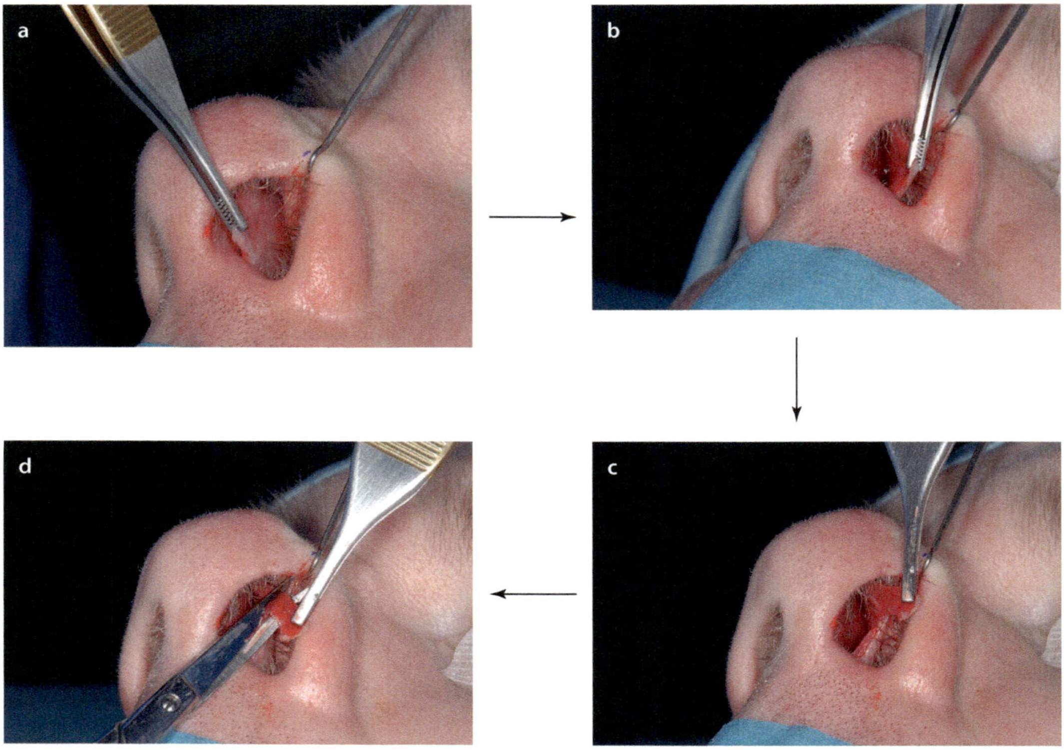

Fig. 11.9 **a–d** Soft tissue columelloplasty to reduce the columellar mucosa which has been stretched due to long-standing septal dislocation

(Fig. 11.11a–f). This can be used to correct both the vertical height and the horizontal length of the existing nasal septal cartilage. These are ideally indicated in a short, less projected caudal septum with columellar shortening causing a grossly retracted nasal tip, with a secondary over rotation of the tip. This procedure is done through open approach or through a hemi-transfixation incision. The graft is harvested either from the posterior part of the septal cartilage leaving an "L" strut or costal cartilage. The graft to be used should be straight and not more than 2–4 mm in thickness. Existing caudal septal dislocations and deviations should be corrected before any form of septal extension can be considered. The graft is secured to the posterior edge of the existing septum with figure of 8, pivot sutures to prevent vertical movements and to withstand torsion forces. The ends can also be overlapped if there is enough cartilage harvest. But this can cause thickening in the external nasal valve region. The medial crus can then be sutured to the new anterior caudal septal graft, thus creating a single tip complex.

11.10 "Tongue-in- Groove" Medial Crural Advancement

This is indicated when there is a prolapse of the medial crus with a columellar overhang. Before securing the medial crus to the caudal septum, make sure there is no volume loss of the caudal septum. Also make sure the caudal septum is absolutely straight in the midline. This technique (Fig. 11.12a–c) helps to support and hold the medial crus in a retro position [5, 6].

11.11 Septal Relocation

Sometimes the septum is freed all along the cartilaginous portion ventrally along the maxillary crest and partly dislocated along the posterior bony cartilaginous junction, leaving a small attachment at the mid "K" area. This can be combined with a separation of the dorsal septum from the upper lateral cartilages by a sharp incision,

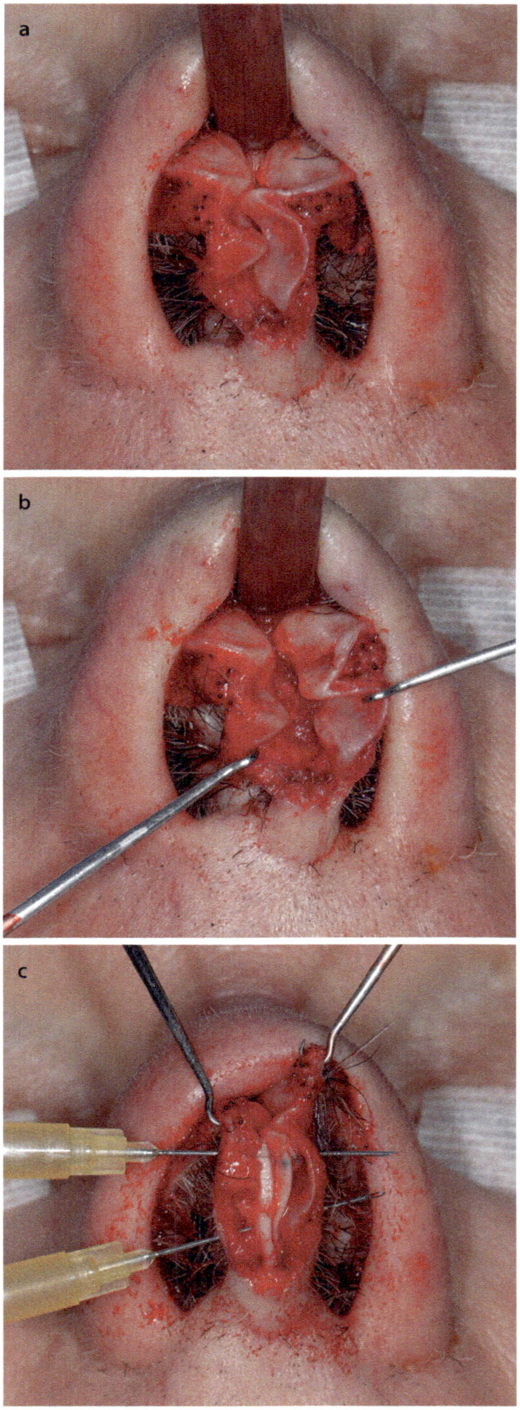

Fig. 11.10 **a–c** The effects of caudal septal Strut. **a** Complex deformity of medial crura. **b** Lack of medial crural support. **c** The role of septal strut to straighten and strengthen the damaged medial crus in the same patient

following which the septum can be relocated back to midline (Fig. 11.13a–c) [7], and sutured to the anterior nasal spine. Separating the upper lateral cartilage from the septum is also another effective technique to straighten a dorsal curvature of the septum and the lower two thirds of the nose. This is usually accompanied by a stabilising spreader grafts to secure the upper lateral cartilage back to the dorsal septum. The use of spreader grafts have been described in detail in ► Chap. 9.

11.12 Use of Non-autologous Material as a Framework

This is gaining more popularity recently with the use of synthetic 0.2 mm perforated or non-perforated PDS (polydiaxonone) sheets and acellular dermal matrix as a scaffold in patients with septal cartilages being in multiple pieces. As with any non-autologous materials, extreme caution is necessary in using them, as any complications such as infection can be difficult to rectify. Also patient's choice and local guidelines should dictate the use of these materials. We have not used these autologous materials on a regular basis apart from patient's own cartilage or fascia, but our advice would be to use this only if necessary and should not be used just to speed up the procedure or due to its ease of availability and reduced surgical time. Septal mucosal flaps should be intact on both sides before using these non-autologous materials, otherwise there is a risk of infection and extrusion. Usually perforated plates are used less than 0.2 mm in thickness so that there is tissue growth in between.

11.13 Extra-corporeal Septoplasty

This is basically a septoplasty performed outside the nose. First described by King and Ashley in 1952 [8]. It is a technique described to correct a very severely deviated septum

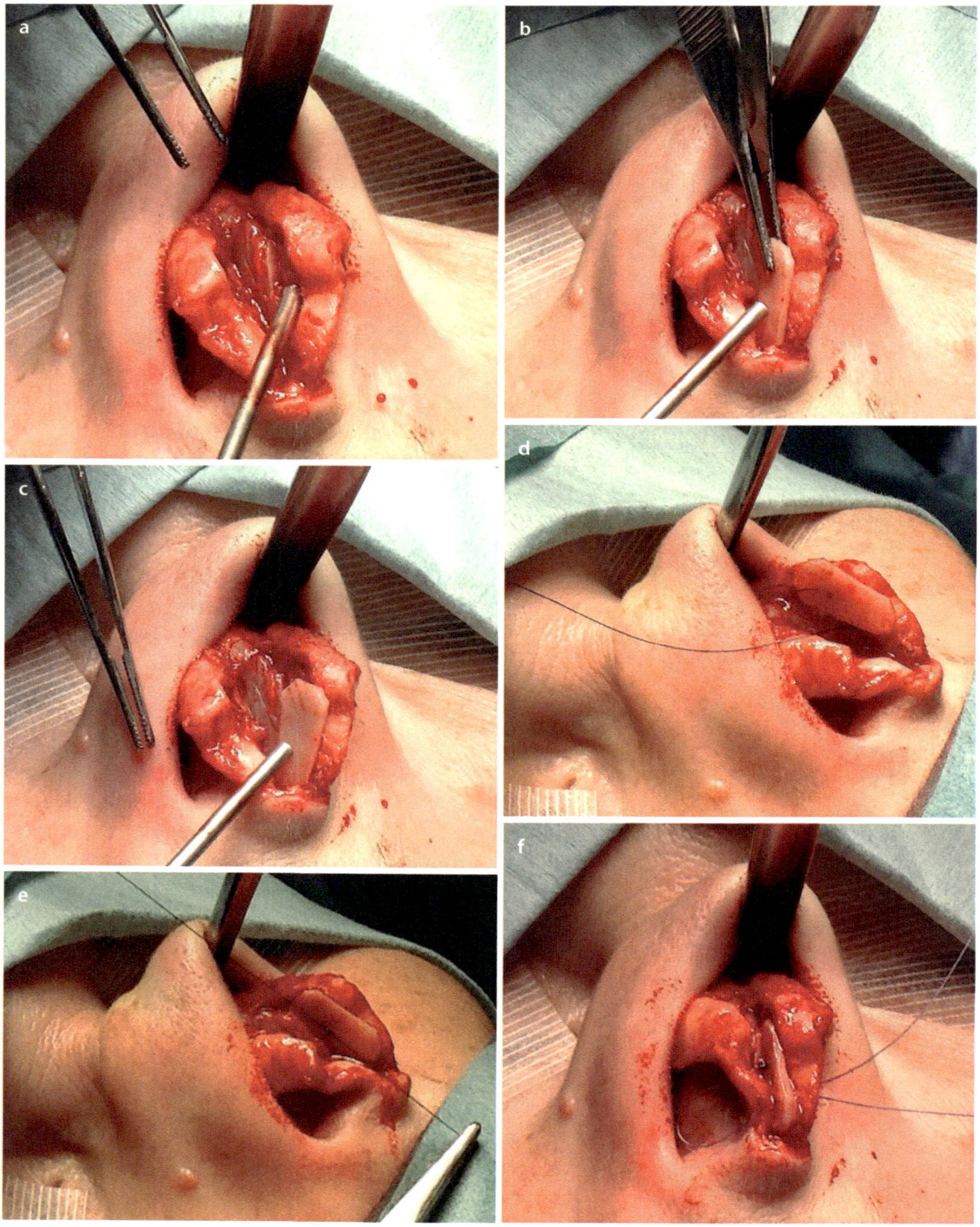

Fig. 11.11 **a–f** The placement of the caudal extension graft and being secured to the remains of the caudal septum

with multiple fractures and gross deformity. Usually performed through an open approach. Dissection is performed between the medial crus and muco-perichondrial flaps raised on both sides. Septum is freed all around. Freed septum is removed after separation from the ULC. The deformed septal cartilage is removed, reshaped either by excision, incision techniques or using non-absorbable sutures and re-inserted into the septal pocket "back

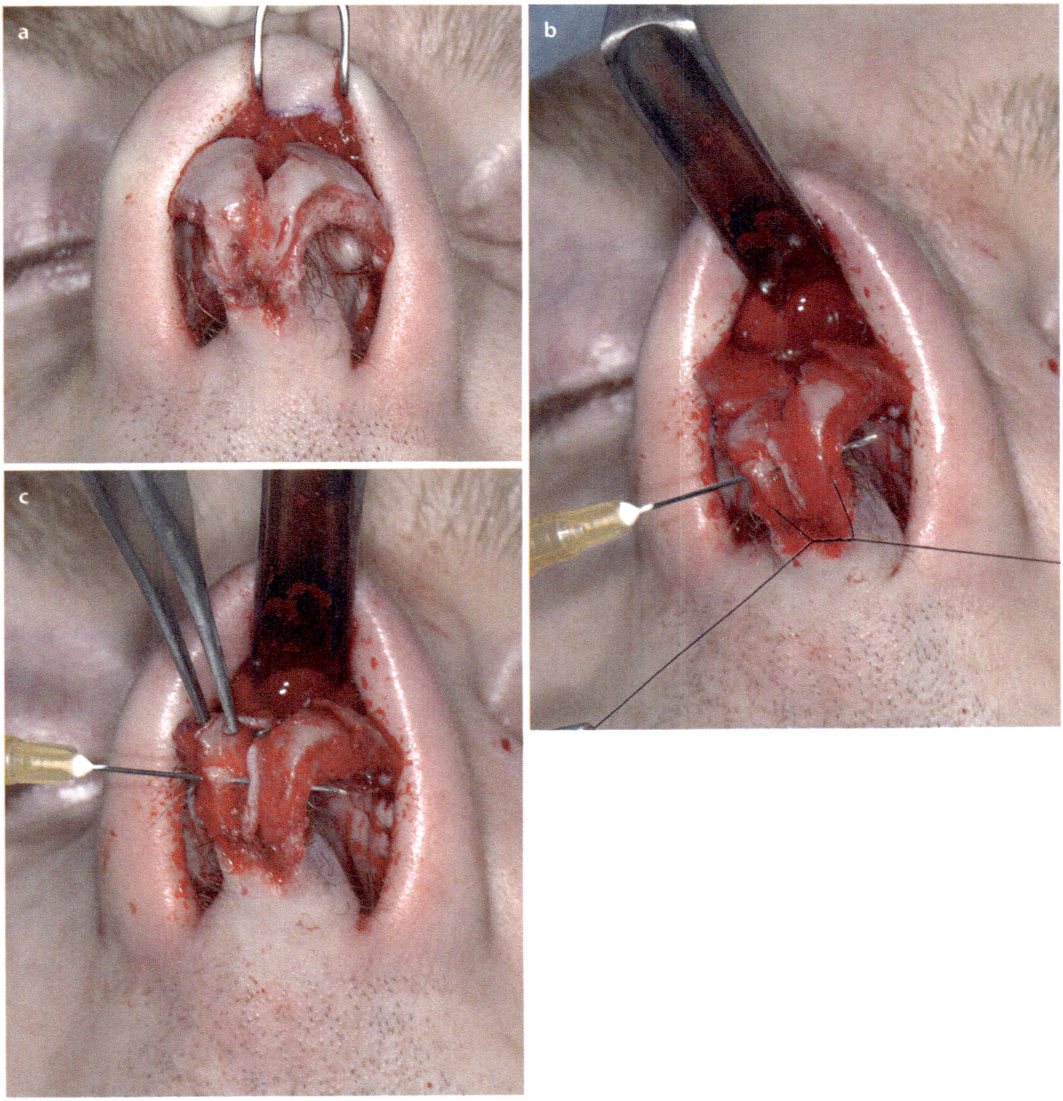

Fig. 11.12 **a–c** The technique of "tongue and groove" advancement of the medial crus on to the caudal septum

to front" as a free graft. This is based on the assumption that any gross nasal trauma would have spared the posterior septum which may still be straighter and can be used for the caudal region by securing it "back to front". This may not be the case all the time. The cartilage is re-sutured back into position, taking care to secure it to the upper laterals at the lateral Key stone area with 5 O′ ethilon sutures. This is the most difficult part of the procedure. The other area which can be difficult is "during the re-insertion" as the dimensions of the cephalic border of the septal cartilage are taller vertically when compared to the entrance of the open approach incision. The re-inserted cartilage would also need to be secured to the anterior nasal spine with non-absorbable sutures [9]. If the septum is not secured dorsally to the ULC and "K" area properly, this can lead to dorsal saddling over the mid dorsum. Dr. Most suggests a modification of preserving the dorsal segment of cartilage and suturing the implanted cartilage back to the left behind dorsal septum [10]. But often this does not

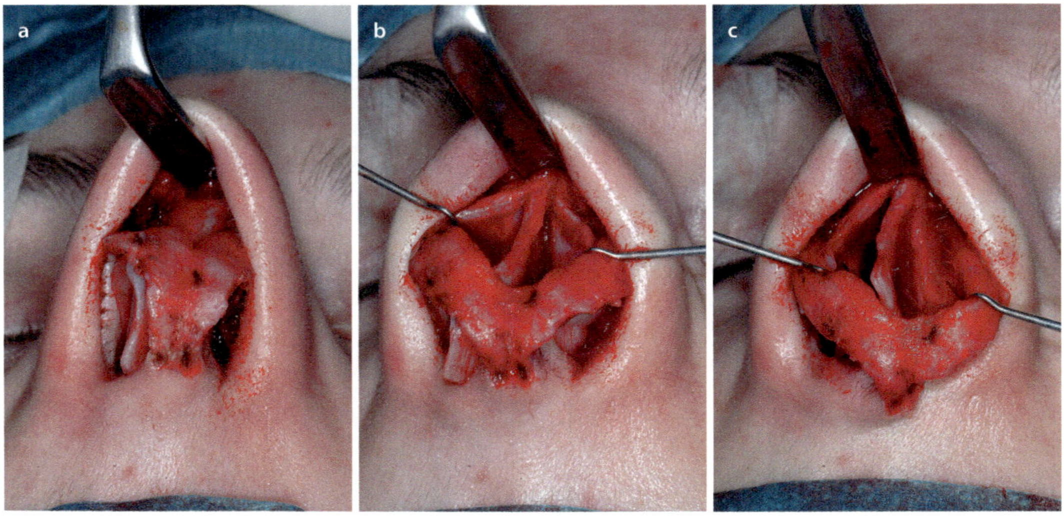

Fig. 11.13 **a–c** The technique of septal relocation. **a** Gross septal dislocation to the right side. **b** The separation of upper laterals from the dorsal septum. **c** The septum relocated to midline following ventral release. (Reproduced with permission from Refs. [5, 6])

apply to our practice, as most of our patients have trauma to the dorsal septal cartilage.

Indications

- Severe deviation of the septal cartilage (Fig. 11.14) with multiple fractures (Fig. 11.14d) and scarring involving predominantly the caudal septum
- Anterior septum lying in the coronal plane
- Complex Cleft lip rhinoplasty
- Complex high dorsal septal deviations
- Recurrent and residual septal deformities in complex revisions

This is a difficult surgery and needs adequate training. Removal of septum without damaging the overlying muco-perichondrial flaps in a severely damaged septal cartilage can be challenging and time consuming. Re-insertion of septal cartilage can be difficult. There could be difficulties in securing the cartilage back to upper lateral cartilages. Sometimes it needs additional support for the columellar region in the form of columellar strut to prevent tip ptosis and dorsal spreader grafts to support the dorsum structurally and to support the internal nasal valve. At the end of the procedure, it is always advisable to put crushed cartilage in the mid dorsum to avoid any postoperative depression at the anchored site and also a shield graft to reconstruct the infra tip lobule segment of the tip.

11.14 Septal Reconstructive Step-Ladder

Thus, apart from septoplasty, there are various ways the septum can be strengthened and medialised. All these steps need not be used in all patients, but may have to be considered and techniques tailored to individual needs with a stepladder approach. The following "step-ladder" approach from one to eight is a useful tool in septal reconstruction.

1. Septoplasty steps including anchoring to the anterior nasal spine
2. Caudal septal cartilage shave, with or without soft tissue columelloplasty
3. Septal resection
4. Septal repositioning
5. Separation of upper laterals from the dorsal septum with dorsal spreader grafts
6. Additional columellar strut
7. Septal extension grafts, dorsal and caudal
8. Finally, extra-corporeal septoplasty

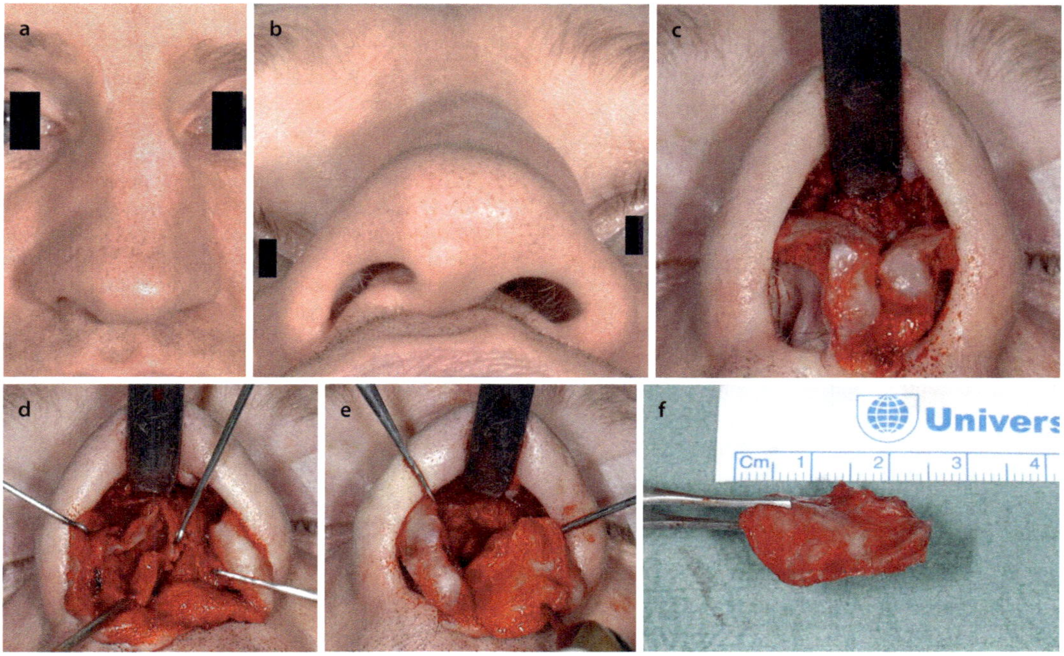

Fig. 11.14 **a–f** The technique of extra-corporeal septoplasty. **a** Frontal view showing gross mid dorsal septal collapse. **b** Basal view showing a collapsed tip. **c** Open approach. **d** Extensive damage to the septal cartilage. **e** Removal of the damaged septum. **f** The removed damaged septal cartilage

Conclusion

Getting the septum "right" is the basis of all rhinoplasty, more so in tip work to achieve long-term stability and can be very difficult to master. Septoplasty is often first taught in the training programme but often last to master. It is advisable to have a mental algorithm, to correct various septal deformities and have a mental step ladder. Should one of them fail to achieve the desired effect, you should have some other technique "up the sleeve" to achieve the desired effects.

Often first in the algorithm is the presence or absence (volume) of the septal cartilage. If it is intact centrally, dorsally and caudally, but damaged due to simple or complex trauma, fracture deviations and dislocations, then it will be worthwhile to start with septoplasty, fracture excision of the segment, relocation, suturing to the anterior nasal spine, cartilage scoring and if worse extra-corporeal septoplasty.

The next scenario being volume loss due to missing septal cartilage either due to trauma or previous resection. This can be central, dorsal or caudal. This will need extra-cartilage to reconstruct in the form of grafts, either spreader or dorsal extension grafts for the dorsum and caudal extension grafts for the columellar region and tip support. But of course, there could be complex deformities involving fractures of septum with volume loss which would require various combinations of reconstructive methods as mentioned above.

Key Points Box

- Septoplasty is the commonly performed nasal valve surgery. Septal correction can be complex particularly in early childhood trauma.
- Correcting nasal septal deformities is the "key" for a successful nasal tip sur-

gery, particularly caudal septum. The height, strength and location of the caudal septum are essential for tip support.

- Be aware that caudal shave of septal cartilage should not be considered in an already short nose with over rotated tips or If tongue and groove advancement of medial crus is planned to control an over hanging columella.
- Generally a "rule of thumb" in septal work and tip work is not to excise cartilage more than 4 mm, and if necessary re-use the segments as a crushed piece.
- Caudal septal shave should never be more than 4 mm as a "rule of thumb" and can be used to decrease projection and alter rotation if necessary.
- Soft tissue columelloplasty should be done in small increments.
- Be aware, that any technique to secure the caudal septum to the medial crus will make the tip rigid and this should be discussed with patients before surgery. Sometimes structure and function cannot be balanced particularly in a traumatic nose.
- One should have a mental algorithm of various techniques to correct the septal deformity, and use them as a "step-ladder" willing to move up one step if one technique does not suffice.

References

1. Guyuron B, Behmand RA. Caudal nasal deviation. Plast Reconstr Surg. 2003;111(7):2449–57.
2. Rohrich RJ, Gunter JP, Deuber MA, Adams WP Jr. The deviated nose: optimizing results using a simplified classification and algorithmic approach. Plast Reconstr Surg. 2002;110(6):1509–23.
3. Metzenbaum M. Replacement of the lower end of the dislocated septal cartilage versus sub mucous resection of the dislocated end of the septal cartilage. Arch Otolaryngol. 1929;9:282–96.
4. Pastorek NJ, Becker DG. Treating the caudal septal deflection. Arch Facial Plast Surg. 2000;2:217–20.
5. Balaji N. Non-suture techniques in nasal tip reconstruction. Rom J Rhinol. 2014;4(13):37–44.
6. Sil A, Ravichandran S, Balaji N. Non- suture techniques in posttraumatic nasal tip reconstruction. ENT Audiol News. 2010;19(2):109–11.
7. Balaji N. Top tips in nasal tip surgery, ENT-FPS UK Newsletter— Feb 2018 –Issue 6.
8. King ED, Ashley FL. The correction of the internally and externally deviated nose. Plast Reconstr Surg. 1952;10:116.
9. Gubisch W. Extracorporeal septoplasty for the markedly deviated septum. Arch Facial Plast Surg. 2005;7:218–26.
10. Most S. Anterior septal reconstruction: outcomes after a modified extracorporeal septoplasty technique. Arch Facial Plast Surg. 2006;8:202–7.

Controlling the Nasal Dorsum

Contents

N. Balaji, *Textbook of Nasal Tip Rhinoplasty*, https://doi.org/10.1007/978-3-030-48157-5_12

Learning Objectives
- To understand the various osteotomy techniques available to control the nasal dorsum.
- To understand the pros and cons of different dorsal reduction techniques.
- To understand the pathogenesis and management of mid dorsal de-projection.
- To learn the principles of managing the nasion and pseudo-humps.

12.1 Nasal Osteotomies

12.1.1 Introduction

Nasal osteotomies as the name suggests involves fracturing (osteotomy) the nasal bones and the frontal process of maxilla to achieve desirable effects to re-establish the nasal dorsum profile line and dorsal projection and symmetry. Osteotomies are helpful in realigning the nose, by dis-impacting the bones from each side and securing them in the midline position. Additionally, they can help to narrow the width of the nasal bony nasal base and hence achieve an increase in dorsal projection. They are also used in closing an "open" roof dorsum after hump removal. The following are the indications for an osteotomy.

12.1.2 Indications

- To correct a deviated nose or a crooked nose deformity [1, 2].
- To close an "open" roof after a bony dorsal hump reduction.
- To reduce the width of bony nasal base and thereby also marginally increase the dorsal projection of the nose.
- To correct an asymmetric thickened and wide lateral bulge in the nasal bones.

12.1.3 Surgical Approach

Osteotomies can be performed either through an external "open" approach using a 2 mm osteotome or through an internal approach using a guarded Joseph's osteotome [3].

It is individual surgeon's preference which method to use. Internal osteotomies are indicated in patients who are not keen on an outside scar, although very hardly noticeable. For internal lateral osteotomies, the osteotome is engaged in the lateral wall of the nose through a small stab incision just lateral and above the anterior attachment of inferior turbinate and using a guarded osteotome the lateral frontal process of the maxilla is osteotomised from "low" in the face to "high" in the nose near the medial canthus [4].

Internal osteotomies have the following disadvantages:

- They can cause potential damage to the underlying mucosa resulting in excess bleeding and long-term scarring at the external valve region.
- The bones are cut as a single large piece along with the periosteum with completely mobile bony segments, which are difficult to control.
- A curved lateral osteotomy cannot be executed properly going from "high to low to high" to preserve the external nasal valve region, without damaging the soft tissues.
- Gently turning the lateral osteotomy to meet the superior oblique osteotomy cannot always be executed satisfactorily from the internal approach.
- They can also restrict the movement of the osteotome while turning medially and in the process frail the edges of the osteotomised nasal bones giving rise to callus formation laterally.

12.1.4 External Osteotomies: Surgical Technique

- In rhinoplasty surgery, "osteotomy" is the most difficult procedure to master and achieve consistent results, based on the author's personal journey. To get good outcomes in osteotomy, you need a good understanding of the pathogenesis of the bony deformity. In our unit, 90% of our own revisions are due to failed osteotomies, but unfortunately this happens to be the first procedure the trainees are taught in rhinoplasty and hence led to believe that it is easy!

- The "KEY" to do good osteotomies is to envisage a three-dimensional "road map" in your mind of the bony deformity and the underlying pathogenesis of the deformity before the surgical procedure. Planning the osteotomies is important. Patients may need a combination of the following osteotomies: lateral oblique, superior oblique, bilateral midline (medial) osteotomies and or intermediate osteotomies. Sometimes patients need a straight lateral osteotomy instead of a lateral oblique osteotomy.
- A surgical plan regarding "sequential" osteotomies and sequential lift is important. Give numerical values (1–4) to the nasal dorsum and the nasal base (▪ Fig. 12.1). Then decide which one you are planning to dis-impact after the osteotomies and in which order to achieve optimum results. Say for example, if there is a bony complex deviation to the left side with a depressed fracture of the right nasal bones, the dorsal aspect of the right nasal bone, (number 1 in the ▪ Fig. 12.1) will be just under the dorsal aspect of the left nasal bone, (number 2 in the ▪ Fig. 12.1), although this may not be very obvious clinically. To reduce such a fracture deviation, it is imperative to do a sequential dis-impaction by moving the site 2 outward laterally and "then only" moving the site 1 laterally and out, followed by pushing the site 4 in ▪ Fig. 12.1 (left nasal base) in and then gently lifting out the site 3 in ▪ Fig. 12.1 (right nasal base) last. By sequentially dis-impacting the bones, there is less soft tissue damage and post-operative bruising. Understanding the pathogenesis of the deformity helps in gentle manoeuvres, without brute force causing less tissue damage. Dis-impaction of the nasal bones is done using the back end of a single freer elevator and use the edge of the instrument to move the dorsal edge of the nasal bones in or out.
- We prefer external osteotomies, as they are more precise with less mucosal trauma, less bleeding and do not cut the entire nasal bones as a single piece. The bones should be broken as multiple postage stamps, where pieces are freely mobile, but able to move as a single piece by the attached overlying periosteum.
- When done externally a 2 mm osteotome is used [5] to make postage stamp breaks in the bone. Hence, these are referred to as micro-osteotomies [6]. These are percutaneous bony perforations without any disruption of the periosteum in between [7]. Osteotomes are preferred than chisels.
- Our choice of external osteotomies include three osteotomies on either side, lateral oblique, superior oblique and a midline osteotomy. These are oblique osteotomies (▪ Fig. 12.2a) and not straight. The two lateral oblique and superior oblique osteotomies preserve three triangles, two at the sides of the nose (▪ Fig. 12.2c) which prevents any airway compromise at the external valve region and one triangle at the root of the nose which prevents rocker deformity. Use wet folded swabs on the skin to apply pressure, so that they do not mark the skin (▪ Fig. 12.2b).
- Start the lateral oblique osteotomy with a stab incision with a 15 blade knife, placed vertically (▪ Fig. 12.2e) midway between the medial canthus and the lateral margin of the pyriform aperture.
- Then with a 2 mm osteotome start low on the face at the mid-point of the maximum curvature (▪ Fig. 12.2f) and move downwards towards the pyriform aperture keep-

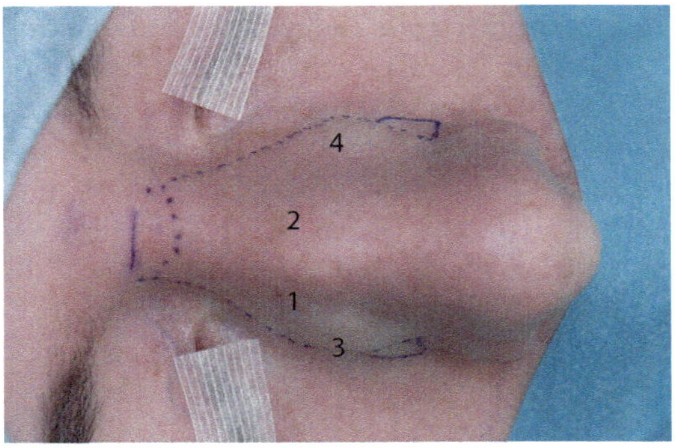

▪ **Fig. 12.1** Frontal view showing the markings of the lateral oblique and superior oblique osteotomies and numbers 1–4 marked on the dorsum of the nose, with number 1–2 at the dorsal edge of the nasal bones and numbers 3–4 marking the base of the nasal bony aperture. These help in planning sequential osteotomy and sequential lifting and dis-impaction of the bony edges

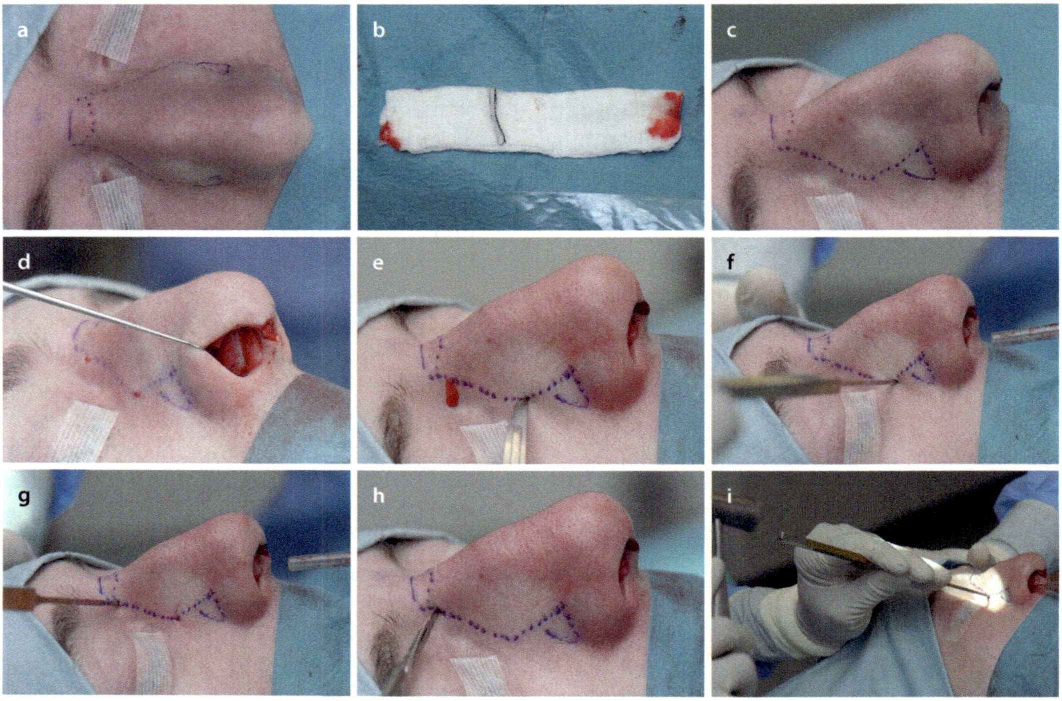

Fig. 12.2 **a–i** Photographs of the nose showing the osteotomy steps. **a** and **c** the osteotomy markings and Webster's triangle. **c** Folded wet swabs used for compression. **d–i** The technique of lateral and superior oblique osteotomies

ing an angle of 30 degrees (Fig. 12.2i) from the frontal plane of the face.

- Keeping the osteotome angle at 30 degrees from the face is important as it helps to "self-impact" each segments for stability, when splints are applied (Fig. 12.3a). If the angle of the osteotome is flat on the cheek with literally zero angle on the face as shown in the schematic Fig. 12.3b, this will result in a free side to side sliding of the cut edges of the bone when splints are applied.
- For stability, it is advisable to start low on the face in the most convex part of the lateral oblique incision and work towards the feet going higher up on the nose preserving a triangle of bone in the region of attachment of the inferior turbinate. Preservation of this lateral triangle (Webster's triangle) prevents medialisation of the anterior ends of inferior turbinates and helps in preventing functional nasal obstruction [8, 9].
- Then, move to superior oblique osteotomy making another stab incision, this time keeping the knife edge horizontally, midway between the medial canthus and nasion. Through this wound execute the superior oblique osteotomy with a 2 mm osteotome again. This osteotomy should connect laterally with the lateral oblique and medially with the midline osteotomies.
- Then bilateral midline osteotomies are done (after raising septal flaps) with 10 mm guarded osteotomes. The osteotome is held vertically and engaged between the bony septum and the nasal dorsum, feeling the edge of the osteotome all the time and asking the assistant to give two taps at a time. Once it has reached the nasion, it is imperative to turn away from the midline laterally to meet the superior oblique osteotomy [10].
- Do not score the periosteum, as this will lead to freely mobile nasal bones adding to instability. Gone are the days when sur-

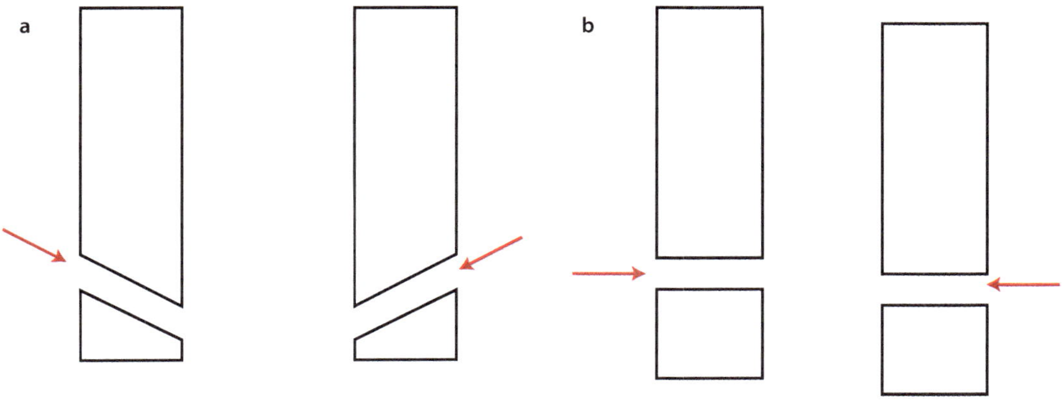

Fig. 12.3 **a** Schematic representation showing the ideal angle (30 degrees) of osteotome on the face to optimise the stability of the reduced fragments. **b** Schematic representation showing if the angle of osteotome on the face is negligible (osteotome being flat on the face), then the bony fragments become unstable

geons used to move the nasal bones side to side before satisfying their ego, that they have broken the nasal bones thoroughly! The bones should be mobile but still attached to the periosteum, so that there is a continuous supportive sheet to mould the bone to the desired position needed.

- Think before using the osteotome. An ideal angle of the osteotome should be around 30 degrees to the face. This not only helps the nasal bones and the frontal processes to be free, but when repositioned the angle of the bony edges is such that the superior complex does not slip laterally under the splint due to the angle of break. If the osteotome is placed horizontally on the cheek, this will create two bony pieces which are sitting squarely one above the other, without any angulation (or opposing forces), which makes the dorsal nasal segment unstable and quite mobile on the nasal base. This can lead to the dorsal bony fragment moving freely laterally or medially under the splint and making it very unstable. Thus an angled osteotomy (30 degree angle) site will be more stable and hence prevent easy displacement.
- *When are intermediate osteotomies indicated?*
  - If the dorsal bony complex is very thick.
  - If the dorsal bony complex is very wide.
  - If the dorsal bony complex is very convex.

If a decision is made to do intermediate osteotomies, it should be done FIRST before lateral or medial osteotomies. This can be either vertically oriented or horizontally oriented. The intermediate osteotomies ideally should be a greenstick fracture and does not have to extend to the entire length and width of the nasal bones and frontal process of maxilla. Intermediate osteotomies should be followed by the lateral and superior oblique osteotomies. Ideally an intermediate osteotomy should be midway between the medial and lateral osteotomies, but can be centred around the most convex portion of the nasal bones. Sometimes in patients with grossly convex nasal bones you may need more than one intermediate osteotomies, and in that case keep the second and the rest osteotomies length shorter than the first one. Thus, if more than one intermediate osteotomies are needed, do the one in the middle first and do the smaller ones either above or below the first one and space it as necessary. Generally the aim of the intermediate osteotomies is to address a localised bony deformity, usually in the form of thickened and convex nasal bones.

- *When do you consider lateral straight osteotomies?*

Lateral straight osteotomies, as the name suggests, run down from "high" in the nose to "low" in the face in a straight line laterally at the naso-facial sulcus, instead of a usual z oblique osteotomy. This is indicated in a small petit nose with dorsal de-projection in a square face requiring the nasal base to be reduced to "gain" some extra projection. The only downside being damage to the lateral bony triangle and medialisation of the anterior end of inferior turbinate, running the risk of narrowing the bony external nasal valve area.

- *What is "high to low to high" osteotomies?*

High or low osteotomies mean the location of osteotomies in relation to the level of the face (maxilla) with the patient lying supine on the operation table. A high osteotomy means starting near the medial canthus at a higher level when compared to the facial plane, and low osteotomy means it is low on the face when compared to the nasal dorsum on the profile view, with the patient lying supine on the theatre table. So a "high to low to high" osteotomy (or low to high) means the osteotomy break is starting higher near the medial canthus and coming down and laterally with a gentle sweep along the frontal process of maxilla and moving up again as it comes down ending near the alar facial groove inferiorly almost in a curved line [11]. Generally this is done to preserve a lateral triangle at the alar facial region of the side of the nose, to prevent any airway compromise. It is simply referred to as lateral oblique osteotomy. On the contrary, a "high to low to low" osteotomy is used to narrow a short and wide nasal complex and to gain extra height and dorsal projection. This is simply a straight lateral osteotomy as mentioned above. The only downside being it will also take the anterior end of the inferior turbinate along with it medially causing potential airway obstruction. Again these nomenclatures can vary between surgeons and they do not matter as long as the surgeon is aware of what, why and how the technique is done.

- *Would you do osteotomies before or after removing the hump?*

We can do both ways, but in our unit we prefer to do the lateral and superior osteotomies *before* hump reduction, although some authors prefer to do after hump reduction [12]. Personal logic in doing a lateral osteotomy first is that, there is no "GIVE" in the nasal bones and hence they break with minimal pressure, avoiding force. As the dorsum is still intact, only a minimal force is required and hence minimal soft tissue damage. If the lateral bones are fractured after the hump removal, there is always a "GIVE" which prevents the bones breaking sharply and always requiring more hits to break the bone. Again this is a personal preference. Small relevant thoughtful steps add to your ultimate outcome and patient satisfaction!

- *The complications of osteotomies include the following:*
  - Irregular dorsum, particularly in patients with thin skin.
  - Rocker deformity, if the superior cut is horizontal.
  - Step deformity laterally, if the bony lateral cut is not low on the cheek.
  - Formation of cysts and callus formation laterally at the osteotomy sites.
  - Collapse of external valve region, if done too low on the lateral aspect.
- *To prevent complications, the surgeon should be aware of the following pearls and pitfalls:*
  - Select 2 mm osteotome, as it causes less damage to the skin and causes less postoperative bruising and swelling [11].
  - Hold the osteotome very lightly and move it over the nasal bones quickly, rather than applying too much force in one place.
  - If too much force is applied, it is more likely that the osteotome will slip in and damage the nasal mucosa and result in bleeding.
  - The aim of the osteotome is to go through the nasal bones, but not through the underlying nasal mucosa.
  - Sometimes the osteotome gets stuck in the osteotomy site. Do not try to pull out the osteotome completely out and go in again, which will damage the skin edges. One way of getting the osteotome out of the bone, but not entirely out of the skin, is to twist the osteotome. This twisting force will make the edge of the osteotome to "jump out" of the cut edges, but will still stay under the skin.
  - Apply soft tissue pressure with a wet swab to reduce the bruising.

12

In conclusion, osteotomy is a key step in the rhinoplasty surgery and if not done properly, it is the major cause of revision surgery in our experience. A three-dimensional mental picture of the pathogenesis of the bony dorsal deformity is a must to achieve good outcomes.

12.2 Mid-Dorsal Augmentation

Mid-dorsal nasal collapse or depression or de-projection can be a part of complex nasal deformity requiring more than one surgical procedure. Dorsal defects are often combined with a loss of support at the middle vault, internal nasal valve obstruction and tip deformities with lack of dorsal and caudal septal support. Often the procedures needed to correct these deformities are not limited to middle vault, but also will involve nasal tip plus or minus spreader grafts at the internal valve for functional reasons. These complex deformities are often poorly treated due to a difficulty in classifying the extent of the deformity and subsequent planning of a surgical solution. There are various classification systems put forward by Tardy [13], Daniel [14], etc. We follow our own *classification* system to assess mid-dorsal defects based on our observation of the combination of deformities as seen in our patients. Our classification has helped us to target specific sites in specific deformities and thereby tailoring the procedures to the deformity.

12.2.1 Glasgow Classification

- Type 1 – Minor dorsal de-projection with *no tip deformity or internal valve issues* requiring only minor dorsal augmentation (e.g. cartilage graft).
- Type 2 – Mid-dorsal de-projection with hour-glass narrowing of mid dorsum causing *internal nasal valve obstruction* requiring additional internal nasal valve surgery (e.g. spreader grafts).
- Type 3 – Mid-dorsal de-projection with *abnormalities of tip* requiring additional nasal tip reconstruction with or without caudal septal reconstruction.
- Type 4 – Mid-dorsal de-projection with *combination of internal valve and tip deformities* requiring complex multiple procedures.

12.2.2 Surgical Planning

Assessment of the deformity is the key step. The patient with dorsal de-projection will invariably need osteotomies to achieve some dorsal height. The plan should be to reconstruct the mid dorsum as much as possible rather than to camouflage, but usually end up doing both. Most patients will need bilateral spreader grafts with or without dorsal septal extension grafts for improving the function and structure of mid dorsum before using dorsal boat grafts for camouflage. This will achieve long-term stability of structure and function. Grafting of the dorsum is usually done with cartilage grafts from either conchal bowl cartilage, posterior septal cartilage or costal cartilage.

12.3 Dorsal Hump Reduction

An over projected dorsal hump will need a hump reduction along with tip work to achieve an aesthetic dorsal profile. Nasal dorsal profile line is responsible for the projection of the nose starting from the nasion at the upper one-third of the nose and extending almost to the anterior septal angle. Dorsal humps can be limited to the upper third of the nose involving the nasal bones or might be limited to middle third where it will be predominantly cartilaginous or both. Rarely in genetic noses the whole dorsal profile line is projecting forward due to a large bony and cartilaginous hump extending from the nasion to the anterior septal angle causing a general over projection of the dorsum. Dorsal humps are made of four components, dorsal nasal bones, upper lateral cartilages, dorsal cartilaginous septum and dorsal bony septum.

12.3.1 Types of Dorsal Hump

Generally the dorsal nasal humps are basically elevations in the nasal dorsum, which can be a true or pseudo hump. Most of the true humps are either genetic or traumatic in origin. True humps can be bony, cartilaginous or both. It should be noted that most dorsal nasal humps are bony and cartilaginous with less bony part and more of the cartilaginous part [15, 16].

Thus "true" dorsal humps can be as follows:

- Bony dorsal humps limited to upper third of the nasal dorsum.
- Cartilaginous humps limited to the middle third of the nasal dorsum.
- Bony and cartilaginous humps involving the upper third and middle third of the dorsum.
- Extensive familial or genetic bony and cartilaginous hump extending right up to the anterior septal angle.

12.3.2 Clinical Presentation

- Nasal dorsal humps can clinically present in various ways. It can be associated with a uniform smooth dorsum where the attachments between the two nasal bones are convex and smooth, as in a non-traumatic genetic hump. This is usually obvious in a "sky view". These are "smooth" curved dorsal humps, where the only issue is profile line elevation.
- Traumatic nasal dorsal humps are usually wide and irregular causing "open book" deformities with loss of smoothness. The dorsal nasal bony edges can be either "parallel" or "diamond" shaped. A "parallel" open book deformity of dorsum causes symmetrical splaying out of the upper lateral cartilage. The junctional zone between the nasal bones and the upper lateral cartilage at the lateral "K" area is usually intact. This is usually due to a fracture line over the nasal dorsum running in the sagittal plane. Prognostically the results following surgery are more predictable as they are not associated with internal nasal valve narrowing.
- The "diamond" shaped open book bony hump deformity as seen in the eyebrow tip line is usually due to severe nasal trauma, secondary to fracture lines extending down along the width of the nasal bones and frontal process of maxilla. Here the caudal border of the nasal bones junction with the upper lateral cartilage, the so-called lateral "K" area can be affected with or without damage to the cephalic border of the upper lateral cartilage causing internal nasal valve problems. There could be dislocation of the upper lateral cartilage at the lateral "K" area. This type of noses may need bilateral spreader grafts to support the internal nasal valve area. This deformity is usually associated with a twisted nose.
- Asymmetric localised bony humps can be associated with a depressed dorsal border of one of the nasal bones with a deviation of complex to the opposite side. This is usually seen in revision surgeries, following asymmetric hump reduction.
- Hump reduction involves removing the dorsal hump and then closing the dorsal open book to achieve a smooth dorsum which is not only lowered in height but also has a smooth dorsal profile.
- The first step before removing a hump is to make sure it is not a pseudo hump. This implies that although the patient may notice that the hump as an issue, the problem is secondary to some other abnormality, usually a de-projected mid dorsum and a de-projected over rotated tip making the bony profile line more prominent.
- Pseudo humps are usually associated with a short nose and over rotated tip. Planning should involve examination and of course discussion with the patient to agree on achievable outcomes. Most pseudo humps are wide and flat, as opposed to a large familial or traumatic hump. Although the emphasis to correct pseudo humps is to address the secondary issue rather than the hump itself, in practice I usually remove a small sliver of the hump as well, particularly if the bony width is excess and then use a longer dorsal graft over the upper and mid third of the dorsum to get a smooth

dorsal profile line [17, 18]. Removing the small sliver of the bony portion of the pseudo hump also helps in splitting the nasal bones in the midline (which in turn helps to narrow the base), but also helps to create a raw surface, which will stabilise a long dorsal graft. This also helps to prevent any depression of the dorsal profile line at the junction of the graft and the pseudo hump.

- Once a diagnosis of a true hump is made, they are generally removed with osteotomes, and minor irregularities are smoothened with a diamond rasp. Although the hump may be limited to the nasal bones, the osteotomy site is in the frontal process of the maxilla. I use a 2 mm osteotome for lateral osteotomies and 10 mms osteotome for the dorsal hump removal. Hump reduction surgery is usually done either alone or in combination with a de-projection of nasal tip. Powered instrumentations are available nowadays for precise cuts with less tissue trauma [19]. Hump reduction can be done through internal approach or open approach, which gives a better access [20].

12.3.3 "Composite" and "Component" Reduction

There are two types of dorsal hump reduction, "composite" and "component" reduction.

- Composite reduction means taking the bony and cartilaginous hump as a "composite" in one step with a 10 mm osteotome [21]. This is usually indicated in a shorter hump which does not extend up to the anterior septal angle.
- Component reduction means taking the dorsum down by reducing the components individually, which takes more time. This involves separation of triangular upper lateral cartilages from the dorsal septum and then stepwise dropping of the cartilaginous septal height first, followed by bony reduction and finally reducing the dorsal septal border of the upper lateral cartilage if necessary. This is indicated if the hump is large enough predominantly involving the cartilage and extending up to the anterior septal angle. This avoids a less common problem associated with a composite reduction namely internal nasal valve collapse due to extensive removal of upper lateral cartilage. This component reduction technique also gives the opportunity to reconstruct the internal valve region with spreader grafts or a spreader flap before closure.

12.3.4 Technique for "Composite" Reduction

- As mentioned before, composite reductions (Fig. 12.4a–f) are done in a smaller dorsal hump, which is predominantly bony with smaller cartilaginous portion and a fairly straight nasal bony and cartilaginous pyramid without any deviation or damage to the "K" area.
- Composite reductions are quicker when compared to component reductions, but they are less helpful in correcting deviations or deformed mid dorsum requiring spreader grafts.
- Stepwise sequential planning is important before hump reduction. I tend to do the superior and lateral osteotomies first before the hump reduction, as it becomes unstable to do the lateral osteotomies after taking the hump.
- Adequate exposure of the bony and cartilaginous dorsum can be done through open approach. Overlying skin flap is elevated, under the SMAS layer and sometimes in the sub-periosteal layer leaving behind the dorsal vestigial muscles on the flap for covering dorsal irregularities.
- Assessing the amount of hump to be excised requires expertise. Either taking too much or too little means that the patient will need revision surgery.
- Once the dorsal osteo-cartilaginous skeleton is exposed either through an open or closed approach, make lateral incision over the frontal process with a sharp blade at the level of the proposed hump removal. Incise the periosteum of frontal process of the maxilla and extend the cut through the ULC and bring it anteriorly and incise

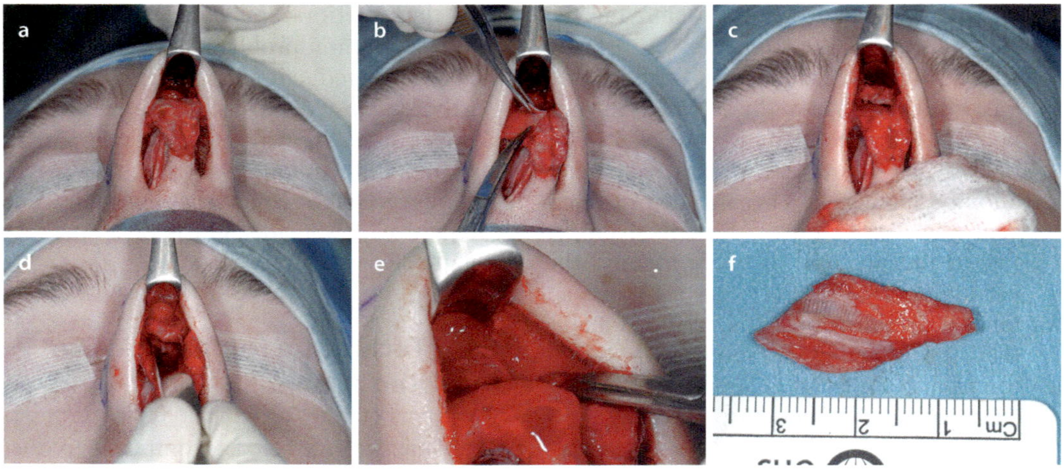

Fig. 12.4 a–f "Open" technique of composite dorsal hump reduction

the anterior cartilaginous septum to create a "fish-mouth" opening that allows the placement of the 10 mm osteotome.

- The orientation of the osteotome should be horizontal and parallel to the bony pyramid taking care not to come out too superficially at the nasion. Also care must be taken not to go too deep.
- Small double tap sequence is used to hit the osteotome with the mallet. The role of the assistant is to tap with the mallet and use the suction under the skin flap to show the surgeon the bony edges.
- Once the dorsal hump is removed, the open roof is closed following the osteotomies laterally and superiorly. The edges of the nasal bones should then be rasped and smoothened with a diamond rasp. Finally crushed autologous septal cartilage (CATS graft) should be used for the dorsum to prevent any minor irregularities showing through.

12.3.5 Technique for "Component" Reduction

- Component reduction, as the name suggests, involves reducing the hump in components and not en masse. The components include the dorsal septum, upper lateral cartilage and bony dorsum. The "component" reduction helps in systematic reduction, the ability to handle various deformities of the dorsum and being able to reconstruct the mid dorsum with spreader grafts if needed. The only downside being it may take more time, but certainly allows for much better outcome.
- The following are the indications for a component reduction of the dorsal hump:
  - Component reduction is advisable in large humps extending lower down up to the anterior septal angle with a poly beak at the tip.
  - Predominantly cartilaginous hump due to excess dorsal septum.
  - In large ethnic noses with genetic dorsal hump involving up to the nasal tip.
  - Large dorsal hump with a twisted nasal bony and cartilaginous pyramid with deviation and squint involving the lateral "K" area.
  - If the dorsal hump is associated with a very thin and narrow nasal dorsum, which may require strengthening of the mid dorsum with spreaders after removal of the hump [22].
- Once component reduction is planned based on the above indications, adequate access is a must through either closed or open approach. Ideally an open approach is preferred for a component reduction, as this cannot be executed properly through a closed approach.
- The septoplasty is performed initially with bilateral septal flaps and the septum

straightened. The dorsal flap is raised and with Aufricht's elevator protecting the dorsal skin, the 11 blade knife is inserted parallel to the septal cartilage on each side and the dorsal septum incised from the triangular upper lateral cartilages under direct vision.

- Note that the dorsal septum does not flush with the upper lateral cartilage, but there is a "T" shaped bar of the dorsal septum joining the upper lateral cartilage. Since the disconnection of upper lateral with the septum is done in a sub-mucosal plane, the mucosa over the internal valve region is protected and hence scarring is prevented later on.
- Once the triangular upper lateral cartilages are separated from the cartilaginous septum, the required amount of the dorsal septal cartilage is removed. This is followed by removal of the dorsal border of the upper lateral cartilage.
- Roughly if the amount of septal cartilage removed is 2 mm, then the amount of upper lateral cartilage to be removed should be 1 mm (a ratio of 2:1 between the septum and upper lateral cartilage). Once this is done, then the bony hump is removed after incising the periosteum and dissecting subperiosteal tunnel and leaving the vestigial muscles over the dorsal skin flap.
- The lateral oblique and superior oblique osteotomies are done before the bony hump removal. Sometimes small superior bilateral midline osteotomies have to be done to separate the nasal bones at the nasion region. The nasal bones are then manipulated depending on the type of deformity, giving due consideration to a sequential reduction of the nasal bones.
- Once the bony and cartilaginous hump is removed, this leaves an "open-roof" which needs to be "closed" to achieve an aesthetic looking smooth dorsum. Inadequate closure of the open roof will lead to a wide "open-roof" deformity with irregular dorsum. Closure of the open roof is aided by lateral, superior and para-median osteotomies as mentioned above.
- Once the bony roof is closed, the dorsum is rasped to get a smooth profile. Despite this the dorsum can never be smooth, particularly when the skin overlying is very thin, it can get stuck down and cause irregular dorsum, which may be more palpable to the patient than visible.
- To avoid this issue in the post-operative period, it is wise to use a septal crushed cartilage (CATS) to cover the dorsal profile line. I usually use a 4-5 mm strip of ventral septal cartilage which I remove during septoplasty.
- In very thin, scarred and pigmented skin or in patients who had multiple revision surgeries, it is better to use a rectangular single layer of fascia lata, measuring 3 cm × 1.5 cm under the skin. This prevents skin sticking to the nasal dorsum and hence prevent small irregular blemishes in the dorsal profile and also improves the pigmentation and vascularity to the skin.
- There are patients with large familial humps who would want the hump to be removed and also de-project the tip. But be aware that some patients may not mention anything about the tip. Be aware of the fact that if the dorsal hump alone is reduced, without reducing the tip, the nasal tip will look longer and projecting from the face more. Sometimes loss of tip support following surgery may even cause drooping of the tip. So dorsal hump reductions may need to be done along with tip de-projection techniques like caudal septal shave or direct tip techniques like intermediate crural resection or a combined lateral crural and medial crural overlap, plus or minus tip anchoring sutures to prevent a post-operative tip drop.

12.4 Managing the Nasion

- One of the important parameters in assessing the nasal dorsal deformity is the root of the nose. "Nasion" is the soft tissue landmark at the root of the nose, where the frontal bone ends and the nasal dorsum starts. The underlying bony suture line where the nasal bones and the nasal process of the frontal bones meet is the "selion". The selion is about 2–3 mm higher than the nasion. When osteotomies are done we take into account the level of the soft tissue nasion than the bony selion. Thankfully this is advantageous to the surgeon as the skull base is above the level of the soft tissue nasion, which helps to prevent any damage to the skull base during osteotomy. The term "radix" is also applied to the nasion. Rhinoplasty surgeons prefer to use the word "radix" instead of nasion, hence grafts used to augment the nasion region of the nose are called radix grafts.

- The length of the nose starts from the radix or nasion superiorly and ends at the nasal tip. The root of the nose is thicker and wider at and above the nasion. The nasal process of the frontal bone does not contribute to the deformity and horizontal fracture at that point can cause a rocker deformity. The length of the nose is longer if the nasion is higher and close to the frontal bone. The "take off" angle of the dorsum of the nose in relation to the frontal bone is an important angle to bear in mind, and this angle is the naso-frontal angle.
- A nasion can be high or low on the face. Normally for an aesthetically balanced nose, nasion is at the level of the interpupillary line. A low-placed nasion gives the impression that the nose is shorter.
- Low nasion is usually due to revision rhinoplasty surgery where excess dorsal bone is removed during surgery or could be secondary to excess fronto-nasal trauma. Sometimes a low nasion can be part of mid-facial dysplasia or hypoplasia syndromes like Binders syndrome.
- A high-placed nasion with "frontalisation of nose", where technically nose looks like starting almost in the frontal bone can be an issue to the rhinoplasty surgeon. A high nasion is usually genetic or familial in origin. Certain racial groups are prone for this. In a patient with a large bony and cartilaginous hump with a high-placed nasion, even if adequate excision of the hump is carried out, the patient might not appreciate the results as it might not be very obvious due to the relative high position of the dorsum.

- All rhinoplasty surgeons should be aware of the scenario where the nasion is low with a pseudo prominence of the mid and lower third dorsum on the profile view giving the impression that the patient has a hump. Here the decision should be made to augment the nasion region rather than removing the mid or lower dorsal hump, even if the patient is complaining of a dorsal hump.
- Patients with shorter nose due to low nasion are ideal candidates for a radix graft to augment the upper third rather than reducing the lower two-thirds. If on the other hand, the lower two-thirds is reduced in patients with low nasion, it can result in a disastrous "washed out" appearance of the nose in the profile view with the nose being in a straight line with the forehead, with a very obtuse naso-frontal angle.
- Radix grafting depends on the available material and whether the procedure is being done in isolation or as a part of a total nasal reconstruction. Pieces of diced or crushed cartilage from the nasal septum or conchal bowl cartilage can be used, packed inside a membranous sheath of either temporalis fascia or fascia lata. Using many layers of fascia lata alone gives a better cosmetic result than using diced cartilage, since it has the added advantage of being able to be moulded into irregular concavities of the radix, particularly when they are done as an isolated procedure. It is advisable to rasp the surface of the bone in the nasion region to create roughness and new vascularity before securing the graft.

Conclusion

Managing the nasal dorsum is key in securing the nasal tip in the right position in the profile line. If a hump reduction is done, always use crushed septal cartilage to buffer the dorsum irregularities after the hump reduction. We suggest using this even if the dorsum is smooth as it will reduce the incidence of dorsal irregularities developing later on in the post-operative period. In very thin and scarred skin due to multiple revision procedures, it is advisable to use also a small graft of fascia lata to cover the nasal dorsum. Also be aware that augmenting or reducing the dorsal hump will have a secondary effect on the tip, and this should be factored in while planning the surgical intervention.

Key Points Box

- Be aware that osteotomies are the most difficult technique to execute and a lot of thought process should be involved. Inadequate osteotomy is the most common cause of my revision surgeries rather than soft tissue nasal tip surgery.
- One of the key and final steps in nasal tip surgery is to secure the reconstructed tip in line with the dorsum to achieve an aesthetic dorsal profile line.

References

1. Murakami CS, Younger RAL. Managing the post rhinoplasty or post-traumatic crooked nose. Facial Plast Surg Clin North Am. 1995;3:421.
2. Bloom JD, Zimmerman SB, Constantinides M. Osteotomies in crooked nose. Facial Plast Surg. 2011;27(5):456–66.
3. Aufricht G. Joseph's rhinoplasty with some modifications. Surg Clin North Am. 1971;51(2):299–316.
4. Hilger JA. The internal lateral osteotomy in rhinoplasty. Arch Otolaryngol. 1968;88:119.
5. Rohrich RJ, Krueger JK. The lateral osteotomy in rhinoplasty: clinical and radiographic rationale for osteotome selection (discussion). Plast Reconstr Surg. 2000;105(5):1817–9.
6. Tardy ME, Denneny JC. Micro-osteotomies in rhinoplasty. Facial Plast Surg. 1984;1:137.
7. Bull TR. Percutaneous osteotomy in rhinoplasty. Plast Reconstr Surg. 2001;107(6):1624–5.
8. Webster RC, Davidson TM, Smith RC. Curved lateral osteotomy for airway protection in rhinoplasty. Arch Otolaryngol. 1977;103:454.
9. Becker DG, McLaughlin RB Jr, Loevner LA, Mang A. The lateral osteotomy in rhinoplasty: clinical und radiographic rationale for osteotome selection. Plast Reconstr Surg. 2000;105(5):1806.
10. Larrabee W. Open rhinoplasty and the upper third of the nose. Facial Plast Surg Clin North Am. 1993;1:23.
11. Murakami CS, Larrabee WE. Comparison of osteotomy techniques in the treatment of nasal fractures. Facial Plast Surg. 1992;8:209–19.
12. Rohrich RJ, Janis JE, Adams WP, Krueger JK. Update on the lateral nasal osteotomy in rhinoplasty: an anatomic endoscopic comparison of the external versus the internal approach. Plast Reconstr Surg. 2003;111(7):2461–2.
13. Tardy ME, Schwartz MS, Parras G. Saddle nose deformity: autogenous graft repair. Facial Plast Surg. 1989;6:121.
14. Daniel RK, Brenner KA. Saddle nose deformity: a new classification and treatment. Facial Plast Surg Clin North Am. 2006;14:301–12.
15. Tardy ME Jr. Rhinoplasty: the art and the science. Philadelphia: W.B. Saunders Company; 1997.
16. Sheen JH, Sheen AP, editors. Aesthetic rhinoplasty. 2nd ed. St. Louis: Quality Medical Publishing; 1998.
17. Gunter JR, Clark CR, Friedman RM. Internal stabilization of autogenous rib cartilage: a barrier to cartilage warping. Plast Reconstr Surg. 1997;100:161.
18. Riechelmann H, Rettinger G. Three-step reconstruction of complex saddle nose deformities. Arch Otolaryngol Head Neck Surg. 2004;130(3):334–8.
19. Becker DG, Park SS, Toriumi DM. Powered instrumentation for rhinoplasty and septoplasty. Otolaryngol Clin North Am. 1999;32(4):683–93.
20. Becker DG, Toriumi DM, Gross CW, Tardy ME Jr. Powered instrumentation for dorsal reduction. Facial Plast Surg. 1997;13(4):291–7.
21. McGregor IA. A nasal osteotome. Br J Plast Surg. 1967;20(2):222.
22. Vuyk HD. Cartilage spreader grafting for lateral augmentation for the middle third of the nose. Faces. 1993;3:159–70.

Alar Base Surgery

Contents

N. Balaji, *Textbook of Nasal Tip Rhinoplasty*, https://doi.org/10.1007/978-3-030-48157-5_13

Learning Objectives

- To understand the anatomy of the alar base and the nasal tip.
- To understand the concept that alar base surgery can be both for "narrowing" a wide alar base and also to "widen" a contracted and scarred alar base.
- To learn the techniques to narrow a wide alar base which can be easier and give consistent results when compared to opening a contracted scarred alar base, which is a more complex surgery.
- To learn to diagnose and manage both alar base contraction and alar base widening.

13.1 Introduction

Alar base surgery as the term denotes is any form of surgery in the alar base complex of the nasal tip. The term "alar base" defines the lateral alar part of the nasal tip complex as it joins the facial sulcus. It is in the "base" of the alar complex as seen in the basal view of the nasal tip. Alar base surgery is *done for two reasons, either to widen a contracted alar base or to narrow a wide alar base*, although for some reason the term alar base surgery is unequivocally seen to be alar base reduction in most surgeons' view. Wider alar base is usually due to genetic reasons and is rare in Caucasian noses, when compared to some ethnic noses as in Afro-Caribbean or Oriental races. It is rare in Caucasian practice. It can also be due to traumatic damage to the nose. In contrast, contracted alar bases are mostly due to trauma and scarring and very few due to congenital issues like secondary to cleft lip noses.

13.2 Anatomy of Alar Base

Alar base is the terminology used to describe the lateral alar part of the nasal tip complex as seen in the basal view (Fig. 13.1). Alar base surgery is a terminology restricted to surgery of the lateral alar base. This is the point of the ala where it meets the facial sulcus. Anatomically alar base is made of skin and soft tissue ONLY and does not have any cartilage, as the lateral crura does not come as lateral and as far down as the alar base. Lack of cartilage makes soft tissue control in the alar base more difficult and any inadvertent move can cause external scarring in the region which will be very difficult to correct. Although there is no cartilage normally in the alar base, sometimes we have to strengthen with additional autologous cartilage to offer support to the alar base, particularly when there is soft tissue scarring. Tardy described the "sil" region as the intra-nostril space between the medial crural footplate and lateral alar facial groove [1]. So, in essence the region around the nostril immediately lateral to the alar-facial groove is the "alar base" and medial to the alar-facial groove is the "sil" region. Relationship of alar columellar margin should be aesthetically pleasing in the lateral view. Normally for an aesthetically pleasing nose, the columellar show should be around 2 mm in the side view. If it is more, it can be a "true" columellar excess show due to the over-hanging columella or "pseudo" columellar show due to upward retraction of the lateral alar margin. The over-hanging columella could be due to excess caudal septum

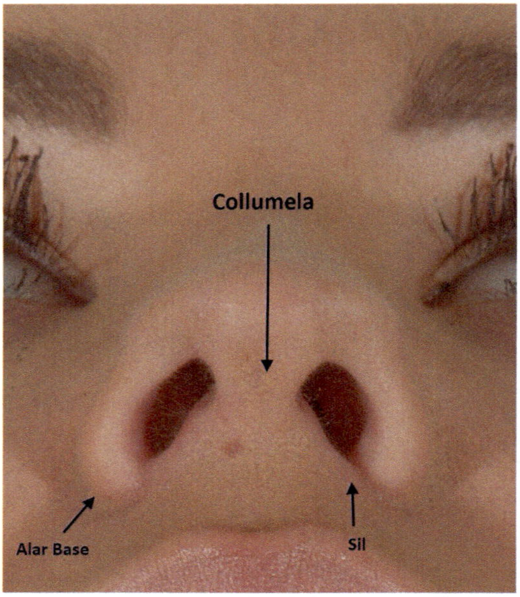

Fig. 13.1 The anatomy of the alar base with arrows showing columella, alar base right side and sil left side

13

or prolapse of medial crural footplates due to disconnection from the caudal septum or both. Similarly upward retraction of ala could be due to cephalic migration of the lateral crus, over resection of cephalic lateral crus or due to soft tissue retraction of alar margin.

13.3 Aetiology and Pathogenesis of Alar Deformities

In recent years, the term "alar base surgery" has come to be synonymous with alar base reduction. This is not so. "Alar base surgery" involves either "narrowing" a wide alar base or "widening" of a narrow and scarred contracted alar base. The surgery for narrowing a wide alar base with alar base reduction is much more simpler and achieve reliable outcomes rather than widening a narrow alar base. Alar base reduction is usually targeted at the site where the alar base meets the facial sulcus, to hide any scar tissue. Thus alar base pathology can be either:

- *A wide alar base* – requiring alar base reduction.
- *A narrow alar base with or without scar contraction* (vestibular stenosis) – requiring surgery to widen the alar base and open up the external nasal valve region.

Both the above types of deformities cause structural and functional issues, but additionally a contracted alar base can pose a challenging surgical conundrum to open the external nasal valve region and keep it open long term. The abnormality may be due to trauma or familial, or due to genetic defects like cleft lip. If it is due to trauma, causing a "wider" alar base, it is vital first to check for de-projection of the nasal tip, which will cause a sagging in the lateral ala thus causing a wide alar base (Figs. 13.2 and 13.3). In most traumatic patients, correcting and increasing tip projection is all that is necessary to narrow the width of the alar base. In genetic noses and certain races the alar base is quite wide, as evidenced by the alar facial sulcus outside the vertical tangent dropped from the medial canthus. Sometimes, this also happens in extremely de-projected traumatic noses with upward rotation of the tip.

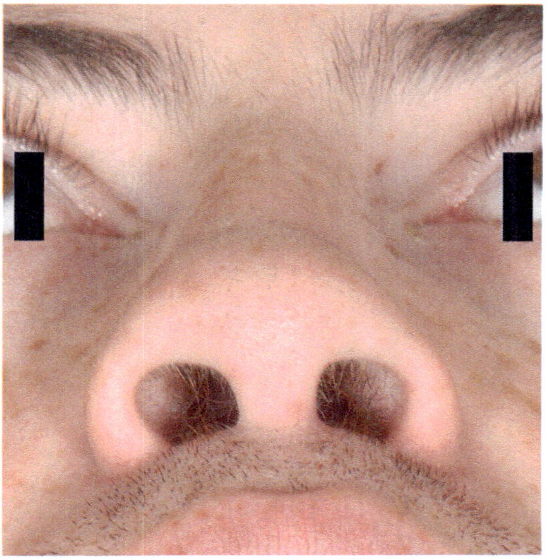

Fig. 13.2 Basal view showing de-projection of the tip causing a wider alar base

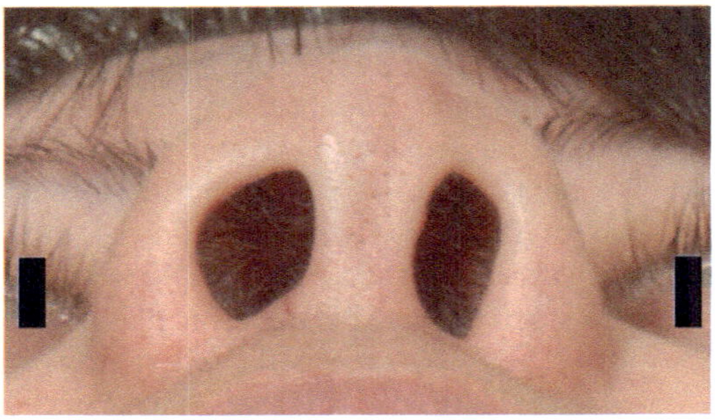

Fig. 13.3 Basal view showing straight columella with negligible sil

13.4 Assessment of Alar Base: Frontal and Basal Views

The following points are important in assessing the alar base.

- *The alar width* – assessed in the frontal view. This is the distance between the maximum point of the alar convexity between the two ala. Ideally this distance should be less than the inter-canthal distance as measured by dropping a vertical line in the medial canthus of the eye. If the alar width is wider than the inter canthal distance, then this may be an indication to reduce the alar width by doing an *alar wedge reduction by excising a wedge of alar*

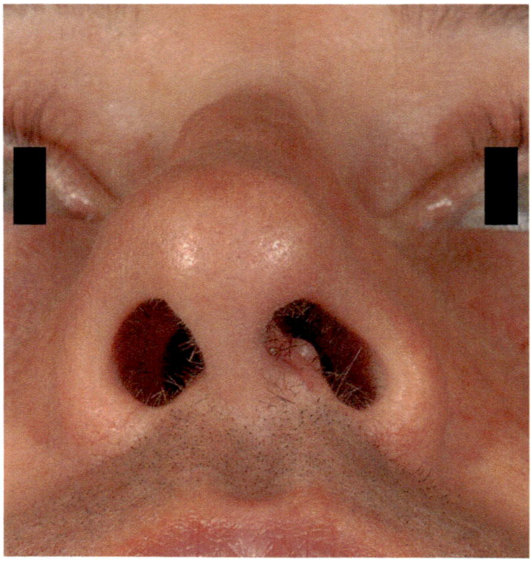

■ **Fig. 13.4** Basal view showing a "doughnut"-shaped nostril on the left side due to prolapse of the medial crural footplate into the nostril

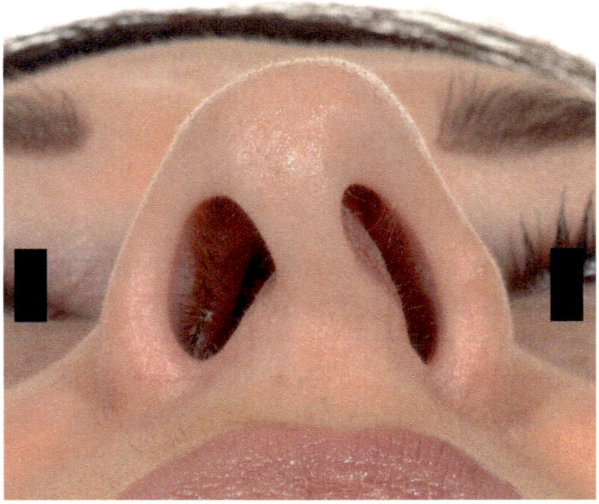

■ **Fig. 13.5** Basal view showing asymmetric excess sil width

base, with the base of the wedge facing outside, taking extreme care not to take the excision edge inside to the alar mucosa.

- The next thing is to look at the "basal" view of the nostrils on both sides. Look at the nostril flare in the basal view. If the intra-nostril space between the alar-facial groove and the columella (sil region) is wider and sloping, this can "show" more of the inside wall of the alar mucosa in the basal view. If this is so, then it may be an indication to reduce the width of the nostril sil region as well. This "intra-nostril sil region" can also be narrower due to a flared medial crural footplates causing thickening of the columella in the lower third and narrowing of the nostril size as well (■ Fig. 13.4). If this is so, then it may be an indication to reduce the width of the medial crural footplates and narrow the columella to widen the intra-nostril space. Excess narrowing of the sil could also be due to caudal dislocation of the septum which may need to be corrected first [2, 3].
- Then look at the shape of the nostril and size of the nostril. Nostrils are pear shaped and slanted 30–45 degrees to the midline [4]. If the nostril shape is rounder and bigger, then there is a possibility that the nostril sil is wider as seen in ■ Fig. 13.2. This type of deformity is usually also associated with a wide alar flare as well, needing alar base width excision as well. The sil width can vary between two sides even in the same patient. If the sil width is unusually more than the width of the columella as seen in ■ Fig.13.5 on the left side, then this might be an indication to reduce the alar sil by a minimal excision keeping the scar line at the alar facial groove, making sure the margins are not extending into the mucosa of the vestibule. The width of the alar sil is dependent on the anatomy of the medial crural footplates and the caudal septal position. ■ Fig.13.6. Before doing anything to the sil region, a thorough assessment and correction of the caudal septum and medial crural footplate anatomy is a must. Any "direct" surgery on the sil should not be taken lightly and rarely done in our practice.
- A diamond-shaped nostril as seen on the right side in ■ Fig.13.7 is due to a wide and high sil, either on one or both sides. A "doughnut"-shaped nostril is due to prolapse of the medial crural footplate into the nostril as seen in ■ Fig. 13.4. On the contrary, If the septum is dislocated into the nostril, then it creates a vertical parallel slit as seen in ■ Fig. 13.8.

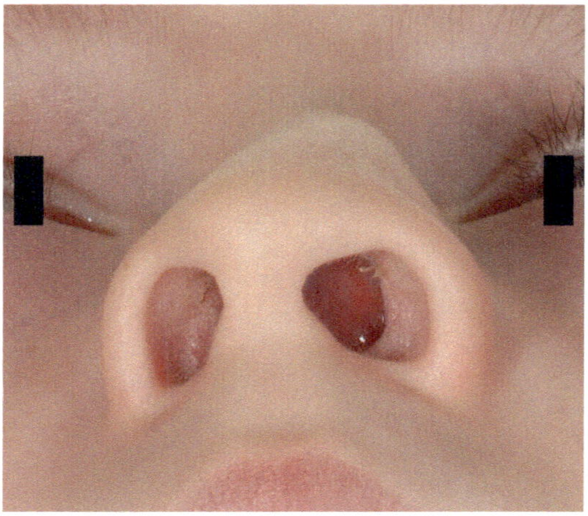

Fig. 13.6 Basal view showing "excess alar show" with the medial wall of the ala seen "more" in the frontal plane due to caudal septal deformity

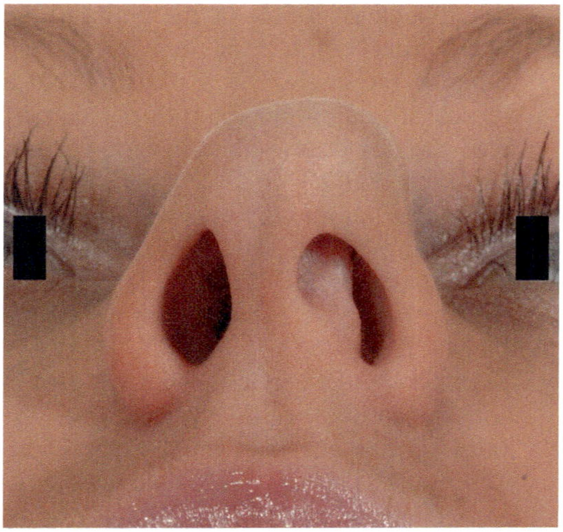

Fig. 13.8 Basal view showing a "vertical slit like" nostril on the left side due to prolapse of the caudal septum into the nostril

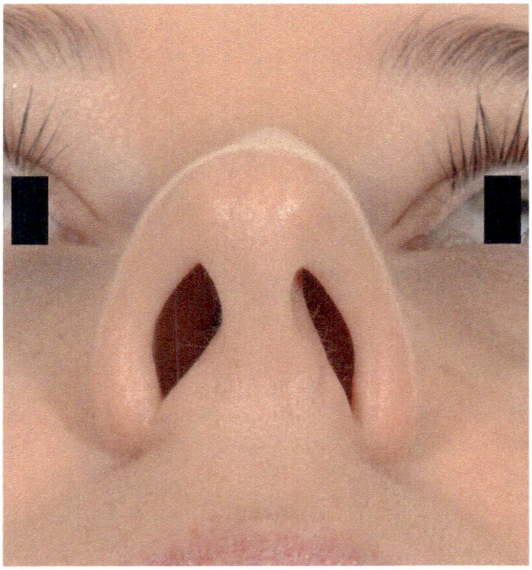

Fig. 13.7 Basal view showing a diamond-shaped nostril on the right side due to a high sil

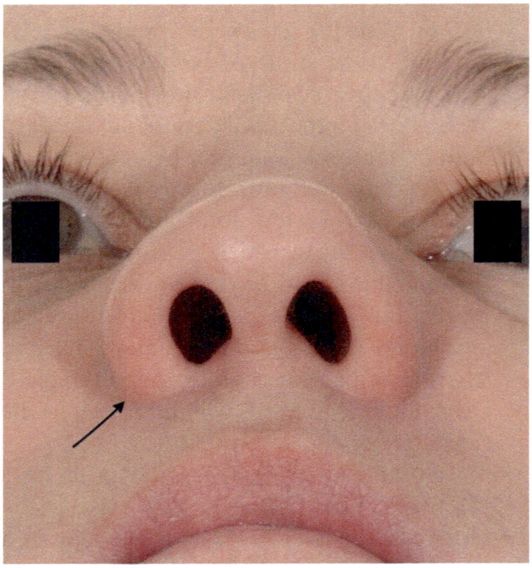

Fig. 13.9 Basal view with the arrow showing a "turned in" alar base causing a rounded nostril

- Then look at the way the alar base is meeting the facial sulcus. It may be coming down straight with little curvature (Fig. 13.7) or maximum curvature (Fig. 13.9). If it is maximum curvature, then an alar wedge resection may be necessary. If the lateral ala is nearly vertical at the naso-alar sulcus, to improve the aesthetics of the nasal base curvature, then a small part of the alar base can still be resected and the alar base turned "in". Be aware this can be an extremely risky manoeuvre to do. Of course an assessment of tip projection should be taken into the algorithm before considering these techniques based on individual deformities [5].
- In the fronto-basal view the junction of the lateral ala to the facial sulcus might also be a fairly straight line coming from above down, akin to various different

attachments of lobule of the pinna to the lateral cheek skin. The gentle outward bulge of the lateral ala is pleasing, but a vertical straight attachment of the ala may need an alar base wedge excision to turn the ala medially.

- But in this situation, you need to be aware that doing an alar wedge excision in a straight ala may narrow the nostril and de-project the tip by a downward pull of the ala as well.
- Then look at the relationship of projection to the alar width. Projection of the nasal tip has an effect on the alar width (Fig. 13.2). *Most often just increasing the projection is all that is needed to narrow the alar base width and improve the alar base aesthetics.* Conversely, decreasing the alar projection can cause alar flaring which may then need an alar wedge resection. In fact, this surgery was first described for this reason by Weir [6]. This is an important relationship to be aware of before considering alar base surgery. When using de-projection techniques on the nasal tip, it is advisable to wait for 6 months or a year before considering alar base wedge excision.
- In the lateral view look for the excess columellar show, which is usually around 2 mm. This could be due to excess downward shift of the columella or upward retraction of the lower alar margin. History of previous surgery or trauma and other clinical findings will direct you to the aetiology of the deformity.
- In a contracted and scarred alar base (Figs. 13.10 and 13.11), assess the extent of the lateral width of the alar skin and assess the static and dynamic movement of the lateral alar base. Also look for the internal scar tissue with an endoscopic examination.

13.5 Management of a "Wide" Alar Base

It is important to understand that the excess lateral alar base width might not be obvious before considering rhinoplasty surgery, but

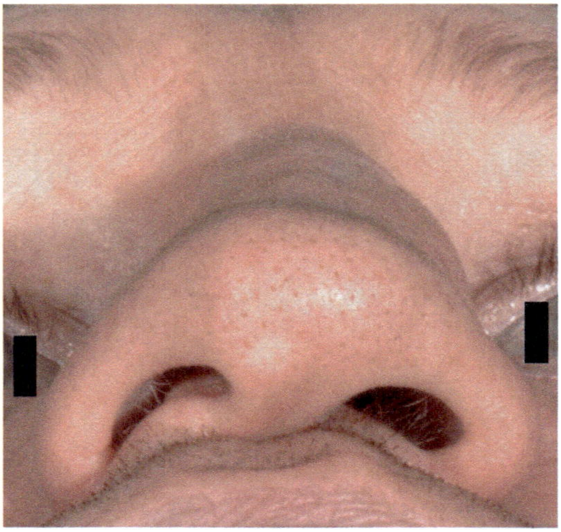

Fig. 13.10 Basal view showing contracted alar base due to abnormal sil on the right side

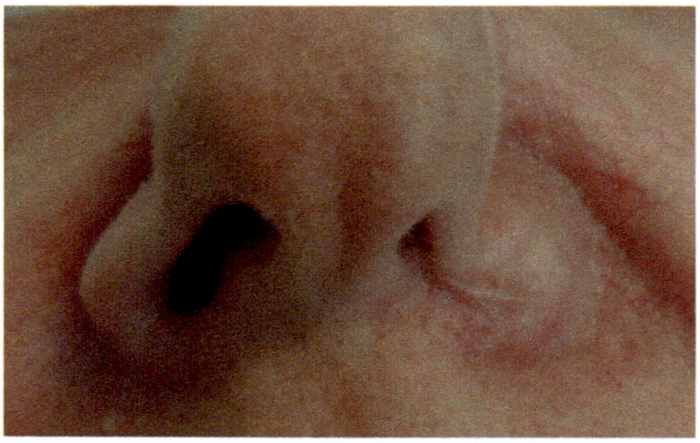

Fig. 13.11 Basal view showing scarred and contracted alar base on the left side due to trauma

once certain tip modifications are done, predominantly any de-projection techniques are done, this can cause secondary widening of the nasal base. Hence it is very important to keep an open mind even in Caucasian noses, particularly revisiting the alar base at the end of the procedure. Wide alar base is usually symmetrical if resulting from iatrogenic surgical de-projection of the tip. Wide alar base can also be asymmetrically placed in a horizontal plane (Figs. 13.12 and 13.13), particularly after non-surgical trauma. These are extremely difficult situations to correct, as they are liable to upward pull and contraction during the healing process.

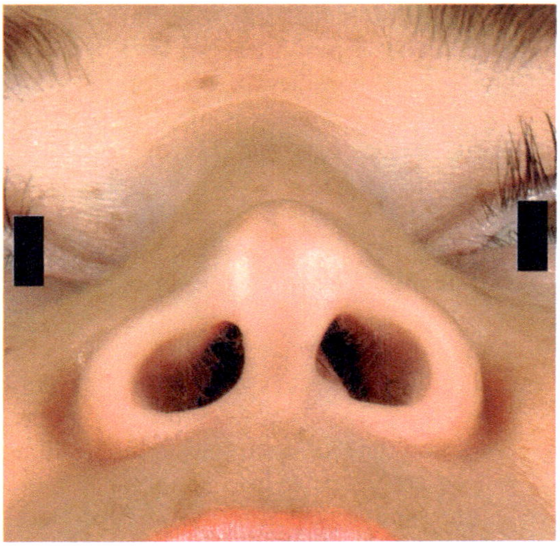

Fig. 13.12 Basal view showing asymmetrically placed alar base following non-surgical trauma

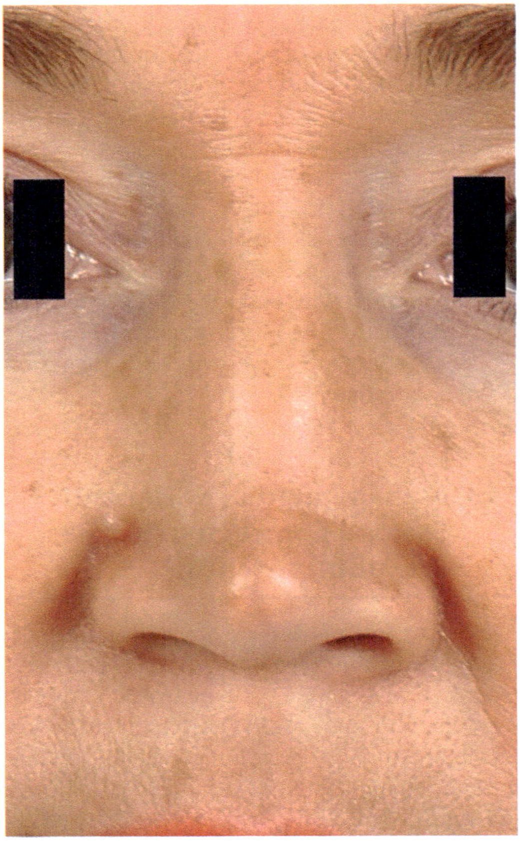

Fig. 13.13 Frontal view showing asymmetrically placed alar base following non-surgical trauma

There are various modifications of alar base reduction described. If the reader is looking for advanced techniques, it is advisable to look into specialised monologues from more experienced surgeons [3, 5, 7].

Even prominent rhinoplasty surgeons have published very limited number of cases over 20 years [8].

The most common technique which we perform (still rare in our practice) to reduce the width of alar base is alar base reduction with or without medial crural footplate surgery. It is very important that doing this operation involves accurate assessment of the deformity [9, 10]. This surgery has got the potential to introduce unwanted variables including scarring at the alar facial crease. The tissues to be excised should be measured and incised with clean sharp cuts and brought together accurately without overlap. At the same time make sure the epidermis is not trapped inside the mucosa of the vestibule to prevent implantation dermoid cysts secondary to poor suturing techniques.

13.5.1 Factors to Consider Before Narrowing Alar Base

- Is it traumatic, familial, racial or genetic due to cleft lip/palate.
- Is it a true deformity or a pseudo deformity secondary to loss of tip projection. As mentioned above, most lateral alar base bulge is due to lack of tip projection, which needs to be sorted before embarking on alar base reduction. On the contrary, any de-projection technique can cause lateral alar widening and hence go back and check the base after tip procedure [11].
- Is it a primary tip problem with damage to lateral crus which can distort the alar columellar relationship.
- Is the rest of the nose, cartilaginous and bony skeleton are in harmony.
- Has all the rest of the deformities corrected before considering nasal base surgery, which should be the last step.

13.5.2 Algorithm to Narrow a Wide Alar Base

- Pseudo or true – if pseudo it is due to loss of tip projection, hence may need a columellar strut or a medial crural fixation suture or a caudal extension graft to lift the tip up. These techniques help to increase tip projection thereby pulling the alar margin inwards to reduce the alar flare and a wide ala.
- If it is a true deformity, check for the alar flare outside the inter-canthal distance and the way the ala meets the alar facial sulcus. If there is a lateral alar bulge, this will need an alar base wedge resection with base of the triangle outside, keeping the incision well away from the internal vestibular mucosa and also well away from the underlying muscles. Take care not to cauterise and damage the underlying muscles.
- If the nostril size is big and rounded associated with a wide nasal sil, this may need a limited excision of nasal sil width without entering the vestibular mucosa.
- Be aware sometimes a very wide and dislocated medial crural footplate can elevate the skin and soft tissue of the "sil" region as a secondary effect and cause pseudo-widening of the sil. This can be addressed by medial crural footplate narrowing procedure rather than any direct sil surgery. Direct "sil" surgery should be approached with extreme caution and is extremely rare in our practice.

13

13.5.3 Surgical Technique of Narrowing a Wide Alar Base

- There are certain basic tenets which need to be followed while considering alar base narrowing surgery: marking the incision and fine dissection with skin hooks and delicate fine closure of the skin avoiding any unwanted damage to the skin margins.
- A decision has to be made if direct alar width excision needs to be done with or without medial crural footplate surgery and caudal septal surgery. Also be aware changing the degree of projection of the tip will affect the alar width. The surgeon needs to be wary of making too many incisions, particularly when someone needs also an open approach involving the columella and there is a risk of destabilising the blood supply to the alar base.
- Meticulous planning of the incision to camouflage the scar is important, particularly when alar wedge resection is planned involving the alar skin. Incisions should be placed at the crease lines [12, 13].
- In alar wedge resection, also called external alar base reduction, a crescent of the alar wedge skin and soft tissues is removed with the medial edge of the skin wedge ellipse (crescent) located in the alar facial groove, so that after excising the wedge of tissue (which should not be more than 4 mm at the external base), the new suture site should be hidden at the alar facial sulcus, thus avoiding unwanted scars on the skin of the alar margin.
- Alar width narrowing can also be achieved by minimal excision of skin and soft tissues on either side of the alar-facial sulcus and re-positioned at the desired level with two layer closure making sure the incisions do not enter the nasal mucosa which can be counterproductive with scar formation at a later date [14].

13.6 Management of a "Narrow" Scarred Contracted Alar Base (Vestibular Stenosis)

There are various causes of narrow nostrils: both genetic and traumatic. Abnormalities in the nasal base is one of the causes of narrow nostrils, although rare. The scar contraction can be involving the columellar skin, medial crus or lateral alar base with mucosal scarring (◘ Figs. 13.14, 13.15, and 13.16) [15]. Caudal septal and medial crural issues are more common to cause nostrils narrowing than alar base abnormalities.

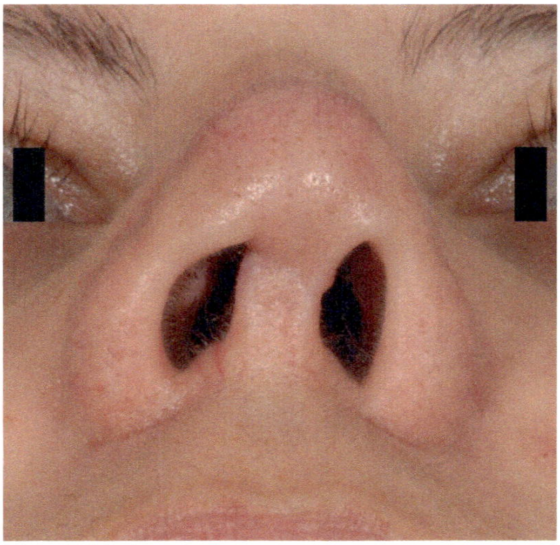

■ **Fig. 13.14** Basal view showing scarred columella

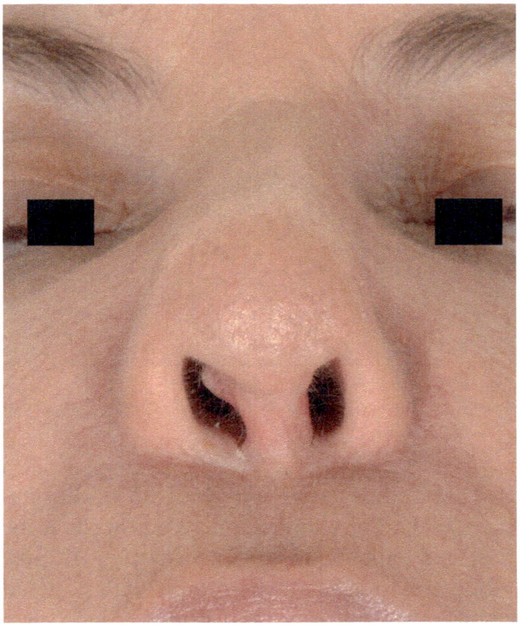

■ **Fig. 13.15** Basal view showing scarred soft triangle

A narrow alar base could be due to a combination of factors, including the skin and soft tissues of the alar base and alar margins, plus damage to lateral alar cartilage and or damage to alar vestibular mucosa. In our experience, the most common reason for a damaged lateral crus is over resection in a primary rhinoplasty or secondary to nasal trauma. Occasionally

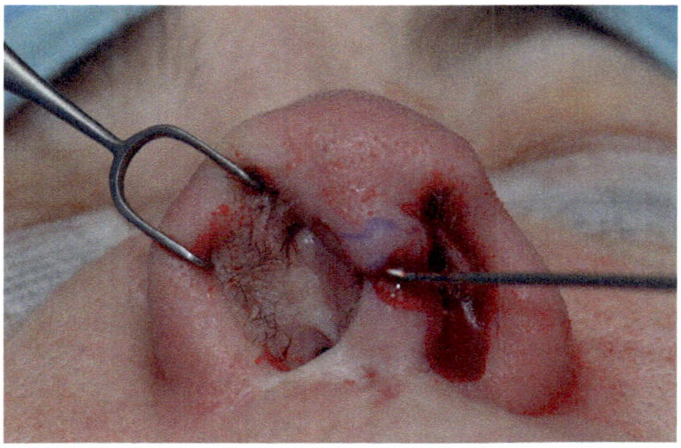

■ **Fig. 13.16** Basal view showing contracted right alar base with mucosal scarring

there are patients with congenital absence or deformity of the lateral crus on one side in cleft lip patients. In patients with nasal trauma with sharp objects, there could be associated mucosal trauma of the vestibule (■ Fig. 13.16), which makes the management very complex. Mucosal scarring may also be due to the use of recreational drugs like cocaine or secondary to granulomatous processes. Loss or damage to external nasal skin of the alar base could be due to surgical excision of skin lesions, without supporting the alar margins.

Ideal graft materials for supporting the alar base would be opposite conchal bowl cartilage. For damaged and scarred internal mucosa, the ideal replacement would be split thickness skin graft taken from inner thigh. We have found that fascia lata can fail dramatically due to avascularity. We do not use fascia lata anymore and use only split thickness skin graft, which has not failed us so far, and they can also be used to cover small defects in the alar skin margins and soft triangles as well, which heals well without any residual defects. Another advantage of split thickness skin graft is to use it as a "wrap" around the alar skin margin defect which usually takes up very well too (■ Fig. 13.17d).

13.6.1 Algorithm to Open a Narrow Alar Base

Clinical examination of both external and internal nasal cavity with an endoscope is necessary. Both structural and functional assessment should be done. It is vital to understand

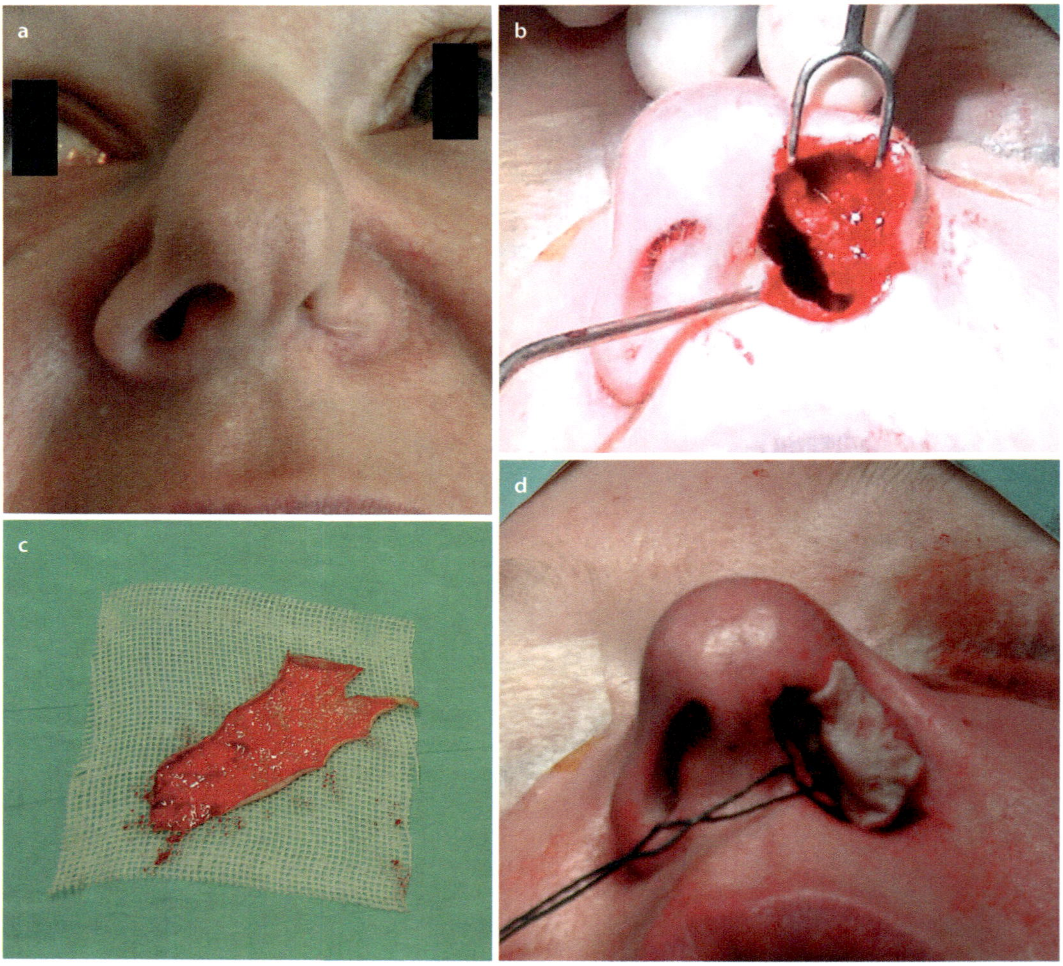

Fig. 13.17 a–d Basal view showing contracted left alar base with mucosal scarring, needing alarotomy and split thickness skin graft

that there are more functional issues with a narrow contracted and scarred alar base than wider alar base. Hence correcting and addressing the functional issues should be taken into account while having a surgical plan to open a structural deformity of a contracted and scarred alar base. Assessment of mucosal scar is the key in achieving long-term results. Be aware that the patient may complain mainly of nasal obstruction rather than cosmetic deformity. Individual assessment of tissues, including the external skin, internal mucosa and the need for cartilage replacement should decide the surgical technique. The approach to the surgery depends on the location of the scar. An alarotomy approach through the scar sometimes is better than an additional scar. If the mucosa is damaged, it needs to be replaced with a split thickness skin graft. Soft tissue collapse has to be rebuilt with conchal cartilage taken from opposite ear.

13.6.2 Surgical Technique of Widening a Narrow Scarred Contracted Alar Base (Vestibular Stenosis)

- A narrow alar base is due to external nasal trauma or over resection of lateral crus or post-surgical after resection of cutaneous malignancies. It is associated with cutaneous and internal mucosal scarring, which can be very extensive (Fig. 13.17a).

- Any technique to open and widen the alar base should also take into account not only structural reconstruction but also consider the functional aspects to open the external nasal valve region.
- Adequate exposure is important, usually through an alarotomy incision (Fig. 13.17b) rather than an open approach incision, which may also be needed of course depending on individual patients.
- After adequate exposure, the vestibular scar tissue should be incised and elevated from the underlying bone. No attempt should be made to excise the scar tissue, as any excision will lead to aggressive recurrence of scar tissue at the vestibular area.
- If necessary cartilage graft should be harvested from the opposite conchal bowl to help the nasal valve function and reconstruct the lateral ala. Use of cartilage graft helps in preserving the nasal function in the external vestibular region.
- Full thickness skin grafts do not work in our hands, particularly getting infected and sloughing away if the defect is very big. We use split thickness skin graft from the inner thigh, which has not failed in our hands so far.
- Split thickness skin graft (Fig. 13.17c) should be harvested from the inner thigh with a dermatome or Hamby's knife. Split thickness skin graft from the thigh gives better long-term results when compared to fascia lata. Use of split skin graft helps in preventing recurrence.
- Ronguering of the bony pyriform aperture is a very important step that is performed to expand the bony pyriform space and also helps in moving the bony edge laterally.
- Then the alar base is repositioned in a more downward and more lateral position and the deformity is "over" corrected.
- Soft triangle scarring is more difficult to handle, and in our experience there is no satisfactory procedure available, apart from excising the scar and leave it to heal by secondary intention.
- Thus surgery of the nasal base in the presence of scarring and vestibular stenosis can be challenging. Adequate over correction is important.
- Sometimes if minimal alar margin skin need to be replaced as well, the split thickness skin graft can be wrapped around the margin, which heals very well (Fig. 13.17d).

Pearls and Pitfalls

- Always check the tip projection before considering alar wedge excision. If the tip is de-projected, improve the projection first before doing alar base work, particularly in Caucasian noses.
- If in doubt wait for the 6 months after tip work before alar base reduction and re-assess the nasal base.
- Be aware that placing the incision in the alar facial crease is very important. Otherwise, the scar can be very obvious.
- Accurate measurements are important with callipers to decide the level of correction avoiding over resection.
- Wedge resection of the alar base should always be base facing outside and the apex of the wedge facing inside but NOT extending to the alar mucosa. Any damage to the smooth vestibular mucosal margins can cause contraction and will be very difficult to correct afterwards.
- Again alar sil narrowing by excision should be carefully planned. The excision margins should be in the middle of the sil and not extending too laterally to the alar facial sulcus and not too much internally into the vestibule. The internal incision should be tapered and should stop short of the vestibular mucosa.
- Fine tissue handling is important. Do not damage the underlying muscle or damage the vestibular mucosa either with knife or diathermy.
- Mucosa over the floor of the nose should be handled with extreme care, over resection should be avoided and

closure should be with mattress sutures and mild eversion of the mucosal edges.
- Alar base widening of vestibular stenosis will involve extensive surgery and the patient should be made aware of this and also the fact that it is difficult to secure the alar base in the right place.
- Surgery of the nasal base in the presence of scarring and vestibular stenosis can be challenging. Adequate over correction is important.
- Use of split skin graft helps in preventing recurrence, and the use of cartilage graft helps in preserving the nasal function in the external vestibular region.
- Patients should be warned of the need for multiple revisions.

Conclusion

Our experience in alar base surgery is very limited, particularly in alar base narrowing procedures. Alar base surgery is rarely needed in Caucasian population. A wide alar base causes structural issues, but a narrow alar base causes not only structural but also functional nasal valve obstruction at the external nasal valve region. Thus alar base surgery can be two fold, either to narrow a wide alar base to widen a narrow alar base. Narrowing a wider alar base is more simpler than widening a narrow alar base. Long-term results of widening a contracted alar base due to scarring is difficult to achieve when compared to alar base reduction surgery. Most of the time, increasing the projection of a de-projected nasal tip is all that is needed to correct an alar width and pull the alar margins "in". Conversely, always remember to look at the alar margins after reducing the tip projection as this may cause secondary alar flare which may need alar width excision. Generally alar sil excision is quite rare until otherwise there is a revision rhinoplasty issues with distortion of lateral alar cartilages. Widening of alar base due to vestibular stenosis may require extensive surgery to achieve favourable outcomes.

Key Points Box

- The term "alar base surgery" is not limited to alar base reduction in a wide ala but also applies to any procedure to widen a contracted alar base.
- In correcting a wide alar base, it is vital first to check for de-projection of the nasal tip, which can cause a sagging in the lateral ala.
- In most traumatic patients, correcting and increasing tip projection is all that is necessary to narrow the width of the alar base.
- Surgery to correct a scarred contracted alar base is more difficult to achieve meaningful long-term structural outcomes.
- In a contracted vestibular stenosis due to scarring, it is best not to "excise" the scar but to "incise" the scar and elevate the scar from the bony surface and re-epithelialise with split-thickness skin graft.
- Contracted alar base is also associated with functional issues, which can be very difficult to address.

References

1. Tardy ME Jr, Patt BS, Walter MA. Alar reduction and sculpture: anatomic concepts. Facial Plast Surg. 1993;9(4):295–305.
2. Daniel RK. Rhinoplasty: nostril/tip disproportion. Plast Reconstr Surg. 2001;107:1454. Davis RE. Diagnosis and surgical management of the caudal excess nasal deformity. Arc Facial Plast Surg. 2005;7:100.
3. Daniel RK. The nasal base. In: Daniel RK, editor. Aesthetic plastic surgery: rhinoplasty. Boston: Little, Brown; 1993.
4. Crumley RL. Aesthetics and surgery of the nasal base. Facial Plast Surg. 1988;5(2):135–42.
5. Gruber RP, Freeman MB, Hsu C, et al. Nasal base reduction; a treatment algorithm including alar release with medialisation. Plast Reconstr Surg. 2009;123:716.
6. Weir RF. On restoring noses without scarring the face. N Y Med J. 1892;56:449–54.
7. Guyruron B. Alar base surgery. In: Gunter JP, Rohrich RJ, Adams WP, editors. Dallas Rhinoplasty: Nasal Surgery by the Masters. 2nd ed. St Louis, MO: Quality Medical Publishing, 2007.
8. Kridel RW, Castellano RD. A simplified approach to alar base reduction: a review of 124 patients over 20 years. Arch Facial Plast Surg. 2005;7(2):81–93.

9. Anderson JR. A reasoned approach to nasal base surgery. Arch Otolaryngol. 1984;110(6):349–58.
10. Adamson P, Litner JA, Dahiya HR. The M-Arch model: a new concept of nasal tip dynamics. Arch Facial Plast Surg. 2006;8:16–25.
11. Warner JP, Chauhan N, Adamson PA. Alar soft-tissue techniques in rhinoplasty: algorithmic approach, quantifiable guidelines, and scar outcomes from a single surgeon experience. Arch Facial Plast Surg. 2010;12(3):149–58.
12. Silver WE, Sajjadian A. Nasal base surgery. Otolaryngol Clin North Am. 1999;32(4):653–68.
13. McCarthy JG, Wood-Smith D. Rhinoplasty. In: McCarthy JG, editor. Plastic surgery. Philadelphia: WB Saunders; 1990.
14. Adamson PA, Oakley S, Tropper GJ, McGraw BL. Analysis of alar base narrowing. Am J Cosmet Surg. 1990;7:239–43.
15. Balaji N, Ravichandran S. Assessment of nasal valve obstruction : a new nasal "wall" subunit concept. ENT Audiol News. 2012;21(4):111–3.

Cleft Lip Nasal Tip Rhinoplasty

Contents

N. Balaji, *Textbook of Nasal Tip Rhinoplasty*, https://doi.org/10.1007/978-3-030-48157-5_14

Learning Objectives

- To understand the anatomy of the alar base and nasal tip cartilages in cleft lip patients before planning surgical treatment.
- To understand the pathology of nasal tip cartilages in patients with cleft lips.
- To understand the surgical principles in correcting the tip deformities in cleft lip noses.

14.1 Introduction

Patients born with cleft lip are more likely to have distortion of the tip cartilages of the nose on the affected side, usually unilateral but can be bilateral. This is a very specialised area of nasal tip reconstruction that requires a combination of various different techniques as described in other chapters. The reader is advised to look into specialised monologues of more experienced surgeons on this topic [2, 6, 7, 9]. The same concepts of tip reconstruction as described for traumatic and congenital noses generally apply to nasal tip reconstruction in cleft lip noses. The key factor in this surgery is to be aware of the various different deformities that are common in a cleft lip nose. Often the same sequence should be applied starting from correcting the septum, then moving on to medial crus and then the dome and then the lateral crural cartilages. The next important factor is the timing of nasal tip surgery as patients present at a younger age due to social pressures of nasal deformity associated with cleft lip. Generally it is advisable to wait till they are 15 or 16 before major surgical intervention. This is not because of the status of tip cartilages, but predominantly because of the opportunity it offers to correct the septum which is more important for long-term stability of tip work in these patients. But based on the surgeon's personal experience and type of patients, primary tip work can also be performed at the time of primary cleft lip surgery [6–8]. Most of these patients in our practice are adults with myriad of deformities, already mentioned in the text, requiring complex reconstructive techniques. These patients can present with primary tip cartilage deformities associated with cleft lip, but also present with deformities secondary to super added nasal trauma and also present with deformity secondary to multiple failed reconstructive attempts.

14

14.2 The Deformities Commonly Encountered Include the Following

- Loss of medial crural height (tip height), usually on the side of the cleft causing asymmetry or equally on both sides in bilateral cleft causing de-projection of nasal tip.
- Lateral crural flattening and loss of lateral alar convexity that cause a pseudo lengthening of the lateral crus (Fig. 14.1). This also results in loss of smooth Intermediate crus, and there is a sharp angulation at the dome between the medial crus and the lateral crus junction [1–4].
- Presents clinically as a Boxy, wide and deprojected nasal tip (Figs. 14.1–14.3). Nostril shape can be abnormal with vertical shortening of nostril axis and superior blunting of the nostril shape, usually on the side of the cleft, but may present with a variety of shapes due to scarring (Fig. 14.4), secondary to surgical trauma of revision surgery or associated non-surgical trauma.
- Nasal sil abnormalities, most commonly being loss of smooth and pleasing sil (Fig. 14.4) on the affected side.
- Lack of caudal septal cartilage with varying degrees of columellar retraction.
- Blunting of the nasal tip due to lack of tip projection either due to loss of anterior septal angle or due to intrinsic loss of lower lateral cartilage height (Fig. 14.5).
- In unilateral patients, there will be asymmetric dome height with affected side dome lower than the other normal side.
- Scarring of the columellar skin due either to previous cleft lip surgery or even previous rhinoplasty surgery (Fig. 14.6).
- Abnormalities of the upper lip with an increase in the vertical height and flattening of the upper lip.

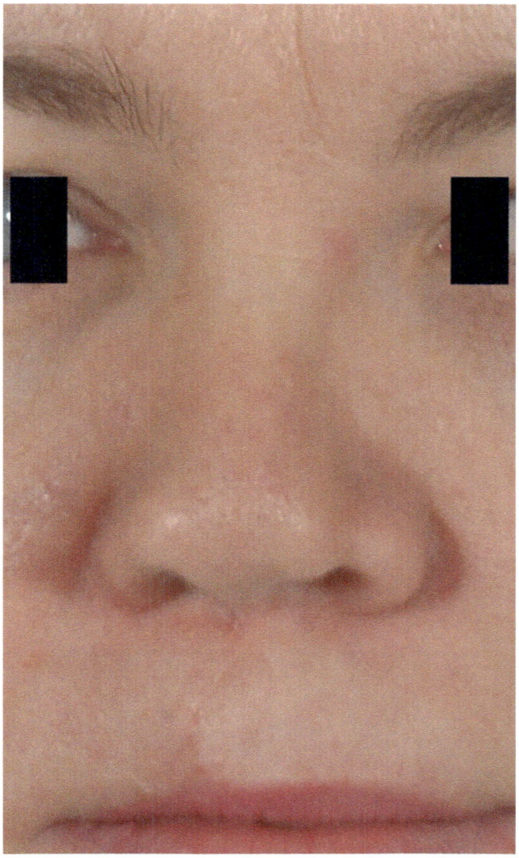

Fig. 14.1 Frontal view showing a de-projected and wide nasal tip in a cleft lip nose with pseudo-lengthening of the left lateral crus

- Vestibular stenosis associated with scarring of the upper lip extending into the nasal floor.
- Functional nasal obstruction could be due to lateral alar weakness, loss of tip height, distortion of nostrils size and shape [5].

14.3 Surgical Principles and Techniques Available to Correct Cleft Lip Nasal Deformity

- The same principles used in correcting a traumatic nasal tip deformity as described in other chapters apply to the cleft lip nose as well, although the results are much more difficult to achieve due to intrinsic weakness of the cartilages.
- The sequence and timing of the surgery is the key for achieving best outcomes. Waiting till the patient is old enough (15 or 16 years of age) is ideal as it helps to do a full septal reconstruction if necessary, which is an important initial step before doing primary surgery on the tip cartilages. But studies have shown earlier intervention during initial cleft lip repair is also beneficial [6–8].
- As the lower lateral cartilages are commonly deformed, an open approach is preferable for adequate exposure and execution of various techniques [9].
- Once the flap is raised the septal cartilage is reconstructed both in the dorsal and caudal segments and repositioned in midline. This may be a simple septoplasty or a spreader graft or a septal dorsal or caudal extension graft depending on the findings.

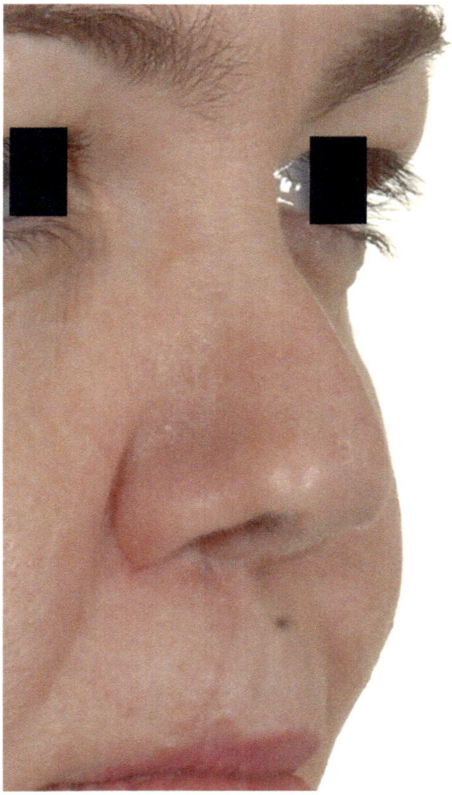

Fig. 14.2 Right three-fourth view showing a de-projected and wide nasal tip in a cleft lip nose

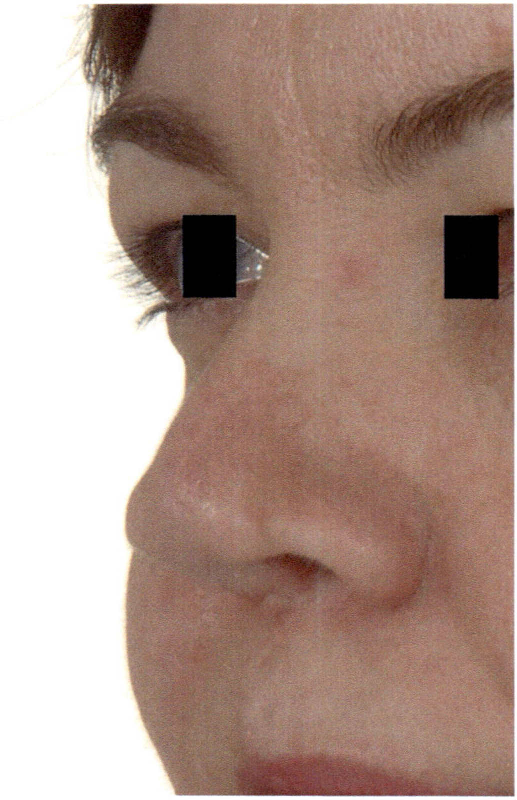

Fig. 14.3 Left three-fourth view showing a deprojected and wide nasal tip in a cleft lip nose

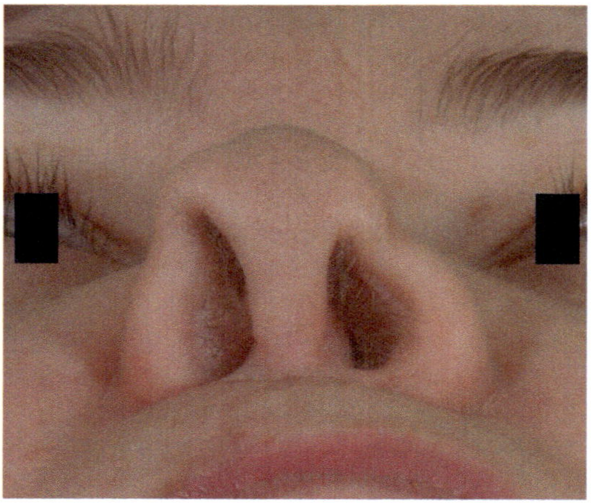

Fig. 14.4 Basal view of the nose showing nostril abnormalities with scarring and asymmetric tip height with loss of tip projection

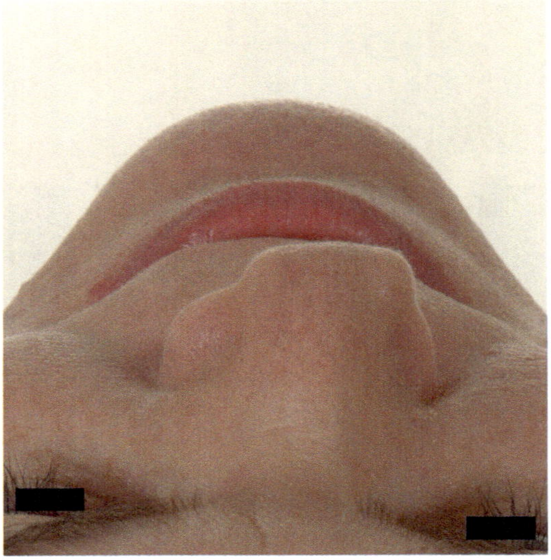

Fig. 14.5 Loss of tip projection and a flat trapezoidal tip

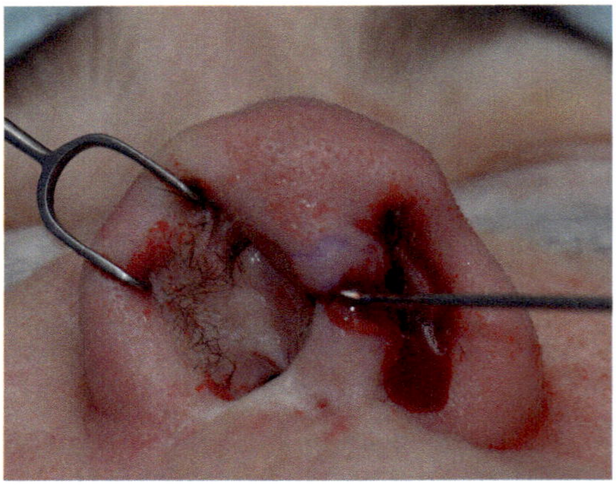

Fig. 14.6 Basal view of the nose showing mucosal scarring after revision surgery in a cleft lip nose

- The tip projection can be established by a lateral crural steel with or without a columellar strut graft.
- Our preferred way of raising the tip projection on the affected side would be to separate the lateral crus from the underlying mucosa, right up to the dome. Ideally separating the lateral crus from underlying mucosa helps in moving the often sagging and flat lateral crus medially towards the centre of the nasal tip and create a new dome at the same height as the other side

with trans-domal sutures. Completely freeing the lateral crus from the underlying mucosa also helps to facilitate lateral crural strut grafting if the lateral crus is weak.
- The next step would be to bring together the two medial crura with medial crural fixation suture as described in the chapter on sutures.
- Then the medial crus in the columella is strengthened by either suturing the two medial crus together by medial crural flare control sutures, if they are structurally strong. If the medial crura is not strong enough, then a columellar strut is used to strengthen the tip and increase tip projection.
- If there is lateral alar weakness, the lateral crus is strengthened with a lateral crural strut graft to prevent functional collapse of the lateral ala region.
- Finally, might need a shield graft to increase projection and soften the infra-tip lobule segment. Also a dorsal supra-tip cap graft may be needed to achieve a desirable dorsal profile line.
- An additional alar rim graft may be needed to correct the alar margin retraction if present.

Conclusion

The surgical techniques used in cleft lip noses are no different from the ones described for traumatic nasal tip deformities, but co-existing issues can make this surgery very complex, particularly cutaneous scarring. Timing of the surgery, adequate planning and sequencing the surgical steps are important to achieve consistent results. It is also important to be aware that these patients may need more than one procedure to achieve acceptable long-term outcomes.

Key Points Box

- Patients with cleft lips can be associated with nasal tip deformities, particularly involving the lateral crura either on one or both sides.
- Wide de-projected and asymmetric tip is the most common tip deformity in a cleft lip nose.
- Timing of the surgery, adequate planning and sequencing of the surgical steps are important to achieve consistent results.
- Patients and family should be counselled well before embarking on this type of surgery. They must be warned that they may need multiple procedures to achieve acceptable long-term cosmesis and functional improvement.
- This is a very specialist area of practice. Although the same surgical principles of tip plasty is applied to cleft lip noses, the presence of co-existing surgical issues, particularly cutaneous scarring can make this surgery very complex.

References

1. Stenstrom SJ. The alar cartilage and the nasal deformity in unilateral cleft lip. Plast Reconstr Surg. 1996;38:223–31.
2. Sykes JM, Senders CW. Pathologic anatomy of cleft lip, palate, and nasal deformities. In: Meyers AD, editor. Biological basis of facial plastic surgery. New York: Thieme Medical Publishers; 1993. p. 57–71.
3. Latham R. The pathogenesis of the skeletal deformity associated with unilateral cleft lip and palate. Cleft Palate Craniofac J. 1969;6:404–14.
4. Park BY, Lew DH, Lee YH. A comparative study of the lateral crus of alar cartilage in unilateral cleft lip nasal deformity. Plast Reconstr Surg. 1998;101:9150919.
5. Jablon JH, Sykes JM. Nasal airway problems in the cleft lip population. Facial Plast Surg Clin North Am. 1999;7:391–403.
6. Sykes JM. The importance of primary rhinoplasty at the time of initial unilateral cleft lip repair. Arch Facial Plast Surg. 2010;12(1):53–5.
7. Sykes JM, Senders CW. Surgical treatment of the unilateral cleft nasal deformity at the time of lip repair. Facial Plast Surg Clin North Am. 1995;3:69–77.
8. McIndoe A, Rees TD. Synchronous repair of secondary deformities in cleft lip and nose. Plast Reconstr Surg. 1959;24:150–61.
9. Sykes JM, Senders CW, et al. Use of the open approach for repair of secondary cleft lip-nasal deformities. Facial Plast Surg Clin North Am. 1993;1:111–26.

Closing the Skin Flap in Open Approach Nasal Tip Rhinoplasty

Contents

N. Balaji, *Textbook of Nasal Tip Rhinoplasty*, https://doi.org/10.1007/978-3-030-48157-5_15

Learning Objectives

- How to close the wound without causing damage to the wound edges.
- How to prevent any unwanted scarring or notching of the wound edges.

15.1 Introduction

Meticulous closure of the skin flap is very important or at times more important than the entire operation, as the patient notices any scar blemishes and equates that with poor outcomes [1–3]. Most of the post-operative scar issues or notching in the wound margins are secondarily due to improper planning, improper closure and damage to the skin margins due to improper use of instruments.

15.2 Surgical Technique

- This is the most important step of the entire operation. It is advisable to close the skin flap in two layers and to reduce the tension on the skin. But over the last 8 years, we have been closing the trans-columellar incision with a single deep skin closure with a non-absorbable 5-0 ethilon suture which has not caused any issues either. There are pros and cons of both.
- Before closing the skin flap, close the septal mucosal flaps first, if it is elevated through a separate incision. This is done with 5-0 absorbable vicryl usually interrupted.
- The FIRST suture in the sequence is closing the alar marginal incision (◘ Fig. 15.1). We suggest the use of one or two absorbable 5-0 vicryl sutures to close the lateral alar marginal incision first, thereby avoiding coming very close to the apex of the nostril to prevent any unwanted notching. Care must be taken to have the bite very close to the cut edges of the lateral alar incision site and not to take a big bite of soft tissues and cause thickening in this area, as it may cause external nasal valve obstruction later. Avoid putting a suture at the apex of the nostril as it will cause distortion and asymmetry of the alar margin. Care is also taken not to take a bite through the lower border of the lateral crus of the lower lateral cartilage. Do not leave any exposed lateral crural cartilage. Sometimes it is easy to forget to close this suture, so always remember to close both lateral alar incision sites first (◘ Fig. 15.2).
- Next the "W" trans-columellar incision is closed with 5-0 non-absorbable ethilon sutures (◘ Figs. 15.3 and 15.4). We usually put only two sutures, one on either side of the apex of the incision. These are the only two sutures to come out in a week's time. The number of sutures can vary with surgeon's preferences, but the key is to keep

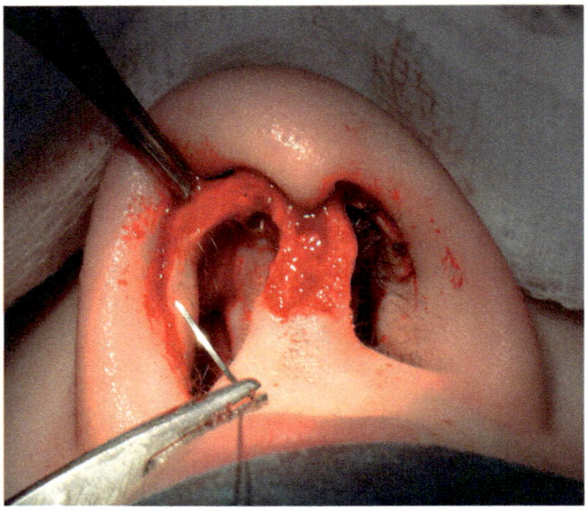

◘ **Fig. 15.1** Closure of the alar marginal incision with 5-0 absorbable suture

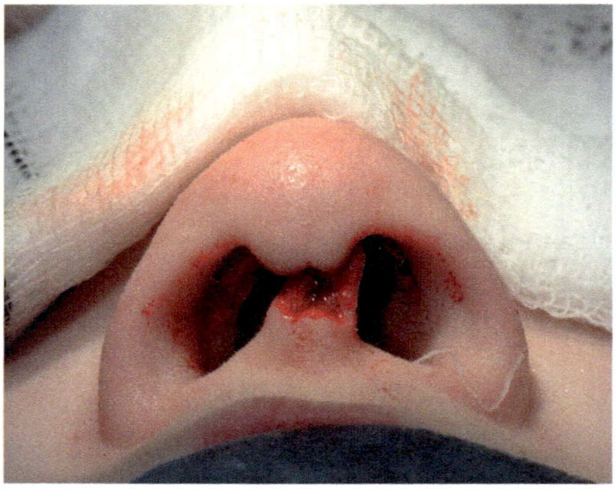

◘ **Fig. 15.2** The flap in place after bilateral placement of alar marginal sutures

15

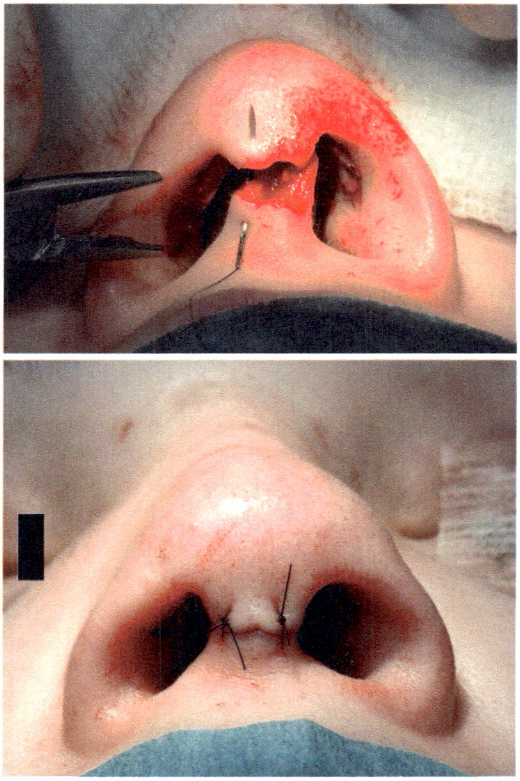

Figs. 15.3 and 15.4 Closing the columellar skin with 5-0 ethilon suture

the tissue trauma to the minimum and not using any forceps [4].

- The last in the sequence is to close the lateral vertical columellar marginal incision. This suture helps to restore the vertical length of the columella which invariably shortens after incision. Use two skin hooks to lift the apex of the nostril to stretch the upper columellar skin flap. The common problem here is the vertical shortening of the columellar marginal incision. This length has to be restored, otherwise there will be fore-shortening and hooding of ala. This suture is done with an absorbable 5-0 vicryl, suture.
- Finally a topical antibiotic and steroid cream of your choice is applied over the skin wound edges and the wound is kept moist and clean over the next 5 days. Be aware that naseptin cream we use in the UK has peanut oil, so contra-indicated in peanut allergy patients. Over the last 5 years, we have been using topical chloramphenicol eye ointment for a week at the suture site, which keeps the area moist and very helpful to prevent any crusts and thus helps in easy removal of sutures a week later.

Pearls and Pitfalls

- We used to start with a 5-0 vicryl single subcutaneous horizontal mattress suture of the trans-columellar incision before closing the skin. We have stopped using this over the last 8 years and have not regretted since. This suture is difficult and takes time to put since the flap is thin and not enough subcutaneous tissue thickness is available. Although this suture can take the tension "off" the skin suture, but the downside being this suture can cause asymmetry in the skin approximation preventing any minor adjustments to the skin margin not possible.
- Make sure there is just approximation of the flaps in the trans-columellar incision, may be with slight eversion of the wound margins in the trans-columellar region. Avoid step deformity where the superior flap overlaps the inferior flap, particularly after a reduction rhinoplasty, when the flap is lax and slightly excess [4, 5].
- Make sure there is no alar notching or disparity while closing the columellar incisions. The junctional areas between the various incisions should be clean and sharp, without any tissue loss or blunting.
- Avoid putting a suture at the apex of the nostril as it will cause distortion and asymmetry of the alar margin.
- Care is also taken not to take a bite through the lateral crural cartilage. Do not leave exposed lateral crural cartilage in the alar region as this will cause granulomas and nasal alar obstruction.
- Meticulous approximation using skin hooks and gentle pressure moulding of the skin edges with wet swabs at the end restores the natural curvatures of the columella.

Conclusion

The importance of closing the skin flap in fact begins at the incision planning stage before opening the skin. Spending time initially planning the incision avoids unnecessary issues later. Fine tissue handling is a must, thereby avoiding the use of destructive techniques.

Key Points Box

- Closing the skin flap should be meticulous, as any abnormality of the wound margins is visible.
- Care must be taken not to distort the alar margins and cause alar notching.
- Care must be taken not to introduce any dents or distortion of the columella, as any scarring or defects in the columella cannot be satisfactorily corrected.
- Do not leave the skin suturing to the trainees, and it is better for the senior surgeon to do the closure.

References

1. Adamson PA, Galli SK. Rhinoplasty approaches: current state of the art. Arch Facial Plast Surg. 2005;7:32–7.
2. Adamson PA, Smith O, Tropper GJ. Incision and scar analysis in open (external) rhinoplasty. Arch Otolaryngol Head Neck Surg. 1990;116(6):671–5.
3. Goodman WS. External approach to rhinoplasty. Can J Otolaryngol. 1973;2:207–10.
4. Adamson PA. Open rhinoplasty. Otolaryngol Clin North Am. 1987;20:837–52.
5. Goodman WS, Charles DA. Technique of external rhinoplasty. J Otolaryngol. 1978;7:13–7.

Post-operative Care and Complications After Nasal Tip Rhinoplasty

Contents

N. Balaji, *Textbook of Nasal Tip Rhinoplasty*, https://doi.org/10.1007/978-3-030-48157-5_16

Learning Objectives

- To understand the issues in the immediate post-operative care.
- To know how best to manage the patients in the immediate post-operative period.
- To be aware of both patient-related and surgeon-related complications.
- To learn how best to avoid these complications as much as possible.

16.1 Post-operative Care

- Rhinoplasty surgery in the UK is mostly done under general anaesthetic and not under sedation. Hence recovering a patient from the rhinoplasty procedure following a general anaesthetic involves a close co-operation between the anaesthetist, recovery nurse and the surgeon.
- The post-operative care begins in the initial consultation. Patient should be seen twice with an interval period, so that they have time to absorb verbal information. This should be reinforced with written material.
- Post-operative care in rhinoplasty begins with adequate preparation of the patient for surgery, both mentally and physically. The immediate family should be kept well informed, although it is sensible to allow only patients to make decisions.
- The patients should be advised to stop smoking before the surgery and up to 2 weeks after the surgery. The patient should be advised not to take any strong painkillers. Be aware of health foods which increases the bleeding time. We advice patients not to take any health foods, which can prolong bleeding time and affect clotting.
- Intra-operatively endotracheal tube or laryngeal mask with throat pack is used in the UK. Surgeons prefer the operative site to be as bloodless as possible, which may conflict with the anaesthetist's views depending on the patient's general health. Ideally hypotension along with low heart rate is preferable, and this should be discussed with the anaesthetist prior to induction depending on the health status of the patient. Be aware a low blood pressure alone may increase the pulse rate and be counterproductive.
- The patient should be nursed in head up position. In the recovery care must be taken not to apply pressure on the splints and avoid displacement of the osteotomised nasal and maxillary bones as they can be very unstable.
- In an open approach surgery, care must be taken not to apply any pressure on the wound by avoiding bolsters.
- If an open approach is planned, or in revision procedures, the patient is given per-operative intravenous broad-spectrum antibiotic during induction. Minimal tissue trauma with gentle handling of tissues is the key for fast recovery.
- Recovery should be smooth without coughing and the patient should be in a head up posture if possible with holding the facial mask upside down with wider section resting on the forehead and the narrower section resting on the chin with no pressure over the nose in the middle.
- Gentle suction in the back of the throat to clear any blood should be done under direct vision without sucking the uvula into the suction tip. Any mucosal damage to uvula will not settle for at least 2 weeks in the post-operative period with swelling and pain on swallowing. This can be very unpleasant to the patient.
- Sometimes patients can wake up aggressive and start rubbing and pulling on the splints and packing. Make sure the patient's hands are held gently preventing him from damaging the nose.
- Gentle constant verbal reassurance from the surgeon, while in the recovery will go a long way, although the patient is drowsy and sleepy as they are aware of surgeon's voice!
- After the patient is extubated and awake, they should be nursed in the upright posture with two pillows under the head.
- Post-operative or intra-operative dexamethasone helps both nausea and vomiting and post-operative swelling.
- There will be nasal packing and splints on the nose. The patients will feel there is something in the nose and may not be able to breath and hence may struggle. The

patient should be adequately reassured that they cannot breathe through the nose after surgery due to the nasal packing, but can breathe through the mouth.
- Extreme caution is important in monitoring patients with sleep apnoea, as their condition can be made worse on nasal packing, and hence their saturation overnight should be monitored and if necessary the nasal packing may need to be removed.
- Put pressure dressing for the ears if conchal or helical graft is harvested, which is usually removed after 12 hours.
- If rib cartilage is harvested, always look out for any post-operative pneumothorax.
- After discharge care is equally important. Patient should be told of their responsibilities to keep the nose safe from any injury. Avoiding trauma in the first post-operative week is important. The nose should be examined before discharge to make sure there is no septal haematoma. The patient should be warned about bruising and advised not to take any medications or food supplements which prolong the bleeding time. Patient should be advised to sleep with two or three pillows.
- The patient should be seen back in a week's time for removal of splints and external skin sutures.
- Finally, more importantly, the surgeon should always be available for any reassurance the patient needs.

16.2 Post-operative Complications

There is no surgical procedure without complications, and nasal tip reconstruction is not an exception. A literature search on the topic not surprisingly shows the maximum number of publications on complications following septorhinoplasty, ranging from simple to serious complications like blindness and brain injury to even death. The post-operative patient may fit into the following four categories:

- A happy patient and happy surgeon.
- A happy patient and unhappy surgeon.
- An unhappy patient and unhappy surgeon.
- An unhappy patient and a happy surgeon.

The first two categories where the patient is happy are acceptable situations. An unhappy patient and an unhappy surgeon is acceptable as the defect may be fixable and the patient can be referred to someone better. But a worrying situation is, if the patient is unhappy and the surgeon is happy with his performance. This means either the patient's psychological status is questionable or the surgeon's skills are questionable! But studies have shown that this is more often due to patient dissatisfaction due to psychological issues rather than to the surgical technique [1, 2].

16.2.1 Rhinoplasty Complications Fall into Two Main Groups

- *True complications* – these are defects which were directly or indirectly related to the surgery and not present before the surgical intervention.
- *Pseudo complications* – these are persistent deformities due to failure in achieving agreed outcomes.

Of course, the concern is more about the "true" complications than failure to achieve the outcomes which can be inherent to this type of surgery despite the surgeon's level of expertise. In our practise, "true" complications leading to revision surgery is around 5%, and majority of them are due to failure of osteotomy techniques [3].

16.2.2 The Following "True" Complications Can Happen After an Open Approach Tip Plasty

- External scar issues – improperly placed incisions (▣ Fig. 16.1), notching, keloid, hypertrophy and external valve issues with scarring at the inter-cartilaginous incision sites [4].
- Erythema and infection at the external scar site in the columella (▣ Fig. 16.2).

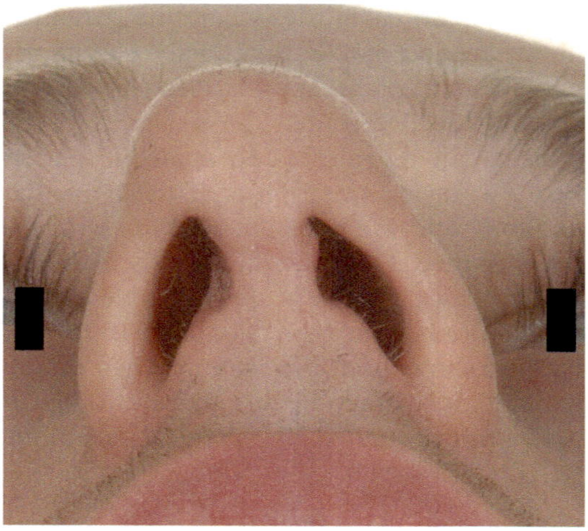

Fig. 16.1 Basal view of the nose showing distorted columellar scar due to misplaced columellar incision

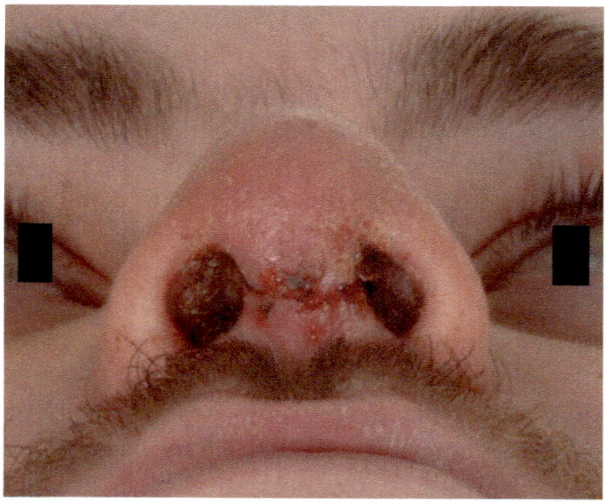

Fig. 16.2 Erythema and infection at the external scar site in the columella

- Septal haematoma, infection, septal perforation resulting in mid-dorsal collapse and delayed cosmetic issues.
- Prolonged oedema of the tip and numbness of tip [5].
- Use of non-absorbable sutures extruding through the overlying skin that causes infection, puckering and depressed scars.
- Minor dorsal irregularities, particularly when the overlying skin is very thin and due to failure to camouflage the dorsum with crushed cartilage or fascia [6].

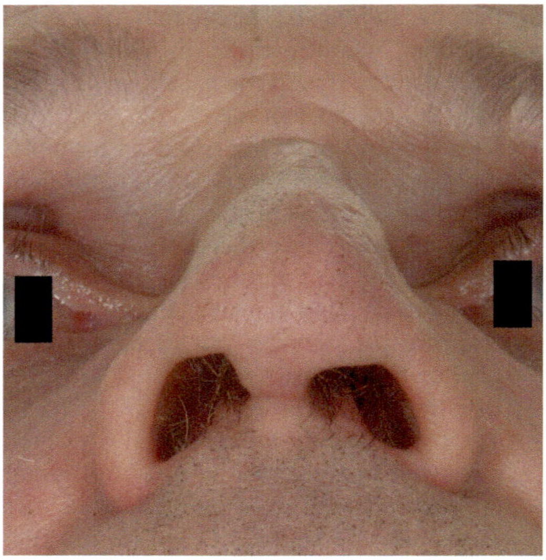

Fig. 16.3 Basal view of the nose showing notching of the columellar scar due to poor technique

- Osteotomy issues with persistent deviation of the complex, particularly when adequate medial osteotomies are not done properly. This is the common indication for my revision surgeries.
- Asymmetric nostril size, columellar notching (Fig. 16.3), alar retraction (Fig. 16.4) and rarely even excess columellar show due to excess cephalic trimming of the lateral crus.
- Tip deviations due to in appropriately placed tip sutures, particularly when the medial crus is sutured to the caudal septum which is not been centralised properly.
- Over rotation of the tip if the tip anchoring suture is tightened too much.
- Skin colour and texture changes in multiple revision surgeries (Fig. 16.5).
- Poly beak deformity due to persistent dorsal septal cartilaginous excess at the anterior septal angle [7].
- Pinocchio type of lower thirds tip over projection, if dorsal hump reduction is performed without addressing the tip over projection.
- Over resection of the lateral crural cartilages that causes lateral alar pinching.
- Damage to soft triangle due to injudicious use of curved scissors while dissecting tis-

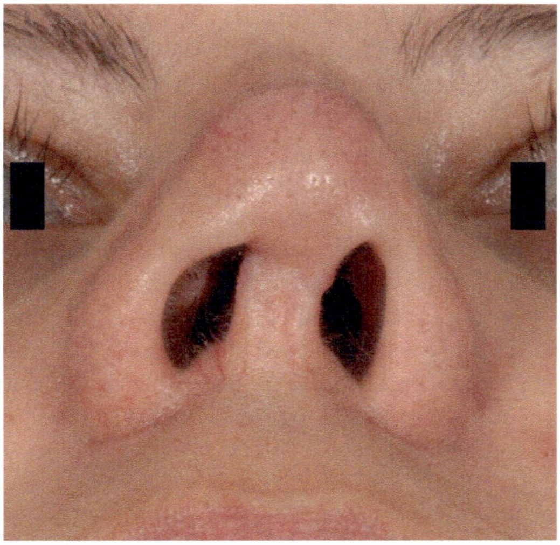

Fig. 16.4 Basal view of the nose showing distorted columellar scar and soft triangle scar and in drawing due to misplaced columellar incision

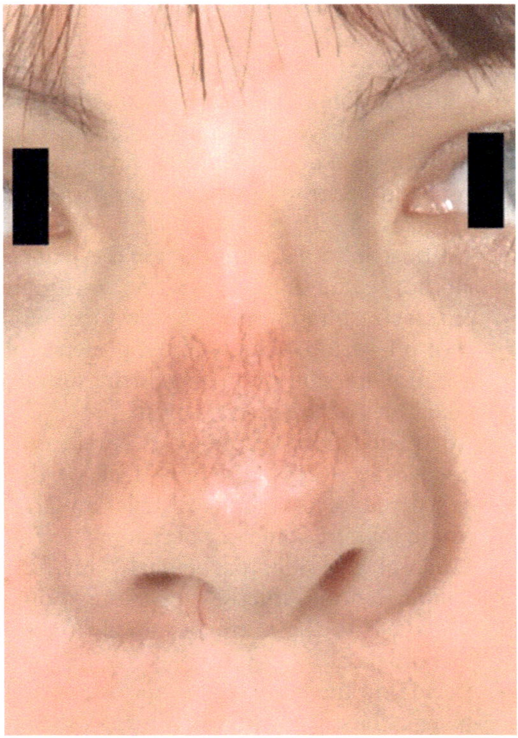

Fig. 16.5 Skin colour and texture changes in multiple revision surgeries

sues at the soft triangle and also due to inappropriately placed alar incisions.
- Over resection of the dorsum with inverted V deformity, with over resection of the upper lateral crus.
- Loss of sense of smell [8].
- Devitalisation of upper incisors [9].
- Extrusion of silastic implants (or any other foreign material) which can be devastating to the patients and extremely difficult to achieve some meaningful outcomes following revision surgery [10, 11].
- Functional issues with persistent or worsening nasal obstruction either due to over resected middle vault causing internal valve issues or excess resection of lateral crus causing external valve issues [12, 13].
- Serious complications have been reported in literature, including blindness, intracranial complication and even death [14, 15].

16.3 Post-operative Clinical Scenarios to Be Aware of to Avoid Unhappy Patients

- Patients usually come alone during the first appointment, but invariably come with the two of the close relatives or friends when the splints comes off in a week's time. It is always wise to see a patient with their relatives during the initial discussion so that everyone is aware of our identified goals and outcomes. Otherwise when the splints comes off, an accompanying relative or a friend whom you have not seen before can pass a negative comment as soon as the splints come off. This sets a chain of events which can lead to an unhappy patient.
- Most patients complain about very obvious deformities like deviation or a large hump, but not complain of associated minor deformities. As a surgeon, you need to point out the other minor deformities like nostril asymmetries prior to surgery. Otherwise despite achieving the major outcomes, you will end up in an unhappy patient.

- Do not operate on a psychologically disturbed patient. These are patients to be avoided or counselled properly before surgery. Even an experienced surgeon can miss a difficult patient if not constantly on guard. Always listen to third sense that you may be dealing with a difficult demanding and over expecting or unrealistic patient.
- Some patients in the post-operative period may raise a concern that they were not aware of such a complication. Hence record keeping is vital. Written material is better than verbal advice. An informed consent with written leaflets is a must.
- Seeing patients twice or even thrice is important. A "cool-off" period is important for both the patient and the surgeon. Please do not operate on patients before you are convinced that they are fully aware of the consequences and results of surgery. Having said that most patients have decided whether they like you or have confidence in you at the very first appointment.
- Agree a set of goals or outcomes which are practical and easy to quantify before you proceed for surgery. Make sure you give written post-operative instructions. This is an important phase where patients should feel well supported.
- When dealing with functional aspects of septorhinoplasty, the surgeon needs to explain that the functional improvement in breathing will not be better for at least 6 weeks and may take up to 3 months. Otherwise failure to improve the breathing in the immediate post- operative period may be equated as a "failure" by the patient.
- In septoplasty surgery, it will also be worthwhile pointing out that the septum is a midline structure and you can access it through the right nostril or the left nostril and whichever side you access it there will be sutures. This prevents patients to assume quickly in the immediate post-operative period that the lack of improvement in the nasal function is because the surgeon has done the wrong side, simply because they saw the sutures on the opposite side of the nasal obstruction. This has happened to us before!
- Deal with patient's expectations genuinely and sincerely – the surgeon can only improve the deformity by moving the grades down by a point or two, but will never make a nose 100% better.
- Remember while doing the revision procedure, the final surgeon will be in the patients' mind and technically responsible for everything which has happened before. It is not that whether we can technically correct the deformity that matters, but whether we are going to make the patient happy at the end of the procedure is what matters.
- Remember despite all the efforts and care, still an unhappy patient can cause trouble which can last for years!

16.4 Dealing with Revision Surgery Patients

- Dealing with revision surgery patients, either your own or someone else, please make sure your agreed goals are realistic – it is not what the surgeon can technical achieve which matters, but it is all about how it is going to heal and how happy the patient is going to be after the surgery [16].
- If you think you can make the situation worse, please do not consider revision surgery and better refer to a more experienced colleague.
- Adequate photo documentation is essential.
- Do not see these patients alone. Adequate repeat consultations may be few times with cool-off period, usually in the presence of a senior nursing or management staff to take notes of the conversation.
- Adequate record keeping is essential.
- Assess the overlying skin – thick or thin or scarred, colour changes. This can guide you in making some key decisions.
- Mucosal scarring, particularly any vestibular stenosis, mucosal adhesions should be noted as these are not easily fixable pathologies.
- Decide on the approach either internal or external based on various clinical issues.
- Picking the correct tools – a combination of sutures and grafts are used in revision surgeries. Conchal cartilage, helical rim cartilage, septal cartilage and rib cartilage are preferred. Alloplastic materials should

be avoided in revision surgeries. It is better to use fascia lata or temporalis fascia when the overlying skin is very thin with colour changes.

- Finally any revision procedure in our experience should be kept simple and try to achieve maximum benefit with minimum disruption to the skeleton. To achieve this, it is extremely important to know during the consultation process what exactly will make the patient happier.

Conclusion

A clever surgeon learns from his mistakes and anticipate problems and try to prevent future complications. Meticulous planning, surgical sequence, delicate handling of tissues, correct placement of incisions, aseptic technique and minimal trauma are all important to prevent complications. Try and do the minimum to achieve the maximum benefit. Remember, do not try and use all the techniques which you have seen in a training course or a video. The more techniques you use, there is more risk of introducing variables and increased likelihood of an unhappy patient.

Key Points Box

- Nasal tip surgery has got its own share of complications.
- Meticulous planning and surgical sequence are important.
- Delicate handling of tissues with minimal trauma is important to prevent complications.
- Per-operative single dose of broad-spectrum antibiotic is used in most centres when open nasal tip surgery is contemplated.

References

1. Burgess LPA, Everton DM, Quilligan JJ, et al. Complications of the external (combination) rhinoplasty approach. Arch Otolaryngol Head Neck Surg. 1986;112:1064–8.
2. Padovan IF, Jugo SB. The Complications of External Rhinoplasty. Ear Nose Throat J. 1991;70(7):454–6.
3. Rettinger G. Complication or mistake. Facial Plast Surg. 1997;13(1):1.
4. Rettinger G, Zenkel M. Skin and soft tissue complications. Facial Plast Surg. 1997;13(1):51–9.
5. Thompson AC. Nasal tip numbness following rhinoplasty. Clin Otolaryngol Allied Sci. 1987;12(2):143–4.
6. Sessions RB. Complications of rhinoplasty. Laryngol Rhinol Otol (Stuttg). 1983;62:185–95.
7. Tardy ME Jr, Kron TK, Younger R, Key M. The cartilaginous pollybeak: etiology, prevention and treatment. Facial Plast Surg. 1989;6(2):113–20.
8. Champion R. Anosmia associated with corrective rhinoplasty. Br J Plast Surg. 1966;19(2):182–5. Devitalisation of upper incisors.
9. Sykes JM, Toriumi D, Kerth JD. A devitalized tooth as a complication of septorhinoplasty. Arch Otolaryngol Head Neck Surg. 1987;113(7):765–7.
10. Adamson PA. Grafts in rhinoplasty: autogenous grafts are superior to alloplastic. Arch Otolaryngol Head Neck Surg. 2000;126:561–2.
11. Deva AK, Merten S, Chang L. Silicone in nasal augmentation rhinoplasty: a decade of clinical experience. Plast Reconstr Surg. 1998;102(4):1230–7.
12. Adamson PA, Smith O, Cole P. The effect of cosmetic rhinoplasty on nasal patency. Laryngoscope. 1990;100:358–9.
13. Beekhuis GJ. Nasal obstruction after rhinoplasty: etiology and techniques for correction. Laryngoscope. 1976;86(4):540–8.
14. Cheney ML, Blair PA. Blindness as a complication of rhinoplasty. Arch Otolaryngol Head Neck Surg. 1987;113(7):768–9.
15. Marshall DR, Slattery PG. Intracranial complications of rhinoplasty. Br J Plast Surg. 1983;36(3):342–4.
16. Tardy ME Jr, Cheng EY, Jernstrom V. Misadventures in nasal tip surgery: analysis and repair. Otolaryngol Clin North Am. 1987;20(4):797–823.

Nasal Valve Surgery

Contents

N. Balaji, *Textbook of Nasal Tip Rhinoplasty*, https://doi.org/10.1007/978-3-030-48157-5_17

Learning objectives

- To cover the surgical anatomy of the nasal valve complex area.
- To go through existing concepts of external and internal valve classification and show how the current system of external and internal valve is not helpful.
- To suggest a "Glasgow nasal wall subunit" system [2, 3] to help in the diagnosis and management of nasal valve pathology.
- To understand how the nasal wall subunit system helps to achieve consistency and uniformity in the diagnosis and management of nasal obstruction.

17.1 Introduction

The diagnosis and surgical management of nasal valve surgery have always been shrouded in mystery, even for experienced surgeons [1, 5–8], and pose a big dilemma in getting a uniform consensus in teaching and training the residents, as very few surgeons agree with each other on the aetiology of nasal obstruction in one particular patient. Part of the reason being nose is a subjective organ and many tests available to objectively assess the air flow cannot be related to clinical symptoms. We have done few surveys in big conferences and was surprised how many experienced surgeons disagree with each other regarding diagnosis and management of functional nasal valve disorders. Survey outcomes in Scotland and the UK over the years showed consistent responses with only two-thirds of the qualified surgeons being confident to diagnose clinically external nasal obstruction and internal nasal valve obstruction and that figure drops to one-third when it comes to deciding the surgical plan. This is the same among senior trainees or experienced surgeons. It is rather surprising that despite these findings among experienced surgeons, we are still using the terminology "external and internal" nasal valve surgery. ***Ever since the term "nasal valve complex" was first coined*** [1, 6]***, although anatomically proven, this differentiation between external and internal valve regions is of no practical value in the patient management.***

17

Nasal obstruction is one of the common presenting symptoms to the otolaryngology department. It is a subjective symptom, which can be due either to mucosal problems like rhinitis or structural problems involving the cartilaginous or bony nasal skeleton. The term "nasal valve complex" was first coined by Mink in 1903. He described this site as the narrowest portion of the nasal cavity which offers the greatest resistance to nasal airflow. As per the current literature, the nasal valve complex is bordered ***superiorly*** by the caudal end of the upper lateral cartilages and septum. ***Posteriorly*** it is bordered by the inferior turbinate. The ***inferior border*** is the nasal floor and the ***lateral border*** is the bony pyriform aperture and adjacent fibro fatty tissue of the ala. Traditionally this nasal valve complex is split into the **"internal nasal valve"** and **"external nasal valve"** [1]. The internal nasal valve (INV) is a specific area located superiorly within the nasal valve complex. It is the junctional area between the caudal end of the upper lateral cartilage laterally, and the adjacent caudal nasal septum medially. This usually subtends an angle of between 10 and 15 degrees. Subjects with an internal nasal valve angle of less than 10 degrees tend to present with obstructive symptoms. External nasal valve is the area from the nasal entrance to the internal valve, and it is the alar margin composed of lower lateral cartilages and the floor. It is not as well defined as the internal nasal valve area.

17.2 Why the Current Classification of Internal and External Valve System Is Not User Friendly?

- ***In a patient with nasal obstruction, diagnosing the site of nasal obstruction is paramount***. The current classification of internal nasal valve and external nasal valve, albeit, anatomically proven, has its own drawbacks.
- Traditional teaching regarding nasal valve obstruction as stated above has centred on the categorisation of defects into those affecting the internal nasal valve area

(higher up in the nose) and those affecting the external nasal valve area (lower down in the nose). This categorisation requires drawing ***"an imaginary horizontal boundary line"*** between the superior internal nasal valve area and inferior external nasal valve area. However ***"in practice",*** it is not possible to draw this imaginary line in a deformed nose (◘ Fig. 17.1) and hence not possible to arrive at a tailored surgical solution.

- ***"In practice",*** in a traumatic nose with multiple deformities (requiring complex procedures) the so-called external nasal valve, internal nasal valve and also areas ***"in between"*** are involved making it difficult to accurately define the site of the lesion, hence making it difficult to choose the right surgical option.
- Moreover, not all deformities causing nasal obstruction can be fitted into the classification of internal and external nasal valve problems. For example, based on the above definition of external and internal valve, patients with extensive deformity of the nose (◘ Figs.17.1 and 17.2) will not fit into either external valve or internal valve problems. Another example will be vestibular stenosis which cannot be classified into either internal or external nasal valve problems. Again aging changes with upper and lower lateral weakness with a ptotic obstructive tip cannot be classified into a specific group either (◘ Fig. 17.3).
- The perceptions of the rhinologist regarding anatomical boundaries of what is actually internal and external nasal valve do vary; hence, comparative data of any intervention becomes meaningless.
- Apart from the internal and external valves, there is also literature on "septal valves" and "turbinal valves" [1] which adds to the spectrum of confusion.
- Thus simply drawing an imaginary horizontal line in the middle of the nose and

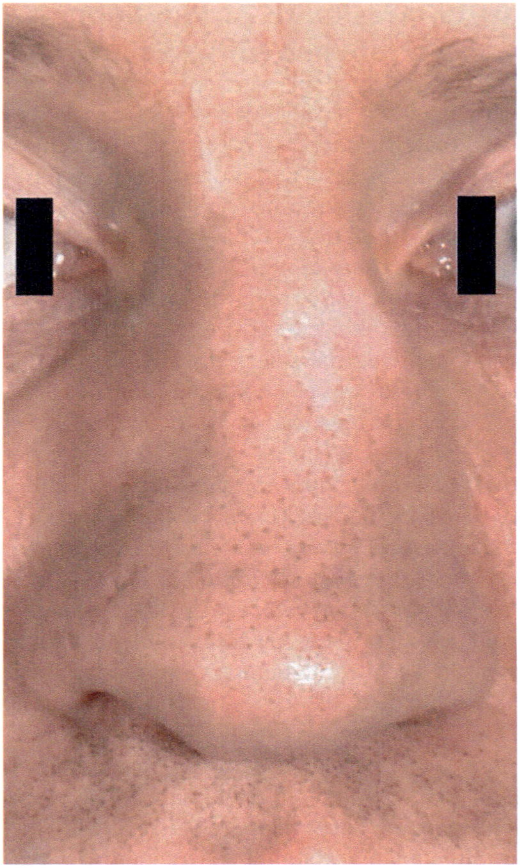

◘ **Fig. 17.1** Frontal view of the nose showing extensive deformity where ***"an imaginary horizontal boundary line"*** cannot be drawn between the superior internal nasal valve area and inferior external nasal valve area

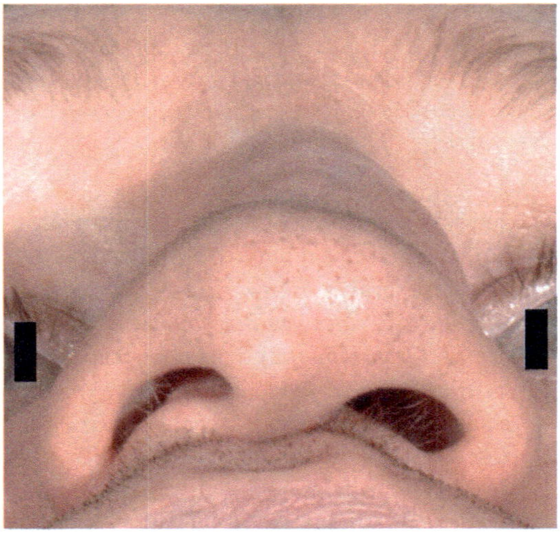

◘ **Fig. 17.2** Basal view showing extensive deformity of the nose, which cannot be classified easily into external and internal nasal valve issues

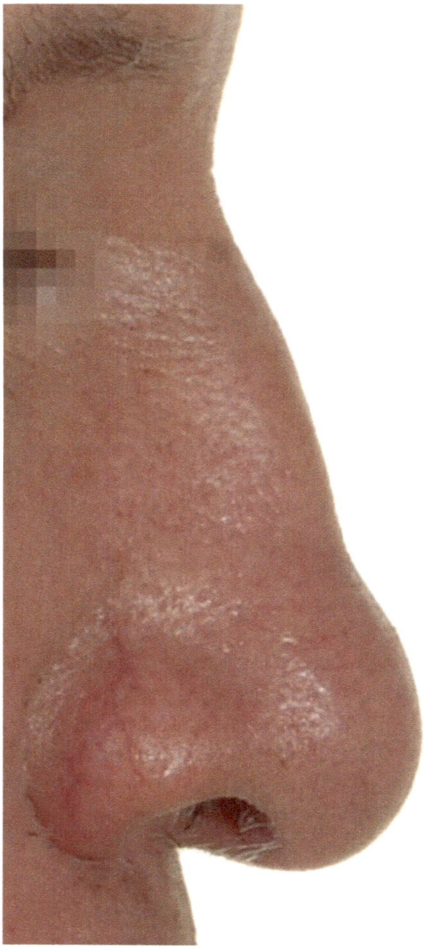

Fig. 17.3 Lateral view showing a ptotic aging nose with upper and lower lateral wall weakness, which again cannot be classified easily into external and internal nasal valve issues

dividing the areas of obstruction into superior internal nasal valve and inferior external nasal valve is ***not always practically possible*** and ***does not help in identifying the site of the problem*** and ***so does not help in the management plan*** either. Hence it is not a surprise that after 100 years since Mink described this area, surgeons still have problems in making an appropriate anatomical diagnosis of nasal valve obstructions and arriving at specific interventions which can be standardised and Mink's classification of nasal valve problems have gone unchallenged for over a century!

17

17.3 Glasgow Nasal Wall Sub-unit Concept

The concept which we use involves a user friendly, clinical classification based on anatomical sub-unit sites in the nose, which the rhinologists are already familiar with and hence can easily visualise a surgical option. Thus, in contrast to the terms, external and internal nasal valves, the concept which we use [2, 3] re-defines the nasal airway into simple, easy to use ***"Anatomical areas and sub-units"*** as follows:

17.3.1 "Medial" Nasal Wall Areas and "Lateral" Nasal Wall Areas with Various Subunit Problems Within Each Area

The **"medial"** nasal wall (MW) area (the so-called internal nasal valve region) is the central area of the nose which is easily seen on nasal speculum examination and diagnostic endoscopic examination of the nose. In contrast, the ***"lateral" nasal wall areas*** (the so-called external nasal valve region) that causing nasal obstruction are paired lateral areas of the nose involving the side walls and also can be seen on nasal speculum examination and diagnostic endoscopic examination of the nose.

The **"medial"** nasal wall (**MW**) is further divided into the following sub-units from above downwards, namely (1) ***high dorsal septum,*** (2) ***anterior membranous and caudal membranous septum,*** (3) ***conjoined medial crural foot plates and*** (4) ***soft tissue columella***. All these medial wall sub-units are easily accessible by examination and hence a diagnostic and management algorithm can be formulated which can be standardised and reproducible. The **"lateral"** nasal wall (LW) areas causing nasal obstruction are more difficult to diagnose and manage. The **"lateral"** nasal wall (**LW**) is further divided into the following sub-units from above downwards, namely (1) ***caudal nasal bones with upper lateral cartilage and "K" area,*** (2) ***junctional areas between upper and lower lateral cartilage including the scroll region,*** (3) ***lateral crus of the lower lateral cartilage and*** (4) ***soft tissue alar***

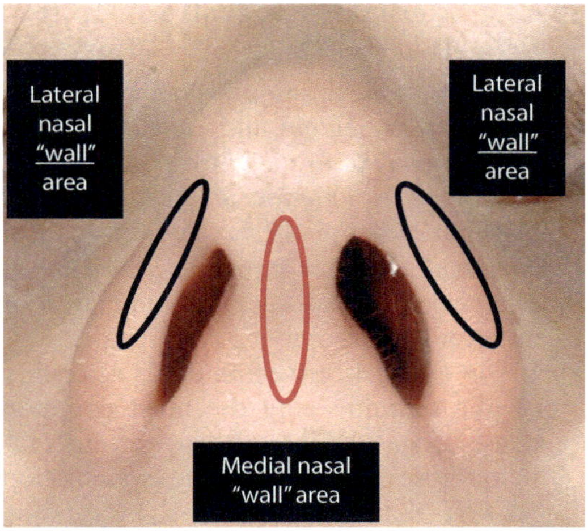

Fig. 17.4 Schematic representation of the New Glasgow nasal wall sub-unit concept with medial nasal wall sub-units and lateral nasal wall sub-units. (Reproduced with kind permission from Refs. [2, 3])

margin, including soft triangle. All these four sub-unit site pathologies in the lateral nasal wall may not be clinically obvious on examination, and sometimes an open approach is the only way to make the right diagnosis, particularly lateral crural issues.

The *main advantage* of classifying the valve areas into "medial and lateral wall sub-units" is that it helps the rhinologist to focus on the ***"aetiological anatomy"*** of the defects, which in turn helps in tailoring the surgery to the particular site. We have been using this form of classification in assessing nasal valve problems, over the past 13 years and this has not only given us the clarity of diagnosis, but also helped in the surgical planning tailored to individual needs (Fig. 17.4).

17.3.1.1 "Medial Nasal Wall" Valve Area

"Medial" nasal wall sub-unit problems are more common in our practice than "lateral" wall sub-unit issues. The problems could be in the following anatomical **"sub-units"** in the "medial" nasal wall region from above downwards, which are easier to diagnose and thus easier to tailor the surgical procedures.

1. High dorsal septum – **MW 1**.
2. Caudal membranous septum and anterior membranous septum – **MW 2**.
3. Conjoined medial crural footplate – **MW 3**.
4. Soft tissue columella – **MW 4**.

17.3.1.2 "Lateral Nasal Wall" Valve Area

"Lateral" nasal wall problems are less common cause of airway obstruction in our practice based on our cohort of patients. The problems could be in the following anatomical **"sub-units"** in the "lateral" nasal wall region from above downwards:

1. Caudal nasal bones with upper lateral cartilage and "K" area – **LW 1**.
2. Junctional area between upper and lower lateral cartilage including the scroll – **LW 2**.
3. Lateral crus of the lower lateral cartilage – **LW 3**.
4. Soft tissue alar margin, including soft triangle – **LW 4**.

17.4 Diagnostic and Management Algorithm of Medial Nasal Wall Pathology

Nasal obstruction is a subjective symptom, and an objective finding in the nose may not subjectively relate to the functional symptoms. Nevertheless the nearest you can come to is to make the right structural diagnosis to account for the functional issues. There is a constant quest for diagnosing anatomical deformities in the nose which we presume is the cause of the functional issues in the nose. The areas of maximum resistance is considered to be internal nasal valve area (high midline nasal region) and external nasal valve area (lower lateral nasal region).

Based on our experience, we suggest an algorithm in the management of patients with nasal obstruction first looking for pathology in the medial nasal "WALL" region working from top down. The "sequence" should always be managing midline abnormalities first and then dealing with lateral nasal wall regions [4]. A description of various sub-unit pathologies in the **"medial nasal wall" areas** and a diagnostic algorithm to arrive at a targeted surgical solution is provided in the following text. **Assessment** begins with history and examination that are aimed at individual areas and sub-units as mentioned above.

17.4.1 "Medial Nasal Wall" Area (MW): Sub-unit Pathology, Diagnosis and Targeted Surgical Solutions

17.4.1.1 Medial Nasal Wall Sub-unit One (MW1)

- This anatomical sub-unit site is a ***high dorsal septum.***
- Pathology is usually ***high dorsal septum deviations*** (Fig. 17.5a, b).
- Diagnosed only by nasal endoscopic examination.
- Can be easily missed on anterior rhinoscopy and one of the reasons for failed septoplasty!
- Surgical options include ***adequate dorsal septoplasty*** with or without ***bilateral spreader grafts***.

17.4.1.2 Medial Nasal Wall Sub-unit Two (MW2)

- This anatomical sub-unit site is ***anterior membranous septum*** and ***caudal membranous septum*** (Fig. 17.5b).
- Pathology is ***anterior and caudal septal deviations*** (Fig. 17.6a–d)***, as seen most commonly together in traumatic noses.***
- Diagnosed by endoscopic examination or anterior rhinoscopy.
- In our experience, we found this deformity of the septum being the most common cause of nasal valve obstruction in traumatic noses. Seen on simple examination (Fig. 17.6d) or tip tilt test by rotating the tip up.
- In the basal view seen as an additional uninterrupted vertical line next to the soft tissue columella on the side of the dislocation extending along the entire length of the columella from the tip to the sil region as seen in the left nostril (Fig. 17.6b).
- This "un-interrupted vertical line" differentiates this from interrupted lines of medial crural footplate dislocations as seen on the left side in Fig. 17.7a.

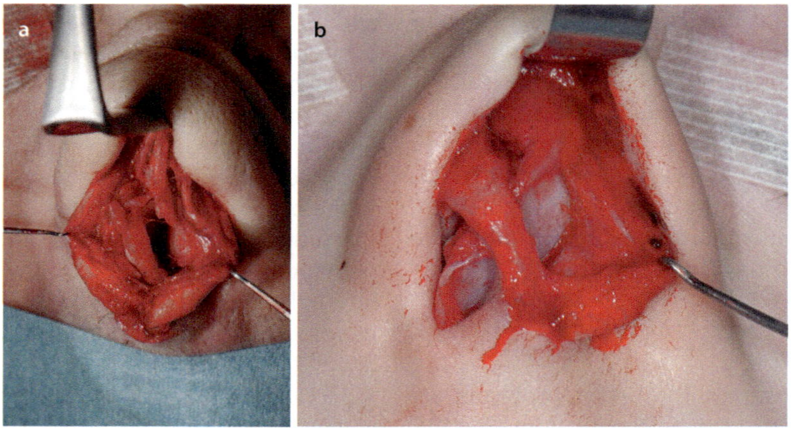

Fig. 17.5 **a** Open view showing high dorsal septal deviation in medial nasal wall sub-unit 1. (Reproduced with kind permission from Refs. [2, 3]). **b** Open view showing high dorsal septal deviation in medial nasal wall sub-unit 1 and anterior membranous deviation in medial nasal wall sub-unit 2. (Reproduced with kind permission from Refs. [2, 3])

17

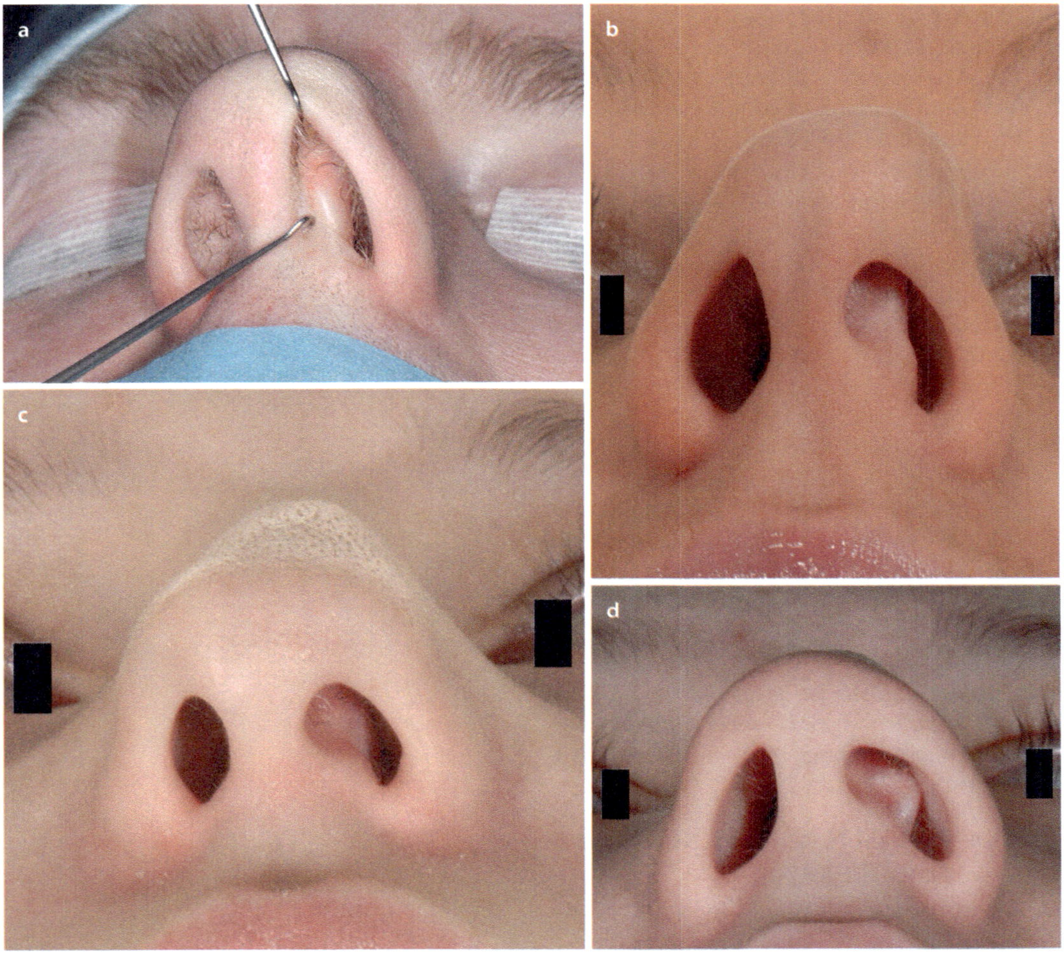

Fig. 17.6 **a–d** Basal view showing medial nasal wall sub-unit 2 issues with anterior and caudal membranous septal deviations

- The deformity is confirmed by palpation of the entire caudal septum by deflecting the conjoined medial crus away from the caudal septum.
- The nostril shape changes on the affected side to a vertical parallel slit, as seen on the left side in Fig. 17.6b.
- On the side of the caudal dislocation, the nostril axis angle is more obtuse than the non-dislocated side thus causing asymetric nasal tip rotation when measured from either side.
- Surgical options being ***septoplasty, anterior columelloplasty and septal extension grafts***.

17.4.1.3 Medial Nasal Wall Sub-unit Three (MW3)

- The anatomical sub-unit site is one or both medial crura in the anterior columellar region.
- Common pathology is ***medial crura footplate prolapse, either unilateral or bilateral***.
- Diagnosed by endoscopic examination or anterior rhinoscopy and confirmed by palpation.
- Medial crural fracture or splaying of the footplate with deviations into the alar

region reduces the inspiratory airflow and causes nasal obstruction.

- If the deformity is bilateral, then it is seen as widening of the width of the columella near the sil region (◘ Fig. 17.7c).
- If unilateral, it is seen as an additional "interrupted vertical line" on the side of the deviation as shown on the left nostril (◘ Fig. 17.7b).
- If unilateral, the nostril shape on the affected side is doughnut shaped as shown on the left nostril (◘ Fig. 17.7a).
- If bilateral, there is a flask-shaped deformity in the basal view (◘ Fig. 17.7c).
- There can be a vertical shortening (base to tip) of the nostril if there are bilateral multiple fractures of the medial crus (◘ Fig. 17.7b). This is also seen in the basal view as a distortion and inversion of the tear-drop appearance of the nostril with the base of the nostril narrower than the apex.
- Surgical options being ***medial crural fixation sutures, medial crural flare control sutures and columellar medial crural strut grafts***.

17.4.1.4 Medial Nasal Wall Sub-Unit Four (MW4)

- This anatomical sub-unit site is the ***soft tissue columella***.
- Pathology is any deformity ***limited to soft tissues of the columella including skin and mucosa***.
- Diagnosed by endoscopic examination or anterior rhinoscopy.
- Infra tip lobule, soft triangle and columellar skin (◘ Fig. 17.8a–c) can all be

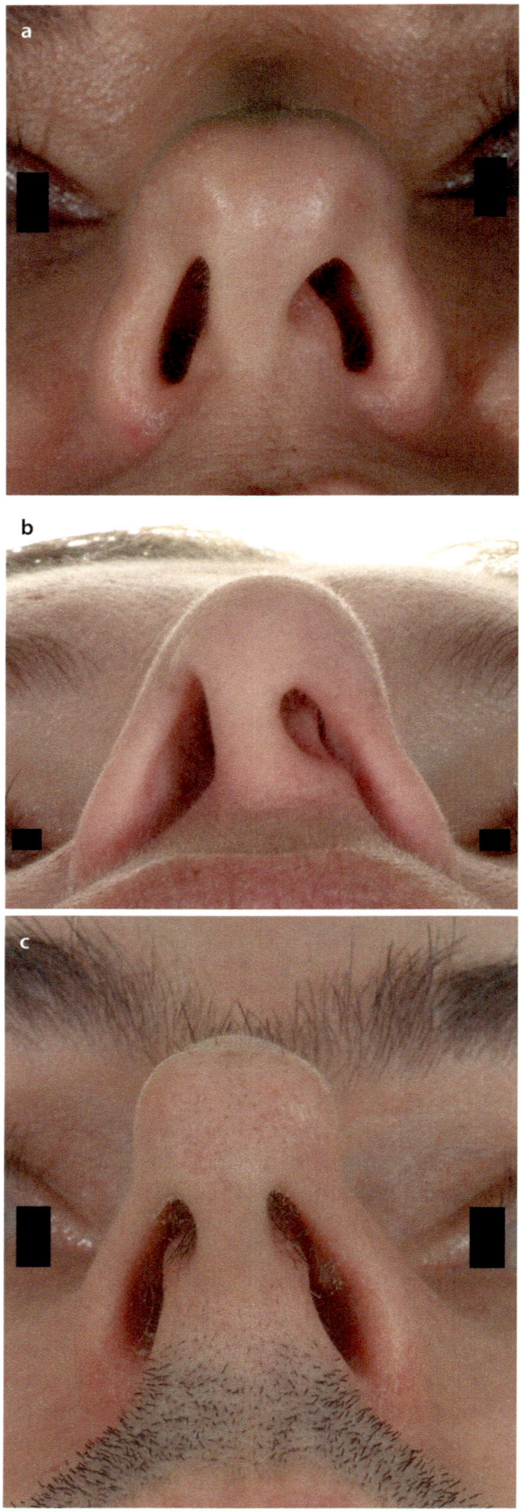

◘ **Fig. 17.7** **a–c** Basal view showing medial nasal wall sub-unit 3 issues with unilateral or bilateral medial crural footplate prolapse. **a** Left medial crural footplate prolapse. **b** Inversion of tear drop nostril due to left medial crural footplate prolapse. **c** Bilateral medial crural footplate fractures and prolapse with hour-glass appearance of nostrils subjected to excess scarring secondary to trauma or revision surgery.

- Aging changes or traumatic changes to the tip skeleton with heavy seborrheic skin and ptotic tip can also result in restricted turbulent airflow.
- Surgical options are limited. Soft triangle scarring in our experience is very difficult to correct and should be excised and left to heal by secondary intention.
- V-Y plasty of the columella skin can be done, and the columella can be lengthened at the expense of width.
- Vestibular stenosis requires incision of scar, skin graft, rongeuring of the bony pyriform aperture with or without excision of the anterior end of the inferior turbinate.

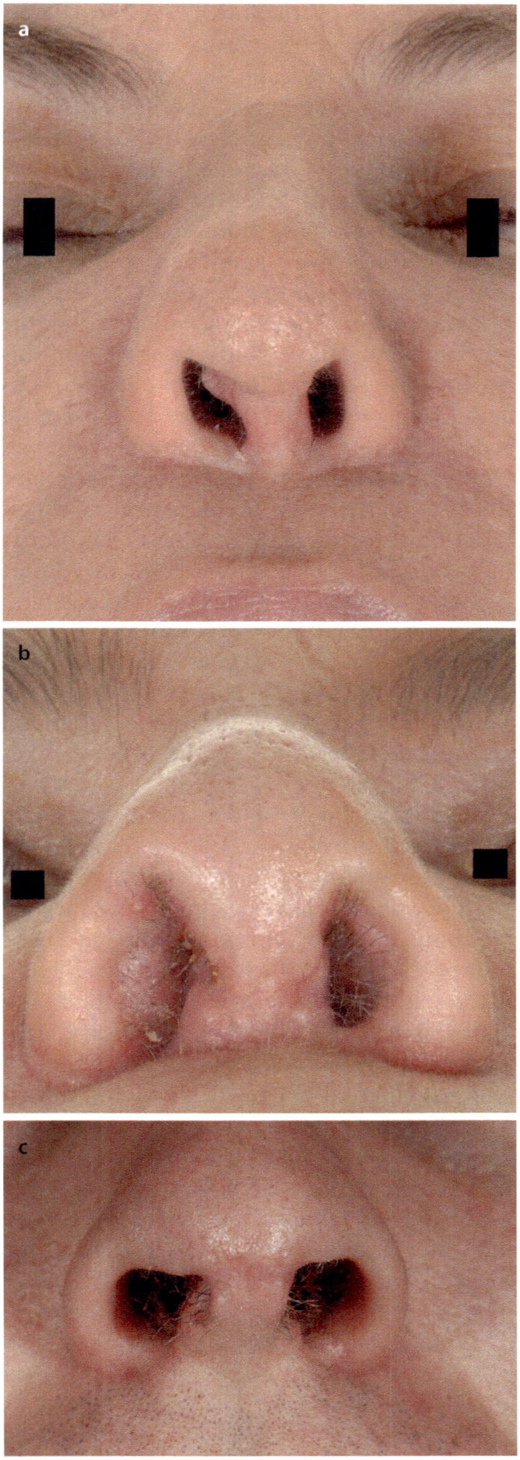

Fig. 17.8 **a–c** Basal view showing medial nasal wall sub-unit 4 issues. **a** Soft triangle scarring. **b** Columellar scarring. **c** Soft triangle and columellar scarring. (Reproduced with kind permission from Refs. [2, 3])

17.5 Diagnostic and Management Algorithm of Lateral Nasal Wall Pathology

Once the assessment of the medial nasal wall region is completed in a patient with nasal obstruction, then the lateral nasal wall units should be examined individually. This nasal wall sub-unit classification [3] helps us in focusing on the anatomical sites so that a diagnosis and a surgical plan can be formulated. Be aware, as compared to the examination of medial nasal wall region (which are usually obvious on clinical examination), ***clinical examination of the lateral nasal wall areas is not a precise science*** and hence difficult to diagnose the exact site of the problem even after clinical examination. *In most situations, the exact anatomical site of the problem in the lateral nasal wall cannot be ascertained until an open approach is carried out.* Experienced surgeons would concur on this fact, which has been highlighted very well by Dr. Most from Stanford [6]. This difficulty in diagnosis explains the high revision rate in correcting lateral alar abnormalities done through a closed approach.

Of course the most important structure responsible for maintaining the nasal function in the lateral nasal alar region is the lateral crus of the lower lateral cartilage. History of nasal trauma or previous rhinoplasty with excess cephalic trim or damage to the lateral crus during the inter-cartilaginous incision gives a clue that the lateral alar weakness could be due to damage to the lateral crus. Apart from the history, clinical examination alone without opening the nose can sometimes give diagnostic clues to lateral crural weakness or dysjunction as the cause of alar collapse. On clinical examination, the severity of the alar collapse is noted and this is directly related to the lateral crural damage. More severe the damage to the lateral crus, the more severe is the alar collapse. Contrary to this, if there is weakness above the lateral crus in the scroll region, alar collapse will not be severe. Also the presence of localised tip abnormalities in the dome, points to structural damage to the lateral crus. The presence of deviation of the tip to the side of the alar weakness is quite a typical pointer for a damaged lateral crus on the same side, since the opposite normal lateral crus pushes the dome to the other weaker side (◻ Fig. 17.11).

The importance of diagnosing the exact anatomical site of the problem in the lateral nasal alar weakness cannot be over emphasised [6], as it not only helps in the surgical planning, but also helps in the informed consent of the patient. Based on our experience, if there is a weak lateral crus causing lateral alar collapse, the use of lateral crural strut grafts is necessary to improve the function and not a batten graft which will add weight to the already damaged lateral crus worsening the symptoms of nasal obstruction. In our experience alar batten grafts do not work, if the weakness is in the lateral crus of the lower lateral cartilage, as it adds to the weight of the damaged lateral crus, akin to building a first floor when the ground floor is already weak. If the alar margin is also weak, an additional marginal rim graft may also be needed. Hence, an accurate anatomical diagnosis of where exactly the problem should be the priority.

17.5.1 "Lateral Nasal Wall" Area (LW): Sub-unit Pathology, Diagnosis and Targeted Surgical Solutions

17.5.1.1 Lateral Nasal Wall Sub-unit One (LW1)

- This anatomical sub-unit site is caudal edge of the nasal bones, cephalic portion of upper lateral cartilage with the junctional "K" area in between.
- Pathology is usually a ***unilateral or bilateral depressed fracture of the caudal nasal bones with unilateral or bilateral collapse of the upper lateral cartilage and "K" area***.
- Usually diagnosed as a depressed nasal bone on the ipsilateral side and deviation to the opposite side (S-shaped) (◻ Fig. 17.9a).
- Associated with depression/collapse of ULC on the same side with "K" area weakness as shown on left side in ◻ Fig. 17.9a.
- Diagnosed in frontal view as a discontinuity in the eyebrow tip aesthetic line on that side (◻ Fig. 17.9c).
- The width of the mid third of the nose is narrow on frontal view (◻ Fig. 17.9c).
- If the defect is bilateral (◻ Fig. 17.9b), there is a classic hour-glass narrowing of the mid dorsum due to the collapse of the upper lateral cartilage causing the caudal border of the nasal bones to be prominent, usually associated with short nasal bones.
- Diagnosed by nasal endoscopy/assessment done by lifting out the ULC with a hook and subjective improvement in nasal obstruction recorded by a visual analogue score.
- Surgical options being ***sequential osteotomies and reduction, stabilisation of nasal bones with or without bilateral spreader grafts***.

17.5.1.2 Lateral Nasal Wall Sub-unit Two (LW2)

- This anatomical sub-unit site is the ***junctional region between upper and lower lateral cartilage, the "scroll" region***.
- Pathology is usually a ***unilateral or bilateral alar pinching or collapse*** (◻ Fig. 17.10a)

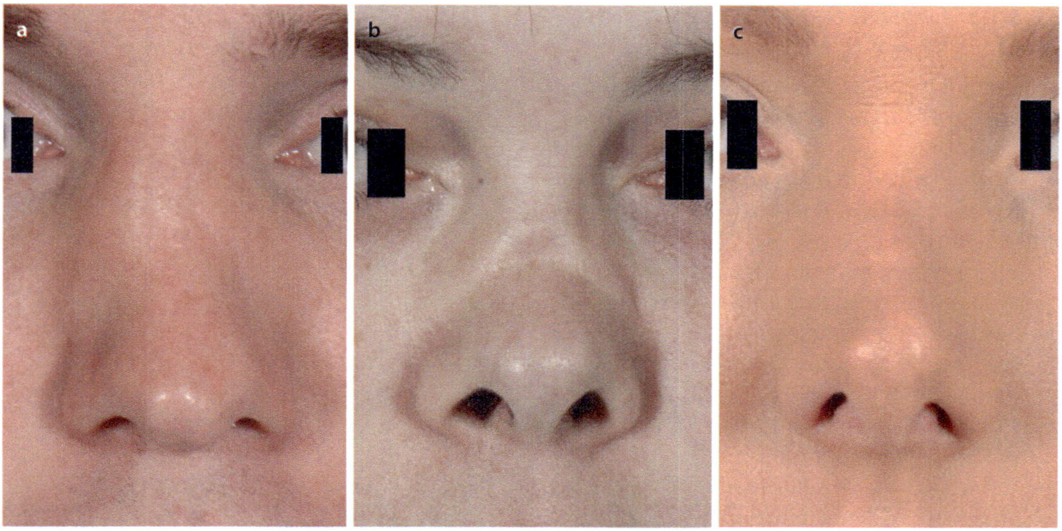

Fig. 17.9 **a–c** Frontal view showing lateral wall sub-unit 1 issues. **a** Unilateral collapse of lateral wall. **b** and **c** Bilateral lateral wall collapse. (Reproduced with kind permission from Refs. [2, 3])

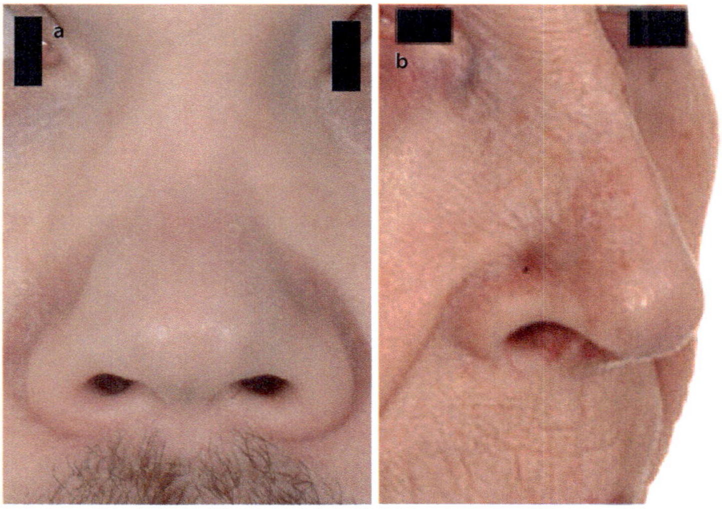

Fig. 17.10 **a**, **b** Frontal view showing lateral wall sub-unit 2 issues

seen on quiet breathing or forced inspiration either due to previous surgery, scarring or trauma.

- There will be alar pinching or in-drawing on deep inspiration just above the lateral crus cartilage involving the junctional region between the lateral crus and upper lateral cartilage.
- More commonly associated with weakness of lateral crus as well.
- These defects involve not only the upper lateral, but also junctional areas below and involve also the lateral crus are not uncommon in revision rhinoplasty patients.
- Surgical options being ***lateral crural strut grafts*** *and/or* ***alar batten grafts***.

17.5.1.3 Lateral Nasal Wall Sub-unit Three (LW3)

- The anatomical sub-unit site is the ***lateral crus of the lower lateral cartilage***.
- Pathology is usually a ***unilateral or bilateral weakness, concavity, scarring or discontinuity of the lateral crus*** with or without alar pinching or collapse seen on quiet breathing or forced inspiration either due to previous surgery, scarring or trauma.
- Severity of the alar collapse, more severe collapse is associated with lateral crural damage.
- Localised sharpness, knobby abnormality of the dome are common.
- External visible deformity – weakness, concavity, discontinuity associated with inspiratory in drawing of the lateral alar region, alar pinching or collapse.
- If the defect is unilateral, the tip gets pushed to the affected side due to the relatively stronger unopposed action of the opposite lateral crus (◘ Figs. 17.11 and 17.12).
- Sometimes the defect can be localised due to interruption of the lateral crus as seen in ◘ Figs. 17.13 and 17.14. This patient

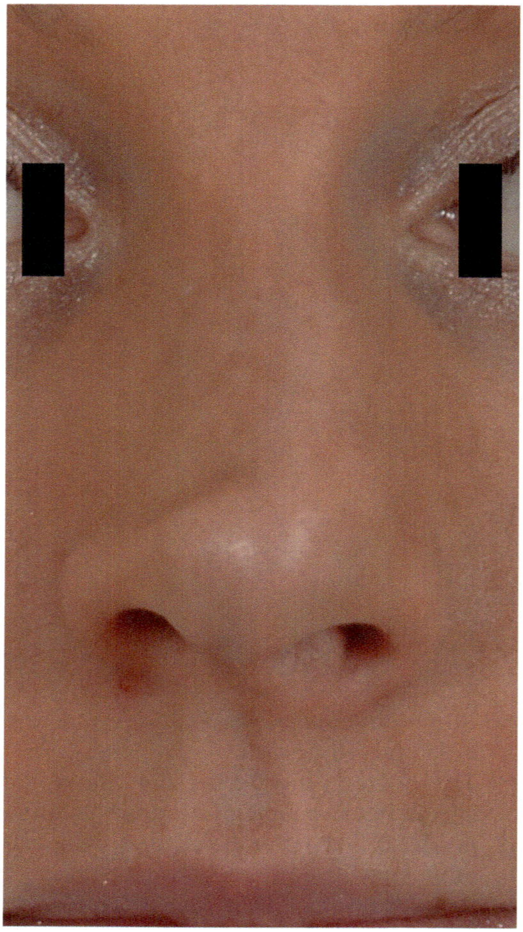

◘ **Fig. 17.11** Frontal view of the nose showing lateral wall sub-unit 3 involvement with lateral crural collapse and tip turn to the affected side

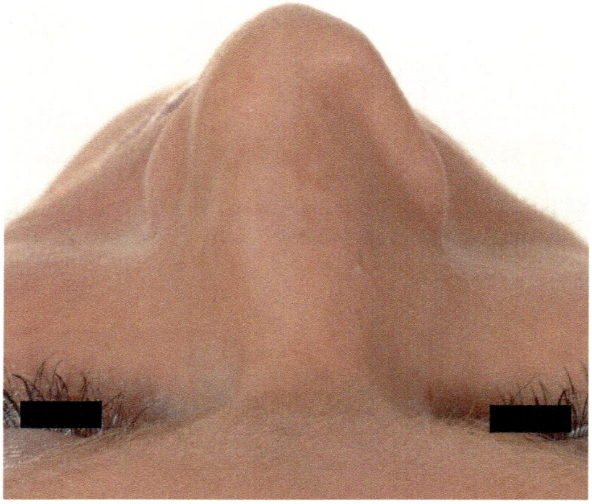

◘ **Fig. 17.12** Sky view of the nose showing lateral wall sub-unit 3 involvement with lateral crural collapse and tip turn to the affected side

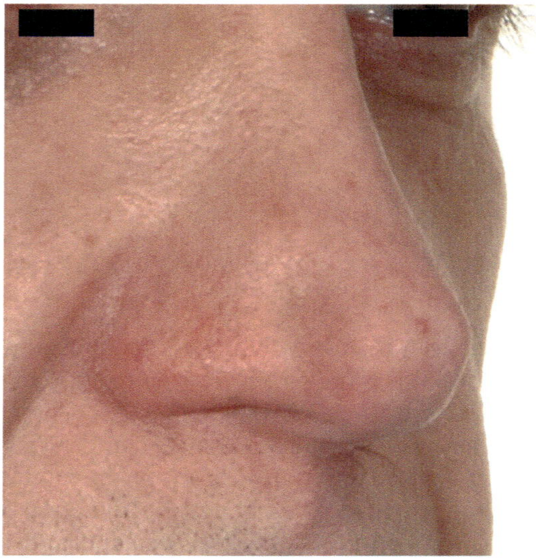

◘ **Fig. 17.13** Three-fourth view of the nose showing localised lateral wall sub-unit 3 involvement with interruption of the lateral crus on the affected side

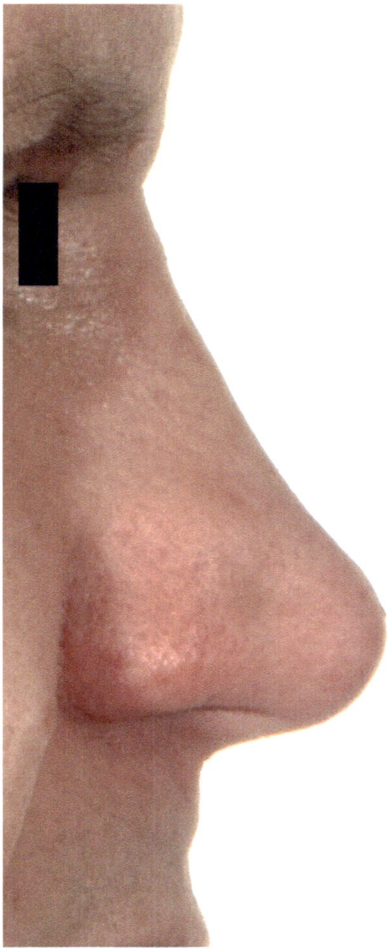

Fig. 17.14 Lateral view of the nose showing localised lateral wall sub-unit 3 involvement with interruption of the lateral crus on the affected side

had bilateral dome division presenting 10 years later with alar collapse localised to the lateral crus just lateral to the dome. This patient had strut grafts with good outcomes.

- Thickness of the alar side wall is a diagnostic sign. Thinner the alar side wall, the more possibility of lateral crural weakness (Fig. 17.15).
- The surgical options being ***lateral crural turn-in flaps or lateral crural strut grafts***.

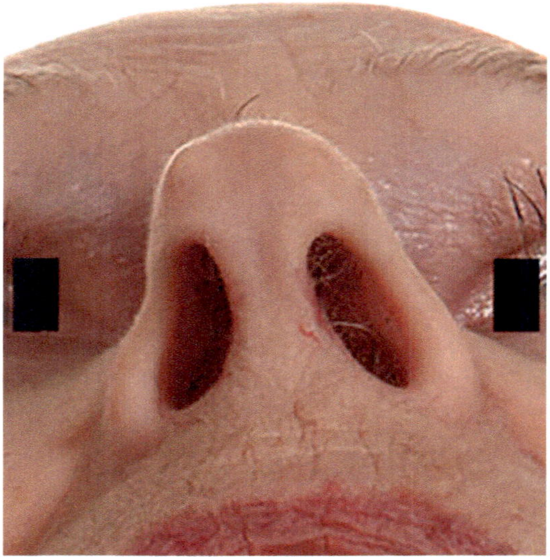

Fig. 17.15 Basal view of the nose showing localised lateral wall sub-unit 3 involvement with thin alar side wall on the affected side

17.5.1.4 Lateral Nasal Wall Sub-unit Four (LW4)

- This anatomical sub-unit site is the ***fibro fatty tissue of the ala and cutaneous alar margins***.
- Pathology could be due to ***previous surgery, scarring or trauma***.
- Marginal alar weakness due to scarring, weakness or damage to fibro-fatty tissue or skin loss.
- Soft triangle scarring (Fig. 17.16) which may be unilateral or bilateral.
- There can be complete collapse of the alar margin as seen in Fig. 17.19.
- Alar marginal "hooding" either bilateral (Fig. 17.17) or unilateral (Fig. 17.18) causing in-drawing during inspiration.
- Soft tissue hooding reduces airflow at the entrance and are best seen in the basal view (Fig. 17.17).
- Surgical options being ***alar marginal rim grafts or composite grafts if there is overlying skin loss as well***.

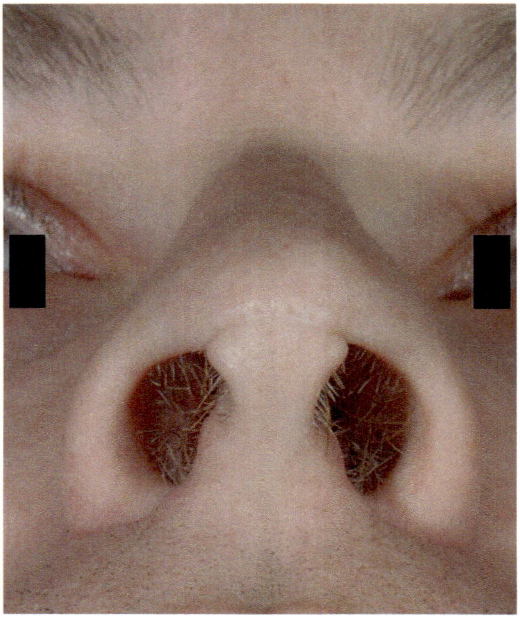

Fig. 17.16 Basal view of the nose showing lateral wall sub-unit 4 involvement with bilateral soft triangle scarring. (Reproduced with kind permission from Refs. [2, 3])

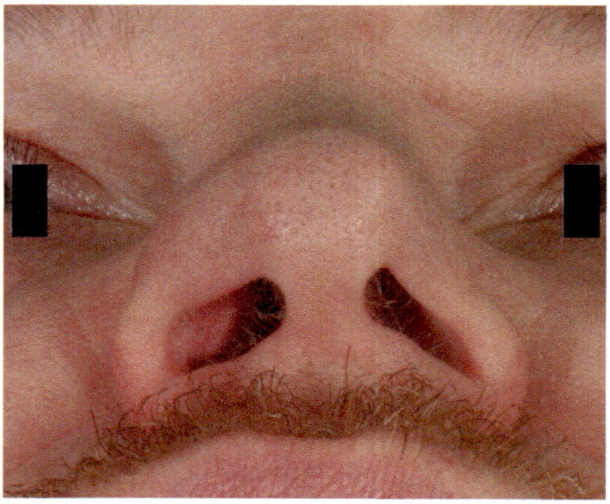

Fig. 17.17 Basal view of the nose showing lateral wall sub-unit 4 involvement with bilateral alar margin hooding. (Reproduced with kind permission from Refs. [2, 3])

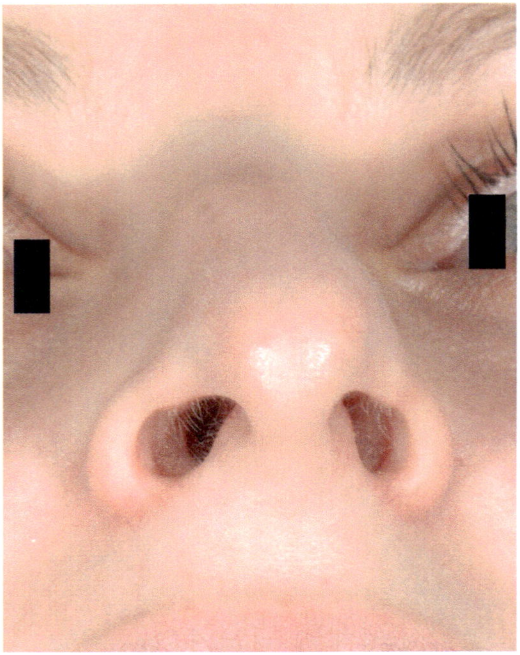

Fig. 17.18 Basal view of the nose showing lateral wall sub-unit 4 involvement with unilateral right-sided alar margin hooding. (Reproduced with kind permission from Refs. [2, 3])

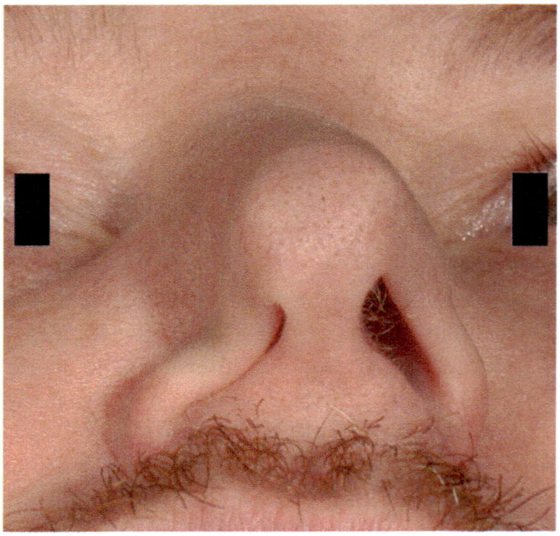

Fig. 17.19 Basal view of the nose showing lateral wall sub-unit 4 involvement with severe collapse of the alar margin. (Reproduced with kind permission from Refs. [2, 3])

Conclusion

Successful outcomes in nasal valve surgery depend on an accurate assessment of the deformity and the selection of the appropriate surgical technique. We suggest an alternative way of assessing valve problems and propose a new classification of lateral and medial nasal wall sub-unit problems which can help in making a precise diagnosis and arrive at a specific tailored surgical procedure.

Key Points Box

- In a patient with nasal obstruction, diagnosing the exact site of nasal obstruction is paramount. This is not an easy diagnostic exercise even for the trained eye. The current classification of internal nasal valve and external nasal valve although anatomically proven has its own drawbacks.
- Categorisation of defects and accurately defining the site of the lesion into those affecting the internal nasal valve area (higher up in the nose) and those affecting the external nasal valve area (lower down in the nose) in a traumatic nose with multiple deformities (requiring complex procedures) is not possible, hence making it difficult to choose the right surgical option.
- We suggest an alternative user-friendly way of assessing nasal valve issues and propose a clinical classification of lateral and medial nasal wall problems with various sub-unit issues rather than vague internal valve and external valve problems. This nasal wall sub-unit concept has helped us in making a precise diagnosis with less inter-observer variations, and also to arrive at a specific tailored surgical procedure.

References

1. Apaydin F. Nasal valve surgery. Facial Plast Surg. 2011;27:179–91.
2. Balaji N, Ravichandran S. Assessment of nasal valve obstruction : a new nasal "wall" subunit concept. ENT Audiol News. 2012;21(4):111–3.
3. Balaji N, Ravichandran S. Assessment of nasal valve obstruction : a new Glasgow nasal "wall" subunit concept. ENT Audiol News. 2012;21(5):86–7.
4. Ghidini A, Dallari S, Marchioni D. Surgery of the nasal columella in external valve collapse. Ann Otol Rhinol Laryngol. 2002;111(8):701–3.
5. Spielmann PM, White PS, Hussain SS. Surgical techniques for the treatment of nasal valve collapse: a systematic review. Laryngoscope. 2009;119(7):1281–90.
6. Vaezeafshar R, Moubayed SP, Most SP. Repair of lateral wall insufficiency. JAMA Facial Plast Surg. 2018;20(2):111–5.
7. Tsao GJ, Fijalkowski N, Most SP. Validation of a grading system for lateral nasal wall insufficiency. Allergy Rhinol (Providence). 2013;4(2):e66–8.
8. Ziai H, Bonaparte JP. Reliability and construct validity of the Ottawa valve collapse scale when assessing external nasal valve collapse. J Otolaryngol Head Neck Surg. 2018;47:15.

Surgical Algorithms in Nasal Tip Rhinoplasty

Contents

N. Balaji, *Textbook of Nasal Tip Rhinoplasty*, https://doi.org/10.1007/978-3-030-48157-5_18

Learning Objectives

- To learn the surgical algorithms for addressing various tip deformities, including a bulbous tip, and addressing over and under projection and rotation.
- To learn the algorithms for addressing the length of the nose and how to approach revision rhinoplasty surgery patients.

18.1 Algorithm to Correct a "Bulbous" Nasal Tip

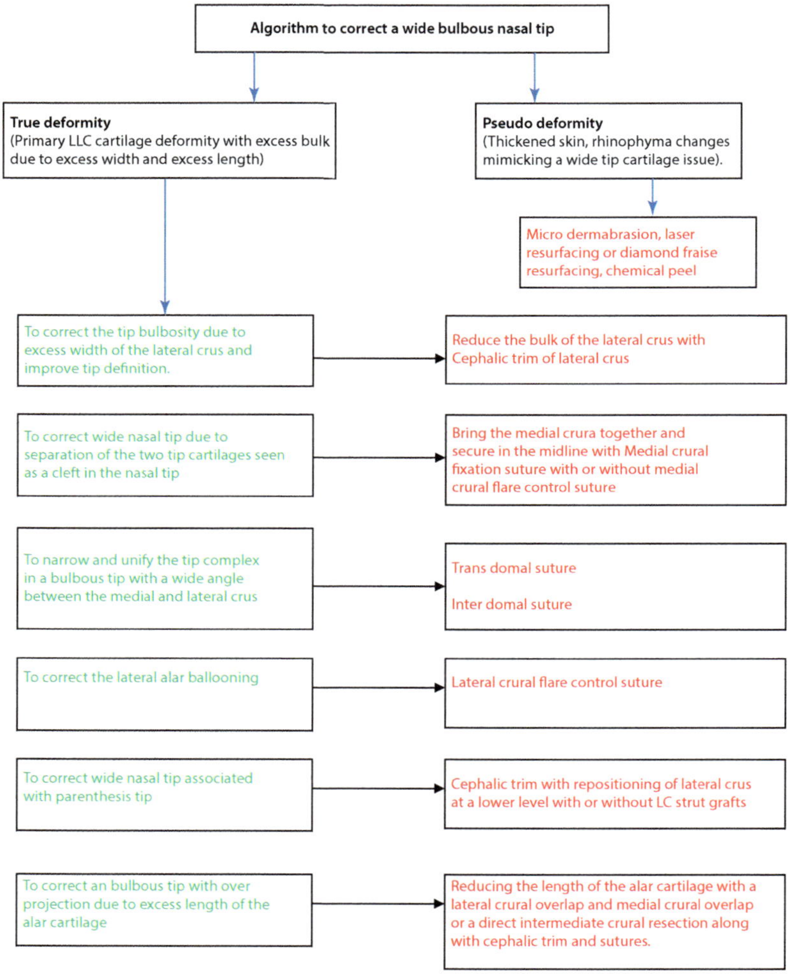

18.2 Algorithm to Correct a "Thin" Nasal Tip

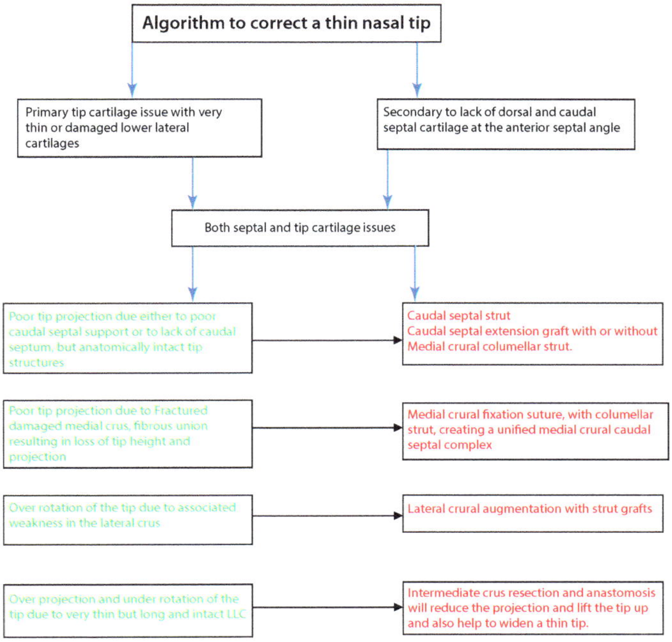

18.3 Algorithm to "Increase" the Tip Projection

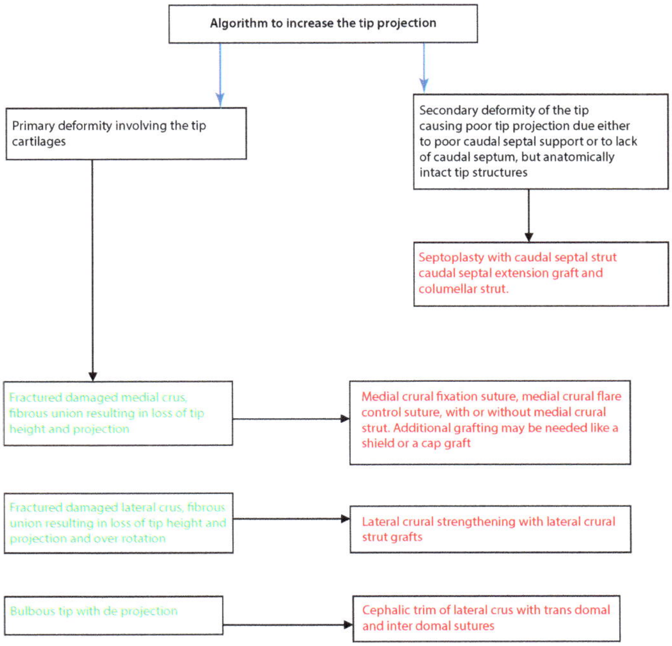

18.4 Algorithm to "Decrease" Tip Projection

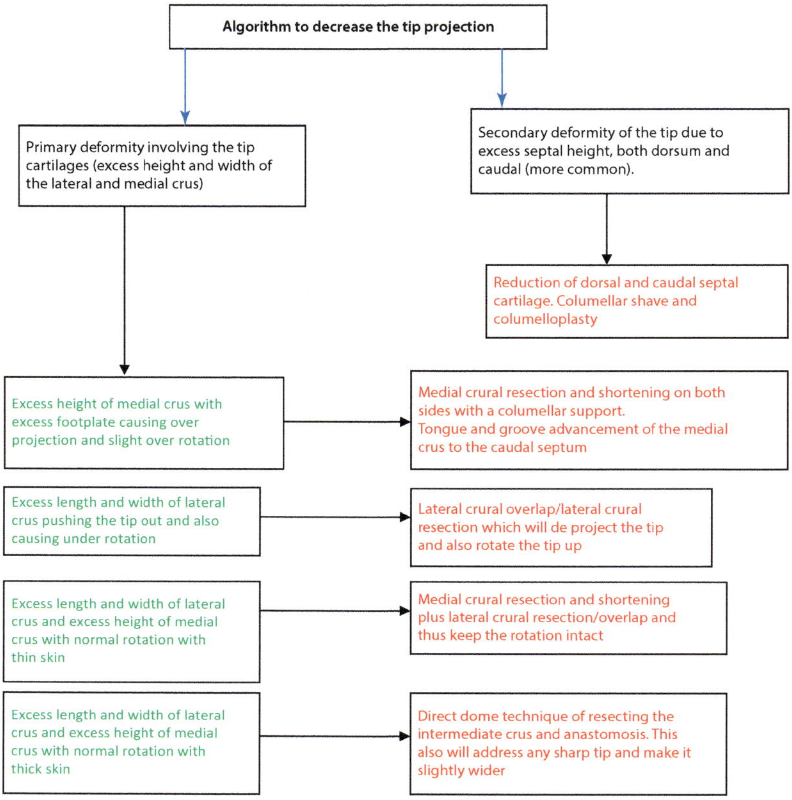

18.5 Algorithm to Correct an "Over Rotated" Nasal Tip

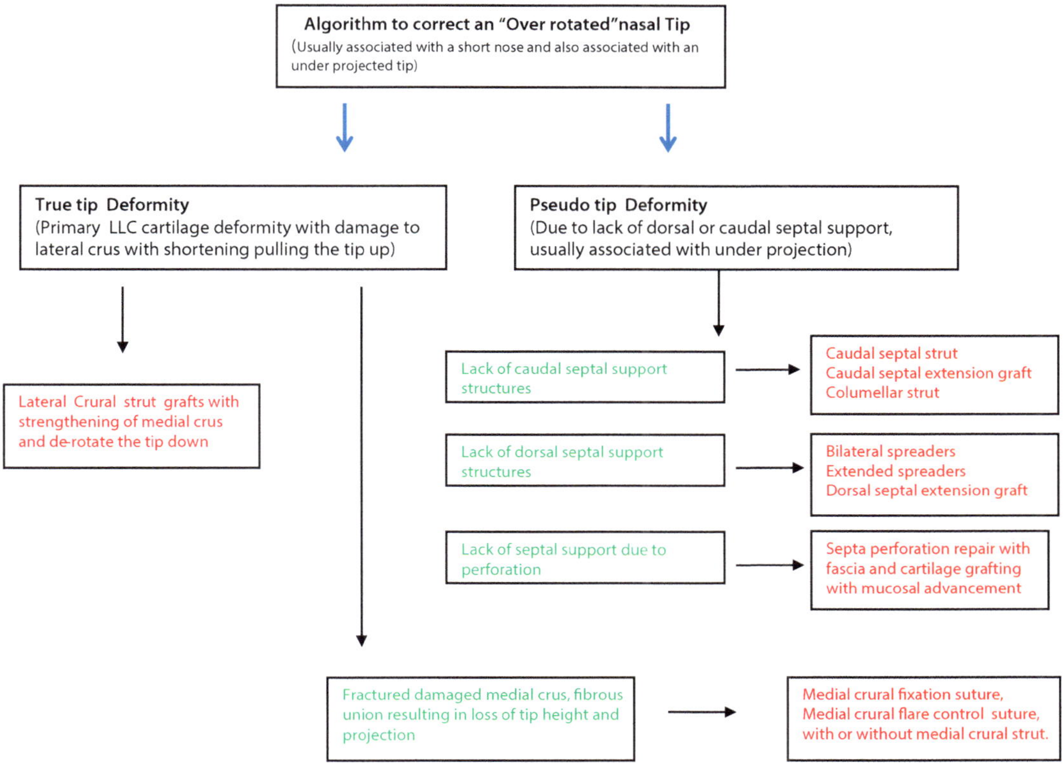

18.6 Algorithm to Correct an "Under Rotated" Nasal Tip

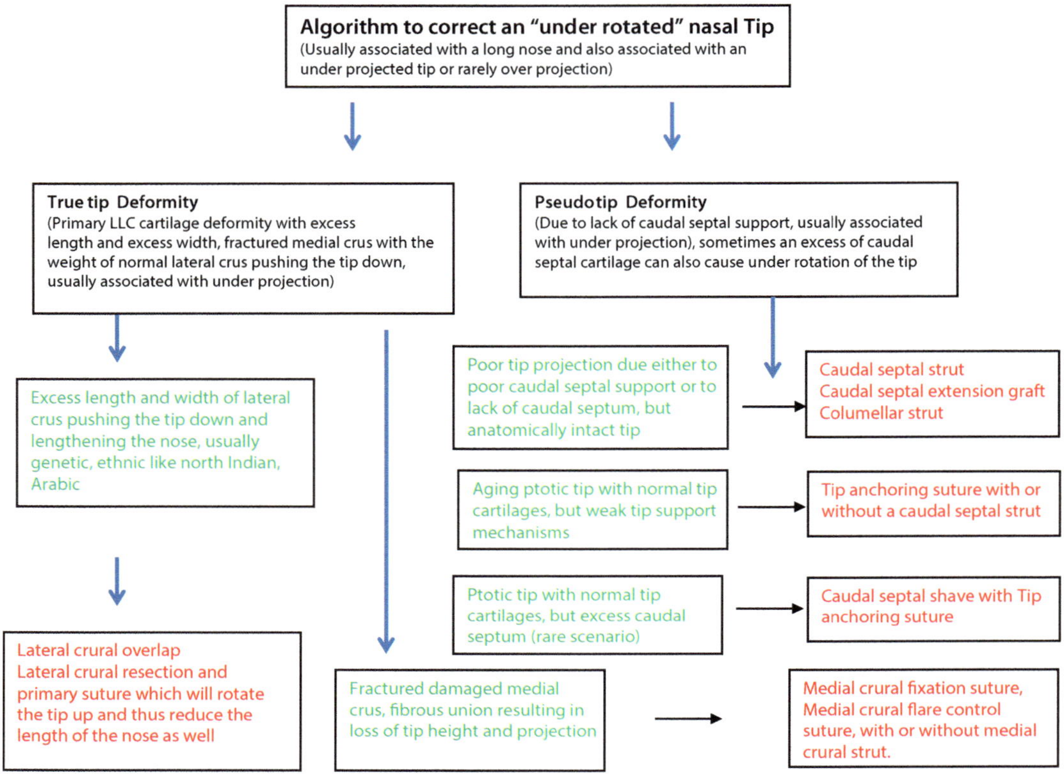

18.7 Algorithm to Reduce a "Long" Nose

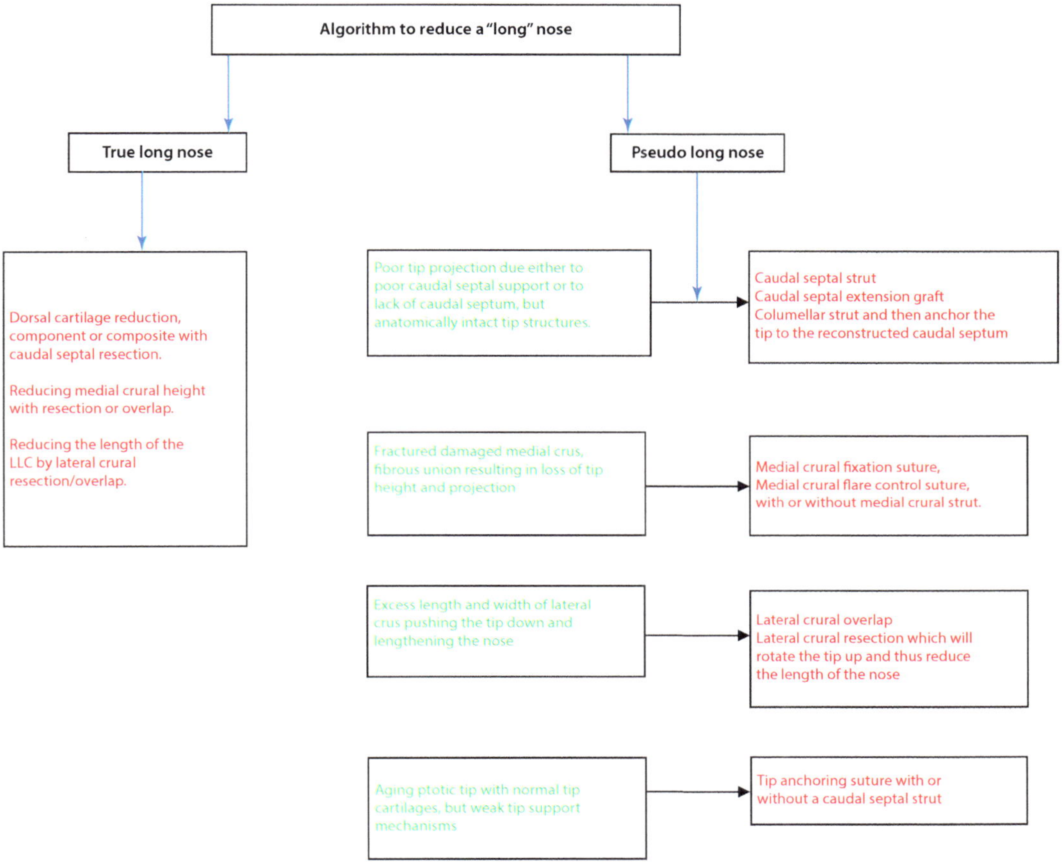

18.8 Algorithm to Correct a "Short" Nose

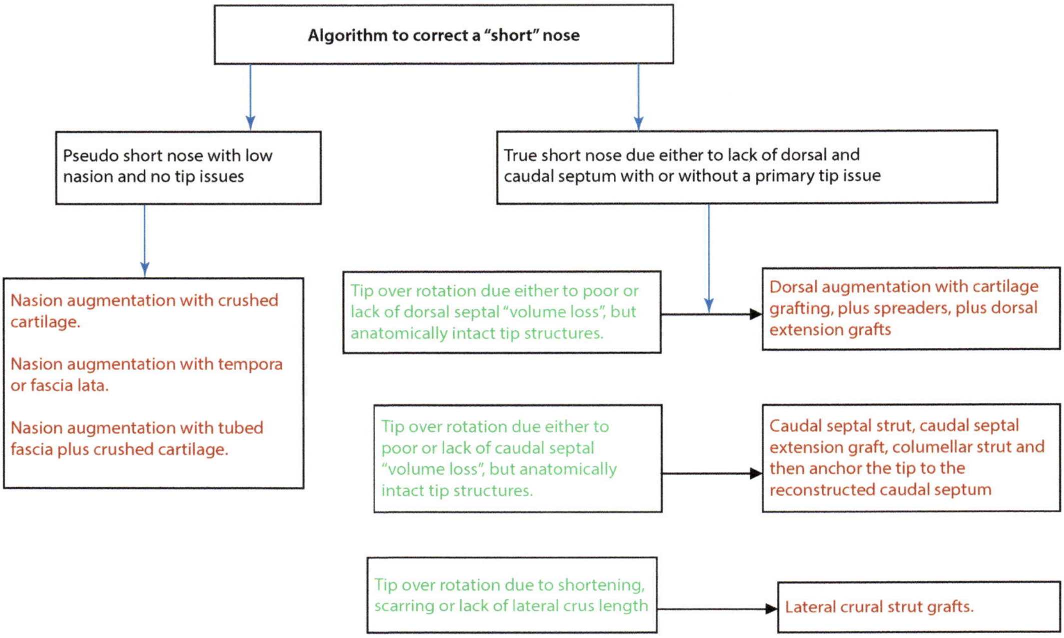

18.9 Algorithm to Correct a "Lateral Crural Pathology" of the Lateral Alar Region

The following algorithm has been published by the author (Fig. 18.1) and has been reproduced with kind permission of the editor of *ENT Master Class* journal [1].

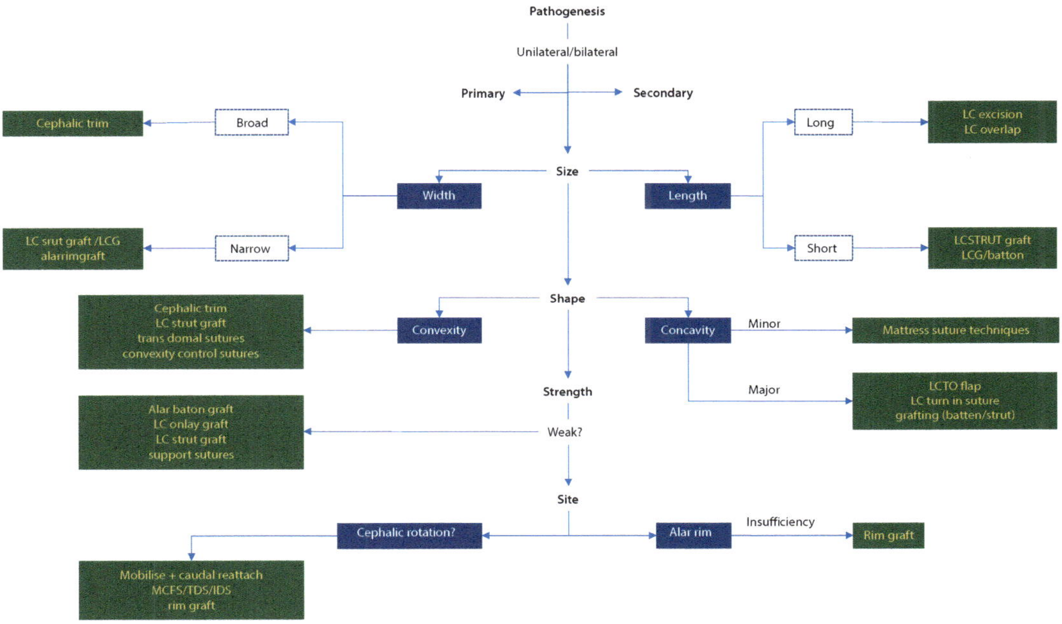

Fig. 18.1 An algorithm to correct a "lateral crural pathology" of the lateral alar region. (Reproduced with kind permission from Ref. [1])

18.10 Suture Algorithm Techniques in Nasal Tip Rhinoplasty

Non-absorbable sutures can be used in a variety of ways to achieve nasal tip definition, projection and rotation. They can be used together with cartilage grafts or stand-alone sutures in primary tip plasty. We suggest the use of the following algorithm [2, 4, 6] for the stand-alone suturing techniques in nasal tip plasty:

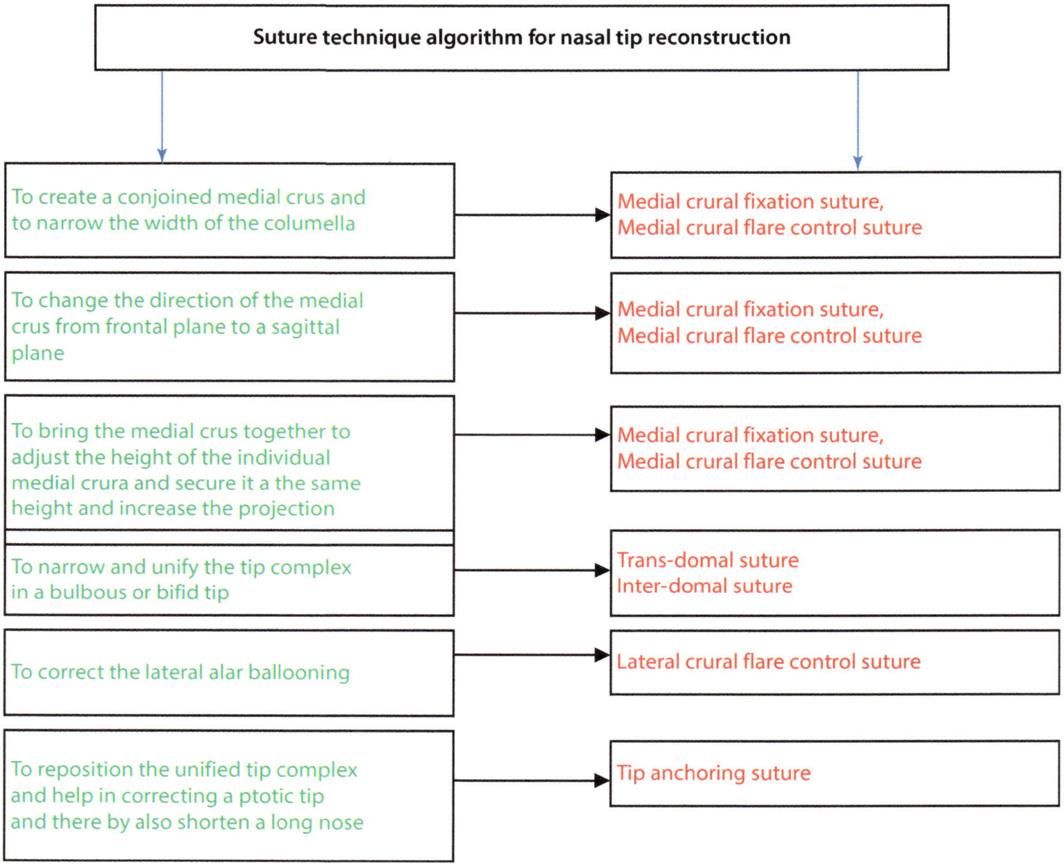

18.11 Non-suture Algorithm

Non-suture techniques can be used in a variety of ways to achieve nasal tip definition, projection and rotation. Please note they are used in conjunction with suture techniques and grafting techniques. We have separated the algorithm just to help in the thought process. We suggest the use of the following algorithm [3, 5, 6] for the appropriate non-suture techniques in nasal tip plasty:

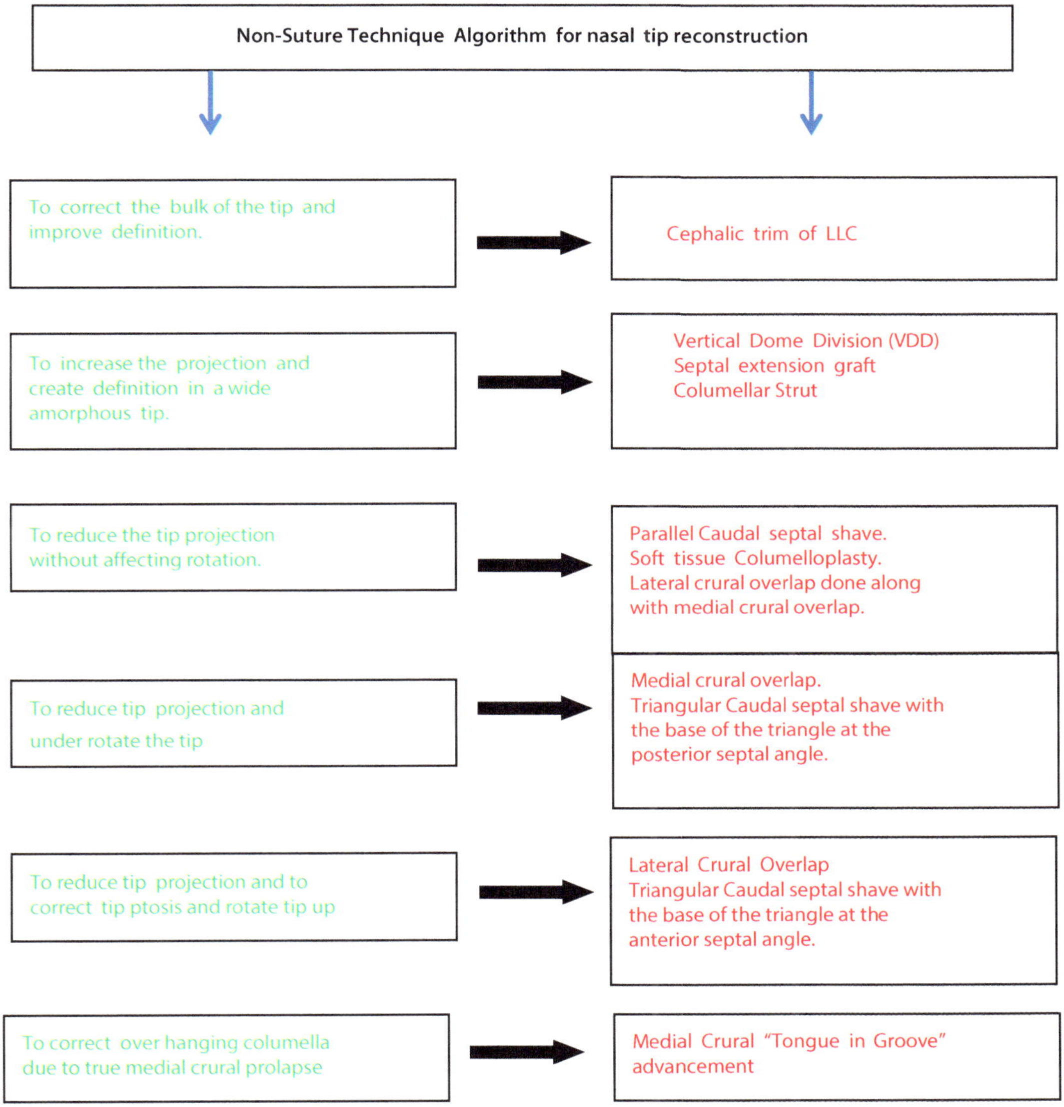

18.12 How to Approach a Revision Rhinoplasty

1. Repeated pre-operative consultations with adequate "cool-off" period.
2. Getting previous records. Any details of previous complaints or litigations.
3. Make sure your goals are realistic – it is not what the surgeon can technically achieve which matters, it is all about how happy the patient is going to be after the surgery which matters.
4. Adequate record keeping.
5. Adequate photo documentation.
6. Assessing the overlying skin – thick or thin or scarred, colour changes.
7. Loss of lateral crural cartilages, damage to ULC or loss of bone, callus formation.
8. Presence or absence of mucosal scarring, vestibular stenosis, mucosal adhesions.
9. A decision has to be made whether the patient will need an "open" approach or a "closed" approach, based on the complexity of the deformity and the presence

or absence of any coexisting muocsal scarring. It is better to keep the revision surgery as simple as possible and avoid destructive techniques.
10. Selecting the "right" tools – conchal cartilage, helical rim cartilage, may be septal cartilage or rib cartilage. Alloplastic materials are not advisable in revision procedures. The patient may need fascia lata or temporalis fascia when the overlying skin is very thin with colour changes.
11. Give more than 100% post-operative care. Be there to answer all their concerns.
12. Good communication goes a long way.

Conclusion

We have separated the flow-charts into different sections for ease of understanding, but be aware that these techniques are all used in conjunction and they are not "stand-alone" techniquues. Thus, surgical algorithms are surgical flow charts helping to guide the surgeon to formulate a treatment plan. They serve as a "route map" to correct complex noses like twisted noses [7–9] and complex tips. We have put forward surgical algorithms for various anatomical abnormalities of the tip with flow-charts. These flow-charts will be easier to understand depending on the experience of the surgeon. The more experienced the surgeon is, the more they will be able to understand the clinical significance of the flow-charts. Algorithms should not be considered as a "rule", and they are at best considered as "guidelines" which helps the surgeon in the thought process to achieve a better surgical outcome.

Key Points Box
- Surgical algorithms are a useful tool in the understanding of the pros and cons of various techniques in dealing with complex deformities of the nasal tip.
- Algorithm helps to critically analyse the effects of each procedure and come to a reasonable rationale in addressing a deformity.

References

1. Okhovat S, Balaji N. An algorithm for the management of lateral crural pathology. J ENT Master class. 2018;11(1):45–53.
2. Sil A, Ravichandran S, Balaji N. Suture techniques in posttraumatic nasal tip reconstruction. ENT Audiol News. 2009;18(5):98–102.
3. Sil A, Ravichandran S, Balaji N. Non- suture techniques in posttraumatic nasal tip reconstruction. ENT Audiol News. 2010;19(2):109–12.
4. Balaji N. Suture techniques in nasal tip reconstruction. Rom J Rhinol. 2014;4(14):105–10.
5. Balaji N. Non-suture techniques in nasal tip reconstruction. Rom J Rhinol. 2014;4(13):37–44.
6. White PS, Ross PD. Open structure rhinoplasty. 2nd ed. Endo Press GmbH, P.O.Box 78503 Tuttlingen, Germany; 2012.
7. Farzad R, Nahai MD. A surgical algorithm using open rhinoplasty for correction of traumatic twisted nose. Aesthetic Plast Surg. 2007;31:757–8.
8. Hwang PH, Maas CS. Correction of the twisted nose deformity: a surgical algorithm using the external rhinoplasty approach. Am J Rhinol. 1998;12(3): 213–20.
9. Hsiao YC, Kao CH, Wang HW, Moe KS. A surgical algorithm using open rhinoplasty for correction of traumatic twisted nose. Aesthetic Plast Surg. 2007;31(3):250–8.

Case Studies in Nasal Tip Rhinoplasty

Contents

N. Balaji, *Textbook of Nasal Tip Rhinoplasty*, https://doi.org/10.1007/978-3-030-48157-5_19

Learning Objectives

Individual case studies are one of the better tools to understand the pathogenesis and the surgical techniques needed to correct a particular nasal deformity pertaining to an individual patient. We will discuss some examples of common nasal tip problems in relation to tip bulbosity, projection, rotation and size of the nose, going through a standard format of the history, patient's expectations, assessment, thought process and surgical steps. The pre-op photos are then compared with post-op photographs to assess the outcomes.

19.1 Management of a Bulbous Nasal Tip

19.1.1 History

This young lady presented with symptoms of left-sided nasal obstruction and nasal deformity with a bulbous tip, requesting surgery to improve the breathing and possibly to narrow the nasal tip. She gave a history of nasal trauma. She had no other issues and was sensible and realistic in her expectations with good general health.

19.1.2 Pre-op Photos (Fig. 19.1)

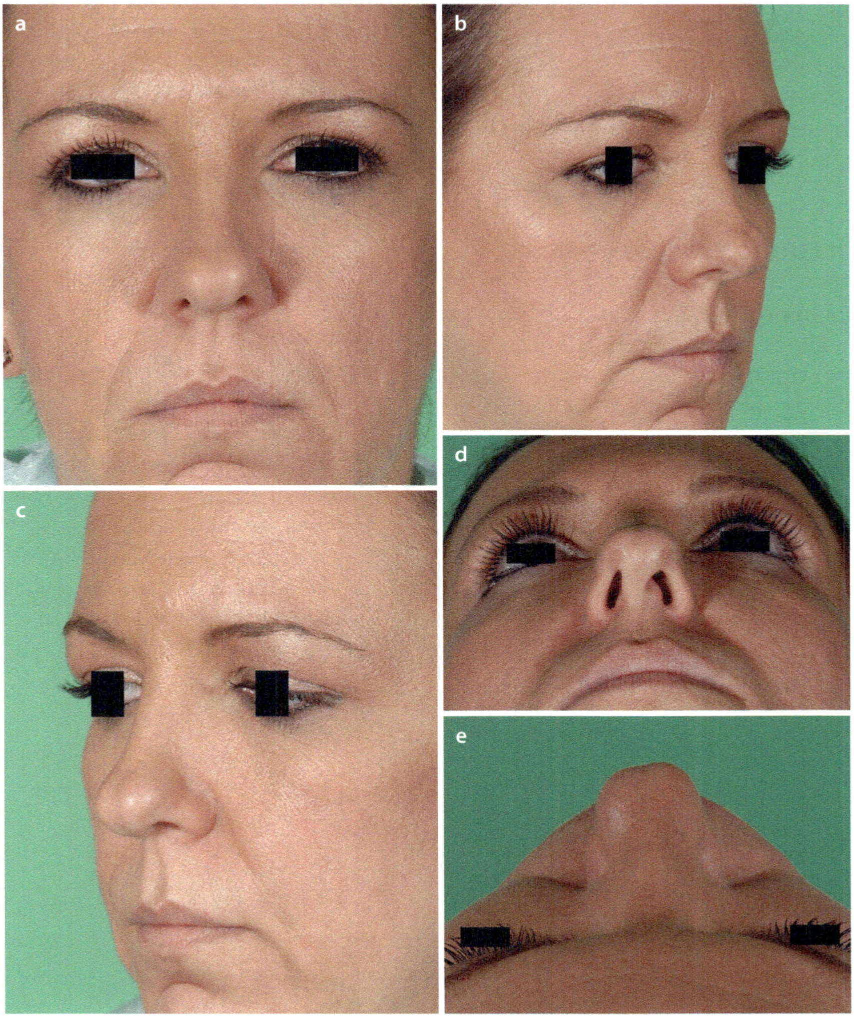

Fig. 19.1 **a–e** Bulbous nasal tip – pre-operative photographs. **a** Right ¾ View. **b** Frontal view. **c** Left ¾ View. **d** Basal view. **e** Sky view

19.1.3 Patient's Expectation

To have the nasal septum straightened and nasal tip less bulky.

19.1.4 Assessment

On examination, in the basal view and the sky view, she has a wide nasal tip with a trapezoidal base and a slightly thicker seborrheic skin. Basal view also shows the dislocated caudal septum on the left side. In the frontal view, there is a "thumb" impression of the two domes with a small cleft between the tip cartilages. Lateral dorsal profile line showed a dip in the supra tip region, particularly in the ¾ view with a slightly over projected tip, which if narrowed will cause more projection. She also has a slightly shorter length of the nose when compared to the projection, due to the slight over rotation of the tip.

19.1.5 Thought Process

Apart from improving the breathing, be aware that although the patient requested narrowing of the nasal tip, the surgeon needs to discuss how narrowing the tip might not show up on the outside due to a thicker skin. There is a strong thumb impression of the alar cartilages on the outside skin envelope with a cleft in the dome. This suggests that the underlying cartilage is still wider and stronger. It is also worth discussing with the patient that any narrowing of the tip will result in increase in tip projection, which can make the dip in the supra tip region more obvious in the lateral profile view. So there should be a plan to correct and augment the supra tip region with crushed cartilage. Our plan was to do a bulk reduction of the cephalic portion of the lateral crus and narrow the tip with tip sutures and use the extra piece of the cephalic lateral crural cartilage to augment the supra tip dorsum to create a uniform dorsal profile.

19.1.6 Surgical Steps

The surgery was performed through an open approach, raised the flap, did a septoplasty and then bilateral cephalic trim of the lateral crus, leaving only 8 mm of symmetrical rim strips, high medial crural fixation suture to bring the two medial crura together (to correct the cleft seen in the skin), followed by trans-domal and inter-domal sutures and a lateral crural flare control suture. Finally covered the supra tip region with a small cap graft taken from the cephalic portion of excised lateral crus to smoothen the dorsal profile line.

Conclusion

Comparing pre-and post-op photographs and subjective assessment of improvement in the shape and breathing, patient was happy with the structural and functional outcome. Extreme care is necessary in selecting the right patient for a tip narrowing procedure. Particularly skin thickness should be taken into account and adequate counselling about the possible outcomes in your hand should be discussed and documented in the records.

19.1.7 Post-op (◘ Fig. 19.2)

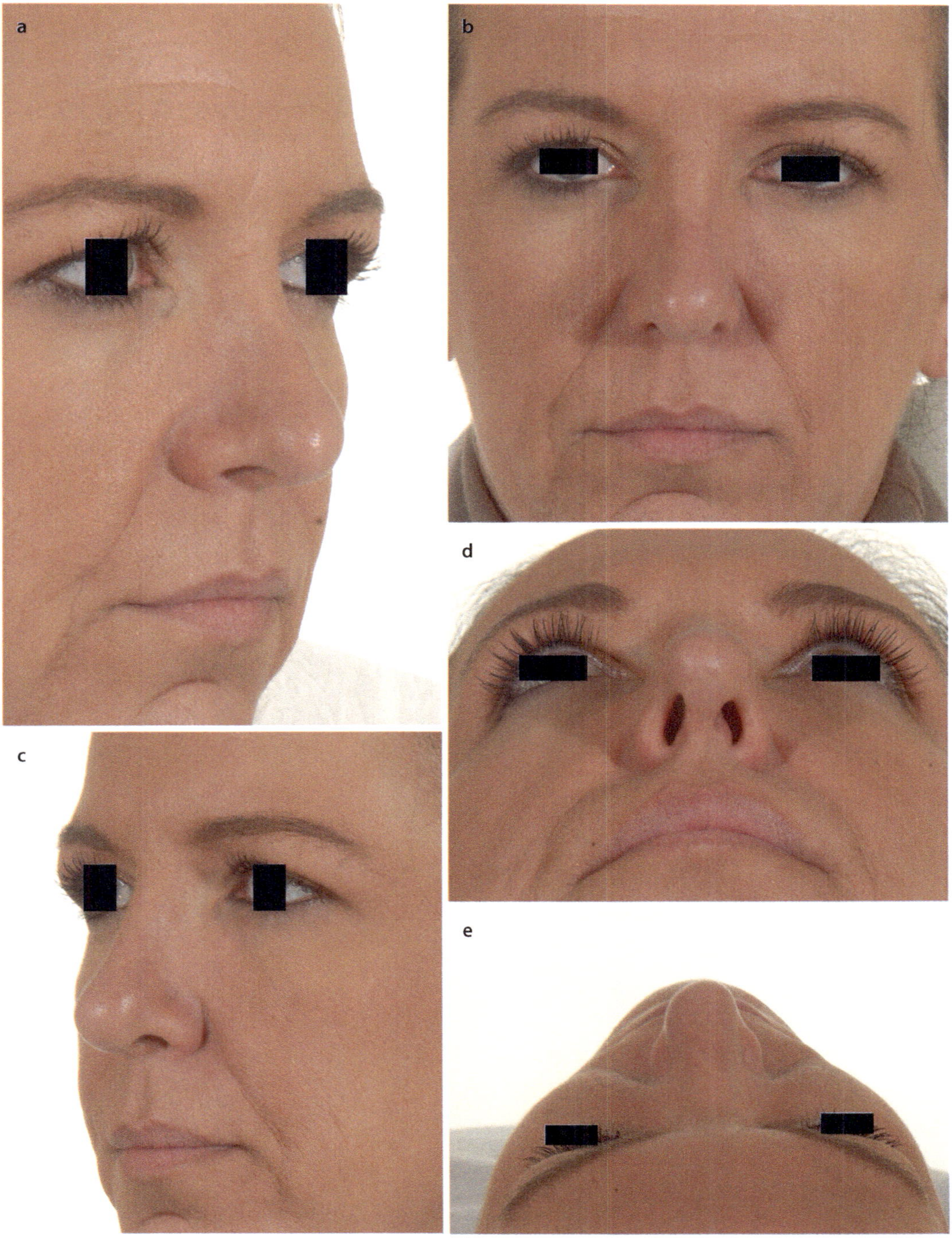

◘ **Fig. 19.2** **a–e** Bulbous nasal tip – post-operative photographs. **a** Right ¾ view. **b** Frontal view. **c** Left ¾ view. **d** Basal view. **e** Sky view

19.2 Management of Dorsal Hump – "Component" Reduction

19.2.1 History

This patient complained of nasal dorsal deformity and nasal obstruction following nasal trauma. He would like to have the breathing improved and the hump addressed. He felt that his hump is more prominent after the trauma.

19.2.2 Pre-op Photos (◘ Fig. 19.3)

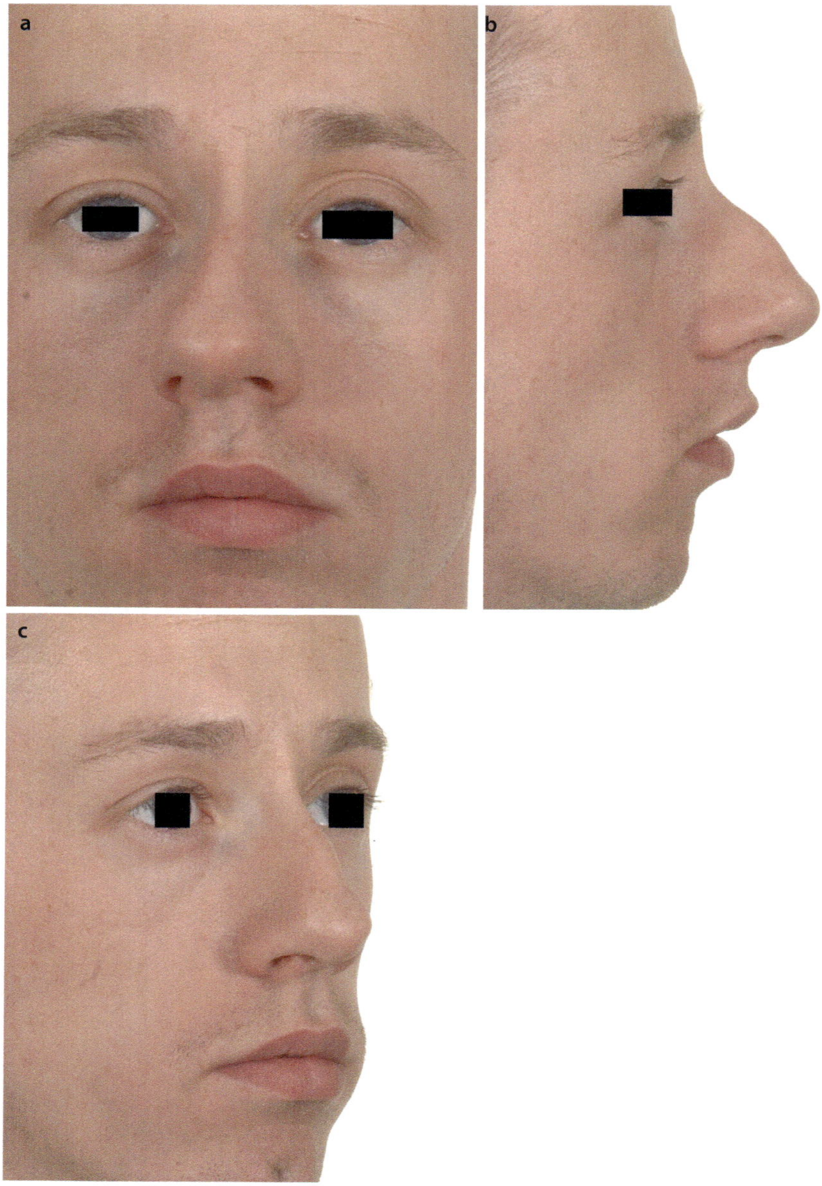

◘ **Fig. 19.3** **a**–**c** Dorsal nasal hump – pre-operative photographs. **a** Frontal view. **b** Right lateral view. **c** Right ¾ view

19.2.3 Assessment

Frontal and lateral views showed an *over projected and very thin nasal dorsum* with a degree of micrognathia. He had *tension nose* with excess caudal septal and dorsal septal cartilage with a longer stretched upper lip. The nasal pyramid is generally shifted to the right side with a split in the tip cartilages and very thin dorsal bony and cartilaginous hump. The columella is wider due to splaying of both medial crural foot plate, distortion of soft triangle, with a bifid tip.

19.2.4 Patient's Expectations

To improve the breathing and removal of the hump to make the nose smaller if possible.

19.2.5 Thought Process

Correcting the septal deviation is a key for a successful rhinoplasty in this patient. Also in view of the extremely narrow, but large bony and cartilagenous hump and overlying thin skin, any hump reduction can collapse the internal valve, and hence be careful not to over excise and also preferably to do a prophylactic spreader graft or an auto-spreader to prevent any post-operative nasal obstruction. Also for this reason, in long thin over projected dorsal humps, we prefer to do a "component" reduction instead of composite reduction preserving the internal valve junction which also helps us in doing the spreader grafts or spreader flaps if necessary.

19.2.6 Surgical Steps

The surgery was performed through an open approach, septoplasty, component reduction of the cartilagenous and bony dorsum and a bilateral spreader grafts to support the internal valve.

Conclusion

The patient was happy with the outcome in terms of both the shape and breathing improvement. Note he is also a candidate for chin implants which we did not do. Hump reduction can be done through either a "composite" reduction or a "component" reduction. The indications for both can be varied depending on the surgeon's choices. One specific indication for "component" reduction in our experience is a large narrow and thin dorsal hump with more cartilage component like this patient. Septal cartilage height is reduced first, then upper lateral, then dorsal nasal bones in that sequence. This technique prevents any damage to the septal-ULC junction and helps to reconstruct this region either with free spreader grafts or turn in the dorsal ULC to form an auto-spreader.

19.2.7 Post-op Photos (Fig. 19.4)

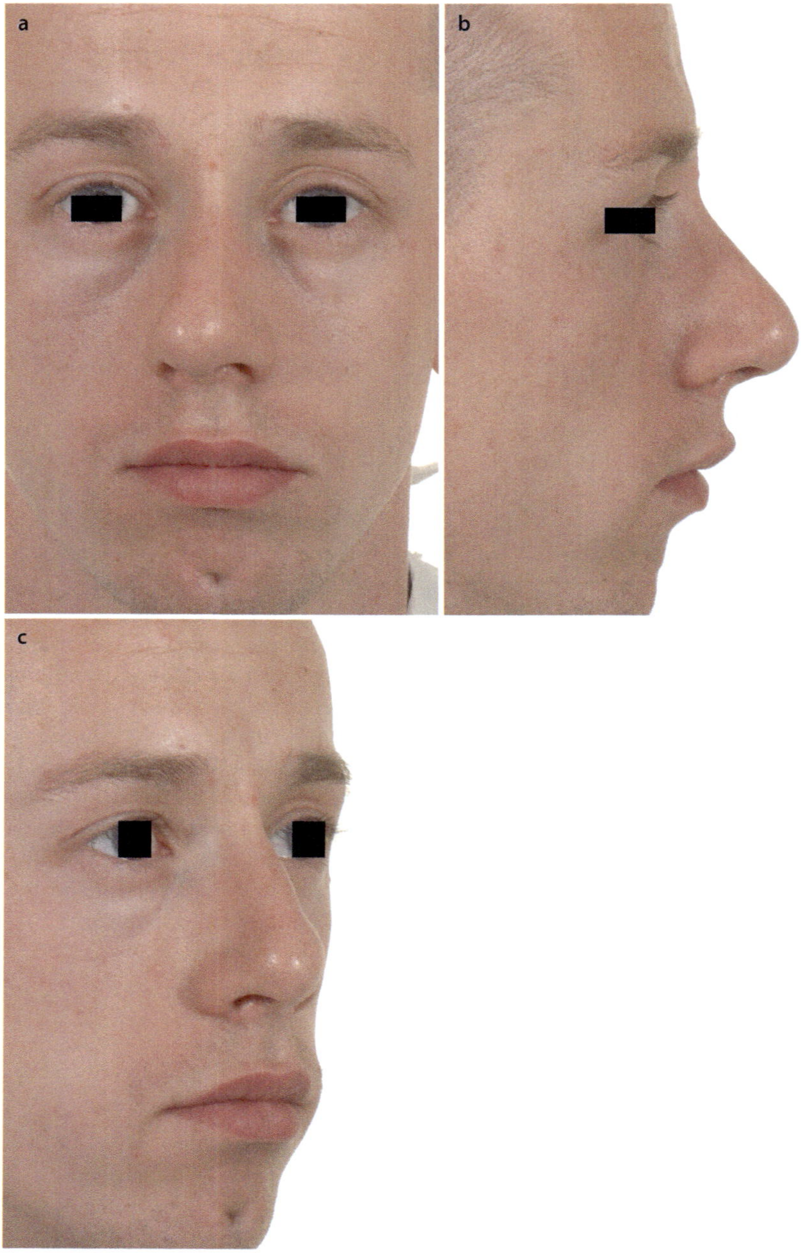

Fig. 19.4 **a–c** Dorsal nasal hump – post-operative photographs. **a** Frontal view. **b** Right lateral view. **c** Right ¾ view

19.3 Management of Dorsal Hump – "Composite" Reduction

19.3.1 History

Similar to the above patient, this patient also complained of nasal dorsal deformity in the form of hump and nasal obstruction following nasal trauma. He would like to have the breathing improved and the hump reduced. He felt that his hump is more prominent after the trauma.

19.3.2 Pre-op Photos (Fig. 19.5)

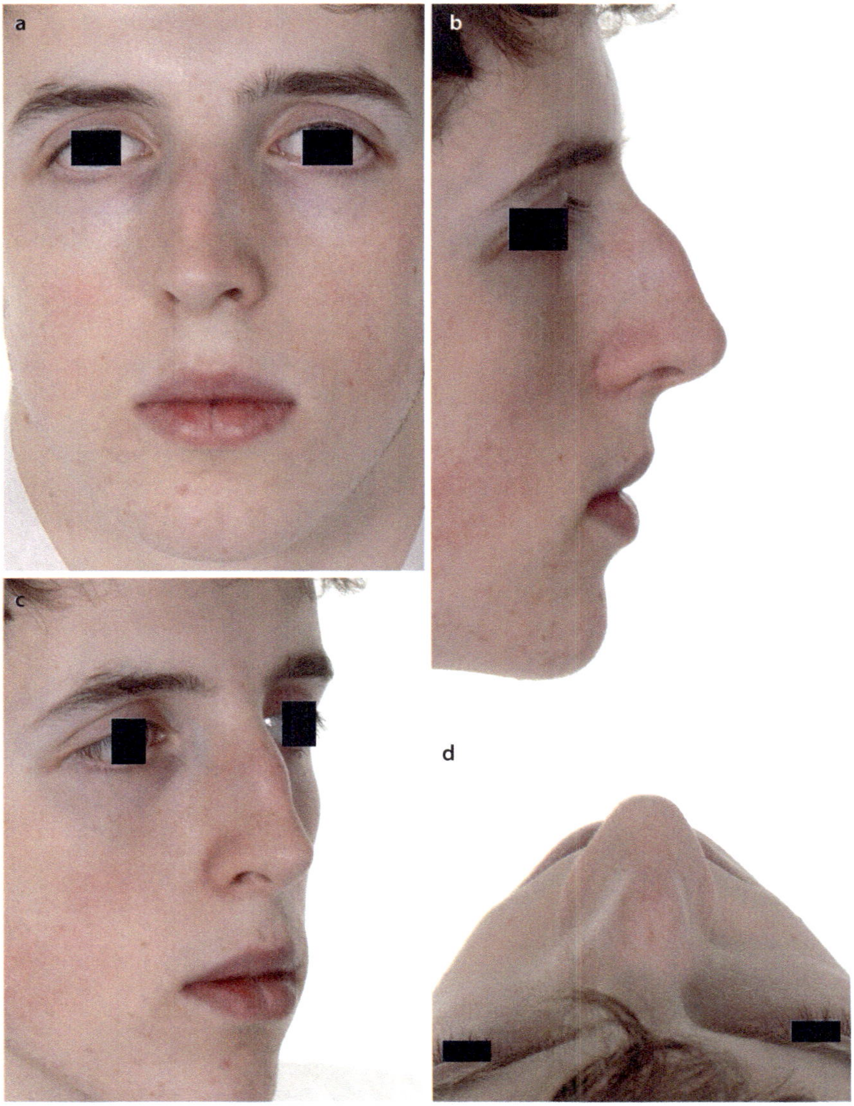

Fig. 19.5 **a**–**d** Dorsal nasal hump – pre-operative photographs. **a** Frontal view. **b** Right lateral view. **c** Right ¾ view. **d** Sky view

19.3.3 Assessment

Frontal and lateral views showed an over projected wider nasal dorsum with "diamond-shaped open book" deformity, involving the bony dorsal pyramid. He had a tension nose with over projection of the tip. He has a dorsal scar.

19.3.4 Patient's Expectations

To straighten the nasal septum and removal of the dorsal hump.

19.3.5 Thought Process

Correcting the septal deviation is a key for a successful rhinoplasty in this patient. Also in view of the fact that the dorsal hump is wider and limited to the bony dorsum, a composite reduction was planned as ideal. The tension nose is more commonly due to excess caudal septum at the posterior septal angle or less commonly due to excess anterior nasal bony spine. Be aware that the new technique of "preservation rhinoplasty" popularised recently does not work in these patients when there is an open book dorsum with external scar.

19.3.6 Surgical Steps

The surgery was performed through an open approach, septoplasty, composite reduction of the cartilagenous and bony dorsum and a caudal triangular septal shave of 4 mm with the base of the triangle at the columellar labial junction.

Conclusion

The patient was happy with the outcome in terms of both the shape and breathing improvement. Thus hump reduction can be done through either a "composite" reduction or a "component" reduction. The indications for both can be varied depending on the surgeon's choices. One specific indication in our experience for a "composite" reduction is a patient like this with a limited bony hump with a wider open book deformity as opposed to a very thin cartilagenous dorsal hump as discussed in case report 2.

19.3.7 Post-op Photos (Fig. 19.6)

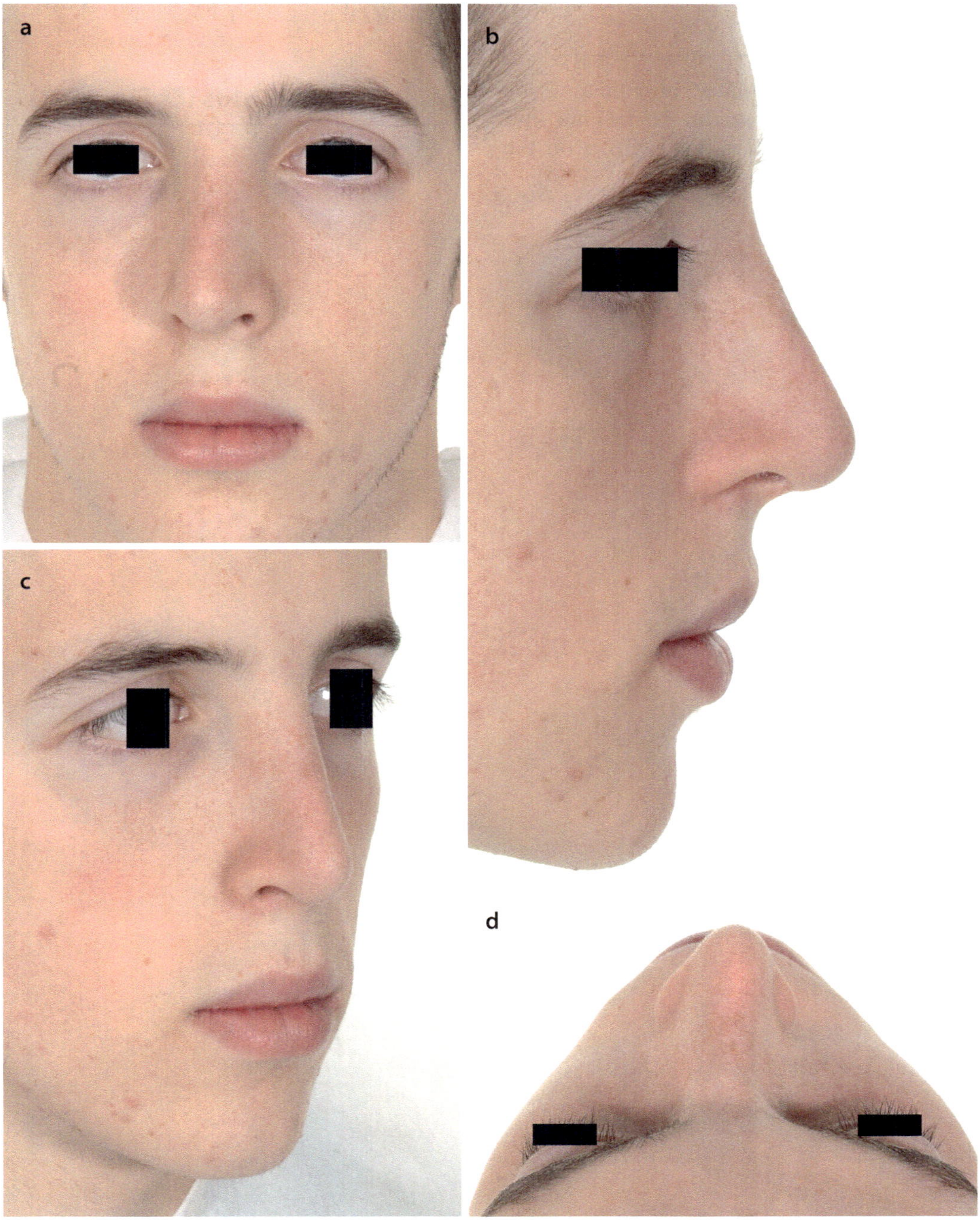

Fig. 19.6 **a–d** Dorsal nasal hump – post-operative photographs. **a** Frontal view. **b** Right lateral view. **c** Right ¾ view. **d** Sky view

19.4 Management of Collapsed Dorsum – Bilateral Spreader Grafts

19.4.1 History

The following two patients illustrate the issue of mid-dorsal collapse due to trauma and previous surgery with varying effects on the tip and internal nasal valve function. Both these patients had dorsal reconstruction without rib graft and had satisfactory, and stable long term results with bilateral conchal and bilateral helical cartilage grafts.

19.4.2 Pre-op Photos (◘ Fig. 19.7)

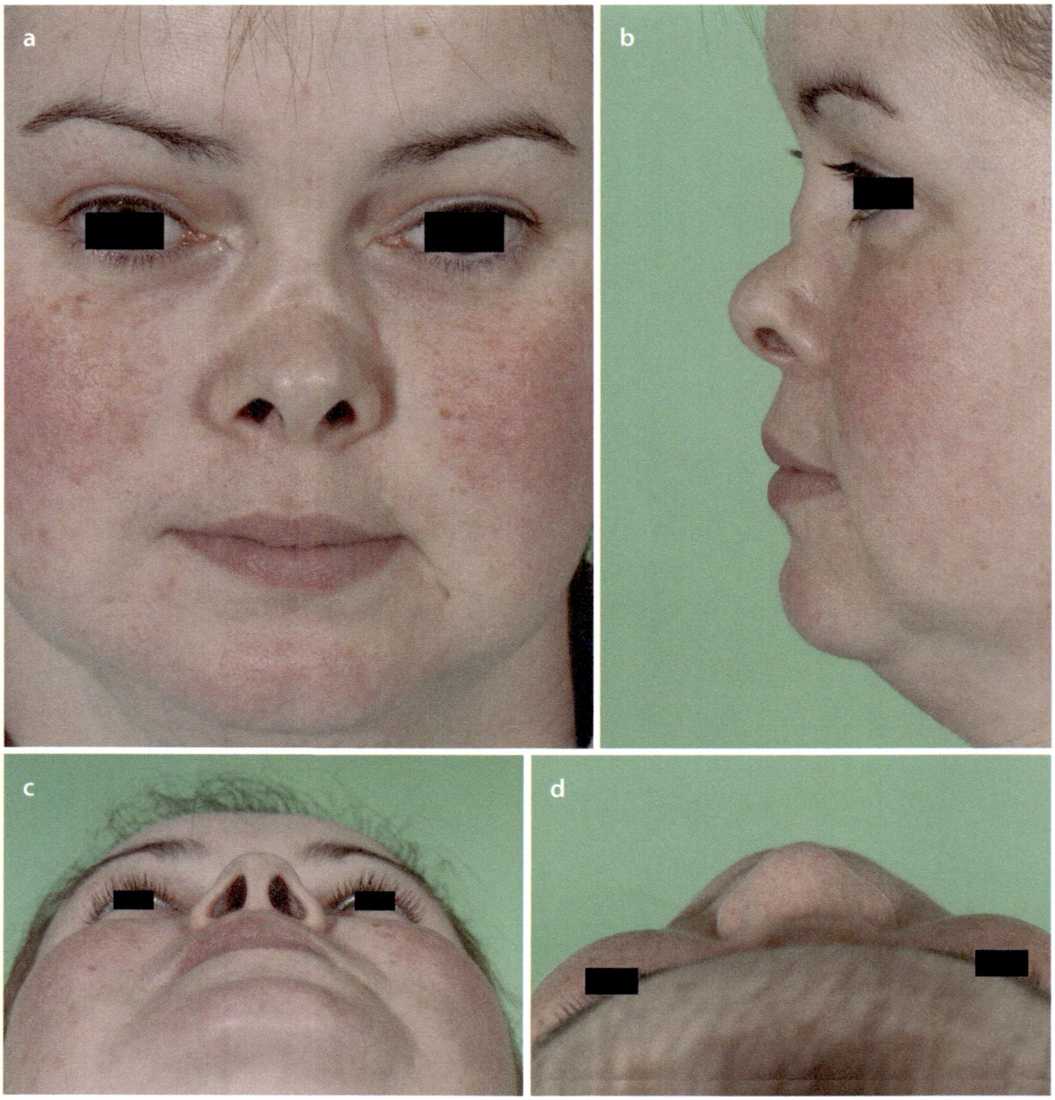

◘ **Fig. 19.7** **a–d** Collapsed nasal dorsum – pre-operative photographs. **a** Frontal view. **b** Left lateral view. **c** Basal view. **d** Sky view

19

19.4.3 Pre-op Photos (Fig. 19.8)

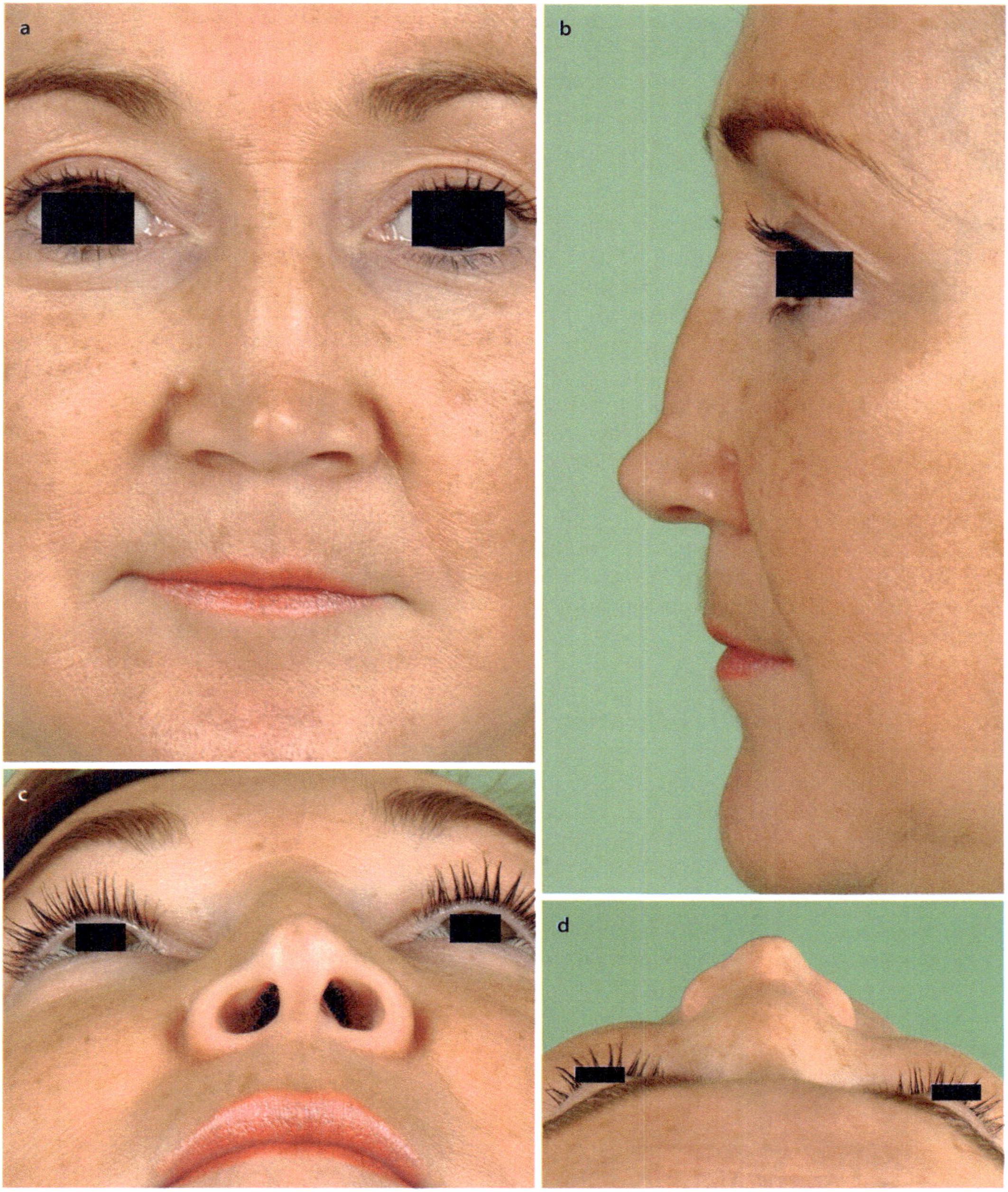

Fig. 19.8 **a**–**d** Collapsed nasal dorsum – pre-operative photographs. **a** Frontal view. **B** Left lateral view. **c** Basal view. **d** Sky view

19.4.4 Assessment

Both have extensive dorsal collapse with pinched lateral alar segments with over rotated tip worse in one patient and very thin and contracted skin, with no septal perforation.

19.4.5 Thought Process

Mid-dorsal nasal depression can be part of a complex deformity requiring more than one surgical procedure. Dorsal defects are often combined with a loss of septal support at the middle vault, internal nasal valve obstruction and tip deformities with lack of columellar septal support. This complex deformity is often poorly treated due to a difficulty in classifying the extent of the deformity and subsequent planning of a surgical solution. Existing classification systems do not address the different co-existing deformities and hence we use our own Glasgow classification as described below.

19.4.6 The Glasgow Classification

Type 1: Minor dorsal de-projection requiring minor dorsal augmentation (e.g., cartilage graft plus or minus bony lateral osteotomies).

Type 2: Mid-dorsal de-projection with hourglass narrowing of mid dorsum causing *internal nasal valve obstruction* with *no tip deformity* – requiring additional internal nasal valve surgery (e.g., spreader grafts).

Type 3: Mid-dorsal de-projection with *abnormalities of tip* – requiring additional nasal tip reconstruction with or without caudal septal reconstruction (e.g., medial crural strut, extension graft).

Type 4: Mid-dorsal de-projection with *combination of internal valve and tip deformities* – requiring complex multiple procedures.

These patients have thin and contracted skin with poor soft tissue cover. As soon as you see these pictures, please do not consider rib grafts straight away. If so, then most probably you have not had much experience or not practising long enough! If ear cartilage is available, then it should be the first choice rather than rib graft due to poor skin cover. We harvested conchal and helical cartilage in both patients. This can be time consuming, results slightly sub-optimal, but certainly long lasting without any issues and without the need for any further surgery, which the patients appreciate. The alternative is a rib cartilage graft (either irradiated or autologous). Be aware that rib cartilage does not do well in these types of patients as the skin envelope is tight and thin and contracted with tip over rotation. Rib cartilage is rigid and do not integrate with the underlying nasal dorsal tissues and move about and easily get dislocated. Moreover rib cartilage failures are extremely difficult to tackle. (We would be very happy to learn from any surgeon who can show us their long-term results of using rib cartilage in these types of patients). Although the reconstruction might be sub-optimal with ear cartilage in these patients, the long-term stability is quite good with ear cartilage graft, provided there is enough material for reconstruction.

If there is no ear cartilage in these types of patients, instead of rib cartilage graft, I have two options, one to send the patient to someone who can give better results with rib grafts or do a simple camouflage grafting with multiple layers of fascia lata, which gives better long-term cosmetic improvement, although sub-optimal. In our experience, rib cartilage grafts are suitable for septal reconstructions, including septal extension or caudal extension grafts and not for dorsal grafting in these patients. Of course the other consideration is the presence or absence of septal perforation. The presence of septal perforation adds to the issues of reconstruction, and it is impossible to provide functional and structural improvement in these patients. The management of these types of deformities are individualised based on what the patient wants and what the surgeon can provide. In our experience given the choice, patients are happier to undergo the procedure which will make the appearance of the nose better than the functional symptoms of a septal perforation, particularly patients with other comorbidities including underlying granulomatous conditions.

19.4.7 Surgical Steps

Based on our classification of the mid-dorsal collapse, these patients may need simple dorsal grafting for type 1 deformities. Type 2 deformities will need additional work in the internal valve region with dorsal extension grafts and spreaders. Type 3 and 4 will need additional tip work which may range from simple to complex procedures, to rotate the tip down with lateral crural strut grafts and also rim grafts to support the alar margin. We prefer an open approach in these patients in view of the complexity of the deformities. Both patients underwent open approach bilateral spreader grafts, dorsal augmentation with ear cartilage graft and tip plasty. Again the grafts were taken from both ears rather than rib cartilage.

Conclusion

Reconstruction of a mid-dorsal collapse can be complex and requires an understanding of the pathophysiology of the defects and the hence the surgery is varied and tailored to individual patients based on their needs and the surgeon's experience. Severity of the dorsal collapse should not be the only factor to make a decision for a rib graft, and adequate augmentation of the dorsum can be achieved with bilateral conchal and bilateral helical grafting in these types of patients.

19.4.8 Post-op Photos (◘ Fig. 19.9)

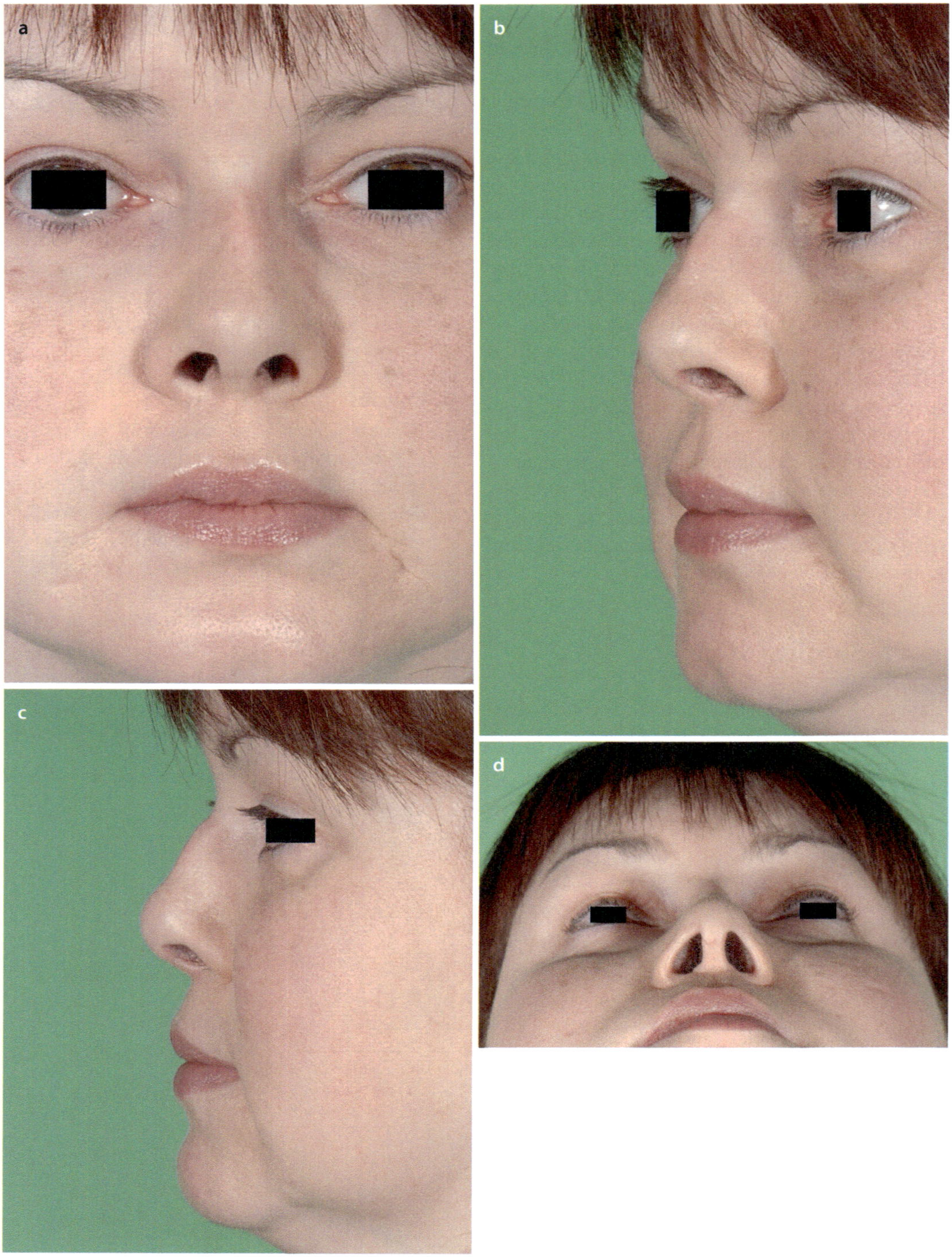

◘ **Fig. 19.9** **a–d** Collapsed nasal dorsum – post-operative photographs. **a** Frontal view. **b** Left ¾ view. **c** Left lateral view. **d** Basal view

19.4.9 Post-op Photos (Fig. 19.10)

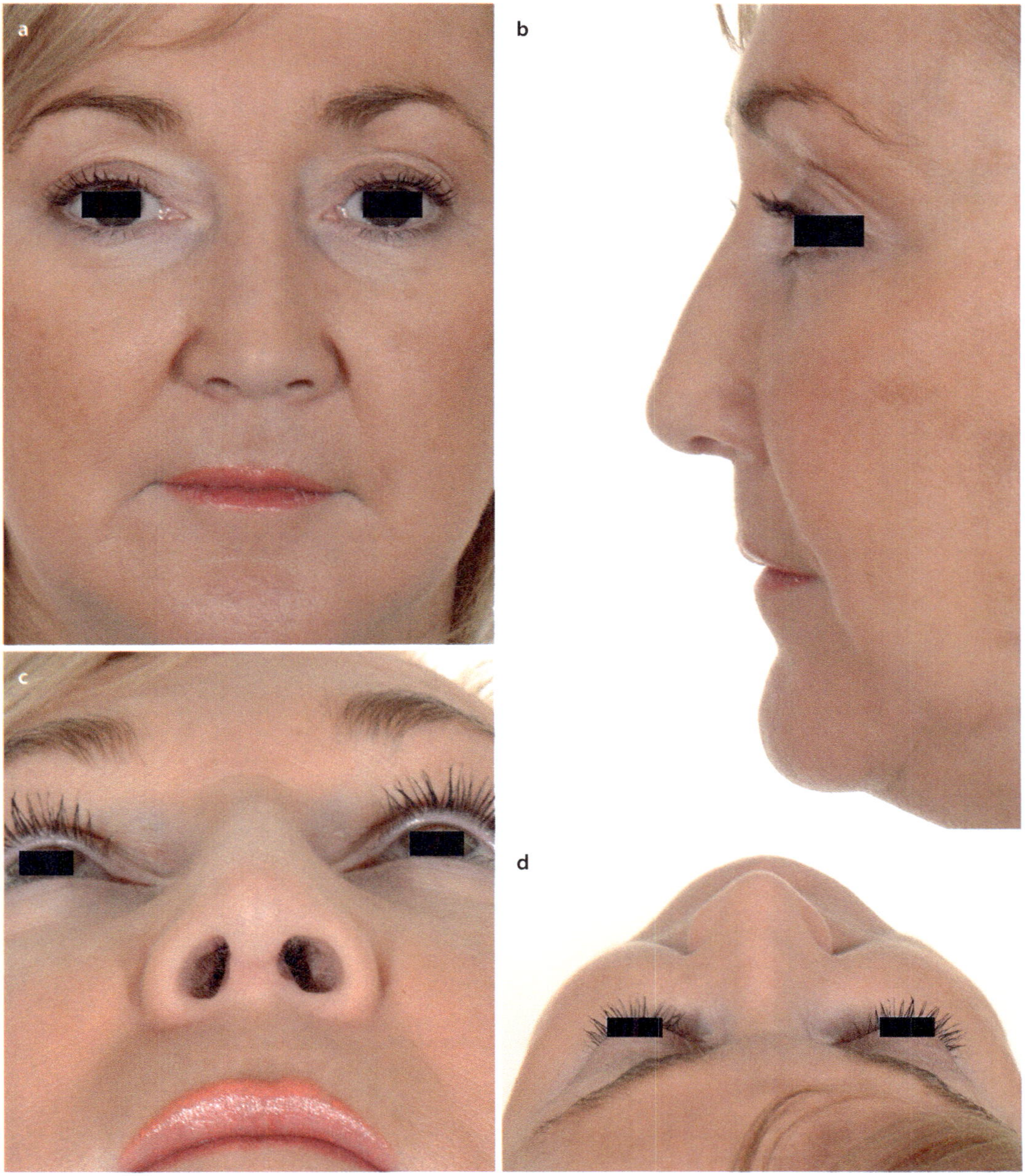

Fig. 19.10 **a–d** Collapsed nasal dorsum – post-operative photographs. **a** Frontal view. **b** Left lateral view. **c** Basal View. **d** Sky view

19.5 Management of Collapsed Dorsum – Septal Extension Graft

19.5.1 History

This young girl presented with a history of early childhood fronto-nasal trauma and nasal obstruction and a depressed and a twisted nasal dorsum. The nasal deformity was getting worse as she grew older. She was requesting septorhinoplasty to improve the breathing and the shape. She was generally fit and well otherwise, with sensible expectations.

19.5.2 Pre-op Photos (◘ Fig. 19.11)

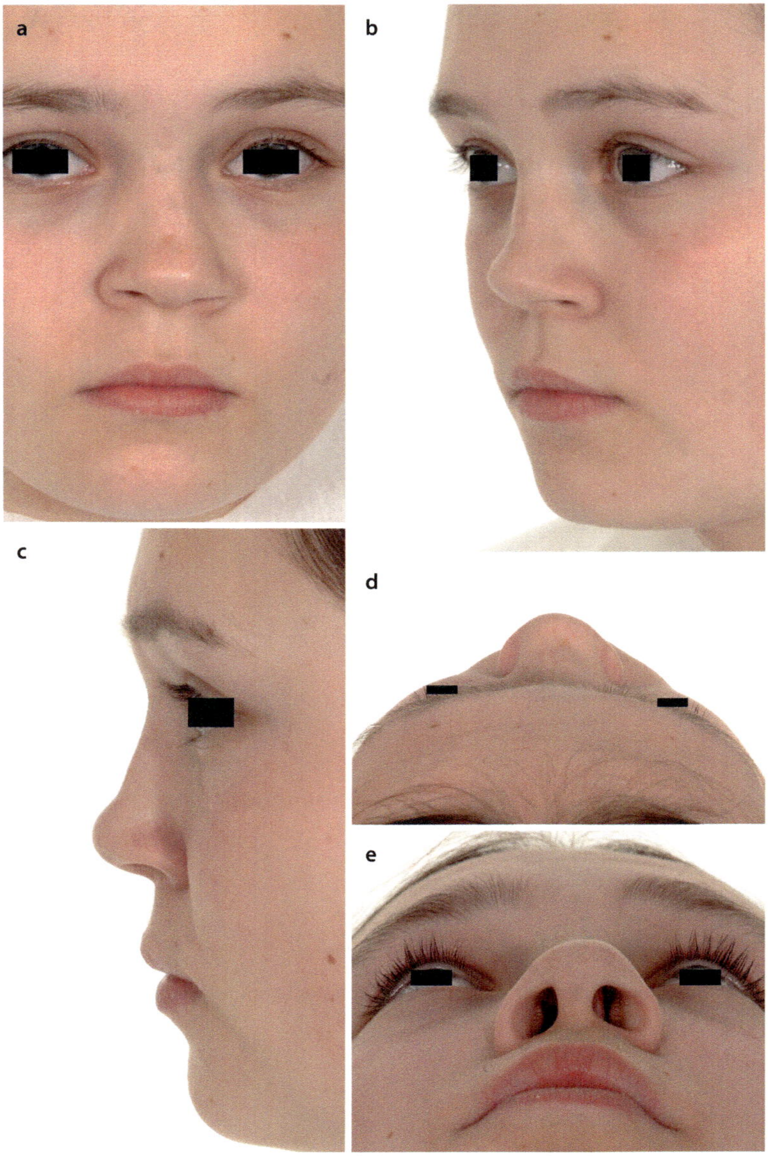

◘ **Fig. 19.11** **a**–**d** Collapsed and twisted nasal dorsum – pre-operative photographs. **a** Frontal view. **b** Left ¾ view. **c** Left lateral view. **d** Sky view. **e** Basal view

19.5.3 Assessment

She has moderate dorsal collapse more towards the right side with a slight deviation of the dorsum to the left with a small de-projected tip. Her septum was grossly deviated with lack of mid dorsal and caudal septal support. Length of the nose was shorter with an over rotated tip. Position of the two ala were asymmetric with right side higher than the left.

19.5.4 Thought Process

Mid-dorsal nasal depression can be part of a complex deformity requiring more than one surgical procedure. In this patient, mid-dorsal defect is due to a loss of septal support at the middle vault, internal nasal valve obstruction with no primary issues with tip cartilages. Straightening the dorsal septum and strengthening the dorsal and caudal septum is the key in this lady to achieve long-term results. Septal extension grafts also help to increase the length of the nose. The patient should be warned that the position of the ala cannot be corrected satisfactorily.

19.5.5 Surgical Steps

This patient underwent an open approach, septoplasty, dorsal and caudal septal extension grafts taken from the septum leaving an "L" strut.

> **Conclusion**
>
> Reconstruction of a mid-dorsal collapse can be complex and requires an understanding of the pathophysiology of the defects, and hence the surgery is varied and tailored to individual patients based on their needs and the surgeon's experience. Although the patient was happy with the reconstruction and the nasal function has improved as well, it was sub-optimal with persistent asymmetry of nostril position which we find very difficult to correct.

19.5.6 Post-op Photos (◘ Fig. 19.12)

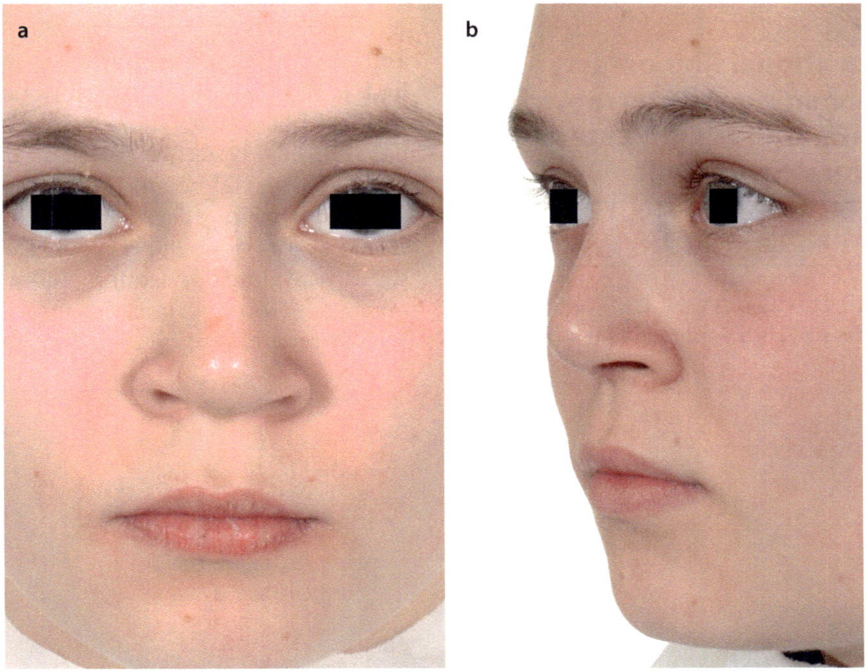

◘ **Fig. 19.12** **a**–**d** Collapsed and twisted nasal dorsum – post-operative photographs. **a** Frontal view. **b** Left ¾ view. **c** Left lateral view. **d** Sky view. **e** Basal view

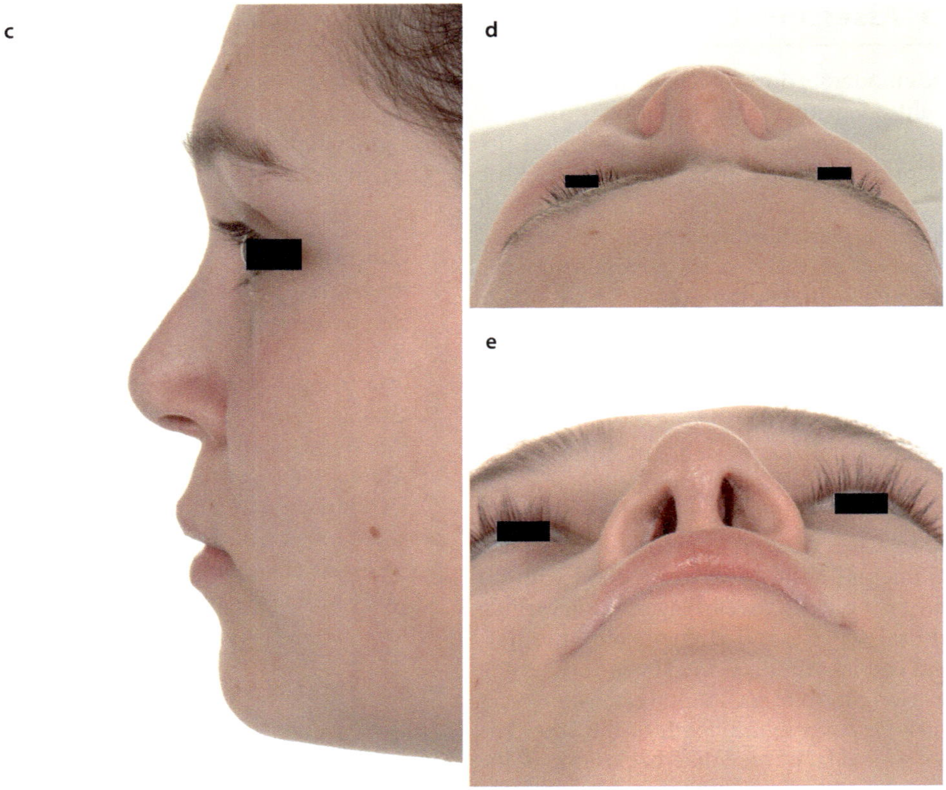

Fig. 19.12 (continued)

19.6 Functional Rhinoplasty – Managing an Interrupted Lateral Crus with Lateral Crural Strut Graft

19.6.1 History

This patient was referred from another unit up north, for right-sided nasal obstruction and collapse on inspiration after having had a vertical dome division done some 15 years back. Since then, nasal obstruction has been slowly getting worse on both sides, with right side being the worse. Patient was happy with the tip projection he got from the previous surgery. He had a classic vertical dome division including the alar mucosa. (Goldman procedure) (There was a good record kept by the patient.)

19.6.2 Pre-op Photos (■ Fig. 19.13)

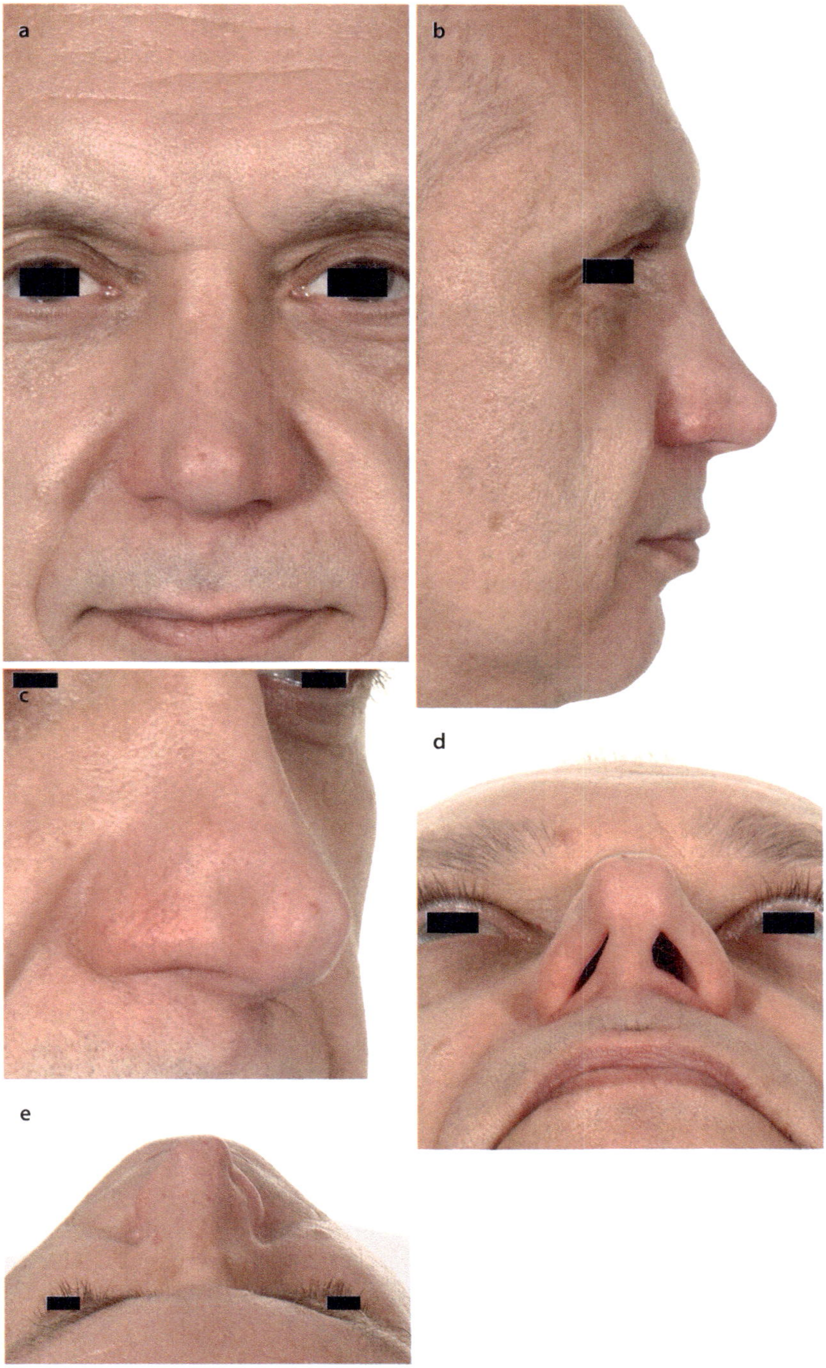

■ **Fig. 19.13** **a–e** Functional rhinoplasty, interrupted lateral crus – pre-operative photographs. **a** Frontal view. **b** Right lateral view. **c** Right ¾ view. **d** Basal view. **e** Sky view

19.6.3 Patient's Expectation

To have functional improvement in breathing on both sides and to correct the concavity in the right alar region if possible. Patient's expectations were realistic.

19.6.4 Assessment

Frontal and right lateral and basal views show narrowing of the right nasal ala with a localised area of concave defect about 4 mm wide in the right lateral ala oriented vertically across the horizontal lateral crus just lateral to the dome, typical findings following a vertical dome division. Please note in the "sky view", the tip is turning to the same affected side (right). This is due to the relatively stronger lower lateral and tip cartilages on the left side (better side) pushing the tip to the more affected side. This is a good sign to diagnose defects involving ONLY the lateral crus and not the soft tissues of the lateral alar region. The tip of the nose is also very sharp and pointing in the frontal view due to the increased projection got in the previous dome division.

19.6.5 Thought Process

Vertical dome divisions as originally described was a powerful technique to divide the dome lateral to the tip and turning them towards each other to increase the tip projection. The down side being lateral alar collapse or weakness developing later on, as seen in our patient. Intranasal examination and palpation showed a straight septum with enough cartilage for reconstruction. Open approach was planned as it offers superior exposure for diagnosis of the pathology. Please remember we do not have the luxury of an MRI scan to diagnose the exact pathology in the cartilage and hence we can't give an informed choice to the patient before surgery. We need to be prepared for all eventualities. The patients should be made aware of these diagnostic dilemmas at the consultation stage, and pros and cons of all the possibilities should be discussed as structure and function cannot be complementary to each other at most times.

This patient's main concern was functional with right nasal obstruction, getting worse progressively. The patient was not concerned with the shape of the nose. If you apply our new Glasgow Nasal "wall" classification, it is the right lateral wall subunit (LW3) is weak. A focussed surgical approach to the lateral crus is needed depending on the damage to the lateral crus.

External nasal tip deformities secondary to weak and damaged lateral crus is one of the difficult scenarios to correct in tip rhinoplasty practice. A damaged lateral crus is ideally reconstructed with a strut graft which goes between the lateral crural remnants and the underlying alar mucosa.

The other choice being a "batten" grafts which is not suitable if there is a fractured or damaged lateral crus. As we mentioned before, batten grafts are good only, if the lateral alar region is weak due to defects either above or below the lateral crus. In this patient we did bilateral lateral crural strut grafts with cartilage harvested from the nasal septum leaving behind an "L" strut. Be aware that batten graft will make symptoms worse if used on a damaged lateral crus.

19.6.6 Surgical Steps

Open approach showed missing 4 mm vertical strip of lateral crus more on the right close to the dome. The rest of the width of the lateral crus was very reduced and moth eaten. Straight septal cartilage grafts were harvested leaving an "L" strut. The remnants of lateral crus were lifted by hydro dissection from the underlying alar mucosa. Then the strut grafts were placed and secured under the lateral crus. The position of the graft was adjusted to prevent alar margin retraction. The graft was secured with 5 o Vicryl since the stitch has to go through the alar mucosa.

Conclusion

Patient was happy with a Visual Analogue Score improvement in airway and patient satisfaction. This patient illustrates the typical indication for a lateral crural strut graft where the weakness is exactly in the lateral crus as evident by a vertical narrow strip of defect in the lateral crus causing functional narrowing of the external nasal valve region. On the contrary batten grafts should not be used when the lateral crus is weak or damaged or fractured and missing. In our experience, sometimes clinical examination alone is not possible to diagnose satisfactorily lateral crural damage until otherwise the nose is opened. Hence open approach is our preferred option for lateral crural deformities. Particularly in a traumatic patient, since we can't make an exact anatomical diagnosis of the deformity without opening the nose, the surgeon should be aware of various different surgical options to correct the lateral crural deformities.

19.6.7 Post-op Photos (Fig. 19.14)

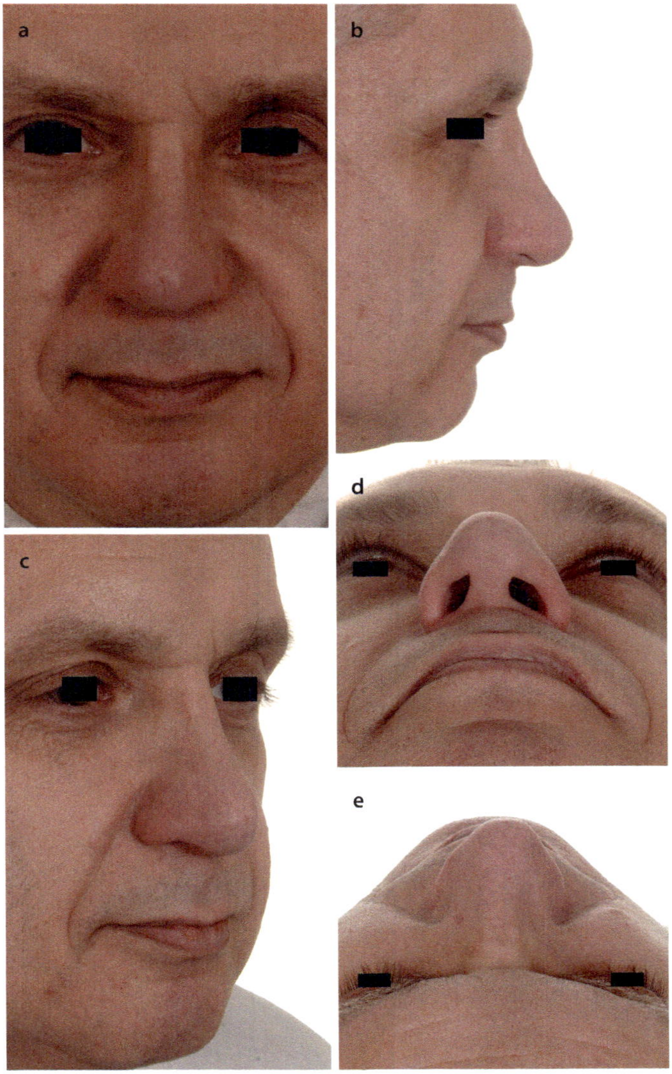

Fig. 19.14 **a–e** Functional rhinoplasty, interrupted lateral crus – postoperative photographs. **a** Frontal view. **b** Right lateral view. **c** Right ¾ view. **d** Basal view. **e** Sky view

19.7 Functional Nasal Valve Surgery – Bilateral Concavity of Lateral Crus

19.7.1 History

This gentleman presented with bilateral nasal obstruction requesting to improve the nasal airway. He had bilateral alar concavity, pinching on inspiration with a straight septum. Symptoms have been there for many years, getting worse recently. History of non-specific nasal trauma in youth. We did see him few times before surgery, and he was keen to pursue surgery to improve his nasal function and if possible correct the alar pinching and concavity. Although he had some dorsal hump and over projected tip as well, he was not concerned with the rest of the nasal structure. He was sensible and realistic in his expectations with good general health.

19.7.2 Pre-op Photos (■ Fig. 19.15)

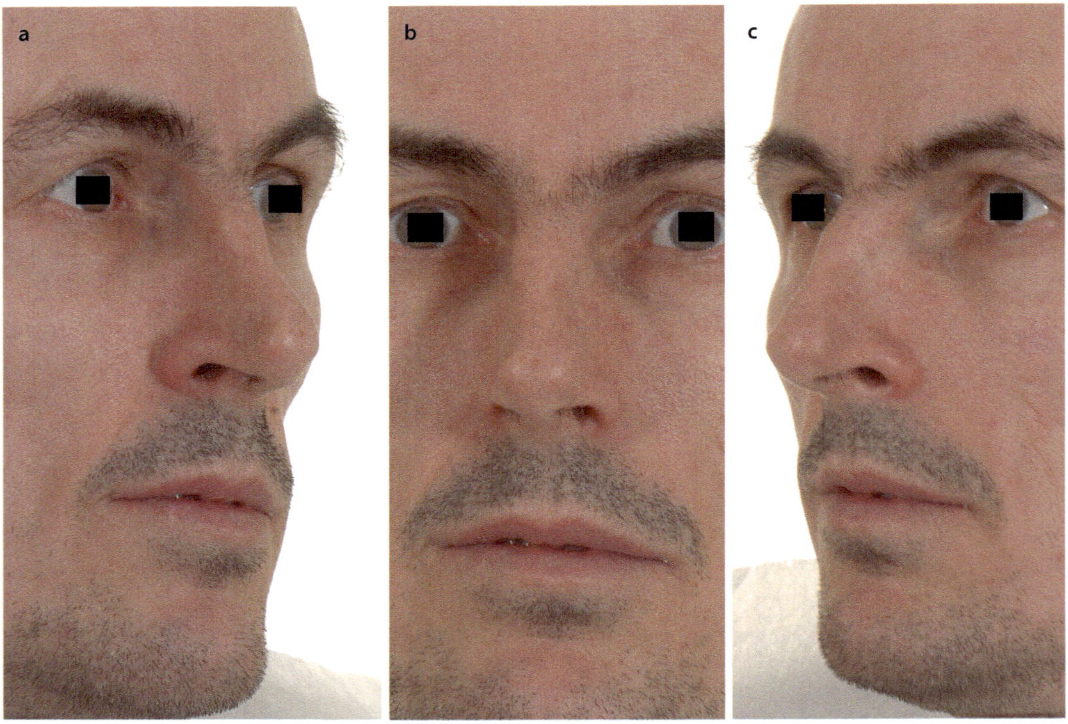

■ **Fig. 19.15** **a–e** Functional rhinoplasty, concave but intact lateral crus – pre-operative photographs. **a** Right ¾ view. **b** Frontal view. **c** Left ¾ view. **d** Sky view. **e** Basal view

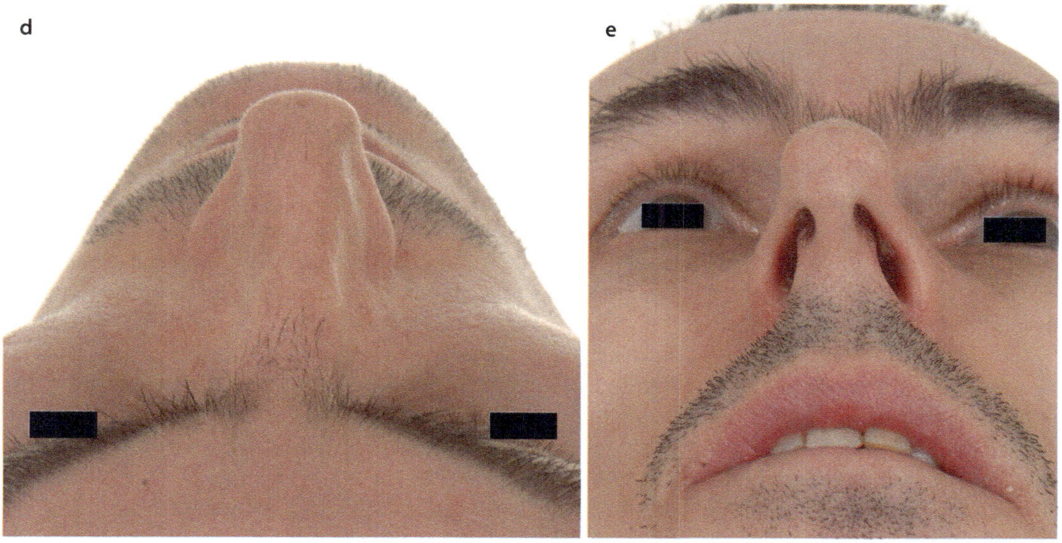

Fig. 19.15 (continued)

19.7.3 Patient's Expectation

To have functional improvement in breathing and to correct the concavity in the ala if possible.

19.7.4 Assessment

On examination, in the frontal view, there is an over projected nose with a narrow dorsum and an over projected tip with concave lateral crus worse on right side. Basal view shows an over projected nasal tip lobule with a uniformly wide columella, with a narrow slit like nostrils. One can see the inverted hour glass widening of the columella from the tip lobule to the sill. This is due to the flaring of the two medial crural footplate as it approaches the nasal base. This is causing unusual thickening of the columella causing narrowing at the external valve region. There may be in addition an excess caudal septum causing this extra width. The septum was straight. The lateral crus on both sides were weak and concave at rest and worse on forced inspiration.

19.7.5 Thought Process

The patient's main concern is functional with bilateral nasal obstruction, getting worse progressively. Not concerned with the shape of the nose. Using the current classification of external and internal nasal valve, most surgeons will agree that the area of narrowing seems to be at the external valve region. But there ends the agreement. The next step of what exactly the pathology is and how to arrive at a surgical plan to help the patient breath better is difficult to agree upon between different surgeons.

Applying our functional New Glasgow Nasal "wall" sub-unit classification, we can figure out that the width of the columella (Area MW 3 sub unit) is too wide which need to be narrowed. Furthermore it helps our thought process to focus on individual sites. This thickened columella could be due to excess caudal septum as seen in this patient with an over projected long nose and or be associated with a bilateral medial crural flaring. These findings can be confirmed on open approach.

In this patient there is also a concavity and alar pinching at the lateral crus level (Area LW 2 subunit), which need to be addressed based on the findings (see algorithm in ► Chap. 18 addressing lateral crural pathology). Any long standing thickening of the columellar region, decreases the airflow and over the years gradually "pulls in" the lateral crus due to negative inspiratory forces, causing concavity of the lateral crus which in turn causes more obstruction at the external valve region. This is more so when they are born with excess width and length of the lateral crus with an over projection of the tip. The Sky view confirms bilateral lateral crural concavity. Any surgical procedure should be aimed at dealing with both the lateral crural concavity and also to reduce the width of the columella to achieve a good structural and functional outcome. This patient illustrates an important concept of addressing the medial nasal wall obstruction as a cause of lateral crural "indrawing" in a young patient with no specific trauma or surgery.

19.7.6 Surgical Steps

External nasal tip deformities secondary to weak and concave lateral crus are one of the difficult scenarios to correct in tip rhinoplasty practice. There are various techniques like batten graft, lateral crural strut graft, lateral crural turn in flap, lateral crural reciprocating grafts have being described to address various individual deformities of the lateral crus. If the lateral crural width is wider, but anatomically intact there is no need for strut grafts. Instead, this patient underwent *Cephalic "lateral crural turn out" flap, which helped both the concavity* and also gave adequate strength to prevent inspiratory collapse. Please see our ► Chap. 18 on algorithms of how to manage lateral crural pathologies.

The surgery was performed through an open approach, confirmed the findings of wide and concave, but structurally intact lateral crus on both sides. There was medial crural footplate flaring on both sides with excess caudal septum extending between the medial crural base just above the anterior nasal spine. He underwent 3 mm excision of the caudal septal cartilage along with medial crural fixation and flare control suture to narrow the columella. This was followed by lateral crural turn out flap leaving an intact lateral crus at the scroll for it to "spring out" to pull the lateral crus out during inspiration.

Conclusion

Patient was happy with an improvement in airway and patient satisfaction. This patient illustrates the typical indication for a lateral crural "turn-out" flap with an intact but wide concave lateral crus causing functional narrowing of the external nasal valve region. Since the width of the lateral crus is in excess, it is more likely the length of the lateral crus will be longer as well causing over projection of the tip as seen in our patient below.

19.7.7 Post-op Photos (◘ Fig. 19.16)

Comparing the pre-op and postop pictures of this patient above, we seemed to have achieved a "balance" between cosmetic appearance of the lateral ala and improvement in the nasal valve function. The patient reported NOSE score 6 weeks post-surgery was 10/10 improvement in the breathing with an improvement of the concave alar deformity. But as mentioned above, we advise this technique in a wider concave lateral crural deformity, *only* when there is no evidence of fracture, scarring or discontinuity of the lateral crus. In our hands, this diagnosis cannot be made for sure, until otherwise the nose is opened. Hence open approach is our preferred option for lateral crural deformities.

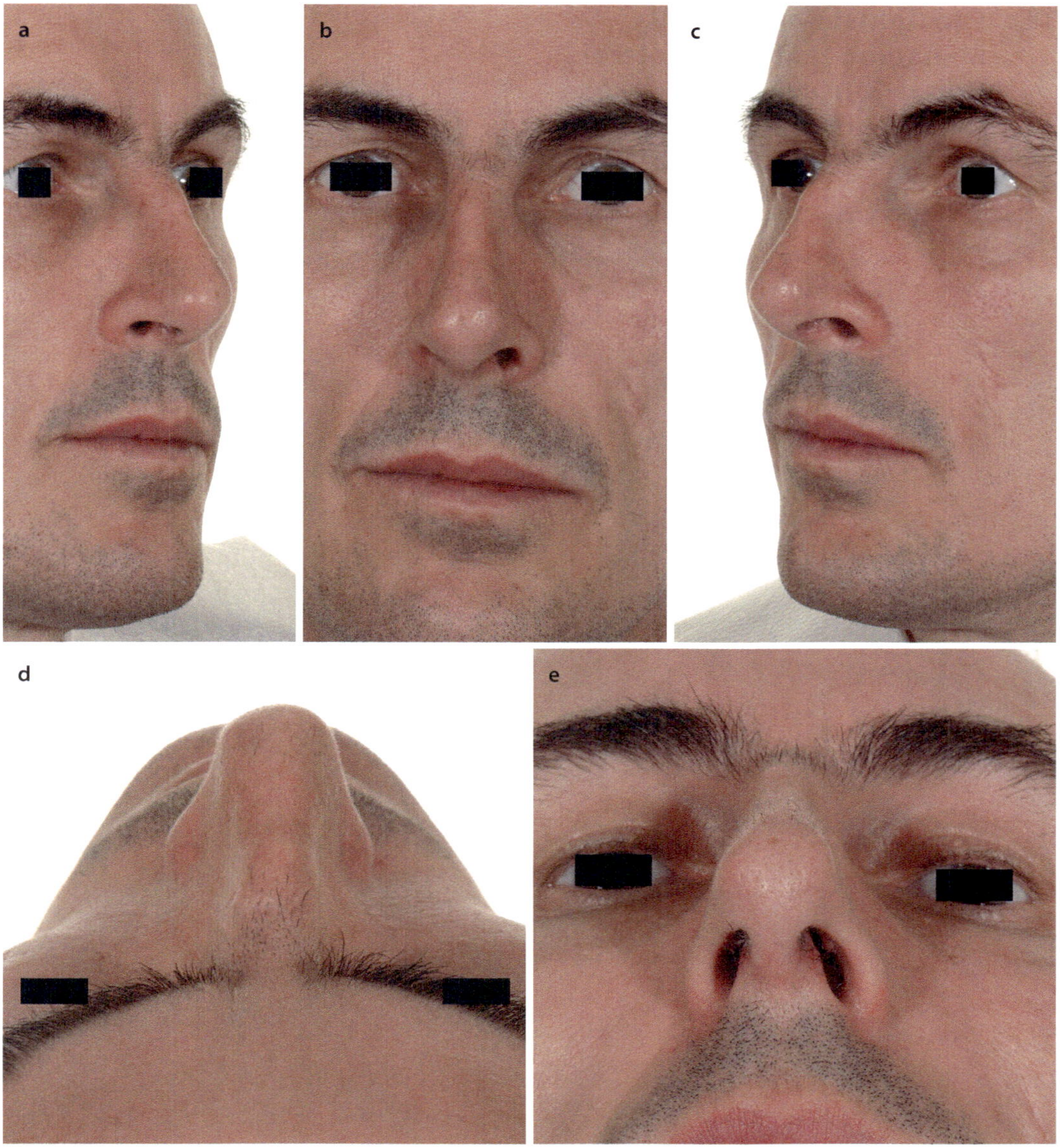

Fig. 19.16 **a–e** Functional rhinoplasty, concave but intact lateral crus – post-operative photographs. **a** Right ¾ view. **b** Frontal view. **c** Left ¾ view. **d** Sky view. **e** Basal view

19.8 Functional Rhinoplasty – Managing Unilateral Lateral Crural Concavity with Reciprocating Graft

19.8.1 History

This young lady presented with right-sided nasal obstruction with a collapsed lateral alar region on the right side following a long-standing repeated nasal trauma, with a twisted nasal tip requesting to improve the nasal airway and the concavity and alar collapse on the right side. There was also a bony twist of the nasal dorsum to the left side.

We did see her few times with a "cool-off" period before surgery and she was keen to pursue surgery to improve her nasal function and if possible correct the alar pinching and concavity on the right side (Area LW3 based on our Glasgow nasal wall sub-unit classification). She also wanted the slight dorsal hump to be reduced and nose straightened. She was sensible and realistic in her expectations with good general health.

19.8.2 Pre-op Photos (◘ Fig. 19.17)

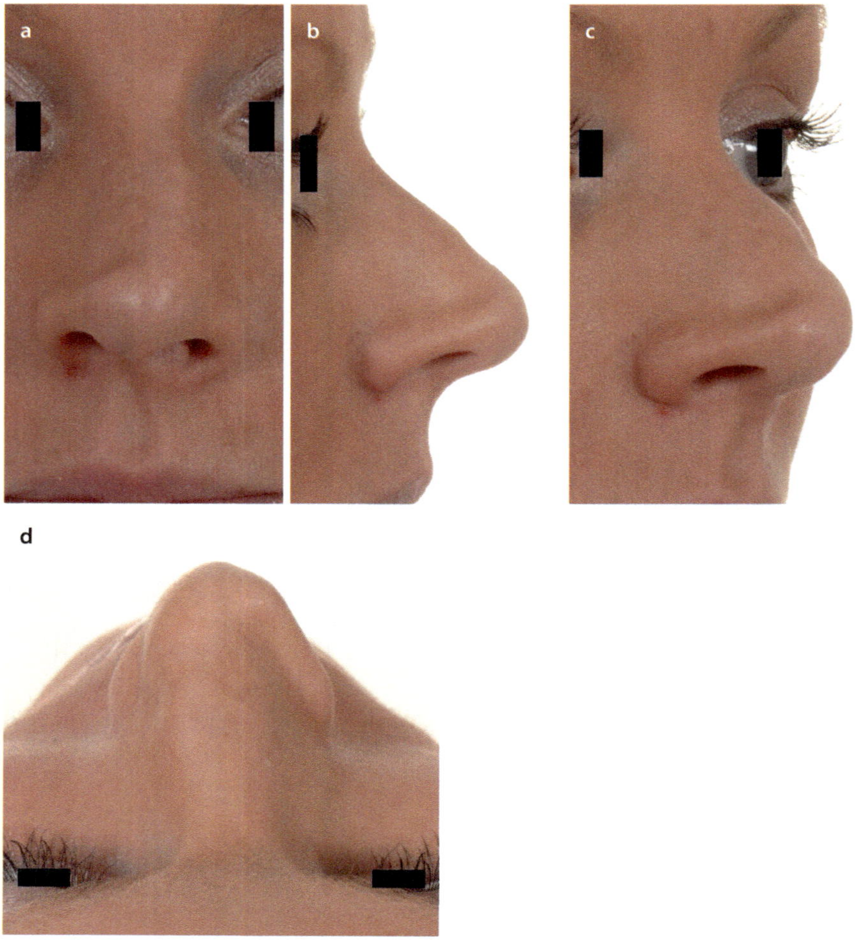

◘ **Fig. 19.17** **a–d** Functional rhinoplasty, unilateral concave lateral crus – pre-operative photographs. **a** Frontal view. **b** Right lateral view. **c** Right ¾ view. **d** Sky view

19.8.3 Patient's Expectation

To correct the concavity of the right ala and to have functional improvement in breathing on the right side.

19.8.4 Assessment

On examination, in the frontal view and in the ¾ view, there is an over projected nose with an over projected tip with concave lateral crus on the right side with tip asymmetry due to weak right lateral crus. There was a tip turn to the same weaker right side due to unopposed action of the left lateral crus. Please note that this tip turn is NOT because of the caudal septum which in fact is to the opposite side! There is also an over projection of the nasal tip lobule with a dip in the lateral crus close to the dome on the right side, with a septal deviation to the left side. There was also a dorsal twist to the left. Medial crural footplate was distorted. This is a primary tip deformity. The sky view confirms lateral crural concavity on the right side (Area LW3 based on our Glasgow nasal wall sub-unit classification). Any surgical procedure should deal with the lateral crural concavity and the worse thing to do in this patient is to put a batten graft on top of a weak and concave damaged lateral crus.

19.8.5 Thought Process

The patient's main concern is functional with nasal obstruction on the right side, getting progressively worse. Using the current classification of external and internal nasal valve, most surgeons will agree that the area of narrowing seems to be at the external valve region on the right side. But there ends the agreement. The next step of where and what exactly the pathology is and how to arrive at a surgical plan to help the patient breath better is difficult to agree upon between different surgeons.

On applying our Glasgow nasal "wall" sub-unit classification, we can figure out that there is a concavity and alar pinching at the lateral crus level (Area LW 3 subunit) on the right side, which need to be addressed based on the findings (see algorithm in addressing lateral crural pathology). Since the width of the lateral crus was adequate and the structure of the lateral crus was intact except a fracture line just lateral to the dome on the left side, we decided to flip the cartilage on its side by releasing the concave cartilage by going through the fracture line on the lateral crus on the right side.

19.8.6 Surgical Steps

This patient underwent *reciprocating LC graft on the right side* which helped both the concavity and also gave adequate strength to prevent inspiratory collapse. The surgery was performed through an open approach, raised the flap, confirmed the findings of wide and concave, but structurally intact with a single fracture in the lateral crus on right side just lateral to the dome. The septum was straightened and bilateral osteotomies done to straighten the bony complex followed by lateral crural reciprocating graft, leaving a convex right lateral crus instead of a concave lateral crus.

Conclusion

Patient was happy with a Visual Analogue Score improvement in airway and patient satisfaction. The following patient illustrates the typical indication for a lateral crural reciprocating graft with a fracture line close to the dome, but otherwise structurally intact and concave lateral crus causing functional narrowing of the external nasal valve region.

19.8.7 Post-op Photos (Fig. 19.18)

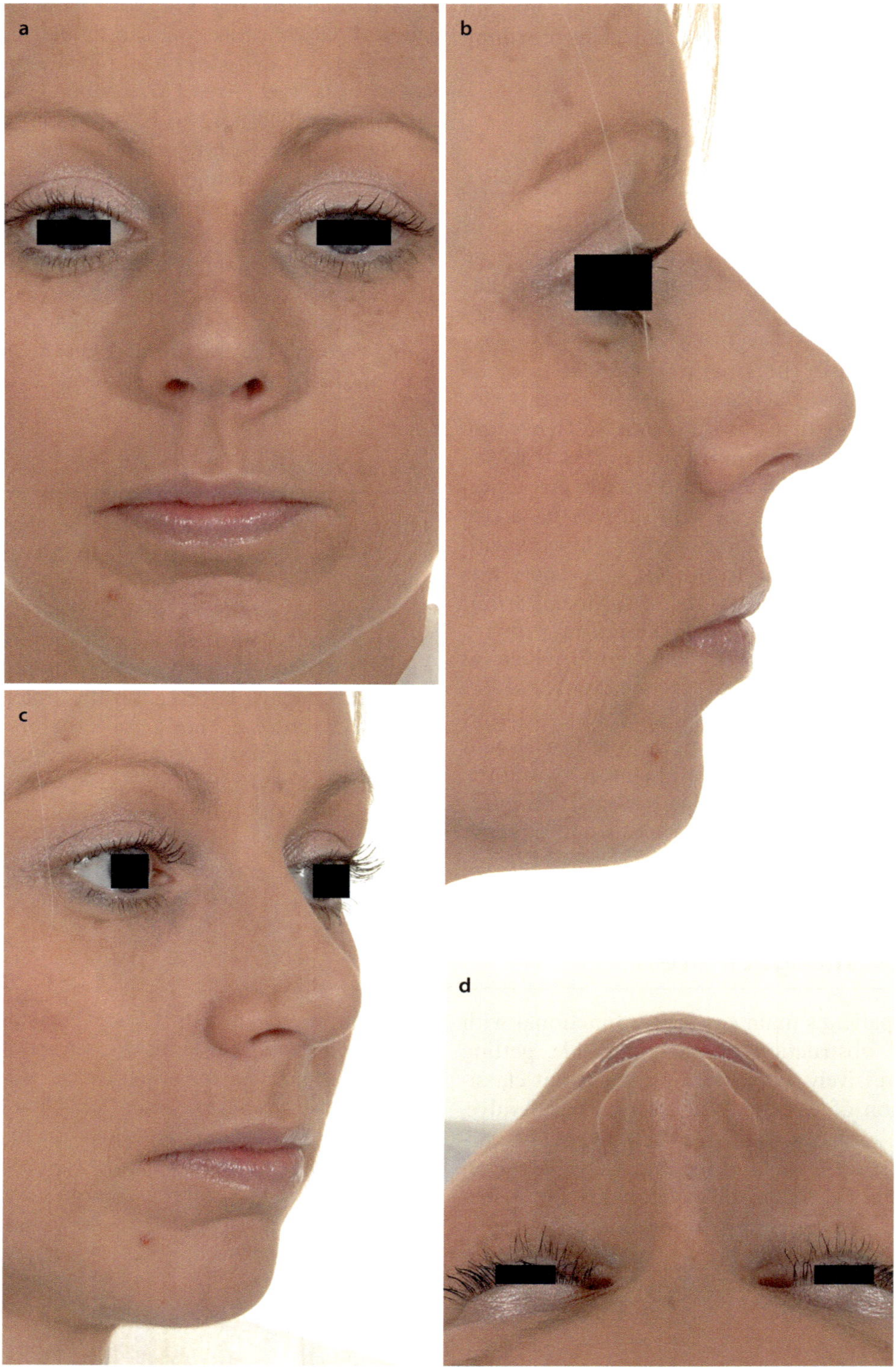

Fig. 19.18 **a–d** Functional rhinoplasty, unilateral concave lateral crus – post-operative photographs. **a** Frontal view. **b** Right lateral view. **c** Right ¾ view. **d** Sky view

19.9 Management of an Under Projected Droopy Tip

19.9.1 History

This patient presented with multiple nasal trauma with a collapsed nasal dorsum and nasal obstruction requesting septo-rhinoplasty to improve the structure and function. He had to lift the nasal tip to make him breath better.

19.9.2 Pre-op Photos (◘ Fig. 19.19)

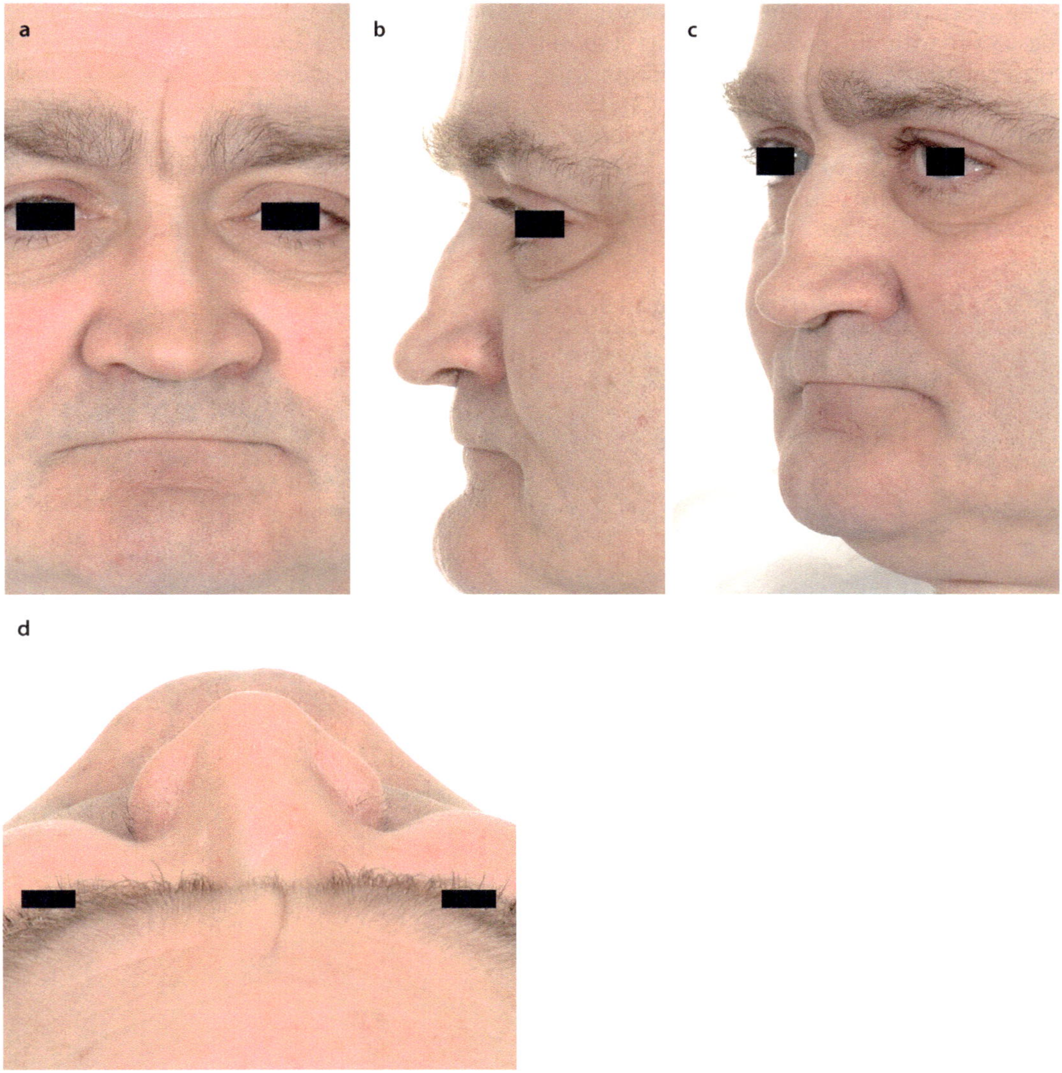

◘ **Fig. 19.19** **a**–**d** Under projected droopy tip – pre-operative photographs. **a** Frontal view. **b** Left lateral view. **c** Left ¾ view. **d** Sky view

19.9.3 Patient's Expectation

The patient was concerned both with nasal obstruction and nasal deformity and wanted the depression to be corrected and also nasal tip droop to be corrected.

19.9.4 Assessment

Frontal, left lateral and basal views shows a de-projected nasal dorsum and a de-projected nasal tip with tip ptosis. This was a post-traumatic nose with a damaged septum with loss of septal height both caudally and dorsally. There was mid-dorsal de-projection. His nasal obstruction was due to both tip ptosis and internal valve narrowing with asymmetric dorsal aesthetic lines.

19.9.5 Thought Process

Intranasal examination and palpation showed a straight septum with enough cartilage for reconstruction. Caudal and dorsal septum was retracted with loss of tip support and tip ptosis. If there was no septal cartilage, then costal cartilage might be needed for septal reconstruction.

19.9.6 Surgical Steps

The surgery was performed through an open approach, septal correction, harvesting of septal cartilage including a piece of ethmoid bone leaving an "L" strut. Caudal septal and dorsal septal extensions done and the medial crus was anchored to the caudal septal extension with a tongue and groove advancement and finally a tip anchoring suture.

19.9.7 Post-op Photos (Fig. 19.20)

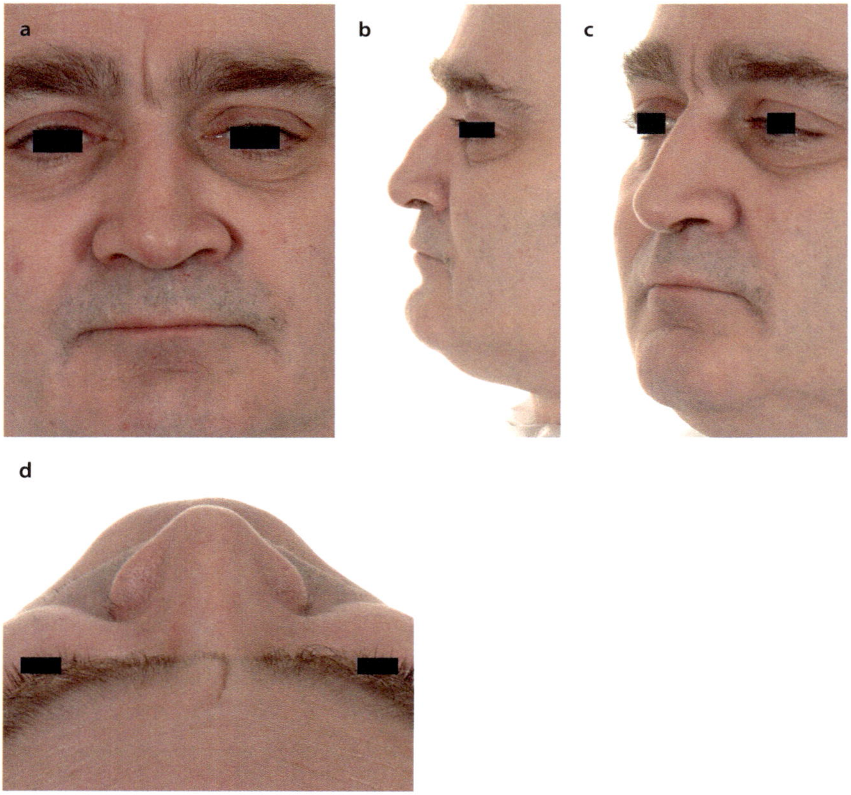

Fig. 19.20 **a–d** Under projected droopy tip – post-operative photographs. **a** Frontal view. **b** Left lateral view. **c** Left ¾ view. **d** Sky view

Conclusion

Patient was happy with the outcome. Any complex septal work is an ideal indication for an open approach as in this patient. It gives the access and the flexibility to achieve all the ancillary grafting and suturing procedures, if necessary.

19.10 Management of a Parenthesis Tip

19.10.1 History

This young lady was referred for nasal tip surgery following a previous septal surgery, which she claims that the appearance of the tip was made worse by previous septal surgery. She has persistent nasal obstruction despite a straighter septum.

19.10.2 Pre-op Photos (Fig. 19.21)

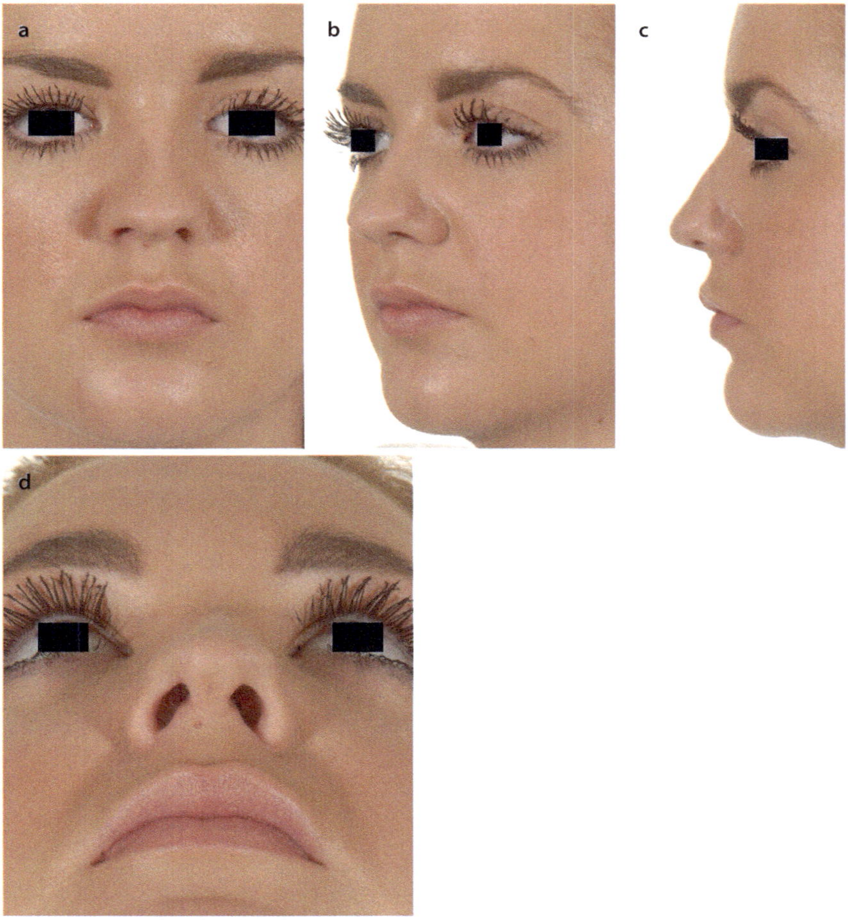

Fig. 19.21 **a–d** "Parenthesis" tip – pre-operative photographs. **a** Frontal view. **b** Left ¾ view. **c** Left lateral view. **d** Basal view

19.10.3 Patient's Expectation

The patient was concerned about nasal tip widening and bulbosity and nasal obstruction on both sides.

19.10.4 Assessment

The tip is wide and typically a parenthesis of the tip is seen with a change in the direction of the lateral crus pointing towards the medial canthus instead of the lateral canthus causing a "thumb" impression on the left ¾ view. Typically the basal and ¾ view of the tip is wider resembling a parenthesis {} symbol. This was causing tip bulbosity and weakness of the lateral alar region due to cephalic migration of the lateral crura on both sides causing weakness in the lateral alar wall. Parenthesis tip is usually associated with under rotated tip, unlike this patient where tip rotation is fine.

19.10.5 Thought Process

This would require de-bulking of the cephalic portion of the lateral crus and tip narrowing sutures with repositioning of the lateral crus in a slightly caudal position.

19.10.6 Surgical Steps

The surgery was performed through an Open approach, cephalic trim of the lateral crus, repositioning of lateral crus caudally and securing to alar mucosa, with trans-domal and inter-domal sutures.

Conclusion

Patient was happy with the breathing and the narrowness of the tip and happy with the projection and tip support achieved.

19.10.7 Post-op Photos (◘ Fig. 19.22)

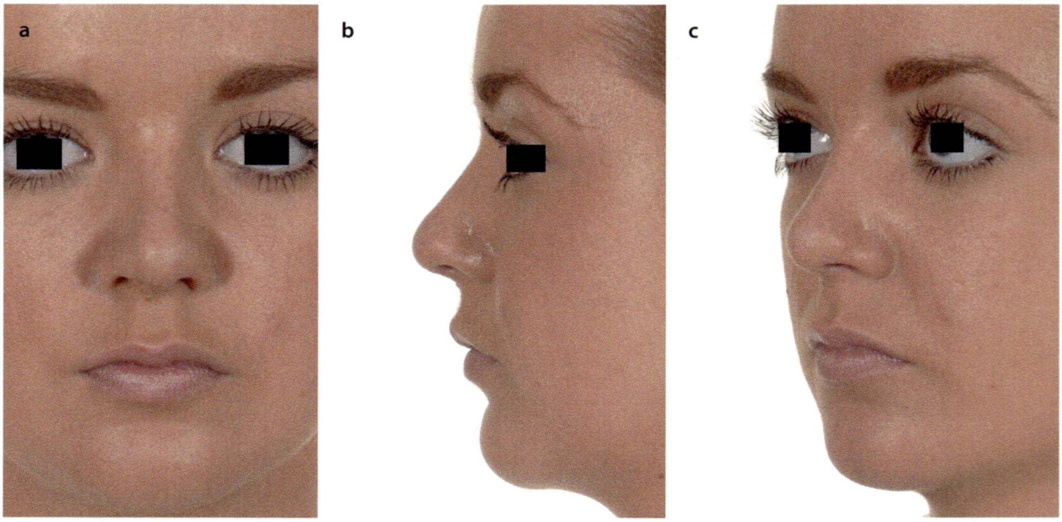

◘ **Fig. 19.22** **a–d** "Parenthesis" tip – post-operative photographs. **a** Frontal view. **b** Left ¾ view. **c** Left lateral view. **d** Basal view

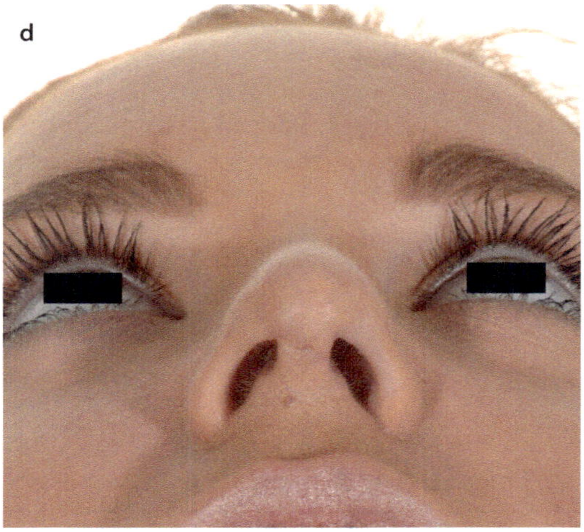

Fig. 19. 22 (continued)

19.11 Managing a Very Wide, Thickened, Convex Nasal Bones

19.11.1 History

This young man had nasal deformity and severe nasal obstruction on the right side due to early childhood trauma. Nose shape was getting worse as he is getting older. He would like the shape and breathing corrected if possible.

19.11.2 Pre-op Photos (Fig. 19.23)

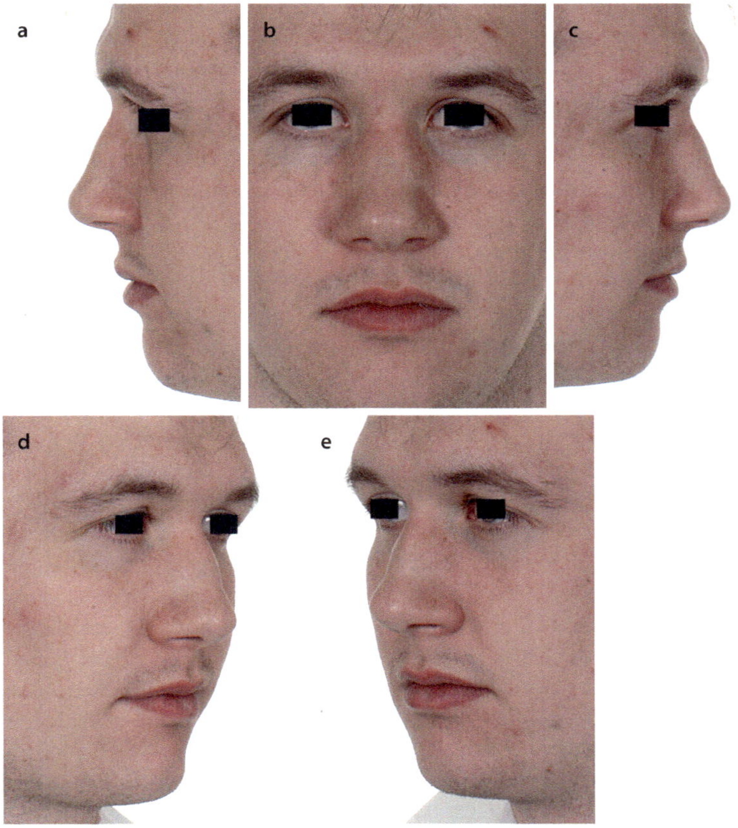

Fig. 19.23 a–g Wide convex nasal bones – pre-operative photographs. **a** Left lateral view. **b** Frontal view. **c** Right lateral view. **d** Right 3/4 view. **e** Left ¾ view. **f** Basal view. **g** Sky view

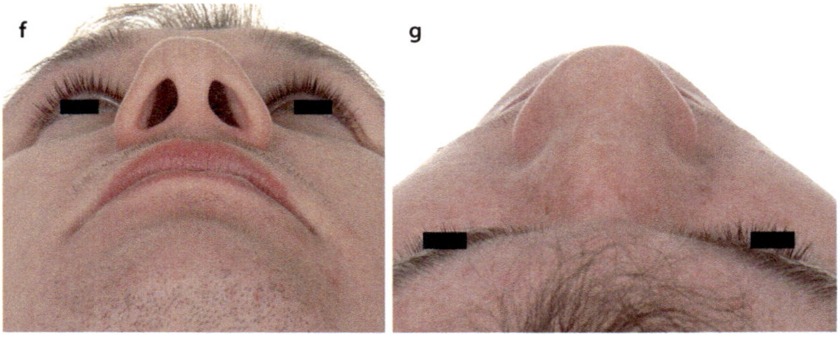

Fig. 19.23 (continued)

19.11.3 Patient's Expectations

This young man wanted nasal obstruction to be corrected and wanted the width of the nose narrowed. There was no history of recent trauma but repeated childhood trauma during the early childhood days.

19.11.4 Assessment

Examination of the frontal view and sky view showed an excessively wide nasal dorsal bony complex with over projection of the dorsal profile line. The "eyebrow tip line" is excessively wide and distorted at the upper third. The bony complex is thickened, wide and convex.

19.11.5 Thought Process

To narrow the dorsal bony width, osteotomies are needed to bring the bones together. But since the dorsal height is already raised on the profile line, this is going to make the profile line more elevated. So to reduce the dorsal width and also not to elevate the dorsal profile further, we have two options, firstly either to do osteotomies associated with bone removal or to do intermediate osteotomies and narrow the dorsum without the need to excise any additional bone width. This deformity of wide, thickened and convex nasal bony dorsum is an excellent indication for intermediate osteotomies. This patient is also an ideal indication for the use of powered instruments.

19.11.6 Surgical Steps

In this patient, the width of the nasal bones was narrowed by two intermediate osteotomies placed vertically between the midline and the lateral osteotomies. The surgery was performed through an open approach to straighten the septum and dorsal osteotomies and tip work to narrow the tip. There was no removal of excess bone from the frontal process of the maxilla, but narrowing the dorsum was achieved purely with osteotomies.

Conclusion

This clinical scenario is quite challenging when the dorsal osseo-cartilagenous framework is convex thickened and forming a dorsal hump. In these circumstances, Intermediate osteotomy is a good tool in achieving a narrow dorsum. Be aware that sometimes, unless excess bone is removed one cannot narrow the dorsum satisfactorily only with osteotomies. Although the post-op pictures are better than the pre-op, the dorsum is still slightly wider and the patient was well informed of the limitations. If a decision is made to do intermediate osteotomies, it should be done first before lateral or medial osteotomies. This can be either vertically oriented or horizontally oriented. The intermediate osteotomies ideally should be a greenstick fracture and does not have to extend to the entire length and width of the nasal bones and frontal process of the maxilla. Intermediate osteotomies should be followed by the lateral and superior oblique osteotomies. Ideally an intermediate osteotomy should be midway between the medial and lateral osteotomies, but can be centred on the most convex portion of the nasal bones. Sometimes, in patients with grossly convex nasal bones we may need more than one intermediate osteotomies, and in that case keep the second and the rest osteotomies length shorter than the first one. Thus if more than one intermediate osteotomies are needed, do the one in the middle first and do the smaller one above and below the first one and space it as necessary. Generally the aim of the intermediate osteotomies is to aid the lateral osteotomies to narrow a very wide and thickened bony osseo-cartilagenous dorsum. Patient was happy with the width of the nose, although not very narrow which shows the realistic outcomes of these surgeries.

19.11.7 Post-op Photos (Fig. 19.24)

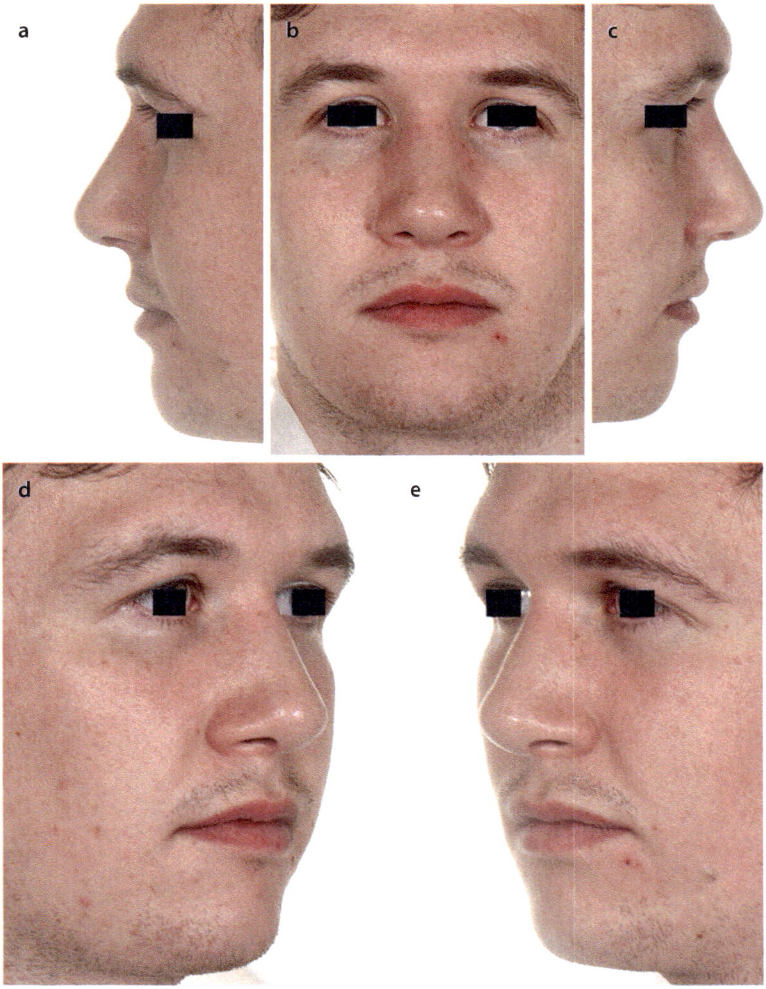

Fig. 19.24 **a–g** Wide convex nasal bones – post-operative photographs. **a** Left lateral view. **b** Frontal view. **c** Right lateral view. **d** Right 3/4 view. **e** Left ¾ view. **f** Basal view. **g** Sky view

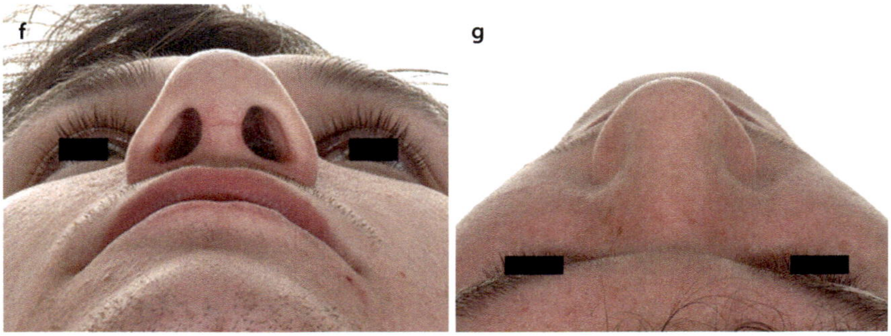

Fig. 19.24 (continued)

19.12 Paediatric Septo-Rhinoplasty

19.12.1 History

This is a very complex subject requiring experience and skill in deciding the management options. Generally a conservative approach is advisable till adolescence is reached. This unfortunate young man presented with gross nasal obstruction and a twisted nose with excessive watering of the eyes, really upsetting his well-being. He was seen few times with a decision to wait before he had any surgical intervention. But his symptoms of nasal obstruction were so severe that he could not sleep due to children being obligatory nasal breathers when compared to adults. An informed choice was made after discussion with the mum that a limited surgery on the septum would be performed. These types of patients are small in numbers even after years of practice and hence my long term experience of any surgical intervention is limited, but what was apparent was the necessity to do something surgical to improve his nasal airway as soon as possible. The mother has given consent to the use of the sons' photographs.

19.12.2 Pre-op Photos (◘ Fig. 19.25)

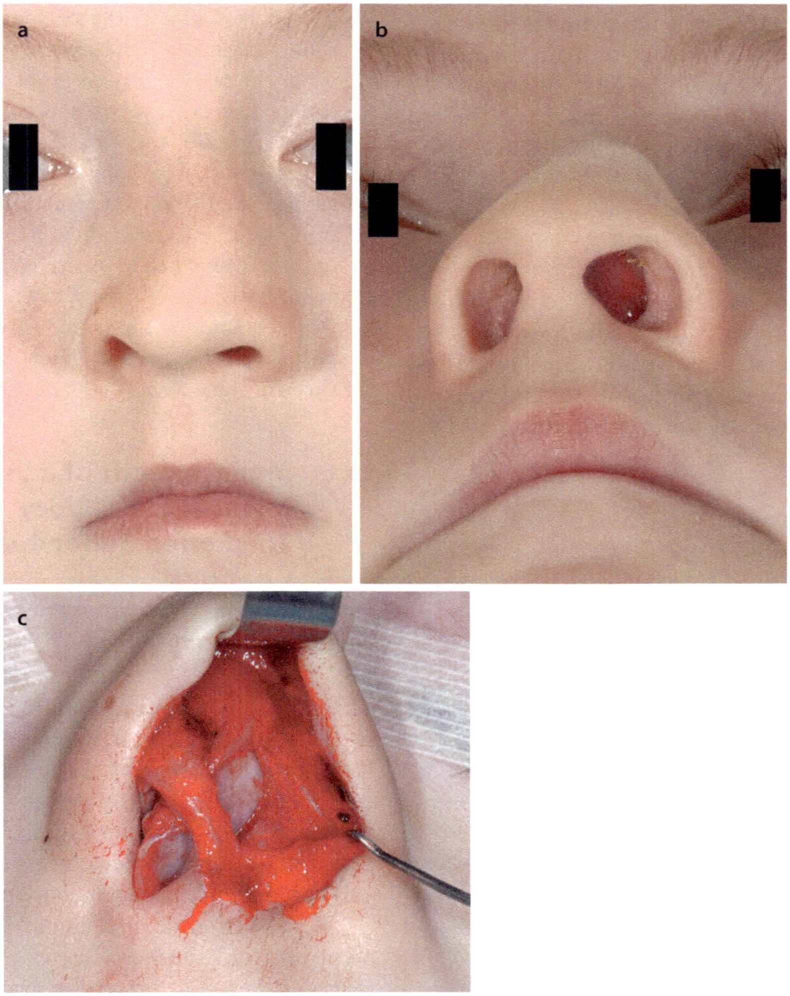

◘ **Fig. 19.25** **a–c** Paediatric septo-rhinoplasty – pre-operative photographs. **a** Frontal View. **b** Basal view showing the septal deviation and de-projected tip. **c** Intra-op view showing the severity of septal deviation

19.12.3 Assessment

Twisted septum with a de-projected nasal dorsum and a twisted nasal tip to right with severe nasal obstruction with no airway on both sides (as seen in the intra-op view). The tip is flat and de-projected due to secondary effects on the lateral crus on both sides.

19.12.4 Surgical Steps

This boy underwent open approach, limited septo-rhinoplasty with medialisation of the cartilaginous septum without excision of any cartilage from the spheno-dorsal and spheno-spinal segments of the cartilaginous septum.

Conclusion

The key points in dealing with children with structural and functional issues of the nose must be based on individual experience of the surgeons. If there is no functional issues, that makes the management algorithm much simpler and the surgery can wait till the skeletal growth is complete.

The issues arise when there is a severe functional impairment like our patient above, necessitating an intervention quickly. The key point to consider in early septo-rhinoplasty in young children is to think about the septal pathology. The cartilagenous septal development starts from the front face of the sphenoid as two "tongues", namely the spheno-dorsal unit growing forward along the dorsal septum and a spheno-spinal units growing inferiorly to the anterior nasal spine region. These are effectively growth centres for mid face development. Try not to damage these areas of the septal cartilages by excision or scoring. Although these are theoretical points to keep in mind, but practically in a severely damaged and bent septum, you cannot figure out these areas clearly. Hence we prefer open approach in these patients. But as a general rule try and avoid surgery in these areas of the septal cartilage growth centres and avoid any bony osteotomy surgical work in young children. Apart from these issues, individual judgements to operate in small children are up to the surgeon based on the patient's symptoms and the experience of the surgeon. We have no post-op photographs in this patient as the shape of the nose was not altered.

19.13 Management of a Bulbous Nasal Tip with Very Thickened Seborrheic Skin Changes

19.13.1 History

This pleasant lady presented in the private sector requesting to the narrow the nasal tip. Patient was referred by a senior and experienced colleague and his letter was cautious and suggested that the outcomes of the surgery will not be as expected due to seborrheic and rhinophyma like skin changes.

We were in total agreement with his assessment and did see her few times before surgery and despite our repeated warnings that the outcome might not be as expected, she was very keen to go ahead. The septum was straight and she was having no other cosmetic or functional issues with the nose and she was sensible and realistic in her expectations with good general health.

19.13.2 Pre-op (◘ Fig. 19.26)

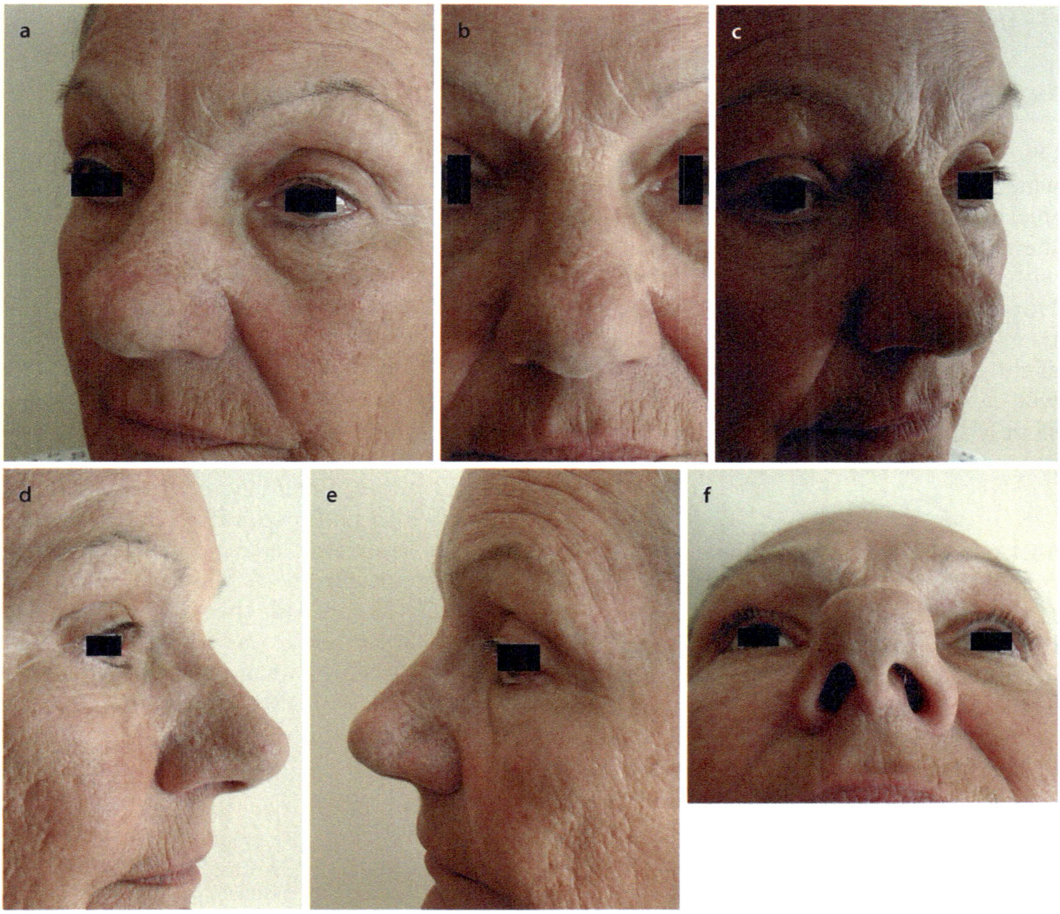

◘ **Fig. 19.26** **a**–**f** Bulbous tip with thickened skin – pre-operative photographs. **a** Left ¾ view. **b** Frontal view. **c** Right ¾ view. **d** Right lateral view. **e** Left lateral view. **f** Basal view

19.13.3 Patient's Expectation

To have the nasal tip narrower.

19.13.4 Assessment

On examination, in the basal view, she has a wide nasal tip with a trapezoidal base and a thicker seborrheic skin. In the frontal view, there is a thumb impression of the two domes with a small cleft between the tip cartilages. Dorsal profile line showed a dip in the supra tip region, particularly in the ¾ view with a slightly over projected tip, which if narrowed will cause more projection. She also has a slightly shorter length of the nose when compared to the projection.

19.13.5 Thought Process

Be aware that although the patient has requested narrowing of the nasal tip only, you need to discuss how narrowing the tip might not show up on the outside due to a thicker skin. The chances of this surgery being successful in achieving a narrower tip are higher due to the fact there is a thumb impression and cleft in the skin. Although the overlying skin is thicker, these findings suggests that the underlying tip cartilage is till wider and stronger causing a thumb impression on the overlying skin, which is relatively thinner when compared to the lower lateral cartilages. This is a good prognostic sign that narrowing the nasal tip may be still successful despite the skin being thicker. It is also worth discussing with the patient that any narrowing of the tip will result in increase in projection, which can make the dip in the supra tip more obvious. So we need to have a plan to correct and augment the supra tip and mid dorsum with some cartilage. Our plan was to do a bulk reduction of the cephalic portion of the lateral crus (which we know is quite big) and narrow the tip with tip sutures and use the extra piece of the cephalic lateral crural cartilage to augment the supra tip dorsum as a "cap-graft" to create a uniform dorsal profile line. We wanted to keep the surgery simple without the need to do a septoplasty for harvesting extra cartilage and hence avoid all the morbidities of septoplasty. One can do this procedure through open or tip delivery techniques.

19.13.6 Surgical Steps

The surgery was performed through an open approach, raised the flap, did a bilateral cephalic trim of the lateral crus, leaving only 8 mm of symmetrical rim strips, high medial crural fixation suture to bring the two medial crura together (to correct the cleft seen in the skin), followed by trans-domal and inter-domal sutures and a lateral crural flare control suture. Finally covered the supra tip region with a small cap graft from the cephalic portion of excised lateral crus to smoothen the dorsal profile line as planned. Patient was extremely happy with the outcome. Post-op photos shown below was taken a week after surgery. Hopefully when the tip oedema goes down it will look even much better a year down the lane.

> **Conclusion**
> Comparing pre-and post-op photographs and subjective assessment of improvement in the shape, patient was happy with a Visual Analogue Score of 10/10 in appearance and patient satisfaction.

19.13.7 Post-op (Fig. 19.27)

Extreme care is necessary in selecting the right patient for a tip narrowing procedure. Particularly skin thickness should be taken into account and adequate counselling about the possible outcomes in your hand should be discussed and documented in the records. Dealing with patient's expectations is very important seeing them few times before surgery and also being realistic with your own skills and outcomes.

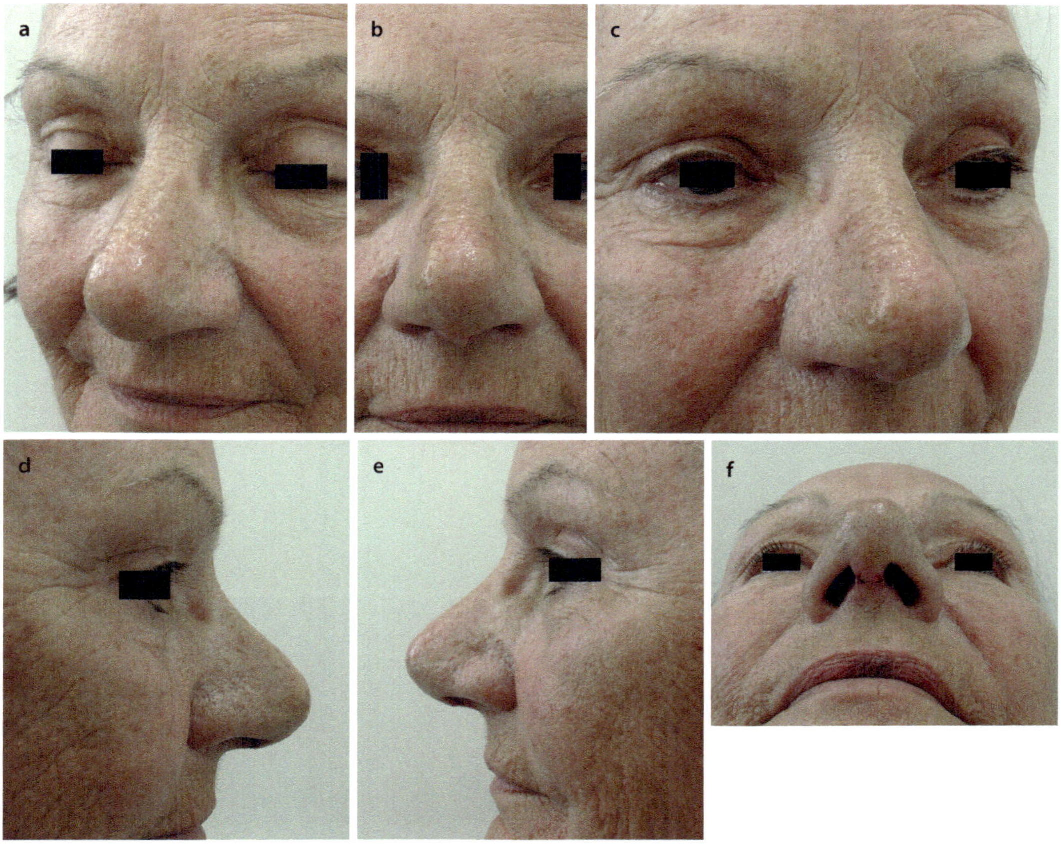

Fig. 19.27 **a**–**f** Bulbous tip with thickened skin – post-operative photographs. **a** Left ¾ view. **b** Frontal view. **c** Right ¾ view. **d** Right lateral view. **e** Left lateral view. **f** Basal view

19.14 Management of an Isolated Over Projected Nasal Tip

19.14.1 History

This lady presented to the clinic with an asymmetrically over projected and over rotated nasal tip following a previous hump reduction with tip being not addressed at the same time. She requested tip de-projection and wanted to decrease the length of the nose. She had bilateral scarring of the inter-cartilaginous incision sites, also causing a degree of alar pinching and airway obstruction at the external nasal valve region.

19.14.2 Pre-op Photos (◘ Fig. 19.28)

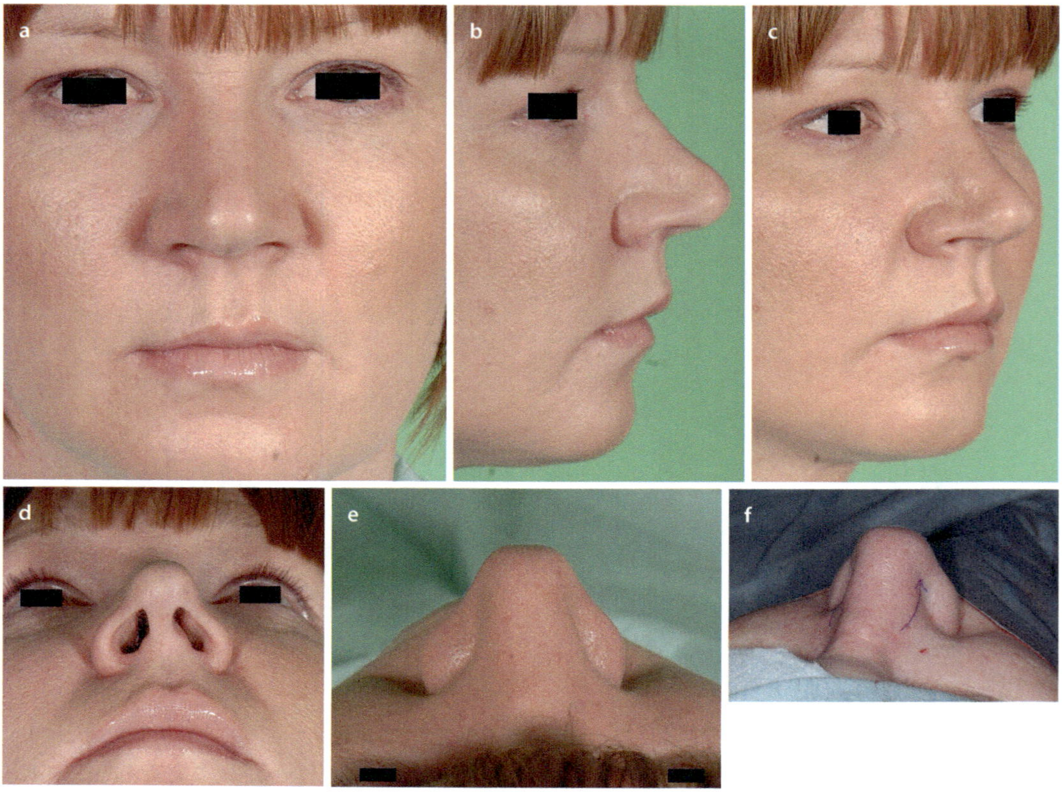

◘ **Fig. 19.28** **a**–**f** Isolated over projected nasal tip – pre-operative photographs. **a** Frontal view. **b** Right lateral view. **c** Right ¾ view. **d** Basal view. **e** Straight sky view. **f** Lateral sky view

19.14.3 Assessment

Three quarters view and sky views showed the deformity better than other views. There was an over projected nasal tip with upward rotation and a ski slope dorsum. She had bilateral mild scarring of the inter-cartilaginous incisions, causing some external lateral alar pinching. Palpation did not reveal any caudal septal excess at the anterior septal angle. There was no alar weakness on inspiration.

19.14.4 Patient's Expectations

Wanted the projection of the tip to be reduced and the nasal tip taken back to the face and establish symmetry between upper half and lower half of the nose.

19.14.5 Thought Process

Sky view and particularly three quarters view showed selective over projection of tip with slight alar pinching. Ski slope appearance to the dorsum with a slight over rotation of the tip as well.

The options to de-project the nasal tip (to take the tip back to the face) can be directed at the tip cartilages or made better by reducing the caudal or dorsal septal excess if there is an issue with the septum. This patient did not have any septal issues. Hence decision was made to do a direct dome technique to address the tip. The options here would be to reduce the length of the two lateral crus equally and also the conjoined medial crus to de-project the nasal tip. This should be done on both sides without affecting tip rotation. The other alternative being direct division (excision) of dome (intermediate crus) and direct anastomosis of medial crus to the lateral crus to establish the continuity of the LC. This is quicker and easier to perform when compared to reducing both lateral crus and the conjoined medial crus, but can show through if the overlying skin is thin. We did this technique in this lady as it was already a revision procedure and she had slightly thicker skin cover. This technique also helps in resecting small localised abnormalities in the intermediate crus. But the surgeon needs to be aware that this procedure may cause small blemishes to be seen through in a young patient with a thin skin. Knots should be carefully placed to avoid eversion of wound edges.

19.14.6 Surgical Steps

The surgery was performed through an open approach. The septum was fine with no septal excess at the anterior septal angle, as expected by clinical examination. 4 mm of the intermediate crus was resected and the medial crus was sutured back to the lateral crus to establish continuity of the alar cartilages (◘ Fig. 19.29a–d). This is an effective alternative for both LC and MC de-projection techniques to achieve nasal tip de-projection but be aware that this will cause some nasal tip blunting. This was helpful in this patient as the sharp tip was made slightly wider and aesthetically pleasing.

Conclusion

Intermediate crural resection is a direct dome technique to address an over projected nasal tip in selected patients, which is consistent in outcomes and less time consuming. Our patient shows acceptable outcomes with a high patient satisfaction score regarding the appearance. Although this is a quick and very effective technique to de-project the nasal tip and take it back to the face, extreme caution is required while planning, as this technique is not advisable in young patient with a very thin skin.

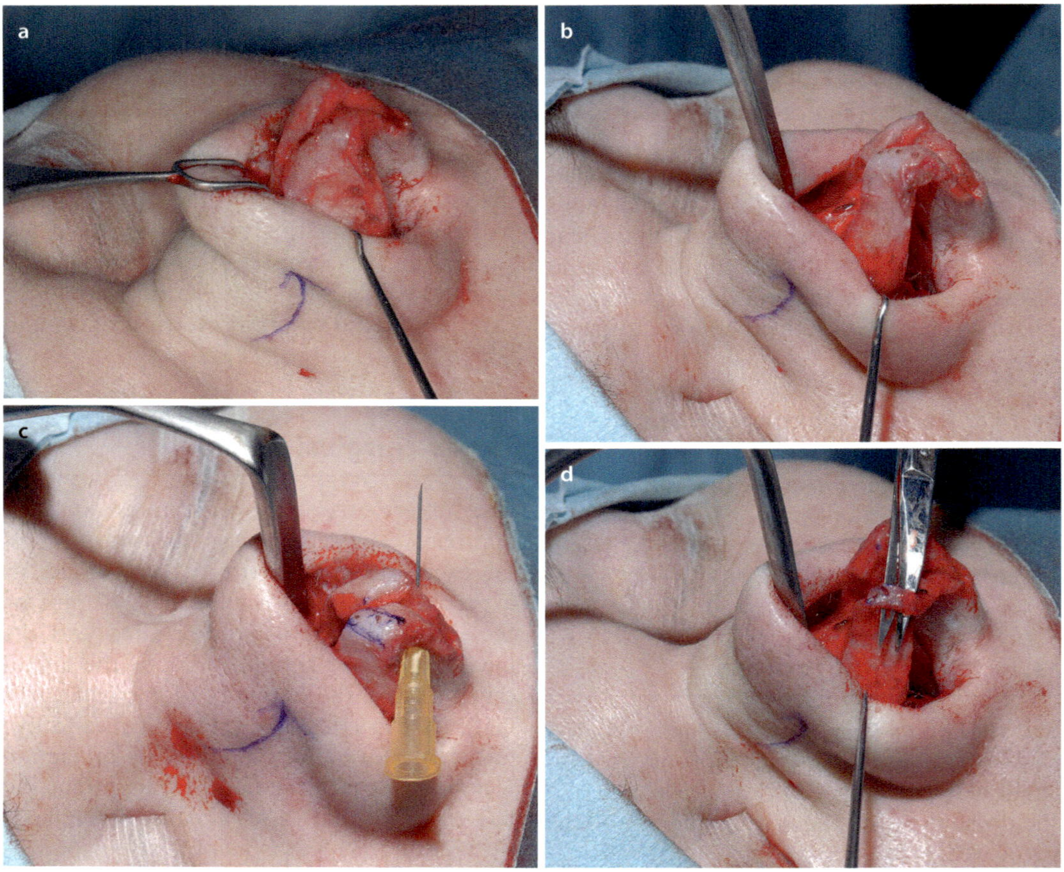

Fig. 19.29 **a–d** Isolated over projected nasal tip – intra-operative photographs. **a** Showing open approach. **b** Over projected intermediate crus. **c** Area of 4 mm excision of IC marked out. **d** IC segment being excised

19.14.7 Post-op Photos (Fig. 19.30)

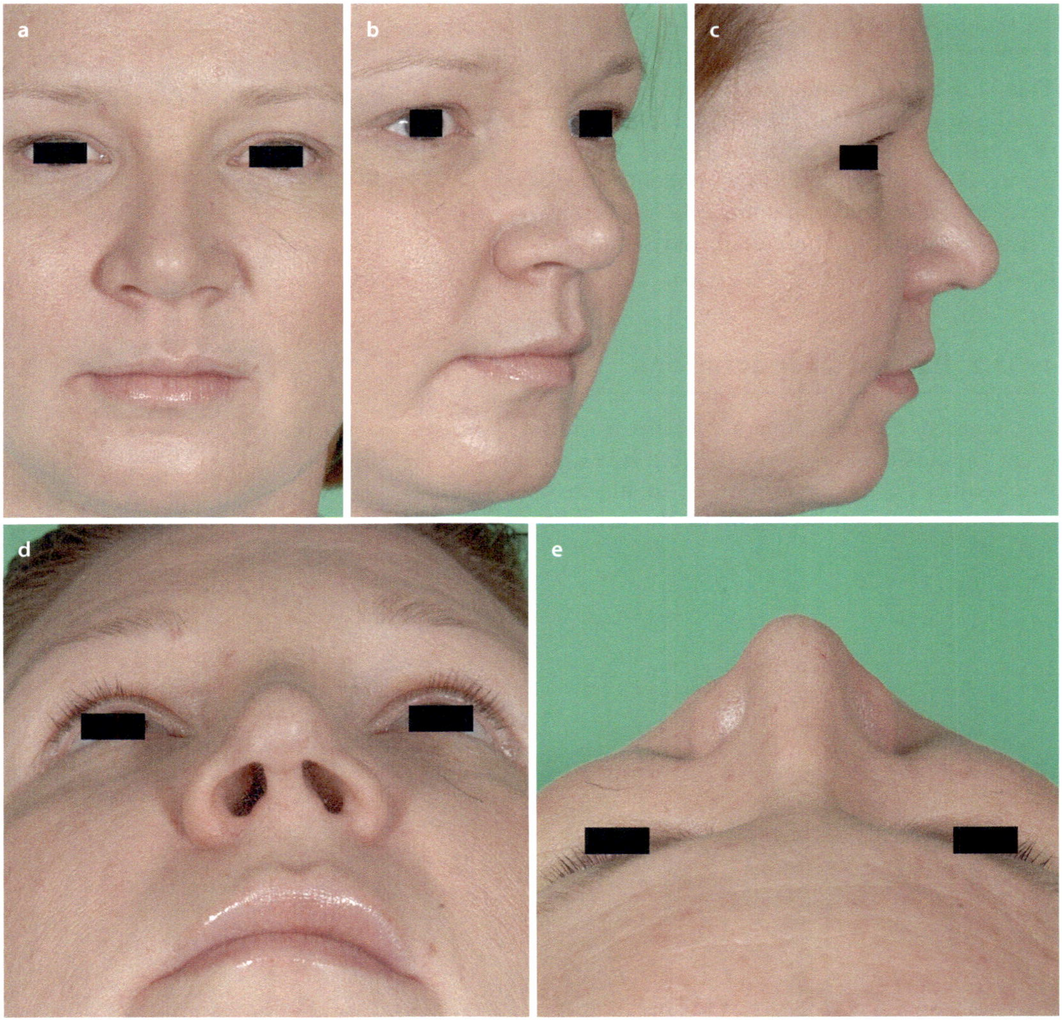

Fig. 19.30 a–e Isolated over projected nasal tip – post-operative photographs. **a** Frontal view. **b** Right lateral view. **c** Right ¾ view. **d** Basal view. **e** Sky view

19.15 Management of Scarred and Contracted Nasal Alar and Vestibular Stenosis

19.15.1 History

This lady had a traumatic damage to the left nasal alar region falling through a sharp piece of glass. Sutured in the emergency department. Over the months, the patient slowly developed a scarred and contracted ala on the left side with both functional and structural issues.

19.15.2 Patient's Expectations

She wanted the breathing to be better and open the nasal passage on the left side and was realistic in her expectations to improve the cosmesis of the alar region on the left side.

19.15.3 Pre-op Photos (Fig. 19.31)

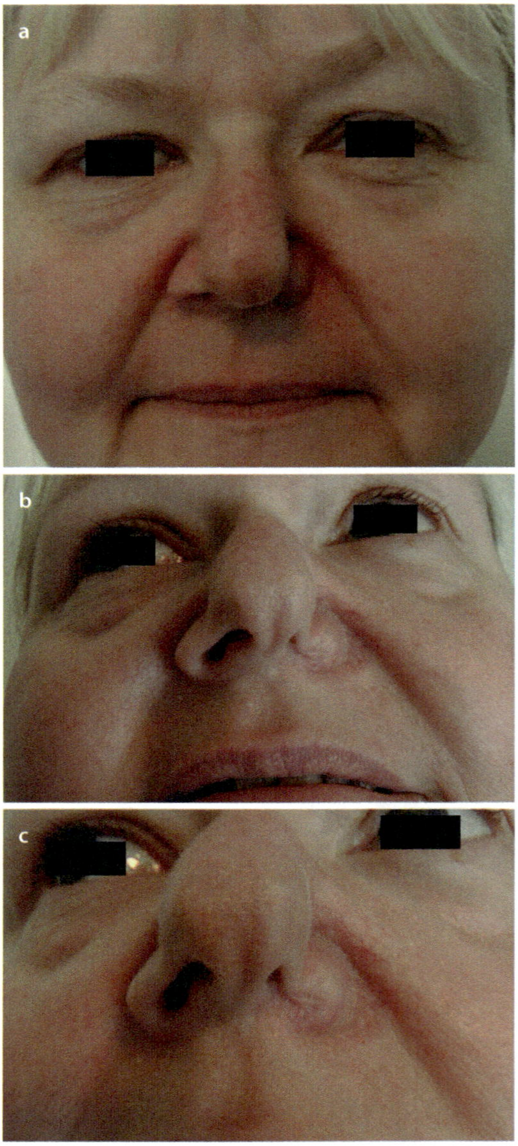

Fig. 19.31 **a–c** Left scarred alar and vestibular stenosis – pre-operative photographs. **a** Frontal view showing collapsed left alar base. **b** and **c** Basal view showing scarred left alar base with vestibular stenosis

19.15.4 Assessment

Left alar region was scarred and contracted with a slit like opening. Endoscopic examination showed adhesions between the lateral wall and the floor of the nose on the left side with scarring and vestibular stenosis extending up to 3 cm inside. There was marked asymmetry of the ala with contracted ala on the left side with extensive scarring. This was causing functional obstruction on the left side plus cosmetic issues. She was very realistic and was made aware that structure and function may not be complementary to each other in this operation and long term outcomes may be not good and scar contraction recurrence is a possibility. She was also made aware that any operation in our hands will not establish symmetry between the two ala.

19.15.5 Thought Process

It is one of the most difficult procedures to achieve some meaningful outcomes in terms of function and structure. Adequate intra nasal examination is important to establish how much scarring is extending inside the nasal cavity. Scarring and adhesion between the lateral soft tissue vestibular wall and the floor of the nose is more common than adhesion between the lateral and medial wall and is more difficult to keep it open post-surgery. Over a period of years we have learnt that "excising" the scar tissue does not work. The scar tissue need to be "incised" and a viable biological layer used in between the scar tissue to keep it open. We used to use fascia lata graft for this purpose in the past with variable success, but now consistently we use split thickness skin graft from the thigh which gives far more consistent long term results, like in this patient. Apart from dealing with scar tissue, it is also important to enlarge the bony pyriform aperture to take the soft tissues laterally to accommodate any scar contracture. This lady also had collapse and damage to the lower lateral crus on the left side which was reconstructed with conchal bowl cartilage taken from the right conchal bowl. The patient should be counselled that the results may not be good and recurrent contracture over a period of time can be a major issue. Patient should also be warned that there can be initial distortion of tissues soon after surgery which will settle down. Slight over correction of the airway by opening the ala a bit more than necessary is important to allow for a degree of post-operative contraction.

19.15.6 Surgical Steps

Adequate exposure of the site is important, and this was done through the alarotomy approach in this lady, and widely incising the scar tissue and opening up the vestibular space. Since the lateral crus was damaged, the conchal bowl cartilage was harvested from the opposite ear and also split thickness skin graft from the thigh. The nasal bony aperture was then enlarged uniformly by ronguering of the bony pyriform aperture. The ala was then repositioned in a more downward and more lateral position to over correct the deformity (▣ Fig. 19.32c) and split thickness skin graft was inserted under the incised scar tissue to cover the bare bone and soft tissue between the lateral wall and the floor of the nose. A small area of soft triangle scarring was excised and left to heal by secondary intention. A small part of the graft was brought out to cover the alar skin, which usually heals very well if it is a split thickness skin graft.

19.15.7 2 Weeks Post-op (◘ Fig. 19.32)

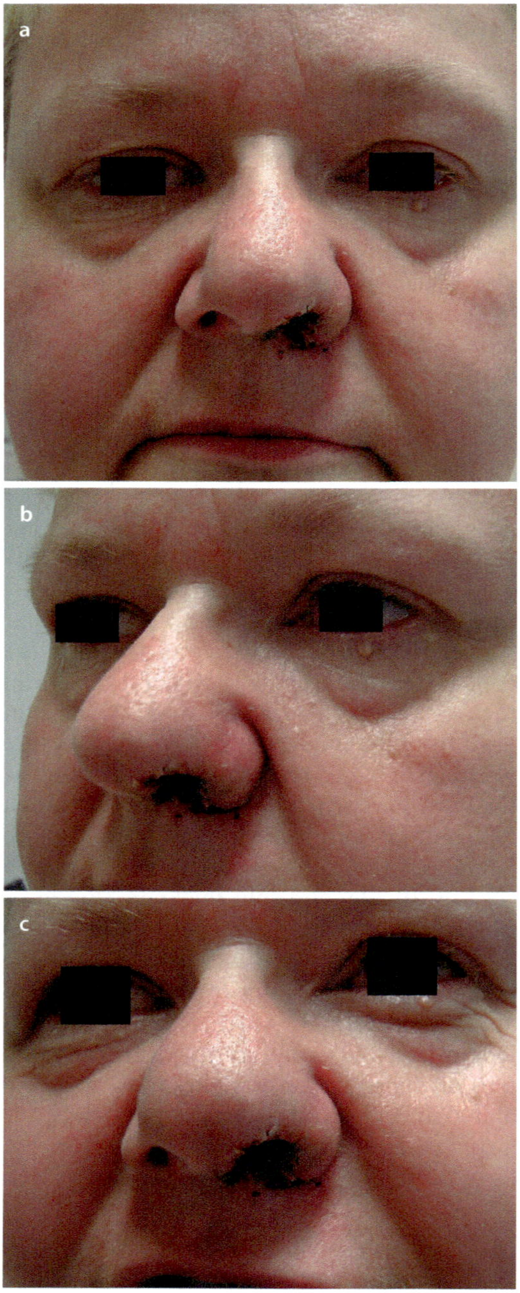

◘ **Fig. 19.32** **a**–**c** Left scarred alar and vestibular stenosis – 2 weeks post-operative photographs. **a** and **c** Frontal view. **b** Left lateral view

19.15.8 3 Years Post-op (Fig. 19.33)

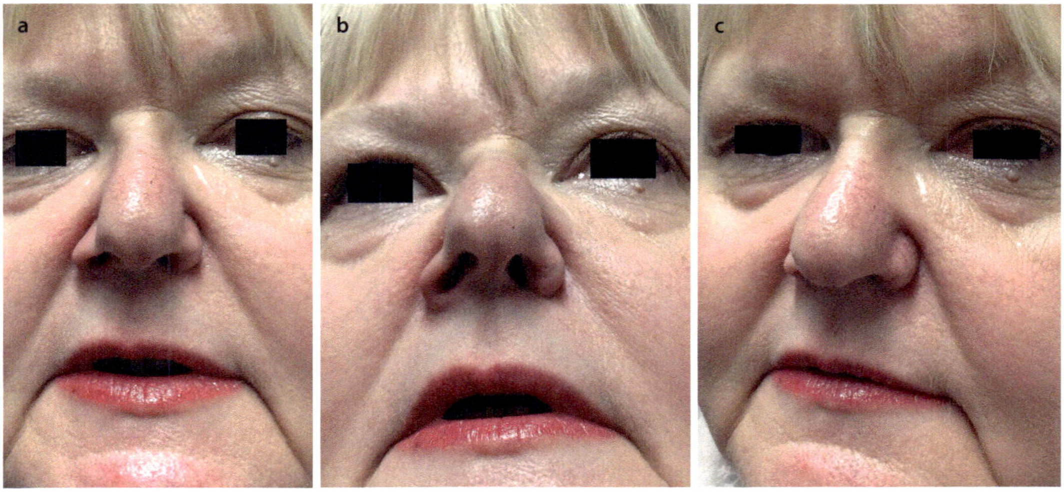

Fig. 19.33 **a–c** Left scarred alar and vestibular stenosis – 3 years post-operative photographs. **a** and **b** Frontal view. **c** Left lateral view

Conclusion

Not an easy condition to correct. The surgical intervention need to be aggressive to get meaningful results. Long-term results are not good particularly with reference to the position of the ala. Hence overcorrection of alar margins is needed to account for post-operative contraction. This may lead to patient's dissatisfaction at an early stage. This patient was seen 3 years after surgery with acceptable outcomes and she was happy with a Visual Analogue Score improvement of 10/10 in improvement in airway and patient satisfaction. The following patient illustrates the need for immediate over correction of the problem and also illustrates that in the immediate post-op period, the wound will look much worse and will take time to settle down. Also long-term results are more important in this operation and the patient should be counselled adequately that results will not be obvious straight away to avoid unnecessary anxiety. Please note that the position of the ala keeps changing in the post-operative period. *Be aware that we cannot achieve symmetry between two sides of the ala, and the patient should be made aware of this as well before surgery. Patient and surgeon should be willing to have a compromise between structural and functional improvement.*

- Thus, our key surgical principles in managing patients with vestibular stenosis due to scarring are as follows:
- Adequate exposure through alarotomy
- Wide incision of scar tissue and not excision of scar tissue
- Widen the bony pyriform aperture by ronguering
- Split thickness skin graft for inside lining
- Cartilage graft for the external nasal alar region
- Repositioning the ala in an over corrected lateral and inferior position

Key Points Box

- Analysing case studies offers a valuable tool in learning the aetio-pathogenesis of the deformity.
- Helps us to arrive at a sensible decision based on the patient's requirements.
- Helps us to understand the surgical algorithm of managing various deformities and the pros and cons of using various techniques.

Ethical Considerations in Rhinoplasty

Contents

N. Balaji, *Textbook of Nasal Tip Rhinoplasty*, https://doi.org/10.1007/978-3-030-48157-5_20

Learning Objectives

To learn the "tenets" of rhinoplasty ethics, based on the author's experience of over the last 23 years as a Consultant in the National Health Service in the UK and 36 years as a doctor.

20.1 Introduction

The word "Ethics" is defined as a set of moral principles that govern a person's behaviour. No type of surgery is as important as rhinoplasty in following strict ethical codes. Holding on to ethical values during the pre-operative, intra-operative and post-operative times are extremely important not only to offer the best care to the patients, but also to give the surgeon piece of mind and avoid lawsuits and further sanctions. The following are the author's ten commandments of rhinoplasty ethics.

20.2 The "Tenets" of Rhinoplasty Ethics

1. Honesty – Being honest to the patients about your outcomes and skill levels is important.
2. Integrity – Both clinical and financial integrity is important. For example not to alter the files/records or not to alter the clinical practice or compromise your principles to achieve financial gain.
3. Maintaining morals and high standards in advertising. Avoiding false information in personal websites.
4. Inadequate clinical examination, failure to obtain an "informed consent", failure to establish the expected outcomes prior to surgery are all considered breaches of standard ethical practice [1]. Establishing clearly the expected outcomes before proceeding for surgery is a must. This is where the initial and subsequent consultation are very important, before proceeding for surgery.
5. There should always be a "cool off" period of 4 weeks between consultations and surgery. A minimum of 2 weeks has been recommended by the British Association of Aesthetic Plastic Surgeons and the GMC guidelines in the UK [2]. If necessary more than two consultations may be necessary. This will enable the patient enough time to understand the implications, pros and cons of the procedure before proceeding with surgery [3]. This time frame will also help to establish a rapport with the patient and the family.
6. Adequate communication with the patients so that they understand what is achievable and more importantly what is NOT achievable. ONLY then proceed with surgery.
7. Financial ethics are important. This does not arise as far as NHS is concerned in the UK, but in private sector the fees should be the same covering all aspects of surgery and the patient should be told of that prior to operation. The surgeon should not be driven to doing unnecessary surgery for financial gain. Do not consider rhinoplasty surgery which is unlikely to achieve the desirable outcomes just because the patient is paying for the procedure.
8. Patient's mental or psychological factors should be taken into consideration. Certainly vulnerable patients with unstable or bipolar disorders with a fixation on the nose should not be put through surgery for monetary gain. Patient's medical co-morbidities, elderly patients who want surgery to help their social lives or very young patients who are not mature enough to handle this operation should not be considered. Of course these are my personal views based on over 24 years of experience.
9. Relationship with other colleagues is important. Undue criticisms of your colleagues should be avoided. An unhappy patient who has come to you for a second opinion will of course criticise the previous surgeon. In this situation, it is very important to stand neutral until you find the facts. It is important to remember that complications can happen to anyone. Beware you will need someone else's help for a second opinion in case your surgery goes wrong, which will happen in your career.
10. Fact finding is important before arriving at a judgement, particularly in revision surgery. Compare before and after pictures.

If possible get the operation notes. Beware of patients who want to tell you their side of the story. Always find out from pre-operative photos and surgeon's operation notes what exactly was the issue before and do not commit to address these issues without knowing the facts. Do not pass derogatory comments about the colleagues.

11. Importance of family support and goodwill is a key factor in patient satisfaction. This operation is very peculiar in that the patient's happiness of the outcome can be related to the family and friend's happiness, although we are classically taught to listen ONLY to the patient and not that of the relatives. A win–win situation would be if the demands of the patient and the immediate family match.
12. Do not be pressurised to operate on a patient the fourth time just because the referral letter is very flattering and you are the best in the region. This is a trap you can fall into even after years of experience. Being technically good is NOT the only factor in achieving patient outcomes in rhinoplasty. Politely refusing to do revision surgery in patients with dubious outcomes in fact raises the respect you hold in the field, both with the patient and the referring surgeon for your honesty and integrity.

Conclusion

This surgery involves maintaining high ethical standards to achieve not only good outcomes, but also protecting you from litigation and of course not losing your sleep!

Key Points Box

- Maintaining honesty and integrity is paramount for the surgeon.
- High morals, financial integrity and maintaining trust are equally important.
- Adequate record keeping is a must.

References

1. Karimi K, McKneally MF, Adamson PA. Ethical considerations in aesthetic rhinoplasty: a survey, critical analysis, and review. Arch Facial Plast Surg. 2012;14(6):442–50.
2. https://www.gmc-uk.org/ethical-guidance/ethical-guidance-for-doctors.
3. Balaji N. Top tips in nasal tip surgery, ENT-FPS UK Newsletter— Feb 2018 –Issue 6.